Essentials of Dentistry

Essentials of Dentistry

Editor: Kaley Ann

FOSTER ACADEMICS

www.fosteracademics.com

www.fosteracademics.com

Cataloging-in-Publication Data

Essentials of dentistry / edited by Kaley Ann.
p. cm.
Includes bibliographical references and index.
ISBN 978-1-63242-542-3
1. Dentistry. I. Ann, Kaley.
RK51 .E87 2018
617.6--dc23

Foster Academics,
118-35 Queens Blvd., Suite 400,
Forest Hills, NY 11375, USA

ISBN 978-1-63242-542-3 (Hardback)

Printed and bound in China.

Contents

Preface

The purpose of the book is to provide a glimpse into the dynamics and to present opinions and studies of some of the scientists engaged in the development of new ideas in the field from very different standpoints. This book will prove useful to students and researchers owing to its high content quality.

Dentistry is a branch of medical science that deals with the prevention, diagnosis, and treatment of ailments affecting the teeth, gum, and oral mucosa. Teeth are an essential part of our total well-being. It comprises topics about root canals, fillings, gum hygiene, etc. This text is a compilation of chapters that discuss the most vital concepts and emerging trends in the field of dentistry. This book discusses the diseases and treatments related to teeth. The book is an essential guide for both academicians and those who wish to pursue this discipline further.

At the end, I would like to appreciate all the efforts made by the authors in completing their chapters professionally. I express my deepest gratitude to all of them for contributing to this book by sharing their valuable works. A special thanks to my family and friends for their constant support in this journey.

Editor

1

Craniomandibular Trauma and Tooth Loss in Northern Dogs and Wolves: Implications for the Archaeological Study of Dog Husbandry and Domestication

Robert J. Losey[1]*, Erin Jessup[1], Tatiana Nomokonova[1], Mikhail Sablin[2]

1 Department of Anthropology, University of Alberta, Edmonton, Alberta, Canada, 2 Zoological Institute, Russian Academy of Science, Saint-Petersburg, Russia

Abstract

Archaeological dog remains from many areas clearly show that these animals suffered tooth fractures, tooth loss, trauma, and dental defects during their lives. Relatively little research has explored the meanings of these patterns, particularly for ancient dog remains from small-scale societies of the North. One limiting issue is the lack of comparative data on dental health and experiences of trauma among northern wolves and dogs. This paper examines tooth loss, tooth fracture, enamel hypoplasia, and cranial trauma in a large sample of historic dog and wolf remains from North America and Northern Russia. The data indicate that the dogs more commonly experienced tooth loss and tooth fracture than the wolves, despite reportedly being fed mostly soft foods such as blubber and fish. The higher rates observed in the dogs likely is a result of food stress and self-provisioning through scavenging. The ability to self-provision was likely important for the long-term history of dog use in the north. Dogs also more commonly experienced cranial fractures than wolves, particularly depression fractures on their frontal bones, which were likely the result of blows from humans. Hypoplastic lesions are rare in both wolves and dogs, and probably result from multiple causes, including food stress, disease, and trauma.

Editor: Michael D. Petraglia, University of Oxford, United Kingdom

Funding: Funding for this project was provided by an ERC Advanced Grant (#295458) to Dr. David Anderson, University of Aberdeen (http://erc.europa.eu). Financial support to Mikhail V. Sablin was provided by the Russian Foundation for Basic Research (Grant 13-04-00203; http://www.rfbr.ru/rffi/ru). The funders had no role in study design, data collection and analysis, decision to publish, or preparation of the manuscript.

Competing Interests: The authors have declared that no competing interests exist.

* Email: robert.losey@ualberta.ca

Introduction

Remains of dogs from across the globe show that these animals experienced traumatic injuries, tooth loss, and disease during their lifetimes. Signs on the skeleton marking these experiences have been shown to have significant interpretive potential for understanding the life histories of dogs, including their relationships with people [1–8]. Research on skeletal pathology is still rare for archaeological dog remains from small-scale societies, particularly those of the North, despite the fact that dogs historically were common across this region's diverse array of hunting and herding cultures. One of the clear limiting factors in interpreting signs of trauma and pathology on the skeletons of northern dogs is a lack of comparative skeletal or documentary data. For example, it is often difficult to ascertain if rates of fracture, tooth loss, or dental defects in archaeological dog remains differ from those observed in local wild canids. Biologists and paleontologists have generated some useful comparative canid trauma and disease data [9–19], but such studies often focus on single highly specific patterns such as tooth fracture, limiting the breadth of their usefulness for archaeological interpretation. Further, most ethnographic accounts of northern groups provide relatively few details about the actual lives of the dogs in these societies, with some notable exceptions [20–22]. To move the study of ancient dog life histories forward, more detailed comparative studies are needed.

Archaeologists working with Late Holocene dog remains from Arctic North America have commented on the occurrence of depression fractures on crania, suggesting they represented "animals sometimes having been severely disciplined as part of their management" [23;24–25]. However, alternative causes of these types of fractures, including kicks from prey animals, should be considered, particularly if similar lesions occur at comparable rates in wolves from the same region. Other lesions on Arctic archaeological dog specimens, typically punctures in the bones of the rostrum, have been interpreted as bite wounds incurred during dog-on-dog fighting [25]. It is unknown, however, how the frequency of such wounds compare to that observed in northern wolves, and how such patterns might be informative about human-dog relationships.

Antemortem tooth loss and fracture patterns may provide insights on the earliest processes of domestication, dogs' food acquisition processes, and even intentional tooth removal. Some scholars have argued that prior to the first intentional human steps towards domestication, a subset of wolves began to regularly scavenge on human kills and other waste, bringing them into close association with people, which in effect preselected these animals for domestication [26]. Tooth fracture and loss during the life of a canid in such settings should be greater than that seen in hunting wolves, as the former would have to masticate much more bone to extract necessary nutrients because of having secondary access to carcasses [15–17].

Tooth loss and fracture frequency in canids might also vary between sexes, and with human husbandry practices. Some studies have indicated that male dogs and wolves tend to out-perform their female counterparts in certain forms of hunting [27–29], and that male wolves appear to be more likely than females to experience traumatic injuries [30]. Research on North American gray wolves also indicated significant differences in tooth size between males and females, and suggested this might relate to different degrees of carcass processing between the sexes [31]. Tooth loss and fracture in dogs also could be affected by human provisioning practices, including the degree to which dogs were fed frozen meat or bony scraps as opposed to softer tissues. Further, historic accounts from Greenland report that the carnassials of dogs were removed to prevent them from chewing their bindings [20–21]. Such practices would leave very visible signs in archaeological specimens.

Enamel hypoplasia is a condition in which defects in the enamel of teeth are produced by disturbances to the process of enamel formation [32]. Enamel hypoplasia has been little studied in archaeological dog remains, despite the many descriptions of such lesions on dog teeth present in veterinary literature [13,33–36]; comparative data on the occurrence of such features in the teeth of wild canids remain rare. Enamel hypoplasia in canid teeth is caused by diseases such as canine distemper, but also by trauma and dietary deficiencies [33,35,37]. Such lesions are potentially informative about food stress, injuries to the facial region, and disease history for dogs and wolves in the first months of life when tooth crowns are forming.

This paper presents comparative data necessary for evaluating the occurrence rates and patterning in cranial trauma and tooth loss, fracture, and enamel hypoplasia in archaeological dog remains. To begin, data are provided for 400 wild wolves from boreal and arctic regions of Canada and Russia. Patterns in this wolf data are compared with those for 144 historic dogs from these same northern regions. We then discuss the meanings of the differences found between wolves and dogs, including how such patterns are informative about dog food stress and provisioning practices.

Materials

Summary demographic data for all canid samples analyzed is presented in Table 1, and catalog numbers are listed in Table S1. Wolf crania and mandibles were examined from three collections. The first is from Alberta (Figure 1), consisting of 177 individuals; all are curated at the Royal Alberta Museum (Edmonton, Canada). Nearly all were obtained through poisoning in the 1960s–80s in northern Alberta, which is largely boreal forest, or in the Rocky Mountains [38]. The second collection of wolves, termed the Nunavut group, was assembled from the 1920s–1980s from Arctic Canada (Figure 1) and consists of 131 specimens; all are curated at the Canadian Museum of Nature (CMN; Ottawa, Canada). The final wolf collection, dating from 1885 to 1984, is from Russia, and is subdivided into Arctic (generally north of 66 degrees north latitude, n = 50) and Subarctic (50 to 65 degrees north latitude, n = 42) groups. All the Russian wolves are curated at the Zoological Institute of the Russian Academy of Science (ZIRAS; St. Petersburg, Russia).

There are nine dog samples from across much of the northern hemisphere (Figure 1). The first set of dog samples includes 24 Inuit sled dogs collected in Grise Fiord, Ellesmere Island (Canada) in 1966–70; most have documented age, sex, and body mass at

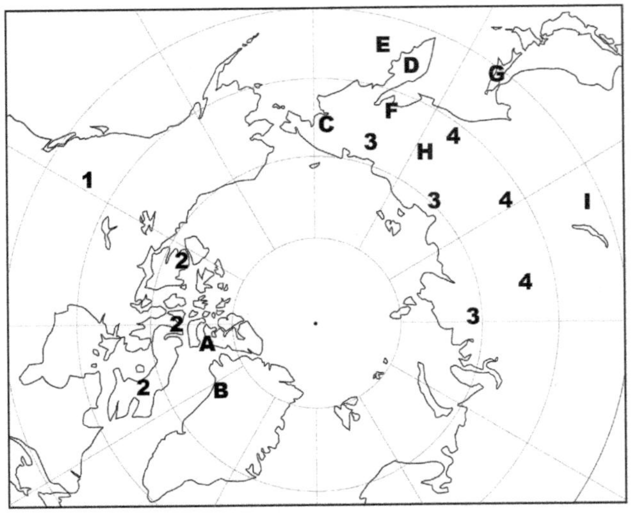

Figure 1. Location of the dog and wolf samples described in this study. Wolves: 1. Alberta, 2. Nunavut, 3. Russian Arctic, 4. Russian Subarctic. Dogs: A. Ellesmere, B. Greenland, C. Chukotka, D. Kamchatka, E. Bering Island, F. Northern Far East, G. Sakhalin, H. Sakha, I. Trans-Baikal.

death and all are curated at the CMN. Dr. M. Freeman, who collected these specimens, was interviewed in 2013. The second dog collection is from northwest Greenland and consists of 13 specimens collected by Robert E. Peary in 1896–7; all are curated at the American Museum of Natural History (AMNH; New York, U.S.A.). All are sled dogs obtained from Greenland Inuit, as reported in Peary's [39] expedition account.

The remaining seven samples of dogs come from the Russian North, and all are housed at the ZIRAS, except for 14 specimens from Chukotka, which are curated at the AMNH. The sample from Chukotka includes 42 dogs collected from 1891 to 1938. The second set of dogs is termed the Bering Island group, collected in 1884. It includes 10 dogs from this island, one of which is listed as a sled dog, and one from nearby Commander Island. The third group includes 11 specimens from unspecified locations on the Kamchatka peninsula in 1884. The fourth group, collected from 1885 to 1928, is from Sakha Republic and includes 21 specimens, with one described as a sled dog, and another as a hare hunting dog. The fifth set of dogs, the Northern Far East group, includes seven specimens collected in 1935. Six are sled dogs, with the seventh being a sled and hunting dog. The sixth group of dogs is from Sakhalin Island, and all were collected from 1882 to 1932. Within this group of nine dogs are six listed as sled dogs. Finally, the seventh group of dogs is from Eastern Trans-Baikal, and consists of six specimens collected in 1914–15.

Methods

Specimens were selected for study only when the permanent dentition was at least partially erupted and the crowns clearly visible. Those classified as adults had no deciduous dentition in place and the permanent teeth were fully erupted, while those classified as juveniles had either partially unerupted permanent teeth or retained some deciduous teeth. Both dogs and wolves obtain their full adult dentition by approximately six months of age, before adulthood, which occurs in both at roughly two years. However, there presently exists no reliable non-destructive means for assessing the age of the crania and mandibles of dogs or wolves.

Table 1. Profile of the specimens analyzed in this study: a. wolves, b. dogs.

Table 1a.

	Alberta	Nunavut	Russian Subarctic	Russian Arctic	Wolf Totals
	(n = 177)	(n = 131)	(n = 42)	(n = 50)	(n = 400)
Males	75	69	20	16	180
Females	89	48	15	8	160
Unknown	13	14	7	26	60
Adult	174	98	42	42	356
Juvenile	3	33	0	8	44

Table 1b.

	Ellesmere	Greenland	Chukotka	Bering Is.	Sakha
	(n = 24)	(n = 13)	(n = 42)	(n = 11)	(n = 21)
Males	13	9	26		5
Females	11	3	8		1
Unknown	0	1	8	11	15
Adult	17	13	39	11	19
Juvenile	7	0	3	0	2
	Kamchatka	**N. Far East**	**Sakhalin**	**Trans-Baikal**	**Dog Totals**
	n = 11)	(n = 7)	(n = 9)	(n = 6)	(n = 144)
Males	0	6		2	61
Females	0	1		1	25
Unknown	11	0	7	3	56
Adult	6	6	7	6	124
Juvenile	5	1	2	0	20

Ideally, assignment of canids as adults versus juveniles would be done using post-cranial skeletal fusion patterns, but in our dataset all but ~50 specimens examined lacked postcranial remains. Our ageing approach is a conservative one, and probably under-represents the number of juveniles present in the collections, but it allows us to treat the specimens in all samples consistently. Notably, 129 of the Alberta wolves have age estimates based on counting of cementum bands in the mandibular 1st premolar, and 18 of the Ellesmere dogs have known ages at death (Table S2). All canid crania and mandibles were scored for traits or conditions using standardized data recording forms (see Figure S1). Where possible, patterns were analyzed by age and sex. The Pearson chi-square statistic is used to evaluate differences between or within sample groups. The four primary conditions recorded were:

1. Antemortem tooth loss (AMTL). Teeth were scored as lost antemortem if no evidence of alveolar remodeling could be observed. If root fragments were present but the crown was missing, the tooth was recorded as absent, as it could no longer function for mastication. Alveoli that were completely filled with new bone were counted as lost teeth. This approach could potentially result in congenitally absent teeth being erroneously counted as lost, a point we return to later. Tooth loss was tabulated by tooth type (incisor, canine, premolar, molar; maxillary or mandibular).
2. Fractured teeth. A tooth was scored as fractured if it was broken and the margins of the break edge showed evidence of wear or the jaw showed signs of related infection; fracture occurrences were tabulated by tooth type.
3. Traumatic lesions. The presence of antemortem fractures (including punctures) was recorded by location on the cranium or mandible using the data recording forms.
4. Enamel hypoplasia. Teeth were scored for presence or absence of hypoplastic lesions by tooth type. We counted the presence of such lesions conservatively, identifying the condition as present only when we were fully confident it was present.

Results

Antemortem tooth loss

Several overarching patterns are apparent in the AMTL data. First, tooth loss occurs in a far greater percentage of dogs than wolves, with 53.47% and 17.00% ($X^2 = 52.85$, $p = <0.0001$) of the total wolf and dog individuals, respectively, having lost at least one tooth (Table 2). Second, dogs of all demographic groups (male, female, adult, juvenile) were more likely to experience tooth loss than their counterparts among the wolves. Third, the overall percentage of teeth lost is also significantly higher in the dogs than in the wolves (4.83% versus 0.91%, respectively; $X^2 = 352.22$, $p = <0.0001$), and is higher in the dogs for each tooth type (Table 3). Fourth, the rank order of the teeth most commonly lost is similar in the dogs and wolves, with the three most commonly lost being the upper and lower premolars and the mandibular molars (Table 3).

Congenital absence of teeth is unlikely to have a significant impact on our AMTL counts. Antemortem tooth loss can generally be distinguished from dental agenesis or delayed tooth

Table 2. Antemortem tooth loss in dogs and wolves by number and percentage of individuals affected: a. wolves, b. dogs.

Table 2a.

		Alberta (n = 177) n (%)	Nunavut (n = 131) n (%)	Russian Subarctic (n = 42) n (%)	Russian Arctic (n = 50) n (%)	Wolf Totals (n = 400) n (%)
Sex	**Male**	14 (18.67)	15 (21.74)	4 (20.00)	2 (12.50)	35 (19.44)
	Female	7 (7.87)	8 (16.67)	5 (33.33)	3 (37.50)	23 (14.37)
	Unknown	1 (7.69)	3 (21.43)	1 (14.29)	5 (18.52)	10 16.67)
Age	**Juvenile**	0 (0.00)	3 (9.09)		0 (0.00)	3 (6.81)
	Adult	22 (12.64)	23 (23.47)	10 (23.81)	10 (23.81)	65 (17.81)
Total		**22 (12.43)**	**26 (19.85)**	**10 (23.81)**	**10 (20.00)**	**68 (17.00)**

Table 2b.

		Ellesmere (n = 24) n (%)	Greenland (n = 13) n (%)	Chukotka (n = 42) n (%)	Bering Is. (n = 11) n (%)	Sakha (n = 21) n (%)
Sex	**Male**	9 (69.23)	9 (100.00)	14 (53.85)		0 (0.00)
	Female	9 (81.82)	3 (100.00)	4 (50.00)		0 (0.00)
	Unknown		1 (100.00)	4 (50.00)	4 (36.36)	3 (20.00)
Age	**Juvenile**	5 (71.43)		2 (66.67)		0 (0.00)
	Adult	13 (54.17)	13 (100.00)	22 (56.41)	4 (36.36)	3 (15.79)
Total		**18 (75.00)**	**13 (100.00)**	**24 (57.14)**	**4 (36.36)**	**3 (14.29)**
		Kamchatka (n = 11) n (%)	**N. Far East (n = 7) n (%)**	**Sakhalin (n = 9) n (%)**	**Trans-Baikal (n = 6) n (%)**	**Dog Totals (n = 144) n (%)**
Sex	**Male**		5 (83.33)		1 (50.00)	38 (62.30)
	Female		0 (0.00)		0 (0.00)	16 (64.00)
	Unknown	5 (45.45)		3 (33.33)	1 (33.33)	21 (37.50)
Age	**Juvenile**	0 (0.00)	1 (100.00)	1 (50.00)		9 (45.00)
	Adult	5 (83.33)	4 (66.67)	2 (28.57)	2 (33.33)	68 (54.84)
Total		**5 (45.45)**	**5 (71.43)**	**3 (33.33)**	**2 (33.33)**	**77 (53.47)**

eruption by the presence of alveolar remodeling, which would occur only when teeth are lost during life. When analyzing the canids, congenital absence was identified by both the lack of alveoli and alveolar remodeling. Bilateral absence was also considered as a strong indicator of agenesis. For both sets of canids, agenesis affected only the upper and lower 1st premolars and lower 3rd molars. First premolars previously were reported as occasionally congenitally absent in 'Eskimo dogs' [13] and these and lower 3rd molars in some wolves, albeit in low frequencies [9,10,40,18]. However, only 15 of the 144 dogs we examined were suspected of having congenitally absent teeth, and of these nine also showed clear evidence from AMTL. Further, ten wolves also showed bilateral absence of the 1st premolars or lower 3rd molars, which may indicate congenital absence. Among these wolves, only two specimens had AMTL.

Tooth loss also varied among the wolf groups, ranging from a high of 23.81% in the Russian Subarctic sample to a low of 12.43% in the Alberta wolves (Table 2). The percentages of AMTL in the wolf groups do not correlate with latitude—slightly higher rates of loss were seen in Nunavut than Alberta ($X^2 = 2.6581$, $p = 0.1030$), while the more northerly Russian wolves had very slightly lower rates than those from further south ($X^2 = 0.1523$, $p = 0.6963$), but this difference is likely due to chance. Note that a previous study on wolves from across the former Soviet Union reported an AMTL rate (# of individuals affected) of 12.4% [18]. In both the Nunavut and Alberta wolves, tooth loss was greater among males than females, but the difference was only significant in the Alberta sample (Nunavut wolves, $X^2 = 0.3705$, $p = 0.5427$; Alberta wolves, $X^2 = 3.7085$, $p = 0.0541$). The opposite pattern is seen in the Russian wolves, but sample sizes are small and the patterns observed are likely due to chance (subarctic wolves, $X^2 = 0.5926$, $p = 0.4414$; arctic wolves, $X^2 = 1.0343$, $p = 0.3091$). No significant difference in AMTL by sex was reported for the previously published Soviet Union wolf sample [18].

For the dogs, tooth loss varied widely between groups, ranging from a high of 100% of the Greenland specimens being affected, to low of 14.29% for the Sakha specimens (Table 2); only this latter group has tooth loss within the range seen among the wolves. Males and females in the total dog sample experienced roughly the same likelihood of having lost teeth ($X^2 = 0.0082$, $p = 0.9278$), and a slightly higher percentage of adults were affected than juveniles,

Table 3. Antemortem tooth loss in dogs and wolves by number and percentage of specific tooth group affected: a. wolves, b. dogs.

Table 3a.

	Alberta			Nunavut			Russian Subarctic			Russian Arctic			Wolf Totals		
Tooth Class	n_a	n_o	%	n_a	n_o	%	n_a	n_o	%	n_a	n_o	%	n_a	n_o	%
Max. incisors	10	1061	0.94	6	786	0.76	1	252	0.4	3	300	1	20	2399	0.83
Man. incisors	9	1062	0.85	4	777	0.51	0	252	0	1	300	0.33	14	2391	0.59
Max. canines	2	354	0.56	1	262	0.38	0	84	0	0	100	0	3	800	0.38
Man. canines	0	354	0	1	259	0.39	0	84	0	0	100	0	1	797	0.13
Max. premolars	2	1412	0.14	19	1044	1.82	3	336	0.89	9	400	2.25	33	3192	1.03
Man. premolars	9	1415	0.64	6	1035	0.58	4	336	1.19	18	400	4.5	37	3186	1.16
Max. molars	0	706	0	1	520	0.19	3	168	1.79	1	200	0.5	5	1594	0.31
Man. molars	5	1060	0.47	21	772	2.72	5	252	1.98	8	295	2.71	39	2379	1.64
Totals	**37**	**7424**	**0.5**	**59**	**5455**	**1.08**	**16**	**1764**	**0.91**	**40**	**2095**	**1.91**	**152**	**16738**	**0.91**

Table 3b.

	Ellesmere			Greenland			Chukotka			Bering Is.			Sakha		
Tooth Class	n_a	n_o	%	n_a	n_o	%	n_a	n_o	%	n_a	n_o	%	n_a	n_o	%
Max. incisors	4	144	2.78	2	78	2.56	0	252	0	8	66	12.12	1	126	0.79
Man. incisors	1	144	0.69	0	72	0	10	234	4.27	6	60	10	1	114	0.88
Max. canines	1	48	2.08	2	26	7.69	3	84	3.57	0	22	0	0	42	0
Man. canines	2	48	4.17	0	24	0	0	78	0	1	20	5	0	38	0
Max. premolars	21	191	10.99	39	104	37.5	13	336	3.87	5	88	5.68	1	168	0.6
Man. premolars	33	190	17.37	25	96	26.04	14	312	4.49	2	80	2.5	1	152	0.66
Max. molars	1	95	1.05	1	52	1.92	6	168	3.57	0	44	0	0	84	0
Man. molars	2	144	1.39	12	72	16.67	12	234	5.13	0	60	0	2	114	1.75
Totals	**65**	**1004**	**6.47**	**81**	**524**	**15.46**	**58**	**1698**	**3.42**	**22**	**440**	**5**	**6**	**838**	**0.72**

	Kamchatka			N. Far East			Sakhalin			Trans-Baikal			Dog Totals		
Tooth Class	n_a	n_o	%	n_a	n_o	%	n_a	n_o	%	n_a	n_o	%	n_a	n_o	%
Max. incisors	3	66	4.55	2	42	4.76	0	54	0	5	36	13.89	25	864	2.89
Man. incisors	0	66	0	0	40	0	0	48	0	2	30	6.67	20	808	2.48
Max. canines	0	22	0	0	14	0	0	18	0	1	12	8.33	7	288	2.43
Man. canines	0	22	0	1	14	7.14	0	16	0	1	10	10	5	270	1.85
Max. premolars	3	88	3.41	2	56	3.57	3	72	4.17	2	48	4.17	89	1151	7.73
Man. premolars	5	88	5.68	2	56	3.57	3	64	4.69	2	40	5	86	1078	8.07
Max. molars	0	44	0	0	28	0	1	36	2.78	0	24	0	9	575	1.57
Man. molars	4	66	6.06	6	42	14.29	1	48	2.08	1	30	3.33	40	810	4.94
Totals	**15**	**462**	**3.25**	**13**	**292**	**4.45**	**8**	**356**	**2.25**	**14**	**230**	**6.09**	**282**	**5844**	**4.83**

Table 4. Antemortem tooth fracture in dogs and wolves by number and percentage of individuals affected: a. wolves, b. dogs.

Table 4a.

		Alberta	Nunavut	Russia Subarctic	Russian Arctic	Wolf Totals
		(n = 177)	(n = 131)	(n = 42)	(n = 50)	(n = 400)
		n (%)	n (%)	n (%)	n (%)	n (%)
Sex	**Male**	30 (40.00)	18 (26.09)	4 (20.00)	5 (31.25)	57 (31.67)
	Female	22 (24.72)	9 (18.75)	1 (6.67)	4 (50.00)	36 (22.50)
	Unknown	1 (7.69)	2 (14.29)	2 (28.57)	3 (11.11)	8 (13.33)
Age	**Juvenile**	0 (0.00)	0 (0.00)		1 (12.50)	1 (2.27)
	Adult	53 (30.46)	29 (29.59)	7 (16.67)	11 (26.19)	100 (28.09)
Total		**53 (29.94)**	**29 (22.14)**	**7 (16.67)**	**12 (24.00)**	**111 (27.75)**

Table 4b.

		Ellesmere	Greenland	Chukotka	Bering Is.	Sakha
		(n = 24)	(n = 13)	(n = 42)	(n = 11)	(n = 11)
		n (%)	n (%)	n (%)	n (%)	n (%)
Sex	**Male**	9 (69.23)	8 (88.89)	11 (42.31)		0 (0.00)
	Female	4 (36.36)	3 (100.00)	1 (12.50)		0 (0.00)
	Unknown		0 (0.00)	1 (12.50)	4 (36.36)	4 (26.67)
Age	**Juvenile**	0 (0.00)		1 (33.33)		0 (0.00)
	Adult	13 (76.47)	11 (84.62)	12 (30.77)	4 (36.36)	4 (21.05)
Total		**13 (54.17)**	**11 (84.62)**	**13 (30.95)**	**4 (36.36)**	**4 (19.05)**
		Kamchatka	**N. Far East**	**Sakhalin**	**Trans-Baikal**	**Dog Totals**
		(n = 11)	(n = 7)	(n = 9)	(n = 6)	(n = 144)
		n (%)	n (%)	n (%)	n (%)	n (%)
Sex	**Male**		1 (16.67)		1 (50.00)	30 (49.18)
	Female		0 (0.00)		0 (0.00)	8 (32.00)
	Unknown	4 (36.36)		3 (33.33)	0 (0.00)	16 (28.57)
Age	**Juvenile**	0 (0.00)	0 (0.00	0 (0.00		1 (5.00)
	Adult	4 (66.67)	1 (16.67)	3 (42.86)	1 (16.67)	53 (42.74)
Total		4 (36.36)	1 (16.67)	3 (33.33)	1 (16.67)	54 (37.50)

but this difference was not statistically significant ($X^2 = 0.1389$, $p = 0.7094$), and varied from group to group. The most commonly lost tooth type also varied widely from group to group (Table 3). Note the very high percentages of premolars lost in the Ellesmere and Greenland dogs, which are several orders of magnitude greater than in the other groups, and far above the total dog average for those tooth groups (Ellesmere versus total dog, $X^2 = 14.8895$, $p = 0.0001$; Greenland versus total dog, $X^2 = 105.4026$, $p < 0.0001$).

Tooth fracture

The tooth fracture data in many ways parallels the AMTL patterns just described. First, the percentage of individuals experiencing tooth fracture (Table 4) is significantly higher among the dogs than the wolves (37.50% opposed to 27.75%, respectively; $X^2 = 2.8812$, $p = 0.0896$). The percentage of wolves with fractured teeth observed here is similar to that previously reported for North American wolves (29%; [15]). Second, all dog demographic categories show higher percentages of tooth fracture than their wolf counterparts. Third, dogs and wolves show the same patterns in which teeth are most commonly fractured; the canines and upper incisors being most commonly affected (Table 5).

Tooth fracture frequency did not always correlate with rates of AMTL. The lowest level of AMTL was seen in the Alberta wolves, but this group has the highest percentage of individuals with fractured teeth, at 29.94% (compare tables 2 and 4). Conversely, the Russian Subarctic wolves had the highest number of specimens with AMTL but have the lowest percentage of individuals with tooth fracture. Overall, more male wolves suffered tooth fracture than females ($X^2 = 2.6022$, $p = 0.1067$), with only Subarctic Russian wolves having more females than males affected (Table 4) but the sample sizes in the latter case are small and the differences likely due to chance ($X^2 = 0.4$, $p = 0.5271$). In all groups where juveniles were present, they are less likely to have broken teeth than adults.

In contrast to the pattern observed in the wolves, the two groups of dogs showing the highest levels of tooth loss, namely those from Ellesmere and Greenland, also show the highest number of individuals with tooth fracture (compare Tables 2 and 4). Males again are more likely to show tooth fracture than females in the total dog sample ($X^2 = 1.1845$, $p = 0.2764$), the single exception

Table 5. Antemortem tooth fracture in dogs and wolves by number and percentage of specific tooth group affected: a. wolves, b. dogs.

Table 5a.

	Alberta			Nunavut			Russian Subarctic			Russian Arctic			Wolf Totals		
Tooth Class	n_a	n_o	%	n_a	n_o	%	n_a	n_o	%	n_a	n_o	%	n_a	n_o	%
Max. incisors	32	1019	3.14	23	732	3.14	4	232	1.72	6	277	2.17	65	2260	2.88
Man. incisors	18	1017	1.77	10	718	1.39	0	236	0.00	1	279	0.36	29	2250	1.29
Max. canines	18	323	5.57	10	237	4.22	2	58	3.45	4	91	4.40	34	709	4.80
Man. canines	11	342	3.22	14	247	5.67	2	84	2.38	2	98	2.04	29	771	3.76
Max. premolars	20	1361	1.47	12	1003	1.20	4	315	1.27	2	376	0.53	38	3055	1.24
Man. premolars	8	1138	0.70	9	991	0.91	1	320	0.31	2	375	0.53	20	2824	0.71
Max. molars	5	703	0.71	6	515	1.17	0	164	0.00	5	198	2.53	16	1580	1.01
Man. molars	12	995	1.21	2	719	0.28	1	230	0.43	2	271	0.74	17	2215	0.77
Totals	124	6898	1.80	86	5162	1.67	14	1639	0.85	24	1965	1.22	248	15664	1.58

Table 5b.

	Ellesmere			Greenland			Chukotka			Bering Is.			Sakha		
Tooth Class	n_a	n_o	%	n_a	n_o	%	n_a	n_o	%	n_a	n_o	%	n_a	n_o	%
Max. incisors	5	140	3.57	8	66	12.12	8	198	4.04	1	34	2.94	2	91	2.20
Man. incisors	2	143	1.40	1	61	1.64	4	184	2.17	1	41	2.44	3	87	3.45
Max. canines	8	47	17.02	7	24	29.17	5	65	7.69	5	15	33.33	0	36	0.00
Man. canines	10	46	21.74	5	26	19.23	13	68	19.12	3	15	20.00	0	34	0.00
Max. premolars	7	170	4.12	6	56	10.71	7	267	2.62	1	70	1.43	2	140	1.43
Man. premolars	2	156	1.28	7	65	10.77	3	266	1.13	0	67	0.00	0	142	0.00
Max. molars	1	92	1.09	1	46	2.17	5	148	3.38	2	41	4.88	0	80	0.00
Man. molars	4	142	2.82	16	47	34.04	1	189	0.53	1	49	2.04	0	98	0.00
Totals	39	936	4.17	51	391	13.04	46	1385	3.32	14	332	4.22	7	708	0.99

	Kamchatka			N. Far East			Sakhalin			Trans-Baikal			Dog Totals		
Tooth Class	n_a	n_o	%	n_a	n_o	%	n_a	n_o	%	n_a	n_o	%	n_a	n_o	%
Max. incisors	2	57	3.51	0	36	0.00	1	50	2.00	2	29	6.90	29	701	4.14
Man. incisors	0	60	0.00	0	35	0.00	0	47	0.00	2	26	7.69	13	684	1.90
Max. canines	3	20	15.00	0	13	0.00	1	18	5.56	0	10	0.00	29	248	11.69
Man. canines	1	21	4.76	0	13	0.00	0	14	0.00	0	9	0.00	32	246	13.01
Max. premolars	1	80	1.25	0	54	0.00	0	69	0.00	2	41	4.88	26	947	2.75
Man. premolars	0	82	0.00	0	53	0.00	0	59	0.00	0	37	0.00	12	927	1.29
Max. molars	2	42	4.76	2	28	7.14	0	35	0.00	1	24	4.17	14	536	2.61
Man. molars	1	56	1.79	0	35	0.00	0	43	0.00	0	27	0.00	23	686	3.35
Totals	10	418	2.39	2	267	0.75	2	335	0.60	7	203	3.45	178	4975	3.58

Table 6. Traumatic lesions in dogs and wolves by number and percentage of individuals affected, and by type of lesion: a. wolves, b. dogs.

Table 6a.

	Alberta	Nunavut	Russia Subarctic	Russian Arctic	Wolf Totals
	(n = 177)	(n-131)	(n = 42)	(n = 50)	(n = 400)
	n (%)	n (%)	n (%)	n (%)	n (%)
Male	21 (28.00)	10 (7.63)	3 (15.00)	3 (18.75)	37 (20.56)
Female	21 (23.60)	13 (9.92)	3 (20.00)	0 (0.00)	37 (23.13)
Unknown	1 (7.69)	0 (0.00)	1 (14.29)	4 (15.38)	6 (10.00)
Juvenile	0 (0.00)	2 (6.06)		1 (12.50)	3 (6.82)
Adult	43 (24.71)	21 (21.43)	7 (16.67)	6 (14.29)	77 (21.62)
Fractures	25 (14.12)	5 (3.82)	3 (7.14)	1 (2.00)	34 (8.50)
Bite marks	18 (10.17)	18 (13.74)	6 (14.29)	6 (12.00)	48 (12.00)
Totals	**43 (24.29)**	**23 (17.56)**	**7 (16.67)**	**7 (14.00)**	**80 (20.00)**

Table 6b.

	Ellesmere	Greenland	Chukotka	Bering Is.	Sakha
	(n = 24)	(n = 13)	(n = 42)	(n = 11)	(n = 21)
	n (%)	n (%)	n (%)	n (%)	n (%)
Male	8 (61.54)	6 (46.15)	5 (19.23)		2 (40.00)
Female	1 (9.09)	3 (100.00)	3 (37.50)		0 (0.00)
Unknown		1 (100.00)	2 (25.00)	10 (90.91)	6 (40.00)
Juvenile	0 (0.00)		0 (0.00)		1 (50.00)
Adult	9 (52.94)	10 (76.92)	10 (25.64)	10 (90.91)	8 (42.11)
Fractures	7 (29.17)	7 (53.85)	9 (21.42)	10 (90.91)	2 (9.52)
Bite marks	4 (16.67)	3 (21.43)	1 (2.38)	3 (27.27)	7 (33.33)
Totals	**9 (37.50)**	**10 (76.92)**	**10 (23.81)**	**10 (90.91)**	**9 (42.86)**
	Kamchatka	**N. Far East**	**Sakhalin**	**Trans-Baikal**	**Dog Totals**
	(n = 11)	(n = 7)	(n = 9)	(n = 6)	(n = 144)
	n (%)	n (%)	n (%)	n (%)	n (%)
Male		0 (0.00)		1 (50.00)	22 (36.07)
Female		0 (0.00)		0 (0.00)	7 (28.00)
Unknown	2 (18.18)		1 (11.11)	1 (33.33)	23 (41.07)
Juvenile	1 (20.00)	0 (0.00)	1 (50.00)		3 (15.00)
Adult	1 (16.67)	0 (0.00)	0 (0.00)	2 (33.33)	50 (40.32)
Fractures	1 (9.09)	0 (0.00)	1 (11.11)	0 (0.00)	37 (28.68)
Bite marks	1 (9.09)	0 (0.00)	0 (0.00)	2 (33.33)	21 (16.28)
Totals	**2 (18.18)**	**0 (0.00)**	**1 (11.11)**	**2 (33.33)**	**53 (36.81)**

being the Greenland sample, which contains too few females to be meaningful. Substantial variability in the number of individuals with tooth fracture is also present among the dog groups, with three (Sakha, N. Far East, and Trans-Baikal) having percentages within the range of that observed in the wolves. Finally, the Ellesmere, Greenland, Chukotka, Bering Island, Kamchatka, and Sakhalin groups all have canines more commonly fractured than other tooth types; for the remaining samples, incisors or molars are most commonly fractured (Table 5). Overall, canines are by far the most commonly fractured teeth in the dogs.

Traumatic lesions

Lesions on the crania and mandibles consistent with trauma were grouped into two categories: bite wounds and other fractures (Tables 6 and 7). Traumatic lesions characterized as bite wounds were round to oval shaped punctures less than 1 cm in diameter. These were sometimes partially healed and nearly refilled with new bone. Most often such marks were found on the snout, which we subdivided into palate and outer rostrum, while a small number were observed on the frontals. The other fractures recorded were larger depression and radiating fractures.

As with the previous two dental trauma indices, dogs were more likely than wolves to have traumatic lesions (36.8% versus 20%, respectively; $X^2 = 12.22$, $p = 0.0005$), and this pattern was found

Table 7. Traumatic lesions in dogs and wolves by position: a. wolves, b. dogs.

Table 7a.

	Alberta		Nunavut		Russian Subarctic		Russian Arctic		Wolf Totals	
	n	%	n	%	n	%	n	%	n	%
Bite mark location										
External rostrum	8	4.52	7	5.34	3	7.14	1	2.00	19	4.75
Palate	10	5.65	13	9.92	4	9.52	5	10.00	32	8.00
Frontals	4	2.26	4	3.05	1	2.38	0	0.00	9	2.25
Other fracture location										
Rostrum	16	9.04	3	2.29	1	2.38	0	0.00	20	5.00
Frontals	3	1.69	2	1.53	2	4.76	1	2.00	8	2.00
Occipital	5	2.82	0	0.00	0	0.00	0	0.00	5	1.25
Mandible	3	1.69	0	0.00	0	0.00	1	2.00	4	1.00

Table 7b.

	Ellesmere		Greenland		Chukotka		Bering Is.		Sakha	
	n	%	n	%	n	%	n	%	n	%
Bite mark location										
External rostrum	2	8.33	1	7.69	0	0.00	0	0.00	1	4.76
Palate	3	12.50	2	15.38	1	2.38	3	27.27	6	28.57
Frontals	0	0.00	0	0.00	0	0.00	0	0.00	0	0.00
Other fracture location										
Rostrum	1	4.17	2	15.38	4	9.52	5	45.45	0	0.00
Frontals	6	25.00	6	46.15	6	14.29	7	63.64	1	4.76
Occipital	0	0.00	0	0.00	0	0.00	1	9.09	0	0.00
Mandible	0	0.00	0	0.00	0	0.00	1	9.09	1	4.76

	Kamchatka		N. Far East		Sakhalin		Trans-Baikal		Dog Totals	
	n	%	n	%	n	%	n	%	n	%
Bite mark location										
External rostrum	1	9.09	0	0.00	0	0.00	0	0.00	5	3.88
Palate	1	9.09	0	0.00	0	0.00	2	33.33	18	13.95
Frontals	0	0.00	0	0.00	0	0.00	0	0.00	0	0.00
Other fracture location										
Rostrum	0	0.00	0	0.00	0	0.00	0	0.00	12	9.30
Frontals	1	9.09	0	0.00	1	11.11	0	0.00	28	21.71
Occipital	0	0.00	0	0.00	0	0.00	0	0.00	1	0.78
Mandible	0	0.00	0	0.00	0	0.00	0	0.00	2	1.55

across all demographic subdivisions (Table 6). When the trauma is divided into bite wounds and other fractures (Table 6), the number of individuals with bite marks differs by only 4.28% between the wolves and dogs ($X^2 = 0.5591$, $p = 0.4546$); this difference may be due to chance. The other fractures, however, are found in over three times more dogs than wolves (28.7% versus 8.5%, respectively; $X^2 = 23.9992$, $p = <0.0001$). When the traumatic lesions are broken down by affected area (Table 7), both wolves and dogs experienced more bite wounds on their palates than in other places on the skull, but only the wolves showed such lesions on the frontal bones, and this only rarely. The patterning in the other fractures differs strongly between the dogs and wolves. Of the 37 wolves with skull fractures, 20 occurred in the rostrum and 8 in the frontals. Among the 43 dogs with skull fractures, 12 were in the rostrum and 28 were in the frontals. Fractures in other portions of the skull were rare in both groups.

Within the wolves, there is little clear patterning in the occurrences of traumatic lesions, other than those just mentioned. Juveniles are always less likely to have such lesions than adults, but there is no consistency by sex. Bite marks were more common than other fractures in all of the wolf groups, with the exception of the Alberta sample. Further, the occurrence of bite marks was fairly similar in all samples, ranging from 10.2% to 14.3%. Both lower latitude samples (Alberta and Subarctic Russia) had higher incidences of individuals with fractures than in the more northerly samples from their respective continents.

Substantial variability in lesion frequency is present between the groups of dogs analyzed. First, four groups of dog (Chukotka, Kamchatka, N. Far East, and Sakhalin) all have traumatic lesions at or below the level seen in the wolves (Table 6). Within this low trauma group, however, the Chukotka group still has a far higher rate of other fractures (bite marks excluded) than the wolves, with 21.42% of the individuals affected compared to only 8.50% of the wolves displaying such lesions ($X^2 = 6.5304$, $p = 0.0106$). The Ellesmere, Greenland, and Bering Islands dogs all have high percentages of individuals affected by fractures (from 29.2 to 90.9%), which accounts for their overall high percentages of trauma. In this set of dogs with high fracture occurrences, the percentage of individuals with frontal fractures is consistently high, ranging from 25% in the Ellesmere group, to 63.5% of the Bering Island group (Table 7). The two remaining groups, from Sakha and Trans-Baikal, both have high rates of trauma due to the number of individuals affected with bite marks.

Enamel hypoplasia

Enamel hypoplasia can be broadly grouped into three categories: furrow-type defects (linear enamel hypoplasia), pit-type defects, and plane-type defects [41–2]. Both pit-type and plane-type defects were observed on the canid teeth (Figure 2) with some affected teeth displaying both types. The defects recorded matched those described in the literature for dogs and wolves [13,33–36]. No cases of furrow-type defects were observed, nor are we aware of such defects being reported in the canid literature. Instances of pit-type hypoplasia consisted of a nonlinear array of pits on the buccal surface of one or more teeth (Figure 2a). Pitting was most common on the mandibular 1st molars and was often asymmetric. Plane-type lesions consisted of two main types: First, isolated hypoplastic lesions exposed broad patches of the underlying enamel (Figure 2b). Like the pit-type defects, these patchy plane-type lesions occurred most frequently on the mandibular carnassials and were generally bilateral. A second, more severe form of plane-type hypoplasia was also observed (Figure 2c). In these cases enamel loss was prolific, affecting multiple teeth with large sections of dentine exposed on all sides of the crowns. All plane-type defects were commonly surrounded by discolored areas of intact enamel.

Overall, occurrences of enamel hypoplasia in the canids were rare, with only 17 dogs and wolves affected in the total sample of 544 individuals (Table 8). A slightly higher percentage of dogs was affected than wolves, but the difference was not significant (4.9% and 2.5%, respectively; $X^2 = 1.8889$, $p = 0.1693$). The greatest number of teeth affected in a single individual was 17 in an Alberta wolf, and 25 in a Chukotka dog. In both dogs and wolves, mandibular canines were the most commonly affected teeth, but the numbers of affected teeth is too small for these patterns to be considered meaningful (Table 9). Within the affected wolves, four individuals displayed hypoplastic lesions on 1-3 adjacent teeth; the antimeres were not affected. Three other wolves had such lesions on both the left and right 1st molars (carnassials), while the remaining four wolves displayed lesions on multiple teeth of the upper and lower dentition. Three of the seven dogs showing hypoplastic lesions had only 1–3 adjacent unilateral teeth affected. Two dogs have lesions on both the left and right lower 1st molars, as seen in the wolves. The remaining two specimens include the Chukotka dog with widespread lesions in its upper and lower dentition, and a Sakhalin dog (which lacked mandibles) with its left and right upper 4th premolars (carnassials) and 1st molars affected.

Discussion

Overall, the dogs examined in this study experienced significantly higher rates of tooth loss, tooth fracture, and traumatic lesions than did wolves living in the same ecological regions. They also exhibited slightly higher frequencies of enamel hypoplasia. These patterns could be tied to a number of canid behaviors and life history parameters, but also human husbandry practices.

As the likelihood of experiencing injury increases with age, it is important to rule out age differences as an explanation for the contrasts observed between wolves and dogs. We do not believe that age is an important factor in our study for two reasons. First,

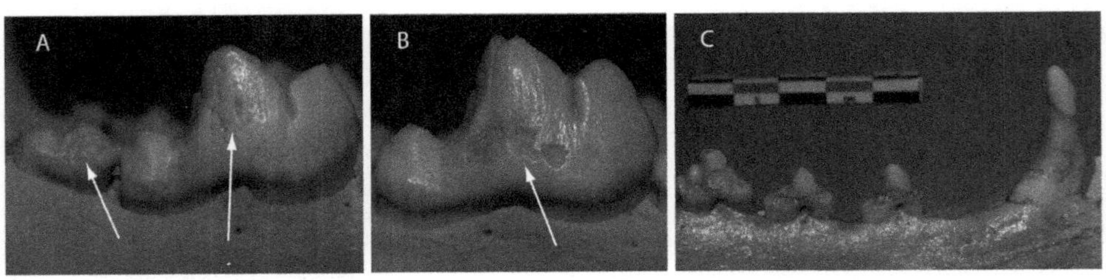

Figure 2. Examples of hypoplastic lesions on wolf and dog teeth. A. Pitted type lesions on the right mandibular 1st and 2nd molars, buccal face. B. Plane type lesion on the right mandibular 1st molar. C. Severe plane type hypoplasitic lesions on the left mandibular canine and 1-3rd premolars.

Table 8. Hypoplastic lesions in dogs and wolves by number of individuals affected: a. wolves, b. dogs.

Table 8a.

		Alberta	Nunavut	Russia Subarctic	Russian Arctic	Wolf Totals
		(n = 177)	(n = 131)	(n = 42)	(n = 50)	(n = 400)
		n (%)	n (%)	n (%)	n (%)	n (%)
Sex	Male	3 (4.00)	1 (1.45)	0 (0.00)	1 (6.25)	4 (2.22)
	Female	4 (4.49)	0 (0.00)	0 (0.00)	0 (0.00)	4 (2.50)
	Unknown	1 (7.69)	0 (0.00)	0 (0.00)	0 (0.00)	1 (1.67)
Age Cat	Juvenile	0 (0.00)	0 (0.00	0 (0.00)	1 (12.50)	1 (2.27)
	Adult	8 (4.60)	1 (1.02)	0 (0.00)	0 (0.00)	9 (2.53)
Total		**8 (4.52)**	1 (0.76)	0 (0.00)	1 (2.00)	10 (2.50)

Table 8b.

		Ellesmere	Greenland	Chukotka	Bering Is.	Sakha
		(n = 24)	(n = 13)	(n = 42)	(n = 11)	(n = 21)
		n (%)	n (%)	n (%)	n (%)	n (%)
Sex	Male	0 (0.00)	0 (0.00)	2 (7.69)		0 (0.00)
	Female	2 (18.18)	0 (0.00)	1 (12.5)		0 (0.00)
	Unknown	0 (0.00)	0 (0.00)	0 (0.00)	0 (0.00)	0 (0.00)
Age Cat	Juvenile	0 (0.00)		1 (33.33)		0 (0.00)
	Adult	2 (11.76)	0 (0.00)	2 (5.13)	0 (0.00)	0 (0.00)
Total		2 (8.33)	0 (0.00)	3 (7.14)	0 (0.00)	0 (0.00)

		Kamchatka	N. Far East	Sakhalin	Trans-Baikal	Dog Totals
		(n = 11)	(n = 7)	(n = 9)	(n = 6)	(n = 144)
		n (%)	n (%)	n (%)	n (%)	n (%)
Sex	Male		0 (0.00)		0 (0.00)	2 (3.28)
	Female		0 (0.00)		0 (0.00)	3 (12.00)
	Unknown	1 (9.09)		1 (11.11)	0 (0.00)	2 (3.57)
Age Cat	Juvenile	1 (20.00)	0 (0.00)	0 (0.00)	0 (0.00)	2 (10.00)
	Adult	0 (0.00)	0 (0.00)	1 (14.29)	0 (0.00)	5 (4.03)
Total		**1 (9.09)**	**0 (0.00)**	**1 (11.11)**	**0 (0.00)**	**7 (4.86)**

the juvenile dogs examined showed rates of tooth loss far higher than those of the juvenile wolves (Table 2); numbers related to tooth fracture are too small to be meaningful, but the percentage affected also is higher in the dogs than the wolves (Table 4). More specific age at death information is available for most of the Alberta wolves and Ellesmere dogs (Table S2). Using this demographic data, half of the Ellesmere dogs can be classified juveniles (two years of age or less), and five of these nine juveniles (55.56%) experienced tooth loss prior to death (excluding cases where congenital absence or non-eruption was suspected), and two of the nine (22.22%) also suffered tooth fractures. The juvenile Alberta wolves showed far fewer individuals affected by tooth loss and fracture (both at 4.34%; Table S2). Second, other modern working dogs seem to have life spans much like those of wolves. For example, sled dogs in Antarctica sharply decline in their working abilities after about 6–7 years of age, if not earlier [43]. Such declining dogs were typically culled, with only a few above this age kept for breeding purposes. Culling of elderly or "worn-out" dogs was also reported in Greenland [21]. Bogoras [44] states that sled dogs in the Chukotka area decline after six to seven years of age, but some work until ten or eleven years old. Detailed quantitative studies of modern Nicaraguan hunting dogs reported an average age at death of 3.7 years, with only 11% of individuals reaching eight years of age [27]; similarly short lives for dogs are reported in other studies [45–48]. Data on average age at death for wild wolves is rare, but it appears that few reach seven to eight years of age [49,50]. Only three of the 129 Alberta wolves reached eight years of age (Table S2).

Differences in feeding practices of dogs and wolves may account for some of the different levels of tooth fracture and loss observed, and perhaps also some of the patterning in traumatic lesions. Relevant aspects of feeding include a series of inter-related factors such as how food is obtained, prey body size, how completely prey/food is being consumed, and the qualities (density, texture) of what is being masticated. We first consider prey size, which might be related to trauma experiences as well as tooth loss and fracture, with larger prey being more capable of striking the canids with forces sufficient to fracture skulls and teeth, and with larger prey having more robust skeletons that would place higher loads on teeth, both during capture and consumption.

Wolves inhabiting the study regions historically have variable diets [49,51], making it difficult to make simple comparisons

Table 9. Hypoplastic lesions in dogs and wolves by specific tooth group affected: a. wolves, b. dogs.

Table 9a.

	Alberta			Nunavut			Russian Subarctic			Russian Arctic			Wolf Totals		
Tooth Class	n_a	n_o	%	n_a	n_o	%	n_a	n_o	%	n_a	n_o	%	n_a	n_o	%
Max. incisors	2	1013	0.20	0	732	0.00	0	232	0.00	2	277	0.72	4	2254	0.18
Man. incisors	0	1005	0.00	0	718	0.00	0	236	0.00	0	279	0.00	0	2238	0.00
Max. canines	1	318	0.31	0	237	0.00	0	58	0.00	1	91	1.10	2	704	0.28
Man. canines	4	335	1.19	0	247	0.00	0	84	0.00	0	98	0.00	4	764	0.52
Max. premolars	9	1354	0.66	0	1003	0.00	0	315	0.00	0	376	0.00	9	3048	0.30
Man. premolars	9	1132	0.80	0	991	0.00	0	320	0.00	0	375	0.00	9	2818	0.32
Max. molars	0	703	0.00	0	515	0.00	0	164	0.00	0	198	0.00	0	1580	0.00
Man. molars	15	995	1.51	2	719	0.28	0	230	0.00	0	271	0.00	17	2215	0.77

Table 9b.

	Ellesmere			Greenland			Chukotka			Bering Is.			Sakha		
Tooth Class	n_a	n_o	%	n_a	n_o	%	n_a	n_o	%	n_a	n_o	%	n_a	n_o	%
Max. incisors	0	140	0.00	0	66	0.00	2	198	1.01	0	34	0.00	0	91	0.00
Man. incisors	0	143	0.00	0	61	0.00	3	184	1.63	0	41	0.00	0	87	0.00
Max. canines	0	47	0.00	0	24	0.00	2	65	3.08	0	15	0.00	0	36	0.00
Man. canines	1	46	2.17	0	26	0.00	3	68	4.41	0	15	0.00	0	34	0.00
Max. premolars	0	170	0.00	0	56	0.00	6	267	2.25	0	70	0.00	0	140	0.00
Man. premolars	0	156	0.00	0	65	0.00	6	266	2.26	0	67	0.00	0	142	0.00
Max. molars	0	92	0.00	0	46	0.00	1	148	0.68	0	41	0.00	0	80	0.00
Man. molars	2	142	1.41	0	47	0.00	8	189	4.23	0	49	0.00	0	98	0.00

	Kamchatka			N. Far East			Sakhalin			Trans-Baikal			Dog Totals		
Tooth Class	n_a	n_o	%	n_a	n_o	%	n_a	n_o	%	n_a	n_o	%	n_a	n_o	%
Max. incisors	0	57	0.00	0	36	0.00	0	50	0.00	0	29	0.00	2	701	0.29
Man. incisors	3	60	5.00	0	35	0.00	0	47	0.00	0	26	0.00	6	684	0.88
Max. canines	0	20	0.00	0	13	0.00	0	18	0.00	0	10	0.00	2	248	0.81
Man. canines	0	21	0.00	0	13	0.00	0	14	0.00	0	9	0.00	4	246	1.63
Max. premolars	0	80	0.00	0	54	0.00	2	69	2.90	0	41	0.00	8	947	0.84
Man. premolars	0	82	0.00	0	53	0.00	0	59	0.00	0	37	0.00	6	927	0.65
Max. molars	0	42	0.00	0	28	0.00	2	35	5.71	0	24	0.00	3	536	0.56
Man. molars	0	56	0.00	0	35	0.00	0	43	0.00	0	27	0.00	10	686	1.46

between typical prey sizes by region. In Alberta, wild prey potentially encountered by wolves range in size from elk (*Cervus elaphus*) and moose (*Alces alces*) to caribou (*Rangifer tarandus*) and deer (*Odocoileus* spp.), but small mammals such as hare (*Lepus* spp.) also are taken. Wolves in Alberta also prey upon cattle, horse, and sheep [38,52]. For the Nunavut wolves, average prey size appears to have been smaller than in Alberta, with the most important prey being caribou, but muskox (*Ovibos moschatus*) are also occasionally taken, as are small mammals [53]. For the Russian Subarctic, diets seem to vary generally by latitude, with wolves inhabiting the northern portions of the boreal forest (taiga) relying primarily on hare (*Lepus* spp.)[49,54]. In the southerly portions of the boreal zone, elk and moose appear to be the most important prey, but smaller deer, wild boar (*Sus scrofa*), rodents, cattle, sheep, and horse also are preyed upon [51]. In Arctic Russia, reindeer (wild or domestic) are the predominant prey, but moose, fox (*Vulpes* spp.), hare, rodents, and ptarmigan (*Lagopus* spp.) also form part of the diet of some wolves [49].

The dogs analyzed in this study appear to have been fed strikingly different diets than their wild counterparts, including substantial quantities of marine mammals and fish. For example, the dogs of Cape York, Greenland subsisted largely on a diet of meat, blubber, and skin of sea mammals (seals (Phocidae) and walrus (*Odobenus rosmarus*))[20]. The dogs were at times fed frozen chunks of these animals, some with pieces of bone in them, which the dogs would gnaw in order to swallow. When the pieces fed to the dogs were unfrozen, they were swallowed as quickly as possible, without being gnawed. Jensen [21] mentions that some Greenland dogs were fed shark meat in summer. Degerbøl and Freuchen [20] further report that in summer, dogs were fed only once a week, or less frequently. In East Greenland, some dogs were left on islands in summer to fend for themselves [55], a practice also reported for other regions of the North American Arctic [56–57]. Peary [39] reports feeding his Greenland sled dogs primarily walrus "meat", but also mentions occasionally provisioning the dogs with seal, polar bear (*Ursus maritimus*), and even other dogs, the latter dying from exhaustion and exposure during his travels. M. Freeman, who collected the Ellesmere dogs, recalled them being fed almost entirely on sea mammal blubber, meat, and skin [see also 58]. Riewe [59] similarly reports dogs at Grise Fiord subsisting primarily on marine mammals. The Inuit of the central Canadian Arctic in the early historic period are said to have fed their dogs seal parts, including internal organs, skins, and bones in winter [56].

Aquatic foods also dominate the diets of dogs from the study regions of Russia represented in the paper. Bogoras [44], who collected a portion of our Chukotka dog sample, states that the "Kamchadal, Koryak, and Russian dogs are fed exclusively on fish – raw, dried, or frozen, according to the season or the locality." Chukchi dogs, by contrast, were fed seal intestines and blubber from seals, walrus, and whales, but rarely received meat, which was reserved for their owners [44]. The solely blubber diet was considered insufficient for the dogs, and the preferred diet also occasionally included some dried fish or marine mammal meat. Bogoras [44] further reports that dogs were not fed in summer, and that during this time they relied totally on killing or scavenging, which in some cases involved catching rodents, and in others feeding on remnants of salmon (*Oncorhychus* spp.). Yukaghir dogs (in Chukotka and Sakha Republic) are described as subsisting predominantly on fish [60]. The Nanai of the Amur River basin fed their dogs mainly fish, but also occasionally parts of land mammals, typically cooked bones or intestines [22].

Overall, ethnographic and historic accounts of dog diets in these regions suggest they were not being intentionally fed substantial quantities of dense bone that might have contributed to the high levels of tooth loss and fracture observed. Some of these dogs clearly were occasionally scavenging, and at some periods were largely self-sufficient and likely under food stress. Scavenging often involves extracting nutrients from remnants of food items such as discarded animal carcasses and individual bones. Extensive mastication of bone and other hard foods to extract nutrients has been shown to correlate with high rates of tooth fracture in carnivores [12,15–17], and has been specifically linked in studies of fossil carnivores to food stress, including high levels of competition between individuals for prey [16–17]. Presumably, high fracture rates would in turn lead to high rates of antemortem tooth loss, as fractures allow bacteria to enter the pulp cavity and can lead to infection of the tooth socket and subsequent tooth loss. Such conditions of periodic food stress and high competition between dogs scavenging for meager and hard to access nutrients might well account for the high levels of tooth loss and fracture observed in most of the northern dog specimens examined. Further, there are no indications that the dogs were commonly encountering larger prey than wolves, which might have led to the higher incidences of trauma observed, including fractures to teeth. Additionally, some of the dog groups (Kamchatka, N. Far East, and Sakhalin) have smaller percentages of individuals with traumatic lesions than seen in all of the wolf groups (Table 6). These dogs nonetheless had higher rates of tooth loss than the wolves (Table 2), which indicates that trauma is not the primary causative factor leading to tooth loss and fracture, at least among these groups.

An additional factor contributing to tooth loss among the dogs from Greenland, and perhaps also Ellesmere Island, is intentional tooth removal. Dogs in these regions are reported to have sometimes chewed and ingested their traces and other items made of hide, causing damage to, or loss of, equipment [20–21,61]. To prevent this, dogs in Greenland were sometimes asphyxiated until unconscious and then their teeth crowns filed away or broken off with a stone or metal hammer. In the specimens examined here, this manifests as the bilateral absence or fracture of the upper 3rd and 4th premolars and the lower 1st molars. In some cases, the sheared-off roots or crown remnants are still in place, and the resulting gaps in the dentition are commonly flanked by unmodified teeth (Figure 3b and 3c). Alveoli of such teeth were commonly filled with remodeled bone, but areas of reactive bone and abscessing also were common. In the Greenland dog sample, twelve of the thirteen dogs were suspected of having intentionally removed teeth, while one of the Ellesmere dogs may be affected. The antiquity of this practice should be relatively easy to assess with archaeological dog remains. We are not aware of tooth removal taking place in the Russian North, nor did we see any evidence for them on the specimens from this region; cutting of the tongue has been reported as a preventative measure for such gnawing in parts of the Russian Arctic [60], which would leave no observable trace on the skull.

Our analyses showed that some groups of dogs (from Greenland, Bering Island, Sakha, and Trans-Baikal) have far greater frequencies of bite wounds than the wolves, while others (Chukotka, Kamchatka, N. Far East, and Sakhalin) have far lower frequencies than the wild canids (Table 6). Such bite wounds are likely from other canids, probably other dogs. High numbers of affected individuals could result from fierce competition over food, which we argue was a likely factor in the tooth fracture and loss patterns observed. Further, a high incidence of bite wounds could occur if there were interactions among large numbers of free-ranging dogs, either in human settlements, or where dogs were left unattended on islands. Unfortunately, there is little historical

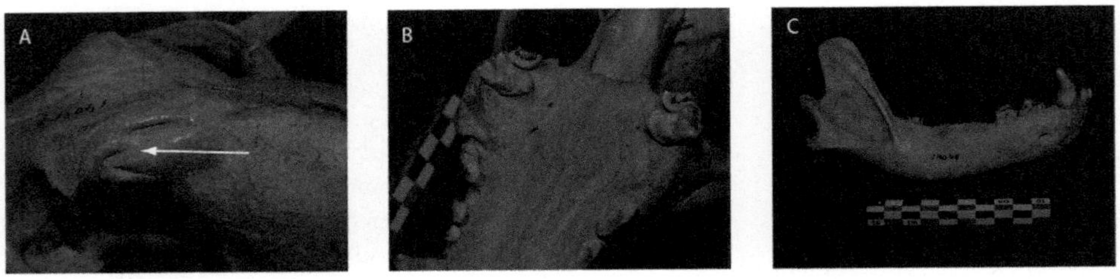

Figure 3. Photographs of a dog crania and mandible collected during the Robert E. Peary expedition in Northwest Greenland in 1897 (specimen #14049, AMNH). A. Healed depression fracture in the left frontal just posterior to the orbit. B. Antemortem loss of the right 4th premolar and antemortem fracture of the left 4th premolar. C. Right mandible with 4th premolar, first molar (carnassial), and 3rd molar lost antemortem. The antemortem tooth loss and fracture observed in this specimen is consistent with intentional tooth removal to inhibit gnawing.

evidence for such practices and behaviors for most of our samples. The Ellesmere dogs were tethered with chains when not pulling sleds, a practice required by law in the 1960s. The percentage of Ellesmere dogs with bite wounds however is similar to that seen in wolves living in this same general region (Table 6). Bogoras [44] mentions that during travel in winter, sled dogs were tethered overnight, but it is not stated whether they were similarly secured during the day. Further, it is unclear which communities he was speaking about, or precisely where he collected the dogs we sampled. Our Chukotka dog sample had some of the lowest rates of bite wounds in the study (Table 6). Overall, no simple correlations between tethering practices and the frequency of bite wounds can be asserted.

Behavioral tendencies in dogs may also influence the frequency of bite wounds and other forms of trauma. Aggressive dogs might be more likely to have traumatic conflicts with other dogs, and perhaps also with humans, resulting in greater numbers of individuals with traumatic lesions. Dog breeds vary in their stereotypical and actual aggressive tendencies [62–63], and for some tasks dogs undertake, aggressiveness can be an asset. Such tasks would include providing protection from other humans and predators, and perhaps also hunting where dogs are used to run down and secure prey. How such tendencies and practices varied across our study region is unknown, but some breeds of northern dogs clearly can exhibit aggressive tendencies [64]. Further, a few dog specimens examined were specifically listed as hunting dogs, and many others likely also were involved in such tasks. Interbreeding with wolves, which is occasionally mentioned in northern ethnographies [20,22,65], might also have produced animals with aggressive tendencies.

Our data also suggest that traditions of animal discipline involving severe physical force are likewise a factor in shaping the traumatic patterns observed. Dogs from Ellesmere, Greenland, Bering Island, and Chukotka all have high occurrence rates of fractures in their frontal bones, the vast majority being depression fractures (Table 7). These fractures and their positions on the crania are very similar to those described on archaeological dog remains from the Canadian Arctic [23–25] and elsewhere [66]. Such fractures are produced by the dogs being struck by blunt objects, and the bone collapsing into the sinuses of the frontal bones (Figure 3a). While such fractures could be caused by kicks from large prey animals, wolves very rarely displayed such lesions (2% of the total wolf population vs. 21.7% across all our dogs). Further, the dogs from Bering Island could not have suffered such lesions as the result of encounters with large terrestrial prey given that, historically, the largest wild mammals on these islands were foxes [67]. This suggests that the depression fractures were caused by people striking the dogs. The groups of dogs with higher rates of frontal fractures also showed higher rates of rostrum fractures than all other dog groups analyzed, and higher rates than in most of the wolves (Table 7). The etiology of these latter lesions is unknown, but blows to the head from humans could also be a cause. Many of these high trauma dogs were used for pulling sleds (the Greenland and Ellesmere dogs) or were from areas where dog sledding was common (Bering Island and Chukotka)[44,67]. However, the dog groups with low occurrences of all fractures were also from areas where sledding was common, and some groups include multiple individuals recorded as sled dogs (see Materials). In short, the patterns in fractures cannot at present be attributed to the ways dogs were utilized.

Finally, the lack of linear enamel hypoplasia in the permanent teeth of the dogs and wolves observed should not be surprising. Hypoplastic lesions are caused by disruptions in ameloblastic function during tooth crown formation. These disruptions can have many causes, including genetic abnormalities, fevers, viral infections, malnutrition, and localized trauma to the deciduous tooth, all of which can affect the developing teeth in the dental crypt [13]. For dogs and wolves, the permanent crowns form almost simultaneously and very rapidly, within ~70 to 120 days, in the first few months of life, beginning with the mandibular 1st molar [68]. By approximately 4 months of age, all of the adult crowns are formed. For a linear lesion to form, the disturbances creating it would have to be very acute and short lived, perhaps a week or less. Stresses that are severe enough to cause hypoplastic lesions, such as disease (canine distemper), dietary deficiencies, and even the infection and inflammation associated with trauma, would all likely be far less acute.

Trauma may best explain the cases where dog and wolf specimens showed hypoplastic lesions on 1–3 teeth adjacent teeth (Figure 2a). Systemic stresses like dietary deficiencies or disease would presumably manifest across multiple bilateral teeth. Where bilateral teeth or the entire dentition are affected, systemic stresses are more likely. As we argued earlier, some level of food stress is evidenced in the dogs, and this too seems a possible cause for hypoplastic lesions observed in some specimens. However, it remains impossible to differentiate such lesions from those produced by diseases such as canine distemper. Canine distemper is highly contagious, typically transmitted by aerolization of respiratory fluids carrying the virus, and can infect dogs without producing noticeable symptoms [69]. It has been shown to pass from dogs to wolves (and other species) [69,70], and has been documented as causing both hypoplastic lesions and lesions on the metaphyses of young dogs [71–3]. This disease was clearly present in northern North American and Russia during the general period in which our specimens were collected [57,60,70], but its longer history in these regions is unknown.

Conclusions

Life for some dogs living in recent northern societies included food stress and violent interactions with humans. This pattern was found in societies where subsistence was primarily based on hunting of marine mammals (Ellesmere Island, Greenland), and where other domesticated animals such as reindeer were common (most of the Russian study areas). Food stress manifests in the dogs as high levels of tooth fracture and loss, likely due to scavenging on hard foods; hypoplastic lesions on the teeth may also sometimes mark food stress in young dogs. Such stresses in these dogs, and in ancient ones, should not be surprising. Working dogs, particularly those used for tasks such as pulling sleds, have very elevated metabolic rates due to high activity levels [74–75]. Correspondingly, such dogs require significant caloric intake to maintain their energy balance [76]. Keeping dogs can be costly for humans in terms of time and energy—one has to purchase, hunt, fish, and forage in order to provision them [58], and at times these efforts may be unsuccessful or insufficient. Dogs' abilities to withstand food stress and feed themselves are rarely discussed in accounts of archaeological dogs, but these abilities clearly lessen their costs to humans, and were critical to their long-term use in the north and other regions. These abilities of dogs were also likely important in their initial domestication.

Our data indicate that dogs were far more likely to experience some types of fractures than wolves. Some injuries may have been due to encounters with prey, but many also were caused by people intentionally striking dogs, or incurred in accidents. The human niche poses a series of hazards to dogs that are more rarely part of the experiences of wolves. These include humans' possessions—sleds, whips, weapons, and other domesticated animals—all of which have the potential to cause bodily harm to dogs. Clearly, humans themselves also were (and are) a serious hazard faced by dogs, but this remains little discussed in archaeological literature. In some cases, humans modified dog anatomy in order to control their behavior, by intentionally removing chewing teeth to prevent gnawing. Overall, the human-dog relationships inferred from the data are complex and unromantic, but clearly had profound effects on these domesticated animals.

Consideration of the long-term histories of the patterns observed in this study raises a suite of further questions. For example, was food stress in dogs long-standing in the north, and how might this have changed with the introduction of new forms of subsistence, including the use of domesticated reindeer? It also seems likely that changing transportation requirements associated with periods of human colonization or dispersal also would have affected the lives of dogs, but this has been largely ignored in archaeology. Looking beyond the historic past, it seems fully worth exploring the levels of tooth fracture, loss, and enamel hypoplasia among the wolves first undergoing domestication. Is their evidence of food stress in wolves prior to the first steps towards domestication, indicating it was a factor in pushing dogs towards the human niche? It might also be intriguing to examine how patterns of trauma and tooth loss and fracture vary in dogs within larger-scale societies, and by various types of dogs, including feral animals and pets. Human violence towards dogs and other domesticates will always be a contentious issue, but exploring how it varies through time and space will provide a more nuanced picture of human-animal relations in the past.

Supporting Information

Figure S1 Data collection forms used in this study.

Table S1 Catalog numbers for specimens analyzed in this study.

Table S2 Age structure of the Alberta wolves and Ellesmere dogs, where known. Antemortem tooth loss and antemortem tooth fracture by age category also shown.

Acknowledgments

Special thanks are offered to the Royal Alberta Museum, Canadian Museum of Nature, Zoological Institute of the Russian Academy of Sciences, and the American Museum of Natural History for allowing access to the materials analyzed in this paper. Our thanks are also offered to Dr. Nancy Lovell for her advice and guidance during data collection and analyses. The comments of the two reviewers are greatly appreciated and significantly improved the manuscript. All necessary permits were obtained for the described study, which complied with all relevant regulations.

Author Contributions

Conceived and designed the experiments: RL EJ MS. Performed the experiments: RL EJ TN. Analyzed the data: RL EJ. Contributed reagents/materials/analysis tools: MS. Contributed to the writing of the manuscript: RL EJ TN.

References

1. Bartelle BG, Vellanoweth RL, Netherton ES, Poister NW, Kendig WE, et al. (2010) Trauma and pathology of a buried dog from San Nicolas Island, California, U.S.A. J Archaeolog Sci 37:2721–2734.
2. Binois A, Wardius C, Rio P, Bridault A, Petit C (2013) A dog's life: multiple trauma and potential abuse in a medieval dog from Guimps (Charente, France). Int J Paleopath 3: 39–47.
3. Lawler DF, Rubin DA, Evans RH, Hildebolt CF, Smith KE, et al. (2013) Differential diagnosis of an unusual shoulder articular lesion in an ancient domestic dog (Canis lupus familiaris L., 1758). Int J Paleopath 3: 282–287.
4. Losey RJ, Bazaliiskii VI, Garvie-Lok S, Germonpré M, Leonard JA, et al. (2011) Canids as persons: Early Neolithic dog and wolf burials, Cis-Baikal, Siberia. J Anthropol Archaeol 30: 174–189.
5. MacKinnon M (2010) 'Sick as a dog': zooarchaeological evidence for pet dog health and welfare in the Roman world. World Archaeol 42 (2): 290–309.
6. MacKinnon M, Belanger K (2006) In sickness and in health: care for an arthritic Maltese dog from the Roman cemetery of Yasmina, Carthage, Tunisia. In: Snyder, L.M, Moore, E.A, (Eds) Dogs and People in Social, Working, Economic or Symbolic Interaction. Oxford: Oxbow Press. pp. 38–43.
7. Warren DM (2000) Paleopathology of Archaic dogs from the North American Southeast. In: Crockford, S.J. (Ed.), Dogs Through Time: An Archaeological Perspective. Oxford: Archeaeo press. pp. 105–114.
8. Zinoviev AV (2010) Study of Medieval dogs from Novgorod, Russia (X-XIV Century). Int J Osteoarchaeol 22: 145–157.
9. Andersone Z, Ozoliņš J (2000) Craniometrical characteristics and dental anomalies in wolves Canis lups from Latvia. Acta Theriol 45 (4): 549–558.
10. Buchalcyzk T, Dynowski J, Szteyn S (1981) Variations in the number of teeth and asymmetry of the skull in the wolf. Acta Theriol 26 (2): 23–30.
11. Dolgov VA, Rossolimo OL (1964) Dental abnormalities in Canis lupus Linnaeus, 1758. Acta Theriol 8 (16): 237–244.
12. Leonard JA, Vila C, Fox-Dobbs K, Koch PL, Wayne RK, et al. (2007) Megafaunal extinctions and the disappearance of a specialized wolf ecomorph. Curr Biol 17: 1146–1150.
13. Miles AEW, Grigson C (1990) Colyer's Variations and Diseases of the Teeth of Animals. Cambridge: Cambridge University Press.
14. Pavlovic D, Gomercic T, Guzvia G, Kusak J, Huber D (2007) Prevalence of dental pathology in wolves (Canis lupus L.) in Croatia – a case report. Veterinarski Arhiv 77 (3): 291–297.
15. Van Valkenburgh B (1988) Incidence of tooth breakage among large, predatory mammals. Am Nat 131 (2): 291–302.
16. Van Valkenburgh B (2009) Costs of carnivory: tooth fracture in Pleistocene and recent carnivorans. Biol J Linn Soc 96: 68–81.
17. Van Valkenburgh B, Hertel F (1993) Tough times at La Brea: tooth breakage in large carnivores of the Late Pleistocene. Science 261 (5120) 456–459.
18. Vila C, Urios V, Castroviejo J (1993) Tooth losses and anomalies in the wolf (Canis lupus). Can J Zool 71: 968–971.

19. Wobeser G (1992) Traumatic, degenerative, and developmental lesions in wolves and coyotes from Saskatchewan. J Wildlife Dis 28 (2): 268–275.
20. Degerbøl M, Freuchen P (1976) Zoology I: Mammals. Reprint of Report of the Fifth Thule Expedition 1921–24, vol. 2, no. 4–5. New York: AMS Press Inc.
21. Jensen B (1961) Folkways of Greenland Dog Keeping. Folk 3: 43–66.
22. Samar AP (2010) Traditsionnoe Sobakovodstvo Nanaitsev. Vladivostok: Dal'nauka.
23. Morey DF (2010) Dogs: Domestication and the Development of a Social Bond. Cambridge: Cambridge University Press.
24. Morey DF, Aaris-Sørensen K (2002) Paleoeskimo dogs of the Eastern Arctic. Arctic 55 (1): 44–56.
25. Park RW (1987) Dog remains from Devon Island, N.W.T.: archaeological and osteological evidence for domestic dog use in Thule Culture. Arctic 40 (3): 184–190.
26. Coppinger R, Coppinger L (2001) Dogs: A New Understanding of Canine Origin, Behavior, and Evolution. Chicago: University of Chicago Press.
27. Koster JM, Tankersley KB (2012) Heterogeneity of hunting ability and nutritional status among domestic dogs in lowland Nicaragua. P Natl Acad Sci USA 109: E463–E470.
28. MacNulty DR, Smith DW, Mech LD, Eberly LE (2009) Body size and predatory performance in wolves: is bigger better? J Anim Ecol 78: 532–539.
29. Mech LD (1999) Alpha status, dominance, and division of labor in wolf packs. Can J Zool 77: 1196–1203.
30. Nielson CA (1977) Wolf Necropsy Report: Preliminary Pathological Observations. Special Report, Federal Aid in Wildlife Restoration Projects W-17-8 and W-17-19. Juneau: Alaska Department of Fish and Game.
31. O'Keefe FR, Meachen J, Fet EV, Brannick A (2013) Ecological determinants of clinal morphological variation in the cranium of the North American gray wolf. J Mammal 94 (6): 1223–1236.
32. Hillson S (2005) Teeth. Second edition. Cambridge: Cambridge University Press.
33. Crossley DA, Penman S (1995) BSAVA Manual of Small Animal Dentistry. 2nd Edition. Gloucestershier: British Small Animal Veterinary Association.
34. Maxie MG (2007) Pathology of Domestic Animals. 5th edition. Philadelphia: A. Saunders, Ltd.
35. Mellanby M (1929) Diet and the Teeth: An Experimental Study. Part I Dental Structure in Dogs. London: His Majesty's Stationary Office.
36. Verstraete FJM (1999) Self-Assessment Color Review of Veterinary Dentistry. Ames: Iowa State University Press.
37. Dubielzig RR (1979) The effect of canine distemper on the ameloblastic layer of the developing tooth. Vet Pathol 16, 268–270.
38. Bjorge RR, Gunson JR (1985) Evaluation of wolf control to reduce cattle predation in Alberta. J Range Manage 38 (6): 483–487.
39. Peary RE (1898) Northward Over the "Great Ice". Volumes 1 and 2. New York: Frederick A. Stokes Company.
40. Räikkönen J, Vucetich JA, Vucetich LM, Peterson RO, Nelson MP (2013) What the inbred Scandinavian wolf population tells us about the nature of conservation. PLoS One 8 (6): e67218. doi:10.1371/journal.pone.0067218.
41. Berten J (1895) Hypoplasie des Schmelzes (Congenitale Schmelzdefecte; Erosionen). Deutsche Monatsschrift für Zahnheilkunde 13, 425–439; 483–498; 533–548; 587–606.
42. Hillson S (1996) Dental Anthropology. Cambridge: Cambridge University Press.
43. Bellars ARM (1969) Veterinary studies on the British Antarctic Survey's sledge dogs. I. Diseases and Accidents. Brit Antarct Surv B 21:1–18.
44. Bogoras W (1909) The Chukchee. Memoirs of the American Museum of Natural History, Volume 11. New York: Johnson Reprint Company.
45. Fiorello CV, Noss AJ, Deem S L (2006) Demography, hunting ecology, and pathogen exposure of domestic dogs in the Isoso of Bolivia. Conserv Biol 20: 762–771.
46. Ikeya K (1994) Hunting with dogs among the San in the central Kalahari. Afr Stud Mono 15: 119–134.
47. Lupo KD (2011) A dog is for hunting. In: Albarella, U. (Ed.), Ethnozooarchaeology. Oxbow: Oxbow Press. pp. 4–12.
48. Koster JM (2008) Hunting with dogs in Nicaragua: An optimal foraging approach. Curr Anthropol 49: 935–944.
49. Bibikov DI (1985) Volk: Proiskhozhdenie, Sistematika, Morfologiia, Ekologiia. Moscow: Nauka. Pp. 609.
50. Stephenson RO, Johnson LJ (1973) Wolf Report, 1971–1972. Federal Aid in Wildlife Restoration Progress Report XI, W-17-4 and 5. Juneau: Alaska Department of Fish and Game.
51. Peterson RO, Ciucci P (2003) The wolf as a carnivore. In Mech, L.D., Botani, L. (Eds.) Wolves: Behaviour, Ecology, and Conservation. Chicago: University of Chicago Press. pp. 104–130.
52. Morehouse AT, Boyce MS (2011) From venison to beef: seasonal changes in wolf diet composition in a livestock landscape. Front Ecol Enviro 9: 440–445.
53. Krizan J (2006) Nunavut wolf morphology and diet study. Final Wildlife Report No. 11, Wildlife Research Section. Igloolik: Department of Environment.
54. Labutin IuV (1972) Geograficheskie osobennosti pitaniia volka i lisitsy. In Zoologicheskie Problemy Sibiri. Novosibirsk: Nauka.pp. 413–415.
55. Weyer EM (1932) The Eskimos, Their Environment and Folkways. New Haven: Yale University Press.
56. Boas F (1974) The Central Eskimo. Toronto: Coles Publishing Company Limited.
57. Bohm J, Blixenhrone-Moller M, Lund E (1989) A serious outbreak of canine distemper among sled dogs in Northern Greenland. Arct Med Res 48: 195–203.
58. Freeman MMR (1969-70) Studies in maritime hunting I. Ecologic and technologic restraints on walrus hunting, Southampton Island N.W.T. Folk 11–12: 155–171.
59. Riewe RR (1977) The utilization of wildlife in the Jones Sound Region by the Grise Fiord Inuit. In: Bliss, L.C. (Ed.), Truelove Lowland, Devon Island, Canada: A High Arctic Ecosystem. Edmonton: University of Alberta Press. pp. 623–644.
60. Chikachev AG (2004) Ezdovoe Sobakovodstvo Iakutii. Iakutsk: SO RAN.
61. Croft A (1937) West Greenland sledge dogs. Polar Rec 2 (13): 68–81.
62. American Kennel Club (1975) The Complete Dog Book. New York: Howell Book House.
63. Duffy DL, Hsu Y, Serpell JA (2008) Breed differences in canine aggression. Appl Anim Behav Sci 114: 441–460.
64. Montcombroux G (1997) The Canadian Inuit Dog: Canada's Heritage. Winnipeg: Whipoorwill Press.
65. MacRury IK (1991) The Inuit Dog: Its Provenance, Environment and History. Masters thesis, Darwin College, University of Cambridge.
66. Baker J, Brothwell D (1980) Animal Diseases in Archaeology. London: Academic Press.
67. Jochelson W (1968) History, Ethnology and Anthropology of the Aleut. New York: Humanities Press.
68. Arnall L (1960) Some aspects of dental development in the dog—I. calcification of crown and root of the deciduous dentitions. J Small Anim Pract 1: 169–173.
69. Deem SL, Spelman LH, Yates RA, Montali RJ (2000) Canine distemper in terrestrial carnivores: a review. J Zoo Wildlife Med 31: 441–451.
70. Elton C (1931) Epidemics among sledge dogs in the Canadian Arctic and their relation to disease in the arctic fox. Can J Res 5 (6): 673–692.
71. Baumgartner W, Boyce RW, Weisbrode SE, Aildinger S, Axthelm MK, et al. (1995) Histologic and immunocytochemical characterization of canine distemper–associated metaphyseal bone lesions in young dogs following experimental infection. Vet Pathol 32:702–709.
72. Dubielzig RR, Higgins RJ, Krakowka S (1981) Lesions of the enamel organ of developing dog teeth following experimental inoculation of gnotobiotic puppies with canine distemper virus. Vet Pathol 18: 684–689.
73. Malik R, Dowden M, Davis PE, Allan GS, Barrs VR, et al. (1995) Concurrent juvenile cellulitus and metaphyseal osteopathy: an atypical canine distemper virus syndrome? Aust Vet Pract 25: 62–67.
74. Hammond KA, Diamond J (1997) Maximal sustained energy budgets in humans and animals. Nature 386: 457–462.
75. Hinchcliff KW, Reinhart GA, Burr JR, Schreier CJ, Swenson RA (1997) Metabolizable energy intake and sustained energy expenditure of Alaskan sled dogs during heavy exertion in the cold. Am J Vet Res 58: 1457–1462.
76. Gerth N, Sum S, Jackson S, Starck JM (2009) Muscle plasticity of Inuit sled dogs in Greenland. J Exp Biol 212: 1131–1139.

Effectiveness of Educational Poster on Knowledge of Emergency Management of Dental Trauma: Cluster Randomised Controlled Trial for Secondary School Students

Cecilia Young[1]*, Kin Yau Wong[2], Lim K. Cheung[3]

1 Private Practice, Hong Kong, 2 Department of Biostatistics, University of North Carolina at Chapel Hill, Chapel Hill, North Carolina, United States of America, 3 The University of Hong Kong, Hong Kong

Abstract

Objective: To investigate the effectiveness of educational poster on improving secondary school students' knowledge of emergency management of dental trauma.

Methods: A cluster randomised controlled trial was conducted. 16 schools with total 671 secondary students who can read Chinese or English were randomised into intervention (poster, 8 schools, 364 students) and control groups (8 schools, 305 students) at the school level. Baseline knowledge of dental trauma was obtained by a questionnaire. Poster containing information of dental trauma management was displayed in a classroom for 2 weeks in each school in the intervention group whereas in the control group there was no display of such posters. Students of both groups completed the same questionnarie after 2 weeks.

Results: Two-week display of posters improved the knowledge score by 1.25 (p-value = 0.0407) on average.

Conclusion: Educational poster on dental trauma management significantly improved the level of knowledge of secondary school students in Hong Kong.

Trial Registration: HKClinicalTrial.com HKCTR-1343 ClinicalTrials.gov NCT01809457

Editor: Michael Glogauer, University of Toronto, Canada

Funding: The study is self-funded by the principal investigator.

Competing Interests: The authors have declared that no competing interests exist.

* Email: ceciliatyp@yahoo.com.hk

Introduction

Prevalence of traumatic dental injuries of primary and permanent teeth is high throughout the world. Statistics from most countries showed that one fourth of all school children and almost one third of adults had suffered trauma to the permanent dentition, with variations among and within countries [1].

Early management is crucial to the prognosis for some dental injuries, especially avulsion [2]. However, most studies showed that teachers or school staff [3–15], parents [15–21], nurses [15,22,23], paramedics [23] and coaches [21] lacked the knowledge to manage traumatic dental injuries appropriately before the injured person reached dental professionals.

Since immediate management of traumatic dental injury does not require special skill but only knowledge, it can be performed by a lay person if one knows the procedures. The ideal situation is that such knowledge becomes everyone's basic practical knowledge. The earlier one learns the appropriate procedure, the higher chance one can save more traumatized teeth. In a literature search conducted before the study and finalized on Sept 21, 2013, there were only 4 studies investigating children's and teenagers' knowledge of traumatic dental injuries [24–27]. The results were that the subjects did not possess adequate knowledge.

Literature search of published studies on education in traumatic dental injuries prior to Sept 21, 2013 using keywords ("promotion*" or "intervention" or "education" or "knowledge" or "campaign" or "seminar" or "lecture" or "pamphlet" or "leaflet" or "banner" or "poster") and ("dental injur*" or "traumatic dental injur*" or "dental trauma") on Pubmed, Ovid, Web of Science and Cochrane Central Register of Controlled Trials resulted in only 14 papers related to education [28–41]. All of them targeted on adults, and there was no information about education in dental trauma for children or teenagers.

All Hong Kong primary school students (US Grade 1–6) are eligible to join the School Dental Care Service and most of them joined voluntarily. Every participant received a handbook for recording dental visits and it contained around 20 pages of dental health information. Since 1994, the handbook contained one page about avulsion and it mentioned that avulsed tooth should be put back into the socket, stored in milk or in mouth. However, in 2011, a survey about the level of knowledge of dental trauma revealed that such knowledge of secondary school students (US Grade 7–12 plus 1 year) in Hong Kong was insufficient [27]. In that survey, only a small portion of secondary school students knew that avulsed permanent tooth should be replanted (23.6%), or stored in cold milk (18.7%), physiological saline (24.2%) or saliva (6.7%), even they were eligible to join the school dental service and received the mentioned handbook in their primary education. Educational campaign on dental trauma management was recommended for secondary school students by the authors.

It is easy to implement poster campaign because of the low cost. In the present study, the effectiveness of dental trauma educational poster on level of knowledge was studied. Secondary school students were chosen and the cluster design was adopted since it is appropriate for the actual school environment as students might discuss with and hence influence each other. Also, since students in the same school may have some unique characteristics, e.g. higher level of health consciousness, the study was randomised at the school level to prevent contamination and improve on comparability.

Methods

Ethical approval

The research project was approved by the Institutional Review Board of the University of Hong Kong and Hospital Authority Hong Kong West Cluster. (HKCTR-1343, ClinicalTrials.gov: NCT01809457)

Subjects

The subjects were secondary school students (US Grade 7–12 plus 1 year) in Hong Kong, who can read Chinese or English. We recruited the secondary schools as clusters. The protocol for this trial and supporting CONSORT checklist are available as supporting information; see Checklist S1 and Protocol S1.

Questionnaire

The questionnaire from a survey of the same series about knowledge of dental trauma among the same target group was used [27]. Chinese and English versions of the questionnaire were constructed. There were 14 questions, divided into two sections. The first section asked for basic demographic information, whether the respondents had received formal first-aid training or acquired dental trauma information and whether they considered themselves able to distinguish between permanent and deciduous teeth. The second part consisted of questions concerning knowledge of dental traumatic injuries, which was for the assessment of dental knowledge in this study. The questionnaire was pilot tested with 59 students. Face validity, length and comprehensibility by secondary school students were pre-tested before the questionnaire was finally adopted. Face validity was established by expert opinion, and a test-retest reliability test indicated that the scores of the first and second questionnaires were positively correlated.

The marking scheme is as follows: for Q9 to Q13, 1 mark would be given for a correct answer, 0 would be given for "do not know" and 1 would be deducted for an incorrect answer. If multiple answers were chosen, 1 would be deducted for that question if an incorrect answer was chosen. There were three correct answers for Q14 as the media for storing avulsed teeth. As avulsion is the most serious type of dental trauma, timely emergency management is critical. Knowledge of more storing media raises the chance of a student being able to find one soon enough to keep the vitality of the periodontal cells on the root surface, which improves the prognosis. Therefore, 1 mark would be given for each correct answer but 1 mark would be deducted for each incorrect answer. Multiple answers were allowed.

Poster

The educational poster was in A3 size, colourful and with pictures. One side of the poster was written in Chinese and the other side in English, The content was constructed by the authors using two publications as reference [3,37]. This poster is the same as the one used in another study for primary and secondary school teachers of the same series [41]. Chinese and English educational posters are available as supporting information S1 and S2.

Sample size calculation

In order to demonstrate a difference in score change of 2 marks (variance 10) between the intervention group and the control group, with a power of 90% and a statistical significance of 5%, 53 individuals are needed in each group under simple random sampling. To account for the cluster design, we assume an intracluster correlation (ICC) of 0.1. No published data on ICC under this setting could be found. However, in general practice studies, ICC takes value commonly between 0.01 and 0.05 [42], so 0.1 would be a conservative estimate. With an average of 40 students per school and a coefficient of variation of cluster size of 0.2 (after realizing that it was difficult in practice to recruit a minimum cluster size of 40 as laid down in the original protocol, we allowed clusters with size smaller than 40, but restricted the coefficient of variation of cluster size to be 0.2), the adjusted sample size is 7 schools, or 266 students, per group. To allow for potential dropouts, we aimed to recruit extra 20% individuals per group (this extra 20% was changed from 30% in the original protocol), yielding a total of 8 schools, or 319 students, per group.

Recruitment

A staff of the principal investigator was invited to act as a voluntary secretary for this study. She was responsible for all mailings, information storage and co-ordination. She was informed that the identities of the participating schools and students should be blinded to all investigators, statistician and clerical staff at the time of appointment. She was the only one who knew the identities of the schools. She kept the information concealed and put them in a locked drawer in her room.

The Education Bureau provided a list of secondary schools upon request. There were a total of 663 schools. Special schools for intellectually disabled students were included in the list. The secretary sent invitation letters with school consent forms and individual guardian consent forms to lots of 50 randomly selected schools beginning on April 29, 2011. In each lot of invitation letters, there were 17 letters for Form 1–3 (US Grade 7–9), 17 letters for Form 4–5 (US Grade 10–11), and 16 letters of Form 6–7 (US Grade 12 plus 1 year). The contact information of the principal investigator was given in the invitation letter.

The secretary followed up with telephone calls. 16 schools with a total of 784 students joined the study after 200 invitations were sent. They replied with both signed school and individual guardian consent forms. The name and contact number of the teacher in charge were given in the school consent form.

Randomisation and masking

The randomisation was performed after both school and individual guardian consent forms were returned. The schools were randomised to the intervention group and the control group at the school level manually using sealed envelopes. The secretary put two pieces of paper bearing the words "intervention group" and "control group" separately into two envelopes. She labelled the sealed enveloped of intervention group as group A and the other as group B. She verified that the envelope was opaque that the words could not be seen through. An independent person who did not know the details of this study were invited to assist the randomisation. The secretary labelled 1 to 16 on separate sheets of paper representing the 16 schools according to the order the consent forms were received. She folded each piece of paper and put it into an envelope and checked that the number could not be seen through, and then put them inside a box.

The independent person, not knowing the identities of group A and B, drew one envelope for group A and then one for group B alternatively until all the envelopes were drawn. The secretary then opened the envelopes and recorded the result of the randomisation. The list was put in a locked drawer that only the secretary could access.

Implementation of the trial

The schools, teachers in charge and students were not informed of the identity of the group (intervention/control) they belonged to, educational material that they would receive and the duration of the trial. The letter of invitation and both consent forms only mentioned that the students needed to fill out two questionnaires (see protocol S1).

The trial began on May 5, 2011 and was completed on Nov 16, 2011. The first set of questionnaires was sent to both groups and hard copies were distributed to the participating students by the teachers in charge. All participating students were asked to fill out the questionnaires and returned them to the corresponding teachers in charge (in class), who then sent the completed questionnaires back to the investigator in 1 week.

A large sealed envelope containing the educational poster along with instructions was mailed to each intervention school. The teacher in charge of each school displayed the educational posters on the notice broad or at an area of similar function in the classroom. No poster was given to the control group.

The posters were removed by the teachers in charge after 2 weeks. The second set of questionnaires was then distributed to schools of both groups and the students were asked to complete the questionnaires in class. The teachers in charge then returned them to the study secretary in 1 week using prepaid envelopes. Educational posters were mailed to the control group after the completion of the study. Every procedure followed that laid down in the protocol after the trial commenced.

Withdrawal from the study

The participating schools or individual students could withdraw from the study at any time, as mentioned in both consent forms. 39 students from the intervention group and 22 students from the control group withdrew from the study by not returning either the first or the second questionnaire.

Data processing

The data entry staff and the statistician were blinded to the group randomisation. The statistician was instructed to analyse under the labels "group A" and "group B" according to the designed method in the protocol. The investigators were blinded to the randomisation. Only after the completion of the whole statistical report and the draft of the article, the study secretary informed the principal investigator the identities of the groups. The principal investigator then relabeled group A as intervention group and group B as control group.

Data analysis

Individual level analysis was performed as our objective and outcome measures pertain to individual level. Our objective is to investigate the effects of the intervention, potentially controlled for some baseline information, on the gain in knowledge. The dependent variable is the score difference between the two questionnaires. To account for potential correlation among students from the same school, a linear mixed model was fitted with a normally distributed random intercept for the school effect.

To select the most appropriate model, a backward elimination method was adopted [43]. It started with including all covariates in the model: group (intervention/control), the score of the first questionnaire, gender, age, form, first-aid training, dental education in first aid, confidence in distinguishing deciduous and permanent teeth, and acquisition of dental injury information from other sources. The covariate associated with the highest p-value was eliminated in each iteration until all p-values were smaller than a threshold value 0.1.

Due to the nature of the data collected and the collection process, we anticipated that the proportion of missing data would not be high. Therefore, we simply discarded subjects who did not provide the demographic or personal information asked in the first section of the questionnaire. Missing answers for questions in the second section of the questionnaire were treated as "do not know", and the total scores were accordingly calculated based on the marking scheme given.

The thresholds of all the statistical tests were set at 5% level of significance. The statistical analyses were performed using a computer software (JMP version 9.0.0, SAS Institute Inc., USA).

Results

There was no unintended effect or harm reported through the teachers in charge or directly to the principal investigator. After removing participants with missing background information, there were 364 individuals (8 schools) in the intervention group and 303 individuals (8 schools) in the control group available for analysis (Figure 1). The basic information for both groups on the school level and the individual level are given in Table 1. Statistical test was not conducted to compare the baseline information of the two groups [44].

The average scores of each question of both questionnaires, along with the average difference in score of the two questionnaires for each group, are given in Table 2.

The result of the multiple linear regression is presented in Table 3. The covariates included in the final model were group (intervention/control) and baseline score only.

From the regression analysis, the group effect is significant. Given the same baseline score, individuals in intervention group had on average a score difference 1.25 (p-value = 0.0407) higher than that of individuals in control group. The baseline score effect is also significant, which indicates that an increase in baseline score of 1 mark would on average reduce the score difference by 0.40 (p-value<0.0001).

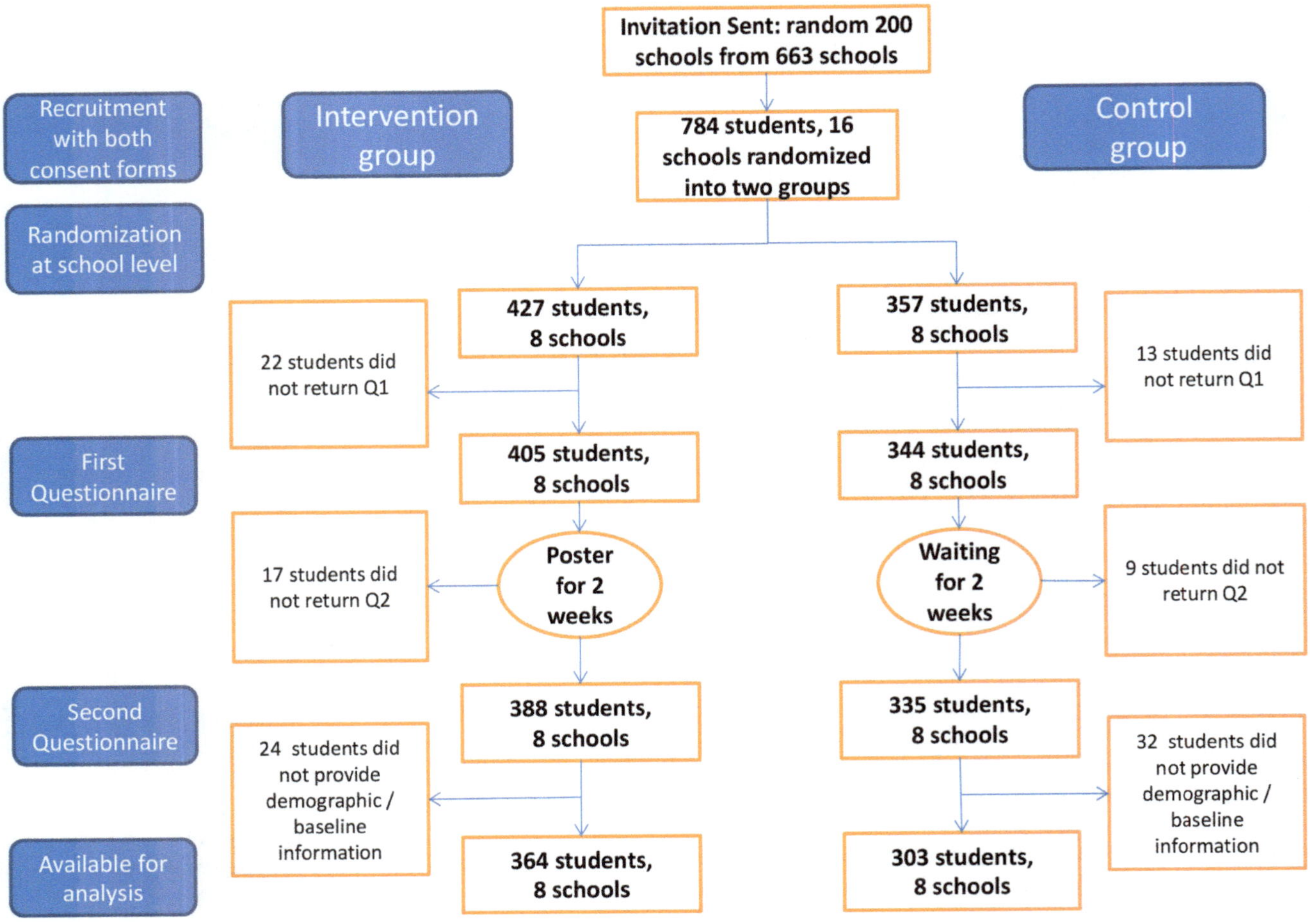

Figure 1. Flowchart of the participants.

Discussion

Effectiveness of educational poster on management of dental trauma on secondary school students was studied. From the statistical analysis, the group effect is significant. It means that the two-week display of the poster improved the score with statistical significance. Given the same baseline score, individuals in intervention group had on average a score difference 1.25 (p-value = 0.0407) higher than that of individuals in control group. However, a score difference of 1.25 marks is smaller than our expectation.

Some questions were not answered any better in the intervention group after the two-week display of poster. It may be that students understood and/or remembered selective portion of the information. Students may be more interested in reading certain area of the poster and may not have gone through the entire poster.

This result reflects whether the students had read, understood and remembered information on the poster. This is the first cluster randomised controlled trial for investigating the effectiveness of educational posters on dental trauma on this age group.

Since a model containing all relevant information collected in the questionnaire is too large under the current sample size, which would make the estimation unstable, we have chosen to adopt a backward variable selection procedure. We are aware that such method would possibly inflate type I error due to multiple testing, and the significant factors remained in the model may just be chosen by coincidence. It means that the p-values of the factors in the model tend to be smaller and the confidence intervals tend to be narrower than they, strictly speaking, should be. One should bear that in mind when interpreting the results. However, under the current setting, the major factor of interest is the intervention effect, which would not be eliminated under the variable selection procedure. The problem of concluding a significant intervention effect by coincidence as a result of variable selection does not exist. Also, besides intervention, there is only one factor remaining in the model, namely the baseline score. Therefore, the inflation of Type I error, if any, is minimal.

With the above being said, one may still be interested in the estimated marginal effect of intervention. Fitting a linear mixed model with only intervention group as independent variable, the estimated effect is 1.26 (p-value = 0.0423), which means that on average students from the intervention group had score improvement of 1.26 more than that of students from the control group. It is, though marginally, significant at 5% level of significance.

The immediate effect of two-week display of poster was investigated, while long term effect is out of the scope of this study. Knowledge, rather than the management of traumatic dental injuries, was tested because long term follow up is necessary for the latter. It is not feasible to carry it out in Hong Kong because the number of cases from the sampling frame may not be large enough to produce a sizable sample that would produce statistically significant results. The list of all primary and secondary schools was exhausted even for the series of short term studies.

Table 1. Demographic information and characteristics of the both groups on cluster and individual levels.

School Level		
	Intervention group ($n=8$)	Control group ($n=8$)
Cluster Size	Mean = 45.5; Median = 45;	Mean = 37.9; Median = 38.5;
	Min = 8; Max = 74	Min = 26; Max = 48
Individual Level		
	Intervention group ($n=364$)	Control group ($n=303$)
	Number (Percentage)	Number (Percentage)
Gender		
Male	122 (33.5)	113 (37.3)
Female	242 (66.5)	190 (62.7)
Age		
10 or below	0 (0.0)	0 (0.0)
11–13	79 (21.7)	45 (14.9)
14–16	145 (39.8)	175 (57.8)
17–19	132 (36.3)	81 (26.7)
20 or above	8 (2.2)	2 (0.7)
Form		
Form 1–3	220 (60.4)	111 (36.6)
Form 4–5	2 (0.5)	128 (42.2)
Form 6–7	142 (39.0)	64 (21.1)
Received First-Aid Training		
Yes	28 (7.7)	49 (16.2)
No	336 (92.3)	254 (83.8)
Learnt Dental Injury Management in First-aid Training		
Yes	4 (1.1)	10 (3.3)
No	360 (98.9)	293 (96.7)
Confident in Distinguishing Type of Teeth		
Yes	83 (22.8)	90 (29.7)
No	281 (77.2)	213 (70.3)
Read or heard dental injury information besides from First-aid Training		
Yes	101 (27.7)	91 (30.0)
No	263 (72.3)	212 (70.0)

No statistical test for comparison of baseline for both groups [43].

From the 663 secondary schools in Hong Kong, with altogether 454244 students, the sample was randomly selected with only the condition that the students were able to read Chinese or English. The results apply to all these students. The generalizability of the results to other countries is unclear since the culture, students' workload, educational system, health consciousness, ability to comprehend the study information and the importance students placed on dental trauma material may differ.

As some schools display a lot of information to students and change the notices or posters quite frequently, display time of longer than two weeks may not be feasible. Classroom is the most suitable location for effectively displaying information to students.

Though they are usable media for storage, Hank's balanced salt solution (or e.g. Save-A-Tooth), Viaspan, eagle's medium and propolis culture medium were not mentioned in the choices explicitly in question 14 because these were not accessible to students in Hong Kong. However, if students mentioned these in the "others (please specify)" option, they would be considered correct. Nevertheless, no student mentioned any of these solutions. These media were not mentioned in the poster for the same reason.

The randomisation of this trial was blinded to the investigator, data entry staff and the statistician. Only the secretary knew the identities of group A and B, and this information was given to the investigators only after the whole statistical report and the manuscript were drafted. Other than relabeling "group A" and "group B" as "intervention group" and "control group", respectively, no information on the figure or results was amended. So doing was to minimize bias and to improve the representability of the statistical analysis result.

Educational posters are relatively inexpensive and easy to distribute. There is no temporal limitation and assembly of students is not needed, as in the case of lectures and seminars. Displaying educational posters in classrooms is practical and effective means to improve students' knowledge of dental trauma.

Table 2. Scores of both questionnaires of both groups.

	Intervention group (*n*=364)		Control group (*n*=303)	
	Number (Percentage)		Number (Percentage)	
	Baseline Score	**Q2 Score**	**Baseline Score**	**Q2 Score**
Q9 Place for treatment				
Correct	126 (34.6)	116 (31.9)	118 (38.9)	102 (33.7)
Incorrect	180 (49.5)	189 (51.9)	150 (49.5)	154 (50.8)
Do not know	58 (15.9)	59 (16.2)	35 (11.6)	47 (15.5)
Q10 Time for treatment				
Correct	216 (59.3)	207 (56.9)	168 (55.4)	150 (49.5)
Incorrect	97 (26.6)	105 (28.8)	110 (36.3)	98 (32.3)
Do not know	51 (14.0)	52 (14.3)	25 (8.3)	55 (18.2)
Q11 Management of fractured teeth				
Correct	99 (27.2)	146 (40.1)	90 (29.7)	92 (30.4)
Incorrect	177 (48.6)	131 (36.0)	137 (45.2)	119 (39.3)
Do not know	88 (24.2)	87 (23.9)	76 (25.1)	92 (30.4)
Q12 Management of displaced teeth				
Correct	79 (21.7)	129 (35.4)	71 (23.4)	84 (27.7)
Incorrect	180 (49.5)	139 (38.2)	175 (57.8)	129 (42.6)
Do not know	105 (28.8)	96 (26.4)	57 (18.8)	90 (29.7)
Q13i Management of avulsed baby teeth				
Correct	221 (60.7)	212 (58.2)	200 (66.0)	172 (56.8)
Incorrect	10 (2.7)	24 (6.6)	10 (3.3)	12 (4.0)
Do not know	133 (36.5)	128 (35.2)	93 (30.7)	119 (39.3)
Q13ii Management of avulsed permanent teeth				
Correct	81 (22.3)	126 (34.6)	72 (23.8)	63 (20.8)
Incorrect	126 (34.6)	95 (26.1)	110 (36.3)	95 (31.4)
Do not know	157 (43.1)	143 (39.3)	121 (39.9)	145 (47.9)
Q14 Mediums for storage of avulsed teeth				
Mean	−0.352	0.310	−0.330	−0.261
Std. Dev.	1.117	1.466	1.155	1.077
Total Score				
Mean	−0.209	1.005	−0.238	−0.076
Std. Dev.	2.414	3.565	2.611	2.616
	Change = 1.214 (SD = 3.447)		Change = 0.162 (SD = 2.265)	

For Question 9–13, 1 mark for each correct answer, 0 for don't know, −1 if it is wrong or any wrong answer if chose more than 1. (−6 to 6); For question 14, 1 for each correct answer, 0 for don't know, −1 for each wrong answer (−7 to 3); Range of total score of the whole questionnaire: −13 to 9.

Table 3. Relationship between score change and intervention, baseline score.

	Estimate	Standard Error	95% Confidence Interval		p-value
Intercept	1.34	0.38	0.59	2.09	0.0049
Group* (Intervention = 0, Control = 1)	−1.25	0.54	−2.30	−0.19	0.0407
Baseline Score*	−0.40	0.04	−0.48	−0.32	<0.0001

Estimated ICC = 0.1193.
* the independent variable is significantly different from zero at 5% significance.

Conclusion

Educational poster statistically significantly improves the student's knowledge of emergency management of dental trauma.

Supporting Information

Checklist S1

Poster S1 Chinese Educational poster.

Poster S2 English Educational poster.

Protocol S1

Acknowledgments

We thank all participating schools and students.

Author Contributions

Conceived and designed the experiments: CY KYW LKC. Performed the experiments: CY. Analyzed the data: CY KYW LKC. Contributed reagents/materials/analysis tools: CY KYW. Contributed to the writing of the manuscript: CY KYW LKC. Wrote the paper: CY KYW LKC.

References

1. Glendor U (2008) Epidemiology of traumatic dental injuries—a 12 year review of the literature. Dent Traumatol 24: 603–611.
2. Andreasen JO, Andreasen FM, Skeie A, Hjorting-Hansen E, Schwartz O (2002) Effect of treatment delay upon pulp and periodontal healing of traumatic dental injuries — a review article. Dent Traumatol 18: 116–128.
3. Young C, Wong KY, Cheung LK (2012) Emergency management of dental trauma: knowledge of Hong Kong Primary and Secondary School Teachers. Hong Kong Medical J 18: 362–370.
4. de Lima Ludgero A, de Santana Santos T, Fernandes AV, de Melo DG, Peixoto AC, et al. (2012) Knowledge regarding emergency management of avulsed teeth among elementary school teachers in Jaboatao dos Guararapes, Pernambuco, Brazil. Indian J Dent Res 23: 585–590.
5. Bayrak S, Tunc ES, Sari E (2012) Evaluation of Elementary School Teachers' Knowledge and Attitudes about Immediate Emergency Management of Traumatic Dental Injuries. Oral Health Prev Dent 10: 253–258.
6. Fux-Noy A, Sarnat H, Amir E (2011) Knowledge of elementary school teachers in Tel-Aviv, Israel, regarding emergency care of dental injuries. Dent Traumatol 27: 252–256.
7. Al-Jundi SH, Al-Waeili H, Khairalah K (2005) Knowledge and attitude of Jordanian school health teachers with regards to emergency management of dental trauma. Dent Traumatol 21: 183–187.
8. Caglar E, Ferreira LP, Kargul B (2005) Dental trauma management knowledge among a group of teachers in two south European cities. Dent Traumatol 21: 258–262.
9. McIntyre JD, Lee JY, Trope M, Vann WF Jr (2008) Elementary school staff knowledge about dental injuries. Dent Traumatol 24: 289–298.
10. Mohandas U, Chandan GD (2009) Knowledge, attitude and practice in emergency management of dental injury among physical education teachers: a survey in Bangalore urban schools. J Indian Soc Pedod Prev Dent 27: 242–248.
11. Mesgarzadeh AH, Shahamfar M, Hefzollesan A (2009) Evaluating knowledge and attitudes of elementary school teachers on emergency management of traumatic dental injuries: a study in an Iranian urban area. Oral Health Prev Dent 7: 297–308.
12. Skeie MS, Audestad E, Bardsen A (2010) Traumatic dental injuries—knowledge and awareness among present and prospective teachers in selected urban and rural areas of Norway. Dent Traumatol 26: 243–247.
13. Al-Obaida M (2010) Knowledge and management of traumatic dental injuries in a group of Saudi primary schools teachers. Dent Traumatol 26: 338–341.
14. Hashim R (2011) Dental trauma management awareness among primary school teachers in the Emirate of Ajman, United Arab Emirates. Eur J Paediatr Dent 12: 99–102.
15. Hamilton FA, Hill FJ, Mackie IC (1997) Investigation of lay knowledge of the management of avulsed permanent incisors. Endod Dent Traumatol 13: 19–23.
16. Ozer S, Yilmaz EI, Bayrak S, Tunc ES (2012) Parental knowledge and attitudes regarding the emergency treatment of avulsed permanent teeth. Eur J Dent 6: 370–375.
17. Raphael SL, Gregory PJ (1990) Parental awareness of the emergency management of avulsed teeth in children. Aust Dent J 35: 130–133.
18. Santos ME, Habecost AP, Gomes FV, Weber JB, de Oliveira MG (2009) Parent and caretaker knowledge about avulsion of permanent teeth. Dent Traumatol 25: 203–208.
19. Sanu OO, Utomi IL (2005) Parental awareness of emergency management of avulsion of permanent teeth of children in Lagos, Nigeria. Niger Postgrad Med J. 12: 115–120.
20. Walker A, Brenchley J (2000) It's a knockout: survey of the management of avulsed teeth. Accid Emerg Nurs. 8: 66–70.
21. Stokes AN, Anderson HK, Cowan TM (1992) Lay and professional knowledge of methods for emergency management of avulsed teeth. Endod Dent Traumatol. 8: 160–162.
22. Hugar SM, Suganya M, Kiran K, Vikneshan M, More VP (2013) Knowledge and awareness of dental trauma among Indian nurses. Int Emerg Nurs http://dx.doi.org/10.1016/j.ienj.2012.12.001
23. Diaz J, Bustos L, Herrera S, Sepulveda J (2009) Knowledge of the management of paediatric dental traumas by non-dental professionals in emergency rooms in South Araucania, Temuco, Chile. Dent Traumatol 25: 611–619.
24. Andersson L, Al-Asfour A, Al-Jame Q (2006) Knowledge of first-aid measures of avulsion and replantation of teeth: an interview of 221 Kuwaiti schoolchildren. Dent Traumatol 22: 57–65.
25. Biagi R, Cardarelli F, Butti AC, Salvato A (2010) Sports-related dental injuries: knowledge of first aid and mouthguard use in a sample of Italian children and youngsters. Eur J Paediatr Dent 11: 66–70.
26. Castilho LR, Sundefeld ML, de Andrade DF, Panzarini SR, Poi WR (2009) Evaluation of sixth grade primary schoolchildren's knowledge about avulsion and dental reimplantation. Dent Traumatol 25: 429–432.
27. Young C, Wong KY, Cheung LK (2014) A survey on Hong Kong secondary school students' knowledge of emergency management of dental trauma. PLoS ONE 9(1): e84406. doi: 10.1371/journal.pone.0084406
28. Holan G, Cohenca N, Brin I, Sgan-Cohen H (2006) An oral health promotion program for the prevention of complications following avulsion: the effect on knowledge of physical education teachers. Dent Traumatol 22: 323–327.
29. Al-Asfour A, Andersson L, Al-Jame Q (2008) School teachers' knowledge of tooth avulsion and dental first aid before and after receiving information about avulsed teeth and replantation. Dent Traumatol 24: 43–49.
30. Levin L, Jeffet U, Zadik Y (2010) The effect of short dental trauma lecture on knowledge of high-risk population: an intervention study of 336 young adults. Dent Traumatol 26: 86–89.
31. Frujeri Mde L, Costa ED Jr (2009) Effect of a single dental health education on the management of permanent avulsed teeth by different groups of professionals. Dent Traumatol 25: 262–271.
32. McIntyre JD, Lee JY, Trope M, Vann WF Jr (2008) Effectiveness of dental trauma education for elementary school staff. Dent Traumatol 24: 146–150.
33. Kahabuka FK, Willemsen W, van't Hof M, Burgersdijk R (2001) The effect of a single educational input given to school teachers on patient's correct handling after dental trauma. SADJ 56: 284–287.
34. Arikan V, Sonmez H (2012) Knowledge level of primary school teachers regarding traumatic dental injuries and their emergency management before and after receiving an informative leaflet. Dent Traumatol 28: 101–107.
35. Al-Asfour A, Andersson L (2008) The effect of a leaflet given to parents for first aid measures after tooth avulsion. Dent Traumatol 24: 515–521.
36. Mori GG, Castilho LR, Nunes DC, Turcio KH, Molina RO (2007) Avulsion of permanent teeth: analysis of the efficacy of an informative campaign for professionals from elementary schools. J Appl Oral Sci. 15: 534–538.
37. Lieger O, Graf C, El-Maaytah M, Von Arx T (2009) Impact of educational posters on the lay knowledge of school teachers regarding emergency management of dental injuries. Dent Traumatol 25: 406–412.
38. Skapetis T, Gerzina T, Hu W (2012) Managing dental emergencies: A descriptive study of the effects of a multimodal educational intervention for primary care providers at six months. BMC Med Educ 12: 103. doi: 10.1186/1472-6920-12-103
39. Skapetis T, Gerzina T, Hu W (2012) Can a four-hour interactive workshop on the management of dental emergencies be effective in improving self reported levels of clinician proficiency? Australas Emerg Nurs J. 15: 14–22.
40. Pujita C, Nuvvula S, Shilpa G, Nirmala S, Yamini V (2013) Informative promotional outcome on school teachers' knowledge about emergency management of dental trauma. J Conserv Dent. 16: 21–27.
41. Young C, Wong KY, Cheung LK (2013) Effectiveness of Educational Poster on Knowledge of Emergency Management of Dental Trauma–Part 1. Cluster Randomised Controlled Trial for Primary and Secondary School Teachers. PLoS ONE 8(9): e74833. doi:10.1371/journal.pone.0074333

42. Underwood M, Barnett A, Hajioff S (1998) Cluster randomization: a trap for the unwary. Br J Gen Pract 48: 1089–1090.
43. Draper N, Smith H (1981) Applied Regression Analysis. New York: Wiley.
44. Froud R, Eldridge S, Diaz Ordaz K, Marinho VC, Donner A (2012) Quality of cluster randomized controlled trials in oral health: a systematic review of reports published between 2005 and 2009. Community Dent Oral Epidemiol 40 (Suppl 1) 3–14. doi: 10.1111/j.1600-0528.2011.00660

3

Relationship between Sponsorship and Failure Rate of Dental Implants: A Systematic Approach

Antoine Popelut[1], Fabien Valet[2], Olivier Fromentin[3], Aurélie Thomas[4], Philippe Bouchard[1]*

1 Department of Periodontology, Service of Odontology, Hôtel-Dieu Hospital, AP-HP, Paris 7 - Denis Diderot University, U.F.R. of Odontology, Paris, France, **2** Department of Biostatistics, Institut Curie, Paris, France, **3** Department of Prosthetic Dentistry, Service of Odontology, Hôtel-Dieu Hospital, AP-HP, Paris 7 - Denis Diderot University, U.F.R. of Odontology, Paris, France, **4** Library of Odontology, Paris 7 - Denis Diderot University, U.F.R. of Odontology, Paris, France

Abstract

Background: The number of dental implant treatments increases annually. Dental implants are manufactured by competing companies. Systematic reviews and meta-analysis have shown a clear association between pharmaceutical industry funding of clinical trials and pro-industry results. So far, the impact of industry sponsorship on the outcomes and conclusions of dental implant clinical trials has never been explored. The aim of the present study was to examine financial sponsorship of dental implant trials, and to evaluate whether research funding sources may affect the annual failure rate.

Methods and Findings: A systematic approach was used to identify systematic reviews published between January 1993 and December 2008 that specifically deal with the length of survival of dental implants. Primary articles were extracted from these reviews. The failure rate of the dental implants included in the trials was calculated. Data on publication year, Impact Factor, prosthetic design, periodontal status reporting, number of dental implants included in the trials, methodological quality of the studies, presence of a statistical advisor, and financial sponsorship were extracted by two independent reviewers (kappa = 0.90; $CI_{95\%}$ [0.77–1.00]). Univariate quasi-Poisson regression models and multivariate analysis were used to identify variables that were significantly associated with failure rates. Five systematic reviews were identified from which 41 analyzable trials were extracted. The mean annual failure rate estimate was 1.09%.($CI_{95\%}$ [0.84–1.42]). The funding source was not reported in 63% of the trials (26/41). Sixty-six percent of the trials were considered as having a risk of bias (27/41). Given study age, both industry associated (OR = 0.21; $CI_{95\%}$ [0.12–0.38]) and unknown funding source trials (OR = 0.33; ($CI_{95\%}$ [0.21–0.51]) had a lower annual failure rates compared with non-industry associated trials. A conflict of interest statement was disclosed in 2 trials.

Conclusions: When controlling for other factors, the probability of annual failure for industry associated trials is significantly lower compared with non-industry associated trials. This bias may have significant implications on tooth extraction decision making, research on tooth preservation, and governmental health care policies.

Editor: James M. Wright, University of British Columbia, Canada

Funding: This study was supported by a grant from the University Paris Diderot, U.F.R. of Odontologie (Paris, France). The funder had no role in study design, data collection and analysis, decision to publish, or preparation of the manuscript.

Competing Interests: The authors have declared that no competing interests exist.

* E-mail: phbouch@noos.fr

Introduction

Despite the paucity of epidemiological studies on edentulism in many countries, partial and/or complete edentulism data indicate that patients eligible to receive dental prosthesis remain numerous worldwide [1]. It has been shown that tooth replacement improves the quality of life in edentulous patients [2,3]. Therefore, tooth replacement is still of paramount importance in health care, even if tremendous efforts have been made by dental researchers in cariology and periodontology to treat and prevent the two main causes of edentulism: dental caries and periodontal diseases [4].

Until the discovery of the osseointegrated implants at the end of the seventies [5], traditional removable dentures or tooth-supported fixed dentures (dental bridges) were universally used to replace missing teeth. However, root-form endosseous dental implants – surgically implantable medical devices aiming to support artificial tooth or group of teeth – have tended to replace the traditional approach. The main reason for the widespread indications of dental implants by practitioners should ideally be the low percentage of annual implant loss, as demonstrated by primary studies and recent systematic reviews and meta-analysis [6–10]. In addition, biological reasons, i.e. the preservation of the integrity of the teeth bordering the edentulous area, and economical reasons, i.e. the cost-effectiveness approach showing that implant therapy could be more cost-effective than traditional dental bridge therapy [11,12], may be advocated. From the patient's point of view, dental implants are more popular than removable dentures or dental bridges because they can offer fixed solutions when traditional tooth replacement therapies cannot.

Therefore, osseointegrated implant discovery has completely changed the therapeutic approach of tooth replacement. Today, 3 journals are integrally dedicated to implant dentistry, and one of them is in the top 10 of the 55 impact factor dental journals. Nevertheless, due to the lack of comparative trials, there is still no evidence that dental implant therapy performs better than traditional therapy, and that one implant brand is more effective than another.

The number of dentists placing dental implants is increasing annually. Estimates indicate that the number of dental implant procedures performed in Europe increased to 3,527,000 in 2008, representing 8.1% growth over 2007 [13]. Markets for dental implants have been estimated at $3.4 billion in 2008, and are anticipated to reach $8.1 billion by 2015 [14]. Implant companies are traded on the stock exchange. Dental implants are manufactured by competing companies. In Europe, 4 companies capture close to 60% of the market [13].

Systematic reviews and meta-analysis have shown a clear association between pharmaceutical industry funding of clinical trials and pro-industry results [15,16]. So far, to our knowledge, the impact of dental industry sponsorship on the outcomes and conclusions of clinical trials has never been explored. As shown above, dental implant therapy appears to be an interesting example when investigating the influence of funding source on study results. A sponsorship bias in oral implant research may have an adverse effect, not only on preventive dental research but also on teeth preservation. Traditional prosthetic approaches such as tooth-supported fixed dentures need to preserve the teeth; whereas, dental implant therapies require edentulous areas, which are the result of tooth loss. Therefore, in light of the high percentage of success of implant therapy, dentists may be incited to extract teeth instead of making efforts to preserve dental organs.

The aim of the present study was to examine financial sponsorship of dental implant articles, and to determine whether research funding source may affect the annual failure rate. We hypothesized that articles exclusively or partially funded by implant companies are more likely to report lower annual failure rates than articles without industry-associated sponsorship.

Methods

Study selection

We included only primary articles from systematic reviews that specifically deal with the length of survival of dental implants. The following factors were examined: publication year (available from Medline), Impact Factor, prosthetic design, periodontal status reporting, the number of dental implants included in the studies, methodological quality of the studies, the presence of a statistical advisor, and the financial sponsorship. Study design, sample size, dental implant brand, corresponding author country, and conflict of interest were recorded for descriptive statistics of the sample. More details on the selection of these factors are given below in the "Data extraction" section. We looked for papers published only in English.

Search strategy

Two independent reviewers (A.P. and O.F.) searched MEDLINE and the Cochrane database of systematic reviews to identify systematic review articles published between January 1993 and December 2008. The MEDLINE search was conducted using the following MeSH terms exploded: "Dental Implants" and "Denture, Partial, Fixed", in combination with 'survival', 'success' or 'complications' (Table S1). The search was limited to "reviews", "meta-analysis", and "humans". In addition, hand searching was conducted in the following dental journals: *Journal of Periodontology, International Dental Journal, British Dental Journal, Journal of the International Academy of Periodontology, Journal Canadian Dental Association, Swedish Dental Journal, Quintessence International, Journal of Clinical Periodontology, Periodontology 2000, Clinical Oral Implant Research, International Journal of Oral and Maxillofacial Implants, International Journal of Prosthodontic, Journal of Prosthetic Dentistry.*

Inclusion and exclusion criteria

Systematic reviews. Systematic reviews with or without meta-analysis, had to report or to allow for the calculation of the pooled survival rate or the estimated survival rate of dental implants. Implant-supported single crown (IS-SC), implant-supported fixed partial denture (IS-FPD) and implant-tooth supported fixed partial denture (ITS-FPD) were the only prosthetic designs that were included in the present study. Studies included in the articles had to have a mean follow-up of at least 5 years and less than 10 years. We choose a minimum mean follow-up of 5 years because it corresponds to the best scientific evidence in implant dentistry [9]. Our data included different types of dental implants studies because there is no evidence that any specific type of dental implant has superior survival [17].

Fully edentulous patients were excluded from our research. The following dental implants were eliminated from the database because of the suggested increased failure rate: immediate and immediate-delayed dental implants; early and immediate load dental implants; dental implants placed after sinus lift procedures [18–20].

Primary articles. The same inclusion/exclusion criteria as those used for the systematic review selection was applied for the primary article selection. Data cleaning was applied to the identification of duplicate publications on the same patient cohorts. When the same cohort was analyzed twice at different follow-up times, the article reporting a mean follow-up closest to 5 years was included.

Data extraction

Data were extracted from the papers included in the final sample. Two independent investigators were involved in the process of extraction (A.P. and O.F.). In the case of disagreement, the two investigators discussed the article and tried to find agreement. When consensus was not reached, a third investigator (P.B.) was involved until agreement was found. The data were extracted on the following publication characteristics:

Journal and authors characteristics. For each article, we documented the name of the journal, the year of publication, and the impact factor for the year prior to publication using the Journal of citation reports. When the journal was not indexed, it was assigned a "0" value. The country of origin of the corresponding author was obtained from the article. The conflict of interest statements were also recorded.

Study characteristics. The study design of each article was identified as retrospective or prospective. Included studies were submitted to quality assessment according to the following three main criteria: (1) Inclusion/exclusion criteria, (2) Blindness of the examiner, and (3) Drop-out rates. Criteria 1 and 2 were categorized as the following: (1) "Yes"; (2) "No", when it was specified that the criteria was not used; (3) "Unclear", when the article did not mentioned the criteria. The third criterion (drop-out rate) was categorized as "Yes" if reported or "Unclear" if not reported. The studies were evaluated as having low risk of bias if at least 2 quality criteria were met; in all other cases the studies were evaluated as having a risk of bias. It was also noted and recorded if an author served as a statistical advisor or if a statistical advisor was indicated in the article. The prosthetic designs were recorded according to three categories: (1) implant-supported single crown (IS-SC), (2) implant-supported fixed partial denture (IS-FPD), and (3) implant-tooth supported fixed partial denture (ITS-FPD).

Studies indicating the periodontal status of the included subjects were recorded.

Sample characteristics. In each trial, the number of inserted dental implants and the number of implant losses, as well as the mean follow-up, were recorded. Dental implant brands were also identified in each article.

Funding source identification. The funding source of each published study was categorized as follows: (1) industry, (2) industry-associated, (3) non-industry, and (4) unknown. The study was categorized as "industry" when it was clearly stated that it was only supported by grants from an implant company, and "industry-associated" when the implant company had a role in the study design (i.e. data collection or analysis, decision to publish, preparation of the manuscript) or in free dental implant providing. The "non-industry" category included studies supported by grants from universities, governmental agencies, independent foundations, and other nonprofits organizations with no industry association. Each institution classified as "non-industry" was carefully verified through Internet searches. When the information was doubtful or not available, the institution was contacted by e-mail. When no information was given on sponsorship, the funding source was categorized as "unknown".

Statistical analysis

Collected data were organized into a spreadsheet using a computer program (Excel, Microsoft, Redmond, WA). After proofing for entry errors, the database was locked and loaded in statistical software program by a statistician (F.V.) blind to the study selection and data extraction. The industry and industry-associated funding-source categories were collapsed for the analysis. All statistical analyses were performed with R 2.10.0 software (R Foundation for Statistical Computing, Vienna, Austria) on PC architecture.

Descriptive statistics were reported as numbers and percentages. The Kappa statistic [21] was used to assess interrater reliability between the two independent reviewers (A.P. and O.F.) using the funding source scale.

The total exposure time of each included study selected from systematic reviews was used for the 5-year estimated survival rate calculation. Failure rate was calculated by dividing the number of events (implant loss) in the numerator by the total exposure time in the denominator [9,10,22]. Implant loss was extracted from the publications. The total exposure time was calculated by the sum of *i)* exposure time of implants followed for the whole observation period, *ii)* exposure time of the implants lost during the observation period, and *iii)* exposure time of the implants that did not complete the observation period. Exact $CI_{95\%}$ for failure rate estimates was calculated using the relationship between Poisson and Chi-square distributions [23]. Five-year survival proportions were calculated via the relationship between event rate and survival function S [$S(T) = \exp(-T \times \text{event rate})$] by assuming constant event rates [24].

The total number of events was considered to be Poisson distributed for a given sum of implant exposure years. The Poisson regression model, with a logarithmic link-function and a total exposure time per study as an offset variable, was used [25]. We used Breslow's recommendation to detect overdispersion [26], and a quasi-Poisson model for handling heterogeneity [25].

Consequently, univariate quasi-Poisson regression models were used to find variables that were significantly associated with failure rates. A multivariate analysis was then performed to identify the variables significantly associated with failure rates. For model selection, a deviance approach with a "drop-one" algorithm was used [27]. An F-ratio statistic was calculated to compare models with and without each of the discarded variables [28].

Results

In the systematic review search, we screened a total of 323 articles and identified 17 articles of which, after full-text reading, 12 articles were excluded (Figure 1). Table S2 indicates the reason for exclusion of these articles. Therefore, a total of 5 systematic reviews were included to serve as the database from which primary articles were extracted [9,10,22,29,30]. Our final sample consisted of 38 published clinical trials. The full list of references which included primary articles is presented in Table S3. Figure 2 depicts the flow diagram for inclusion of the primary articles. Three articles dealt with 2 different prosthetic designs. They were thus each considered as 2 different trials for the analysis, leading to a total of 41 analyzable trials. The Kappa coefficient between examiners (A.P. and O.F.) was 0.90 ($CI_{95\%}$ [0.77–1.00]) demonstrating an almost prefect degree of agreement [31]. The initial Poisson model (with the offset variable only) provided a deviance equal to 161.20, which was much greater than the degrees of freedom (equal to 40), suggesting a strong heterogeneity.

Descriptive data for the extracted trials are shown in Table 1. The funding source was not reported in the majority of the trials (63%, 26/41). Taking into account all years together, the majority of the trials were considered as having a risk of bias (66%, 27/41). The reporting did not mention a statistical advisor in 30 trials (73%), and almost all trials did not report the periodontal status of the patients (83%, 34/41). Implant brands were dominated by one company (59%, 24/41), and Sweden, the company's original country, was the most common country among the corresponding authors (24%, 10/41). In our sample, 22% of the trials (9/41) were published in non indexed journals for the year prior to publication. A conflict of interest statement was disclosed in 2 trials. In both statements, the authors reported that they had no conflict of interest.

Figure 3 indicates that the annual estimated percentages of failures ranged from 0 to 5.56 ($CI_{95\%}$ [0.00–14.76]). The mean annual failure rate of the trials was estimated at 1.09%.($CI_{95\%}$ [0.84–1.42]). The mean annual failure rate calculated for the non-industry trials was equal to 2.73% ($CI_{95\%}$ [1.14–6.55], i.e. almost 3 times the rate for all the trials.

As shown in Table 2, the outcomes of the univariate quasi-Poisson regression models indicate a significant effect of the prosthetic design ($p = 0.023$) and the source of funding ($p = 0.005$). Compared with non-industry associated trials, both industry associated trials as well as trials where the sponsorship was unknown were more likely to report lower annual failure rates, showing ORs of 0.32 ($CI_{95\%}$ [0.17–0.60]) and 0.37 ($CI_{95\%}$ [0.21–0.63]), respectively. The multivariate analysis yields to the selection of publication age ($p = 0.002$) and funding source ($p<0.001$) in the final mode. Given data on funding source, the annual failure rate was 1.12 times higher for a one-year old increase in the publication age. Given information on study age, industry associated ($OR = 0.21$; $CI_{95\%}$ [0.12–0.38]) and unknown funding source ($OR = 0.33$; ($CI_{95\%}$ [0.21–0.51]) trials had lower annual failure rates as compared with non-industry associated trials.

Discussion

The main outcome of this study indicates that the funding sources have a significant effect on the annual rate of failure of dental implants. Given the publication age and when controlling for other factors, the annual failure rate for industry associated trials is significantly lower as compared with non-industry associated trials ($OR = 0.21$). These findings add significant new information to the field of dentistry and contribute to the body of

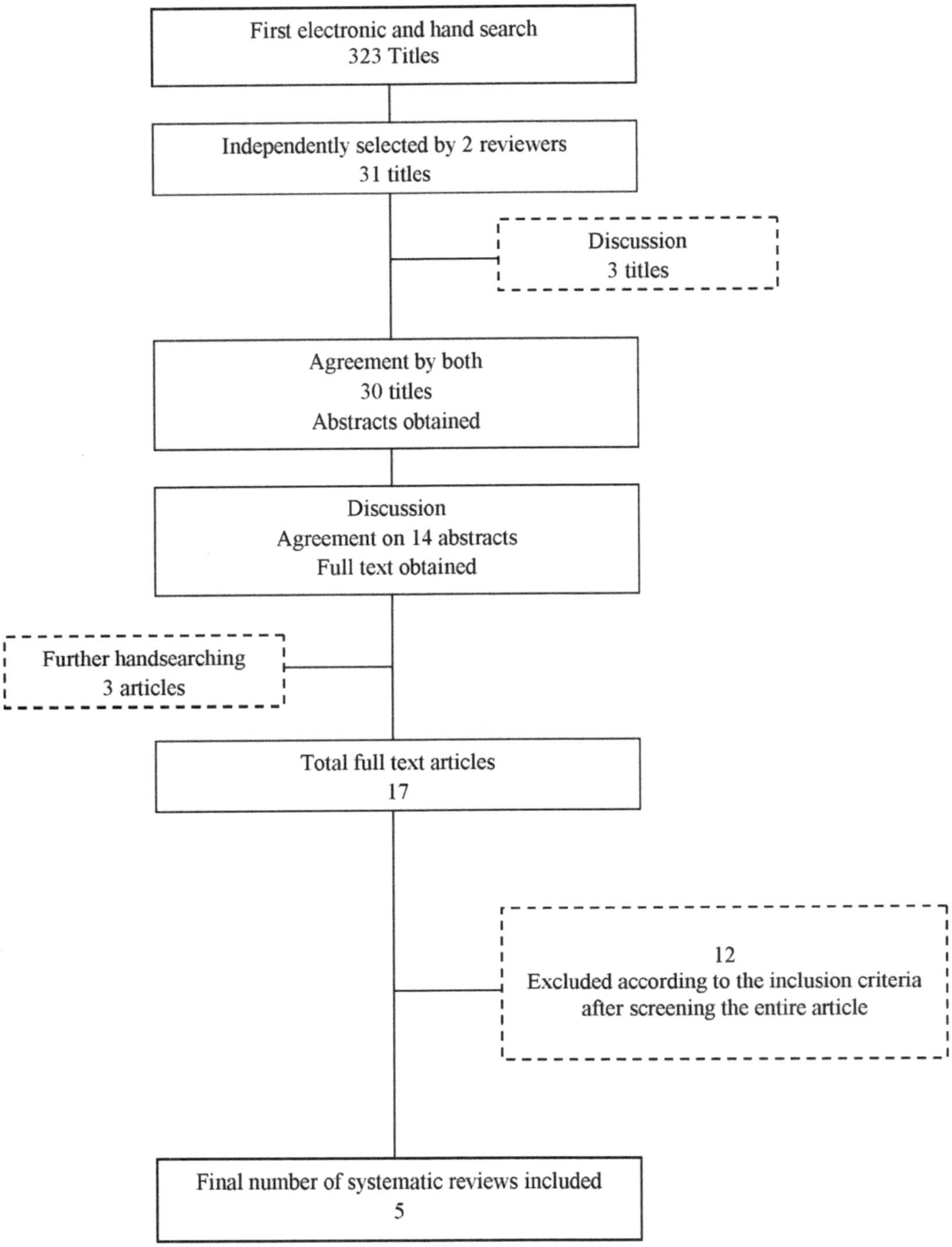

Figure 1. Flowchart of systematic review selection.

literature showing that industry sponsoring may affect biomedical research outcomes [16,32].

Interestingly, the multivariate analysis shows that trials where the financial funding source was not reported had an even lower probability of failure than industry associated trials (OR = 0.33). This outcome is hard to interpret. The trials belonging to this "unknown" category are probably the most biased. The authors deliberately did not report the sponsor. It may indicate that industry involvement in a clinical study implies some quality control to reduce bias in order to maintain company reputation. On the other hand, it is noteworthy that 63% of the trials included in the analysis did not report the funding source. This imbalance between sample size of disclosed and undisclosed funding sources (15/26) may have influenced the statistical results. The multivariate analysis also indicates that the annual rate of failure increases with the article seniority following the date of publication. This outcome may correspond to an improvement in dental implant therapies.

Leaving aside the lack of transparency of the funding source, a number of common weaknesses were identified in the trials'reporting. Lack of inclusion/exclusion criteria, inadequate blinding, and lack of drop-out rates were common, leading to the

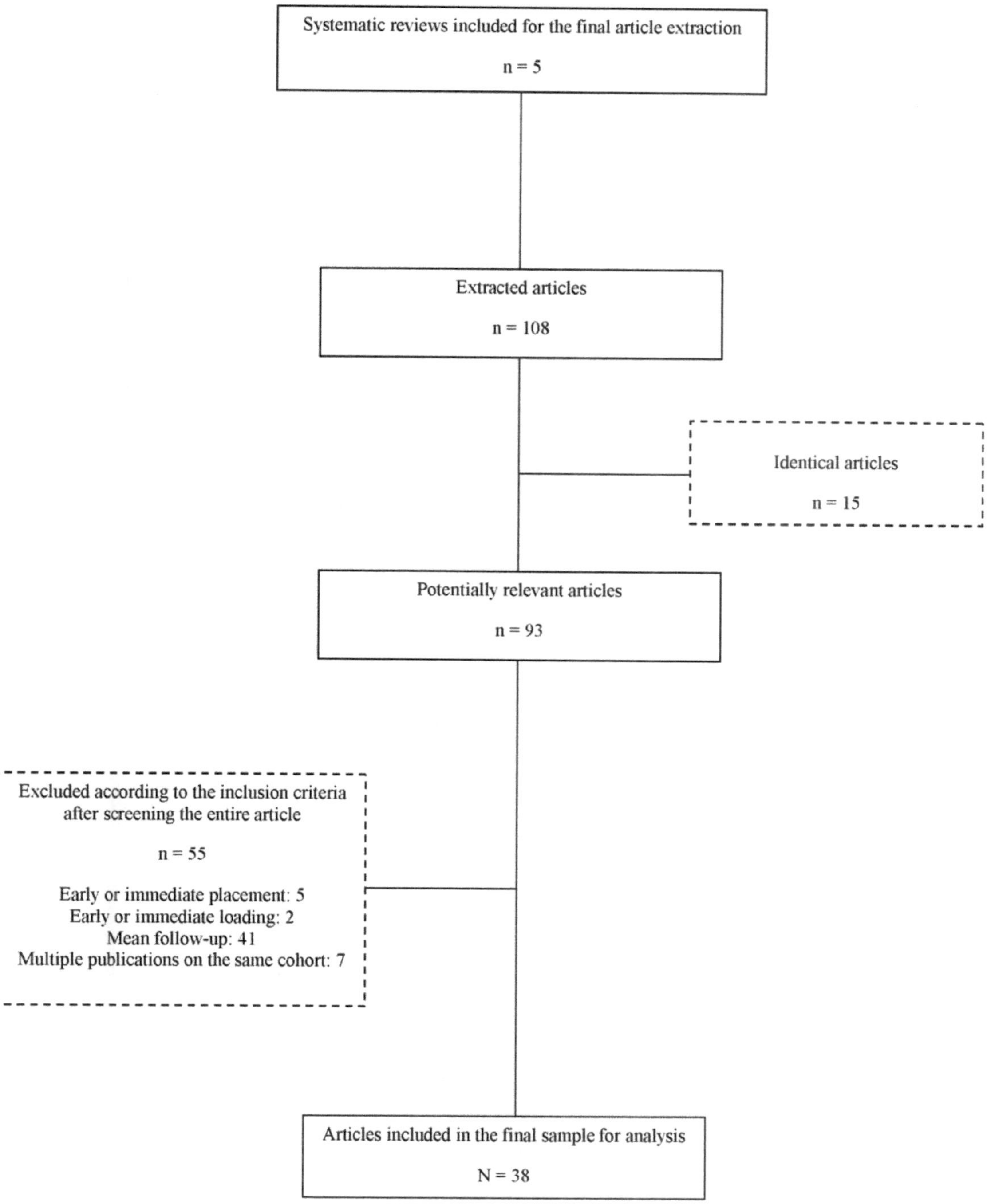

Figure 2. Flowchart of the primary article selection.

classification of 66% of the trials as having a risk of bias using our methodological quality assessment scale. Our intent was not to evaluate the overall quality of the trial, which may imply the rating of each individual feature aimed to reduce bias, but rather to provide a snapshot of the risk of bias of each trial through three items that focus on important aspects of study design. A statistician was identified in only 27% of the trials, rendering the analysis of the data questionable. In addition, the periodontal status of the subjects was reported in only 17% of the trials, although a significant difference in mean peri-implant marginal bone loss between patients with a history of periodontitis and periodontally healthy subjects has been shown [33,34]. These weaknesses suggest that the relevance of the annual failure rates given by these types of trials must be interpreted with caution. However, taken together, these factors could not significantly overcome the impact of the funding source on the annual failure rate when included in the multivariate analysis.

We used the impact factor as the main journal characteristic because the quality of the reporting may vary with the journal. In our sample, only peer-reviewed journals were included. The regression models did not disclose an association between journal impact factors and the annual rate of failure. This finding is similar

Table 1. Sample characteristics.

Characteristics	Category	Total n = 41
Age of publication, tertiles	4–10	31 (76%)
	11–15	9 (22%)
	>15	1 (2%)
Impact factors, tertiles	Not indexed	9 (22%)
	0.52–1.09	8 (19%)
	1.10–1.67	15 (37%)
	1.68–2.24	9 (22%)
Corresponding author country	USA	4 (10%)
	Belgium	5 (12%)
	Sweden	10 (24%)
	Switzerland	5 (12%)
	Italy	2 (5%)
	England	2 (5%)
	Germany	3 (7%)
	Canada	2 (5%)
	Others	8 (20%)
Study design	Retrospective	10 (25%)
	Prospective	31 (75%)
Quality assessment	Low risk of bias	14 (34%)
	Risk of bias	27 (66%)
Statistical advisor	Yes	11 (27%)
	No	30 (73%)
Prosthetic design	IS-SC	18 (44%)
	IS-FPD	15 (36%)
	ITS-FPD	8 (20%)
Periodontal status report	Yes	7 (17%)
	No	34 (83%)
Total number of implants, tertiles	10–347	38 (93%)
	348–685	2 (5%)
	686–1022	1(2%)
Number of failures, tertiles	0–19	37 (90%)
	20–39	2 (5%)
	40–58	2 (5%)
Implant brand	Straumann	8 (19%)
	Astra Tech	3 (7%)
	Nobel Biocare	24 (59%)
	Others	6 (15%)
Funding source	Industry	2 (5%)
	Industry associated	9 (22%)
	Non industry	4 (10%)
	Unknown	26 (63%)

to the outcomes reported by other studies dealing with the sponsorship bias in pharmaceutical trials [16].

Our study is the first, to our knowledge, investigating the impact of sponsorship in the field of dentistry. This study has several strengths. We used dental implant therapy, a model where the market is very competitive as highlighted by the number of implant brands included in the sample. Thus, our findings may be generalizable to other dental products and devices within competitive markets, such as in orthodontics, periodontology or prosthetic dentistry. In addition, the consequences of the widespread use of dental implants have an effect on the health and well-being of the entire population, due to the impact on the extraction indications of the practitioners and on the health-policy aiming to reimburse dental therapies. Our study used the framework of a systematic method to identify the trials, and the annual failure rate as an objective measurable comparator. We decided to use the survival rate as the main variable and not the success rate because biological and technical complications were independently recorded in some systematic reviews [7,8]. The overlap of biological and technical complications, due to the fact that one implant may have more than one complication, precludes any pooled estimate of success rate. Consequently, the number of systematic reviews using the survival rate as the main variable [9,10,22,29,30] was higher than those available using the success rate [30,35].

The primary limitation of our study is the weak transparency of the financial support reporting of the trials included in the analysis. It may be assumed that among the 26 trials where the sponsorship was categorized as "unknown", part of them were in fact partially supported by industry. For example, it is well-known that companies sometimes provide dental implants for free in order to evaluate their products. This may lead to publications and financial support of the companies in a communication plan where the authors are involved.

This "ghost" funding source may affect reporting objectivity. In addition, it was not possible to explore the relationship between a potential sponsor and the authors of the articles, because a conflict of interest statement was mentioned in only 2 out 41 trials. Consequently, it may be assumed that our study underestimated the number of industry associated trials.

Second, our sample is not exhaustive of all the studies dealing with dental implant survival. Systematic reviews were our source of trials because they are presumed to be objective. When done well, they are considered the highest level of evidence for medical decision making [36]. The results and conclusions of systematic reviews are often cited, and are the cornerstones of the decision making process when determining whether or not to insert an implant for tooth replacement. Thus, one can assume that the articles included in these reviews are those responding the best to high quality standards. Interestingly, in our study, 2 out of the 5 selected systematic reviews did not disclose their funding source [10,29]. In the remaining 3 included systematic reviews, 2 of them declared no conflict of interest [9,22].

Third, we were unable to pool meaningful evidences about factors that might be associated with the rate of failure. We thus speculated on variables identifiable in the sample assuming that they could affect the annual rate and be competitive with the sponsorship bias. Among them, the prosthetic design was regularly reported, and we hypothesized that it could be one of the most influential cofactors. We thus excluded trials involving fully edentulous patients in attempt to reduce the heterogeneity of the prosthetic design. Our hypothesis turned out to be strengthened by the significant effect of this variable in the univariate analysis ($p = 0.023$). However, the prosthetic design was not significant in the multivariate models, meaning that, even if strong, this factor could not overcome the funding source variable. Based on the basic principle that the magnitude of the treatment effect is influenced by the sample size, we also speculated that the sample size, i.e. the number of implants per trial, may have an effect on the rate of failure. Indeed, this variable did not show a significant effect in the present analysis.

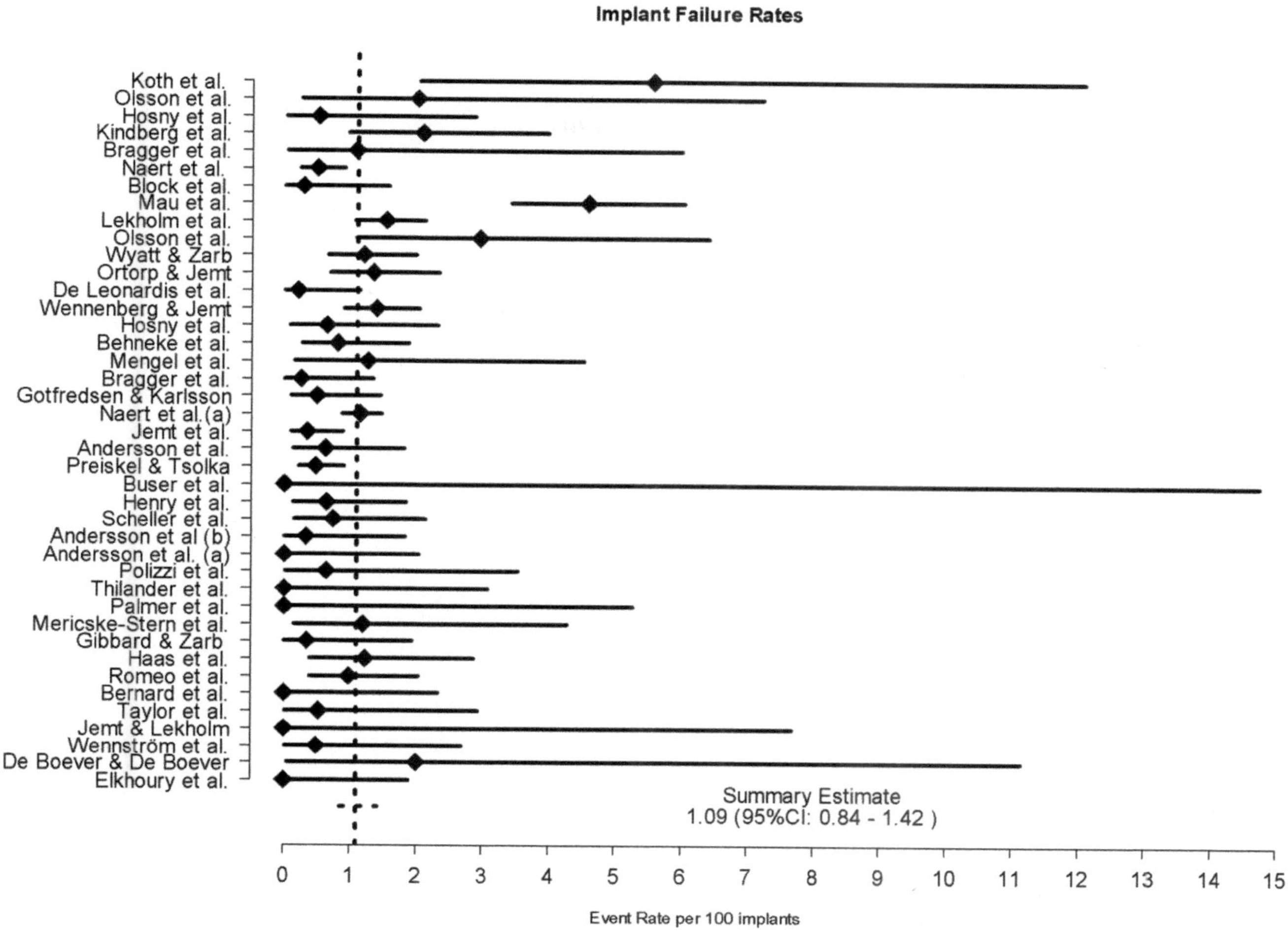

Figure 3. Annual percentages of failures.

Table 2. Regression quasi-Poisson univariate and multivariate models of the effects of independent variables on the annual failure rate of dental implants.

Category		Univariate Quasi-Poisson			Multivariate Quasi-Poisson		
		OR	CI 95%	p-value	OR	CI 95%	p-value
Study Age		1.07	[0.98–1.16]	0.085	1.12	[1.06–1.19]	0.002
Number of Implants		1.00	[0.99–1.00]	0.424			
Impact Factor		0.90	[0.61–1.33]	0.549			
Periodontal Status Report	No	1	–				
	Yes	0.90	[0.33–2.45]	0.812			
Prosthetic Design	ITS-FPD	1	–				
	IS-FPD	0.56	[0.34–0.91]				
	IS-SC	0.34	[0.15–0.77]	0.023			
Quality Score	LRB	1	–				
	RB	0.81	[0.47–1.41]	0.427			
Statistical Advisor	No	1	–				
	Yes	1.54	[0.95–2.50]	0.082			
Funding Source	Non-Industry Associated	1	–		1		
	Industry Associated	0.32	[0.17–0.60]		0.21	[0.12–0.38]	
	Unknown	0.37	[0.21–0.63]	0.005	0.33	[0.21–0.51]	<0.001

Last but not least, all the prospective or retrospective trials that were included in the present analysis had an observational design and not an experimental design. It is well known that observational studies are more vulnerable to methodological problems and must be critically interpreted. They are prone to bias and confounding. Therefore, the real world mean annual failure rate is if anything likely higher than that found here for the non-industry trials (2.73%), given that the study designs have a high risk of bias.

The outcomes of this study strongly suggest the need for more transparency in the sponsorship of trials dealing with dental implant therapy. In the future, details on the financial source should be clearly reported. Dental publications should include at least a conflict of interest statement. So far, only one of the journals quoted in the present study has recently adopted such a statement. This is a first step towards increasing the transparency of the trial funding sources. Our results fully encourage editors of dental journals and authors of future studies in dentistry to be informed of certain initiatives that have been proposed to reduce the sponsorship bias in the biomedical research as well as in the Health Economics studies [15,37]. Ultimately, more studies, including well conducted randomized clinical trials, are needed to identify potentially influential factors that can affect the rate of failure of the dental implants. Efforts should be made to increase the methodological quality of the reporting. So far, only 2 out of 9 dental journals involved in our sample (Journal of Clinical Periodontology and Clinical Oral Implant Research) have adopted the CONSORT guidelines [38]. The conclusions of the present study therefore strongly encourage the implementation of the CONSORT statements in the field of dental clinical research.

Supporting Information

Table S1 MEDLINE (Pubmed) search strategy for systematic reviews selection.

Table S2 List of excluded systematic review articles and the reason for exclusion.

Table S3 List of included articles.

Author Contributions

Conceived and designed the experiments: PB. Performed the experiments: AP OF. Analyzed the data: FV PB. Contributed reagents/materials/analysis tools: AT. Wrote the paper: PB. Designed the study, analyzed data, and drafted the manuscript: PB. Collected data and coded data: AP OF. Revised the manuscript: AP OF FV FT. Advised on analysis and conducted analysis: FV. Advised on the search strategy and supervised the outcomes: FT.

References

1. WHO, Health statistics and health information systems, Disease and injury country estimates, Burden of disease. Death and DALY estimates for 2004 by cause for WHO Member States, 2009. Available: http://www.who.int/healthinfo/global_burden_disease/estimates_country/en/. Accessed 10 January 2010.
2. Hunter JM, Arbona SI (1995) Paradise lost: an introduction to the geography of water pollution in Puerto Rico. Soc Sci Med 40: 1331–1355.
3. Jones JA, Orner MB, Spiro A, 3rd, Kressin NR (2003) Tooth loss and dentures: patients' perspectives. Int Dent J 53: 327–334.
4. Neely AL, Holford TR, Löe H, Anerud A, Boysen H (2005) The natural history of periodontal disease in humans: risk factors for tooth loss in caries-free subjects receiving no oral health care. J Clin Periodontol 32: 984–993.
5. Branemark PI, Hansson BO, Adell R, Breine U, Lindstrom J, et al. (1977) Osseointegrated implants in the treatment of the edentulous jaw. Experience from a 10-year period. Scand J Plast Reconstr Surg Suppl.16: 1–132.
6. Esposito M, Hirsch J, Lekholm U, Thomsen P (1999) Differential diagnosis and treatment strategies for biologic complications and failing oral implants: a review of the literature. Int J Oral Maxillofac Implants 14: 473–490.
7. Berglundh T, Persson L, Klinge B (2002) A systematic review of the incidence of biological and technical complications in implant dentistry reported in prospective longitudinal studies of at least 5 years. J Clin Periodontol 29 Suppl.3: 197–212.
8. Goodacre CJ, Bernal G, Rungcharassaeng K, Kan JY (2003) Clinical complications with implants and implant prostheses. J Prosthet Dent 90: 121–132.
9. Pjetursson BE, Tan K, Lang NP, Brägger U, Egger M, et al. (2004) A systematic review of the survival and complication rates of fixed partial dentures (FPDs) after an observation period of at least 5 years. Clin Oral Implants Res 15: 625–642.
10. Jung RE, Pjetursson BE, Glauser R, Zembic A, Zwahlen M, et al. (2008) A systematic review of the 5-year survival and complication rates of implant-supported single crowns. Clin Oral Implants Res 19: 119–130.
11. Brägger U, Krenander P, Lang NP (2005) Economic aspects of single-tooth replacement. Clin Oral Implants Res 16: 335–341.
12. Bouchard P, Renouard F, Bourgeois D, Fromentin O, Jeanneret MH, et al. (2009) Cost-effectiveness modeling of dental implant vs. bridge. Clin Oral Implants Res 20: 583–587.
13. Millennium Research Group (2009) European markets for dental implants 2009. Available: http//www.mrg.net. Accessed May 2009.
14. WinterGreen Research Report (2009) Worldwide Nanotechnology Dental Implant Market Shares, Strategies, and Forecasts, 2009 to 2015. 335 p. Available:http://www.researchandmarkets.com/reportinfo.asp?report_id=941893&t=d&cat_id=. Accessed 10 January 2010.
15. Doucet M, Sismondo S (2008) Evaluating solutions to sponsorship bias. J Med Ethics 34: 627–630.
16. Bero L, Oostvogel F, Bacchetti P, Lee K (2007) Factors associated with findings of published trials of drug–drug comparisons: Why some statins appear more efficacious than others. PLoS Med 4: 1001–1010.
17. Esposito M, Murray-Curtis L, Grusovin MG, Coulthard P, Worthington HV (2007) Interventions for replacing missing teeth: different types of dental implants. Cochrane Database Syst Rev 4: CD003815.
18. Tonetti MS, Hämmerle CH (2008) Advances in bone augmentation to enable dental implant placement: Consensus Report of the Sixth European Workshop on Periodontology. J Clin Periodontol 35: 168–172.
19. Esposito MA, Koukoulopoulou A, Coulthard P, Worthington HV (2006) Interventions for replacing missing teeth: dental implants in fresh extraction sockets (immediate, immediate-delayed and delayed implants). Cochrane Database Syst Rev 4: CD005968.
20. Esposito M, Grusovin MG, Achille H, Coulthard P, Worthington HV (2009) Interventions for replacing missing teeth: different times for loading dental implants. Cochrane Database Syst Rev 1: CD003878.
21. Cohen J (1960) A coefficient of agreement for nominal scales. Educ Psychol Meas 20: 37–46.
22. Lang NP, Pjetursson BE, Tan K, Brägger U, Egger M, et al. (2004) Systematic review of the survival and complication rates of fixed partial dentures (FPDs) after an observation period of at least 5 years. II. Combined tooth–implant-supported FPDs. Clin Oral Implants Res 15: 643–653.
23. Ulm K (1990) A simple method to calculate the confidence interval of a standardized mortality ratio. Am J Epidemiol 131: 373–375.
24. Kirkwood BR, Sterne JAC (2004) Survival analysis: displaying and comparing survival patterns. In: Kirkwood BR, Sterne JAC, eds. Essential Medical Statistics. Oxford, Malden: Blackwell Science. pp 272–286.
25. Agresti A (2002) Poisson regression for rates. In: Agresti A, ed. Categorical data analysis. New-York: Wiley. pp 385–408.
26. Breslow NE (1996) Generalized linear models: Checking assumptions and strengthening conclusions. Stat App 8: 23–41.
27. Venables WN, Ripley BD (2002) Model selection. In: Venables WN, Ripley BD, eds. Modern Applied statistics with S. New York: Springer. pp 172–177.
28. Zuur AF, Ieno EN, Walker NJ (2009) Model selection in Quasi-Poisson. In: Zuur AF, Ieno EN, Walker NJ, eds. Mixed effects Models and extensions in Ecology with R. New York: Springer. pp 227–230.
29. Lindh T, Gunne J, Tillberg A, Molin MA (1998) Meta-analysis of implants in partial edentulism. Clin Oral Implants Res 9: 80–90.
30. Torabinejad M, Anderson P, Bader J, Brown LJ, Chen LH, et al. (2007) Outcomes of root canal treatment and restoration, implant-supported single crowns, fixed partial dentures, and extraction without replacement: a systematic review. J Prosthet Dent 98: 285–311.
31. Landis JR, Koch GG (1977) The measurement of observer agreement for categorical data. Biometrics 33: 159–174.

32. Lesser LI, Ebbeling CB, Goozner M, Wypij D, Ludwig DS (2007) Relationship between funding source and conclusion among nutrition-related scientific articles. PLoS Med 4: 41–46.
33. Karoussis IK, Kotsovilis S, Fourmousis IA (2007) Comprehensive and critical review of dental implant prognosis in periodontally compromised partially edentulous patients. Clin Oral Implants Res 18: 669–679.
34. Ong CTT, Ivanovski S, Needleman IG, Retzepi M, Moles DR, et al. (2008) Systematic review of implant outcomes in treated periodontitis subjects. J Clin Periodontol 35: 438–462.
35. Salinas TJ, Eckert SE (2007) In patients requiring single-tooth replacement, what are the outcomes of implant- as compared to tooth-supported restorations? Int J Oral Maxillofac Implants 22 suppl: 71–95.
36. PLoS Medicine Editors (2007) Many reviews are systematic but some are more transparent and completely reported than others. PLoS Med 4: 399–400.
37. Bell CM, Urbach DR, Ray JG, Bayoumi A, Rosen AB, et al. (2006) Bias in published cost effectiveness studies: systematic review. BMJ 332: 699–703.
38. Moher D, Schulz KF, Altman DG, Lepage L (2001) The CONSORT statement: revised recommendations for improving the quality of reports of parallel-group randomised trials. Lancet 357: 1191–1194.

4

Using Networks To Understand Medical Data: The Case of Class III Malocclusions

Antonio Scala[1,2*], Pietro Auconi[1,3], Marco Scazzocchio[1], Guido Caldarelli[1,2,4], James A. McNamara[5,6,7,8], Lorenzo Franchi[5,9]

1 Istituto dei Sistemi Complessi Udr "La Sapienza", Roma, Italy, **2** London Institute of Mathematical Sciences, London, United Kingdom, **3** Private Practice of Orthodontics, Rome, Italy, **4** NATWORKS Unit for the Study of Natural Networks, IMT Lucca Institute for Advanced Studies, Lucca, Italy, **5** Department of Orthodontics and Pediatric Dentistry, School of Dentistry, The University of Michigan, Ann Arbor, Michigan, United States of America, **6** Department of Cell and Developmental Biology, School of Medicine, The University of Michigan, Ann Arbor, Michigan, United States of America, **7** Center for Human Growth and Development, The University of Michigan, Ann Arbor, Michigan, United States of America, **8** Private Practice of Orthodontics, Ann Arbor, Michigan, United States of America, **9** Department of Orthodontics, The University of Florence, Florence, Italy

Abstract

A system of elements that interact or regulate each other can be represented by a mathematical object called a network. While network analysis has been successfully applied to high-throughput biological systems, less has been done regarding their application in more applied fields of medicine; here we show an application based on standard medical diagnostic data. We apply network analysis to Class III malocclusion, one of the most difficult to understand and treat orofacial anomaly. We hypothesize that different interactions of the skeletal components can contribute to pathological disequilibrium; in order to test this hypothesis, we apply network analysis to 532 Class III young female patients. The topology of the Class III malocclusion obtained by network analysis shows a strong co-occurrence of abnormal skeletal features. The pattern of these occurrences influences the vertical and horizontal balance of disharmony in skeletal form and position. Patients with more unbalanced orthodontic phenotypes show preponderance of the pathological skeletal nodes and minor relevance of adaptive dentoalveolar equilibrating nodes. Furthermore, by applying Power Graphs analysis we identify some functional modules among orthodontic nodes. These modules correspond to groups of tightly inter-related features and presumably constitute the key regulators of plasticity and the sites of unbalance of the growing dentofacial Class III system. The data of the present study show that, in their most basic abstraction level, the orofacial characteristics can be represented as graphs using nodes to represent orthodontic characteristics, and edges to represent their various types of interactions. The applications of this mathematical model could improve the interpretation of the quantitative, patient-specific information, and help to better targeting therapy. Last but not least, the methodology we have applied in analyzing orthodontic features can be applied easily to other fields of the medical science.

Editor: Angel Sánchez, Universidad Carlos III de Madrid, Spain

Funding: The authors have no support or funding to report.

Competing Interests: Pietro Auconi and James A. Mcnamara work in a private practice of orthodontics, i.e: Studio Auconi in Rome, Italy, and McNamara Orthodontics, Ann Arbor, Michigan, respectively. There are no patents, products in development or marketed products to declare.

* E-mail: antonio.scala@phys.uniroma1.it

Introduction

A general way to understand complex biological systems is to represent them using the simplest units of architecture. Such patterns of local and global interconnection are called *networks*. A network, or in more formal mathematical language, a *graph*, is a simplified representation that reduces a system to an abstract structure capturing the basis of connection pattern of the system [1,2]. The simplest possible network representation reduces the system's elements to *nodes* ("*vertices*") and their pairwise relationships to *links* ("*edges*") connecting pairs of nodes. Links represent functional interactions or anatomical relationships between the nodes, such as "catalyze", or "binds to", or "is converted to", or "shift" [3,4]. The network's inference and analysis refers to information on the identity and the state of the elements of a system to their functional relationships and to the extraction of biological insight and predictions. A multitude of studies have shown that meaningful biological properties can be extracted by network analysis [5,6].

An important advancement in network science has been the possibility of identifying and localizing sub-networks of functional modules (*motifs*) in complex systems [7]. The decomposition of large networks into distinct components, or modules, has to be regarded as a major approach to deal with the complexity of large biological networks. A motif refers to a group of physically or functionally connected components (nodes in graph) that work together to achieve the desired biological function. These organized sets of interactions are capable of local ordering, function, process information, and presumably act as regulators of growth and development in determining auxologic choices between homeostasis and plasticity [8–10].

Already applied in biomedical areas such as genetics, molecular biology, microbiology, and epidemiology, networks often have revealed surprising and unanticipated biological and functional insights, delineating the possibility of a new, holistic approach in scientific investigation. This approach ideally aims to define and analyze the interrelationship of *all* the elements in a biomedical system in order to understand how a system works in ever changing conditions (a new discipline called "*Systems Biology*") [11]. An apparently more modest but not less important task is to apply such an approach to the ordinary data sets used in medical practice; in particular, we will produce an example based on standard orthodontic data.

Network analysis has been applied recently to orthodontics to detect and visualize the most interconnected clinical, radiographic, and functional data pertaining to the orofacial system [12]. In particular, by considering phenotypic, functional, and radiographic characteristics it has been shown that different kinds of dentofacial malocclusions correspond to different network structures (a malocclusion is a misalignment of teeth or incorrect relation between the teeth of the two dental arches).

During the diagnostic process to establish the objectives, strategies, priorities and sequences of treatment, the orthodontist has to identify and locate the critical points of malocclusion [13]. Among malocclusions, the more severe is the so-called Class III malocclusion, often associated with the protrusion of the lower dental arch (Fig. 1). Class III malocclusion in growing subjects is characterized by a complex combinations of skeletal features (*e.g.* a shorter and more retrusive maxilla, an excess of lower anterior face height, a shorter anterior cranial base length, a more acute cranial base angle) with multiple dentoalveolar compensatory processes (*e.g.* proclined maxillary incisors, retroclined mandibular incisors) [14–18]. The management of the architectural and structural Class III network parameters forces the orthodontist to collect clinical and radiographic data sets on craniofacial characteristics, growth, and function. The paradox of daily orthodontic practice is that these data sets may bring more disorientation than understanding of the main problem of the patient [19]. With the aim of identifying pathognomonic traits of severity for Class III malocclusion, Freer [20] found that labiolingual spread and overjet were the most critical variables, while Stellzig-Eisenhauer et al [19] focused attention on the individualized combination of palatal plane angle, inclination of lower incisors, and Wits appraisal, but no morphologic trait was shown to be indicative of potential Class III development [20–23].

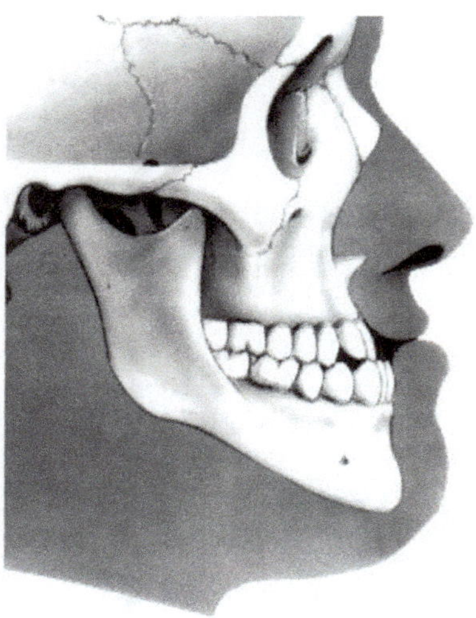

Figure 1. Class III malocclusion with protrusion of the lower dental arch.

The craniofacial region can be regarded as a complex system that grows and remodels itself following an intricate network of auxologic forces, distortive processes and/or compensatory mechanisms [18]. Complex systems are dynamic systems that present with the capacity of self-organizing a large number of interacting elements in a non-linear fashion (*e.g.* forests, ants, flocks of birds, financial markets, the immune system) [3]. In order to understand the function of a biological organization it often is beneficial to conceptualize it as a systems of interacting elements and to define the dynamic behavior of these components [1,11]. The global behavior of complex systems cannot be explained solely on the basis of a single physical law, or the behavior of individual elements. The cooperation of the elements determines the overall behavior and provides properties that can be totally unrelated to the individual components of the system ("more is different"). The system must be analyzed in its entirety, as a coherent unit: it is pattern that matters [24,25].

The aim of this study is to show how "network thinking" and network modeling leads to a systemic analysis of standard diagnostic data under a different perspective that digs out previously undiscovered information. In particular, we will identify the physiological and/or pathological characteristics in a large cross-sectional sample of 532 female Class III subjects on the basis of a model derived from network analysis.

Methods

Objectives

The aim of this study is to apply conjunctly statistical analysis with network tools and methodologies to Class III malocclusion features' longitudinal (i.e. time varying) datasets in order to uncover the systemic importance of such features and to

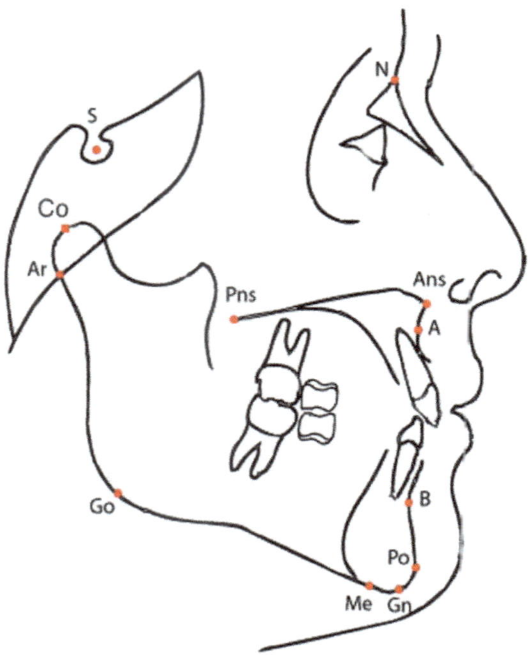

Figure 2. Cephalogram reference points. Most of the cephalometric landmarks are either angles or normalized linear distances. As an example, SN-GoGn is an angle between anterior cranial base and mandibular plane. The 21 cephalometric landmarks analyzed in the paper correspond to the standard set of features analyzed in orthodontics (see Table 1).

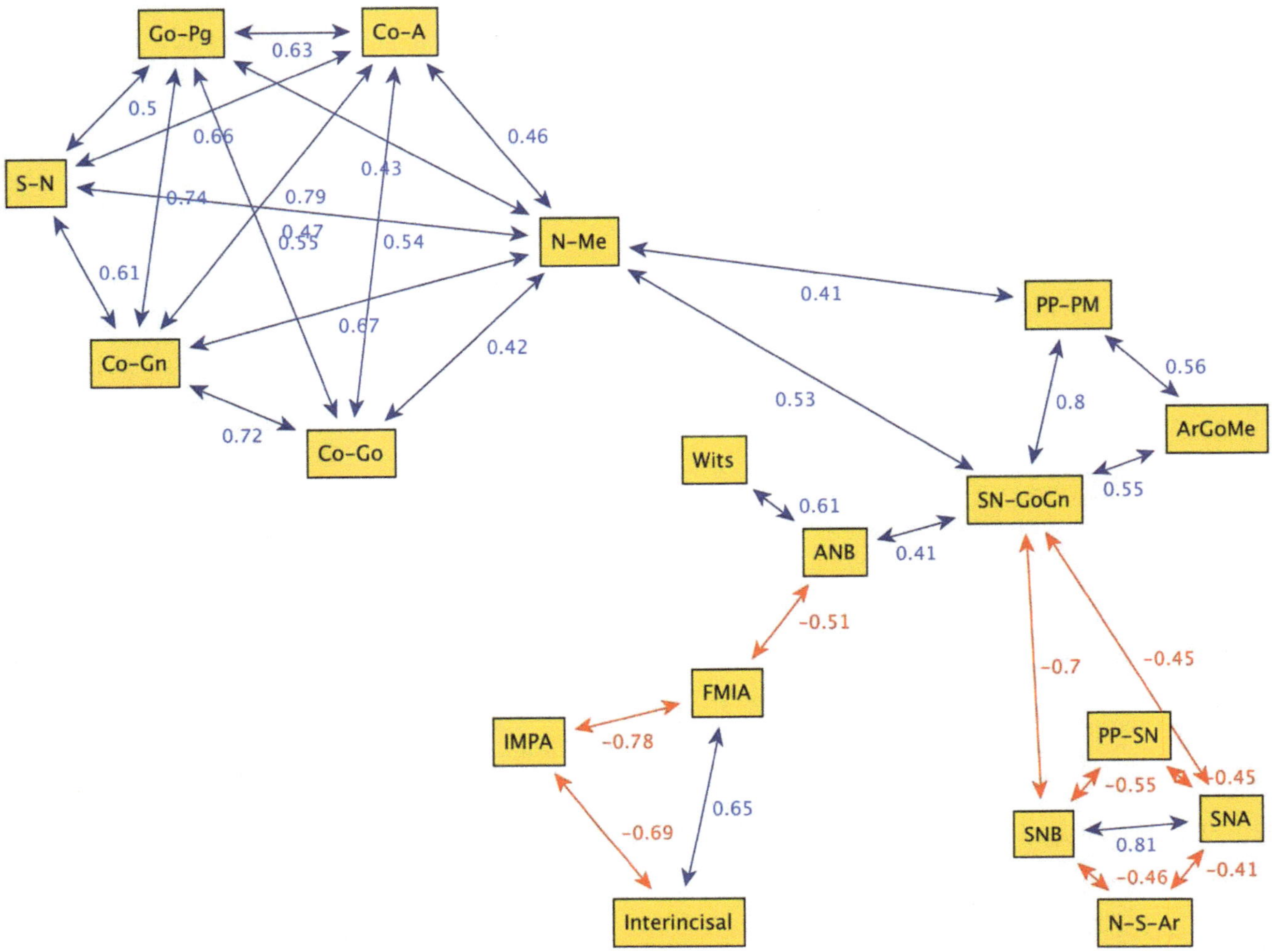

Figure 3. Graph obtained from the cephalometric data of 240 female Class III patients between 7 and 10 years of age (group G1). The highly connected nodes N-Me (anterior facial height) and SN-GoGn (divergence between the anterior cranial base and mandibular body) work as bridges, i.e. they connect separate sub-graphs. The graph highlights a division between the cephalometric parameters: linear (upper left nodes: Go-Pg, Co-A, S-N, Co-Gn, Co-Gn, N-Me), angular parameters (upper right: PP-PM, SN-Go-Gn, Ar-Go-Me) and adaptive dentoalveolar parameters (lower left: IMPA; FMIA, Interincisal).

individuate the possible emergence of features' subset driving the orofacial development of Class III malocclusion

Participants

This study analyzed the pretreatment lateral cephalometric records of 532 untreated Class III Caucasian female patients collected from the Department of Orthodontics of the University of Florence, Italy, and from the Graduate Orthodontic Program at the University of Michigan, Ann Arbor, Michigan. All these subjects was enrolled previously in large descriptive estimates of craniofacial growth in Class III malocclusion [14,23,26]. The age range was between 6 years 4 months to 17 years 3 months.

To be included in this study, the female patients had to satisfy all of the following inclusion criteria:

- Caucasian ancestry;
- no orthopedic/orthodontic treatment prior to cephalogram;
- diagnosis of Class III malocclusion based on anterior cross-bite, accentuated mesial step relationships of the primary second molars, permanent first molar relationship of at least one half cusp Class III;
- no congenitally missing or extracted teeth.

Description of Procedures or Investigations undertaken

The subjects were examined separately in four age groups: Group G1 (from 7 to 10 years) 240 subjects, Group G2 (from11 to 12 years) 89 subjects, Group G3 (from 13 to 14 years) 105 subjects, and Group G4 (from 15 to 17 years) 98 subjects.

The cephalometric analysis required the digitization of 21 landmarks on the tracing of each cephalogram (Fig. 2). The error of the method for the cephalometric measurements was evaluated by repeating the measures in 100 randomly selected cephalograms. Error was on average 0.6° for angular measures and 0.9 mm for linear measures.

Ethics

All data used in this study have been previously published as referenced in the methods section. Written informed consent was obtained from the patients' parents as part of their orthodontic

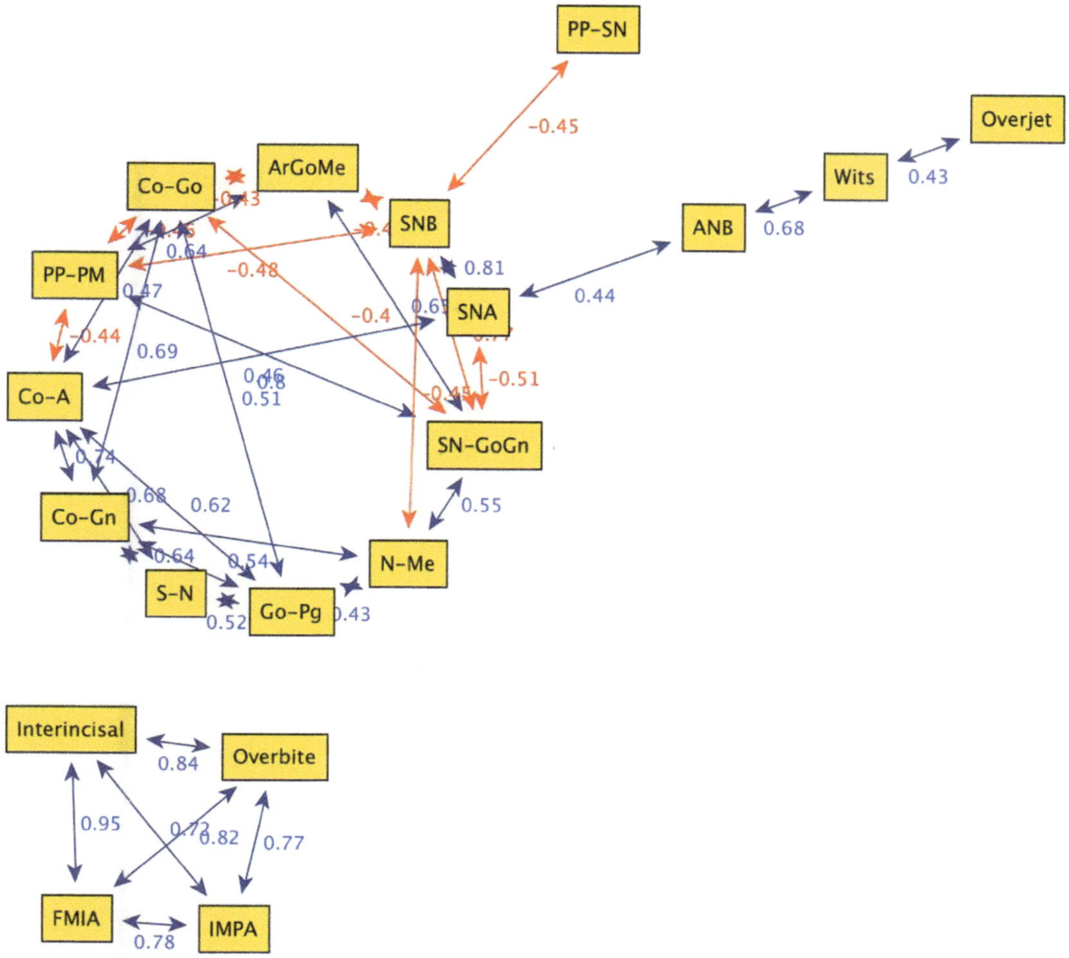

Figure 4. Graph obtained from cephalometric data of 90 female Class III patients between 11 years and 12 years of age (group G2). The graph is composed by two characterized groups: structural (upper group) and dentoalveolar adaptive (lower group of four nodes).

treatment. The approval of an Ethical Committee was not sought as all data analysed were collected as part of routine orthodontic pre-treatment diagnosis.

Statistical methods

We analize the correlation matrices among the 21 cephalographic landmarks considered by using complex netwoks. First we calculate (using KNIME [27]) for each pair of features their sample Pearson correlation coefficient $r_{xy} = (<xy>-<x><y>)/s_x s_y$, where x,y are the numerical values of the landmarks, $<...>$ indicates sample means and s_x, s_y are their sample standard deviations. Each r_{xy} can be considered as the weight of a link between x and y; the associated network therefore is a complete graph, *i.e.* a network where every node is connected to every other node. Such correlation graphs already have been considered in other applications of network theory, like finance and genomics [28,29]; in order to dig out the information present in the whole correlation matrix and sort out relevant features with their global correlations, some filtering has to be applied. Our choice is to use a cutoff to correlation values in order to consider only the most significant correlations [12]; therefore we consider two features (the nodes of our graphs) to be linked if $|r_{xy}|>0.40$. Notice that at difference with most previous studies in networks, we do not discard negative correlations: this is a critical point when analyzing any complex systems where important relations, as a negative feedback, naturally would show up as significantly high negative correlations.

Networks have been visualized using the software yEd [30] with the standard layout; the choice of filtering at $|r_{xy}|>0.40$ reduces the complexity of the system and permitted the identification of many characteristics just by visual inspection. In particular, it is very easy to identify *bridge nodes*, i.e. nodes whose absence would split the graphs in two or more separate parts. Bridge nodes are important both because they allow to detect separate subsystems (sets of highly correlated features) and because they represent the connection among such subsystems.

Furthermore, to investigate the presence of functional modules, we have searched for motifs in our filtered networks. Motifs searches are potentially valuable tools to predict unknown interactions involving 3–5 nodes (rarely more than 6). These organized sets of interactions are capable of higher order functions (such as amplification), and hence probably represent the functional capabilities within the network. They provide balance between modules through signaling gates (*i.e.* negative feed-forward motifs), favoring plasticity (open-gate configuration), or homeostasis (closed- gate configuration). We have focused on the presence of *clicques* (subsets where each of node is connected to every other node) as they naturally represent the presence of a

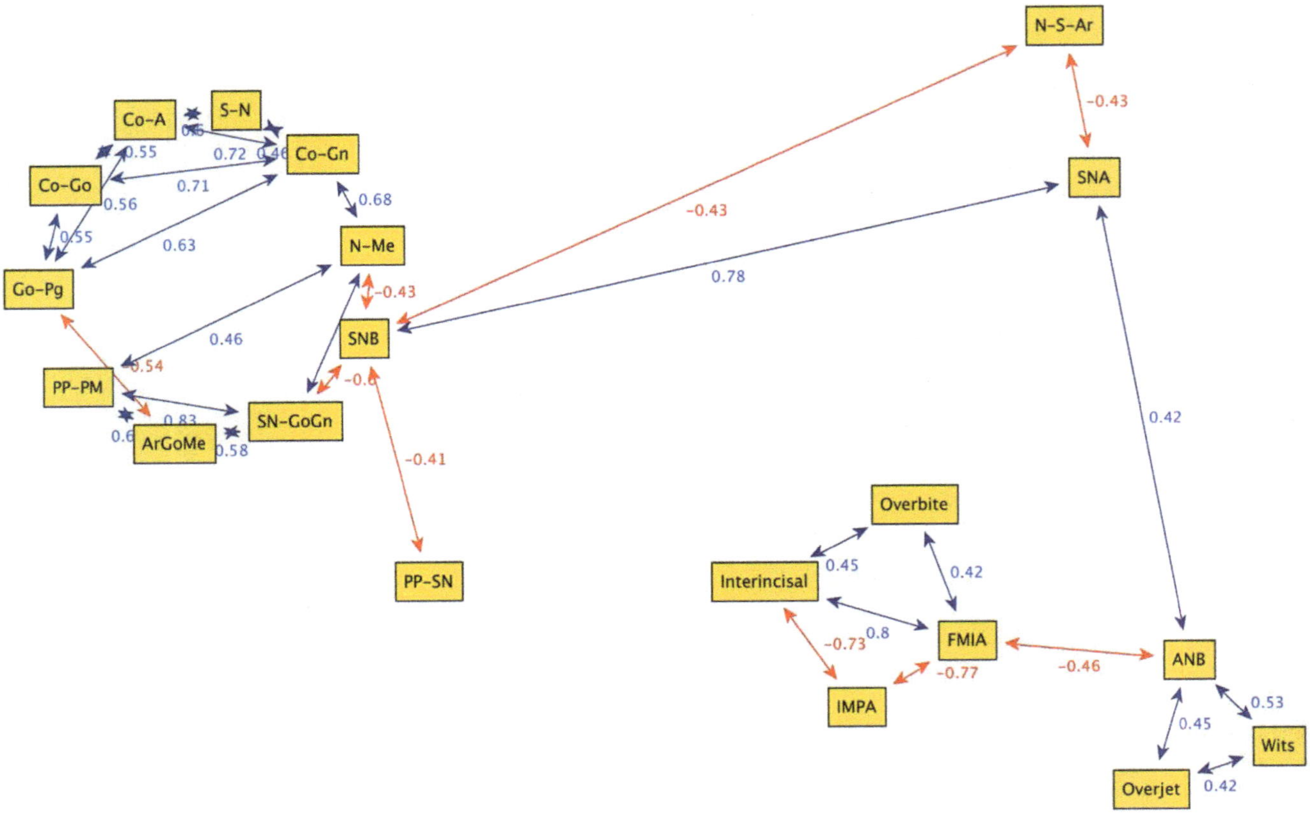

Figure 5. Graph obtained from cephalometric data of 105 female Class III patients between 13 and 14 years of age (group G3). The main bridge node is S-N-B (longitudinal position of the maxillary arch) divides the structural nodes from the ones representing dentoalveolar adaptive and mixed features.

subsystem acting as a whole: in fact, every feature in such a subsystem is interrelated. To individuate the presence of clicques, we have employed the Power Graphs plugin [31] in the software Cytoscape [32].

Results

Figures 3, 4, 5, 6 illustrate the correlation networks of the cephalometric characteristics of 532 Class III female patients, from 7 to 17 years of age. In all ages considered, the most-connected nodes are those related to vertical skeletal features (N-Me, SN-GoGn, PP-PM). These vertical parameters always are connected with those of mandibular sagittal nodes (SNB, GoPg). These strong patterns of interaction are observed for all ages considered. Due to the persistence of such network topology in all age groups, these highly connected nodes can be regarded as the key features in the growth of female Class III subjects.

Further results come from the Power Graph analysis of the networks. With the aim of defining the possible clinical relevance of these orthodontic network patterns, the patients were differentiated into two cephalometric categories using Wits appraisal of jaw disharmony, a simple method whereby the severity of degree of anteroposterior jaw displasia may be measured on a lateral cephalometric head film. The two class consist of "mild" and "severe" Class III patients (Wits appraisal greater than −3 mm and Wits appraisal smaller or equal to −3 mm, respectively) [19]. The visual network inspection of these "mild" and "severe" Class III patients (group G4) reveals several interesting characteristics:

1. the networks of the "mild" patients exhibits a balanced node pattern (Fig. 7a);
2. in the "severe" patients group, we find a preponderance of maxillomandibular divergence nodes (related to the vertical development of the craniofacial system) and mandibular sagittal nodes (related to the horizontal prominence of the chin), with poor balance of adaptive nodes (Fig. 7b).

Discussion

Instead of searching single or multiple dentoskeletal radiographic predictors variables, our work attempts to delineate the overall dentofacial organizing principles, the functional dynamics, and the regulatory growth principles of Class III malocclusion. The cephalometric data of a large retrospective cohort of 532 Class III female subjects, in mixed and permanent dentition, were analyzed through a combination of multivariate computational techniques: networks analysis of correlation matrices and search for regulatory motifs. These high-throughput techniques allow the extraction and identification of new biological insight from data regarding several related topics of importance during the Class III craniofacial growth such as robustness, adaptation, time progression, and structural stability.

Understanding structure-dynamics relationships in networks is a major goal of complex system research. In several biomedical fields, the analysis of interaction dynamics of the components may be useful to capture the essential behavior of the system, to understand higher-order biological function, and also to facilitate prediction responses [9,25].

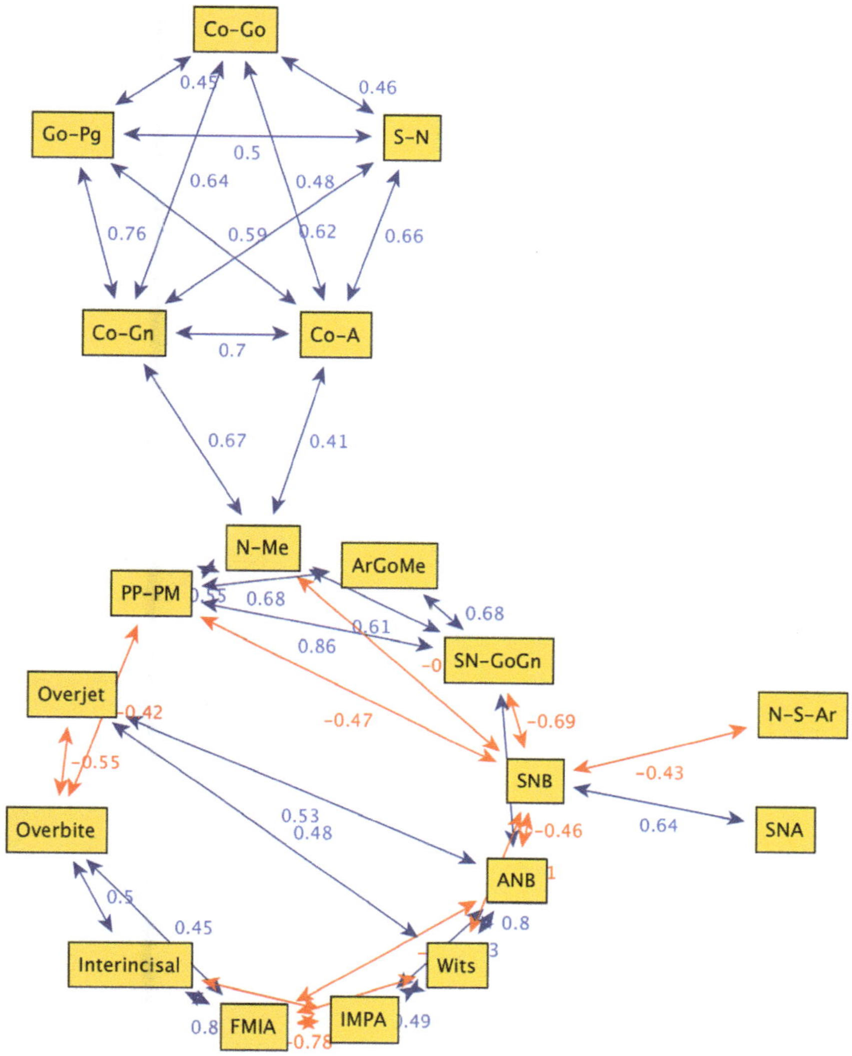

Figure 6. Graph obtained from cephalometric data of 99 female Class III patients between 15 and 17 years of age (group G4). The graph is divided into two groups clearly inter-connected via the bridge N-Me (anterior facial height).

General principles behind the relationships between orthodontic structure and dynamics still are lacking, in part due to the scarcity of sufficiently general formalism to study structure and dynamics within a common framework. When a complex system is investigated using network analysis, the network map often shows groups of nodes only weakly connected, alternating with groups of highly connected nodes. Many aspects of the inherent complexity of nature follow a pattern that is the same in many contexts (from biology to ecology, sociology, financial markets, etc.). Among the network of connections, very few nodes have many links ("*hubs*"), while the majority of the remainder are characterized by few or very few links. These hubs govern the entire system through preferential interactions, facilitating the movement of information, creating shortcuts between distant nodes, helping to create a robust network ("*small world networks*") that can adapt to environmental stresses [4,24].

A previous investigation illustrated the more compact network Class III malocclusion structure as regard to Class I and II when considering phenotypic, functional, and radiographic characteristics [12]. The results of the current study showed that, in the interrelationship of Class III skeletal elements, the "*driver nodes*" that presumably guide the growth of the orofacial system are located in the interplay between maxillomandibular divergence (PP-PM, NS-Go-Gn) and mandibular sagittal nodes (Go-Gn, Co-Gn). This structural organization, reflected in the network topology, probably constrains the range of dynamical behaviors available to the system during the generative process of the malocclusion. Our data confirm the observation of Bui et al. [21] regarding the generative process of Class III malocclusion observed in a retrospective cohort of 309 patients: the most important cephalometric variables reflect the anteroposterior and vertical imbalance during growth, rather than specific Class III craniofacial structures.

Malocclusions are isoforms of biological complexity. The network of functional and morphologic characteristics of the orofacial system causes diffuse connections of strict interdependence. Any therapeutic intervention applied to a part of the system, invariably has an impact on other structures. For example, the decision to open the bite by rotating the mandible clockwise must take into account the concomitant effects on the vertical dimension, on the convexity of face, and on the potential divergence of the occlusal plane [13,17].

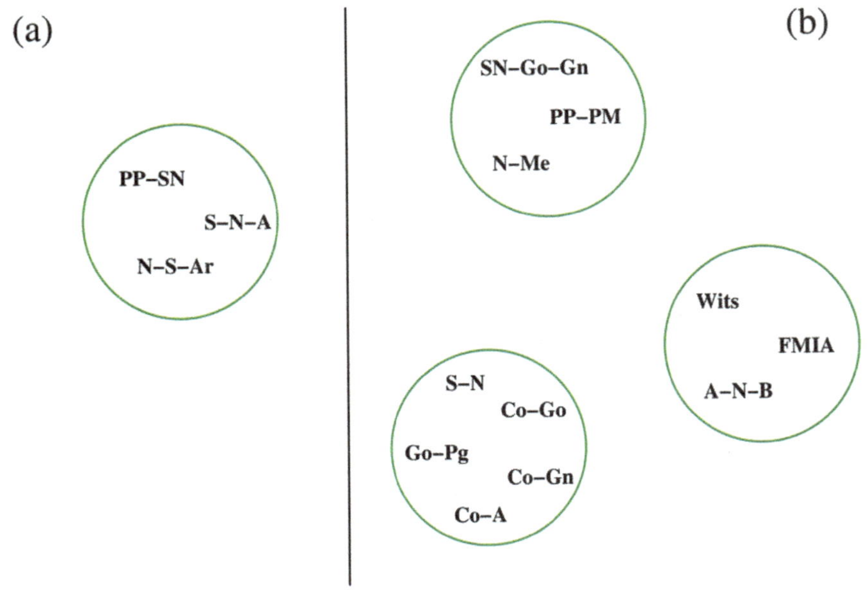

Figure 7. Cliques (motifs) individuated by the Power Graphs analysis for female patients (15–17 years) with mild Class III malocclusion (panel A) and with severe Class III malocclusion (panel B). Mild Class III patients show a single clique of only three structural nodes (SNA, N-S-Ar, PP-SN). Severe Class III patients show the presence of three separate cliques: mandibular sagittal nodes (S-N,...), maxillomandibular divergence nodes (N-Me,...) and adaptive nodes (Wits,..). The comparison between the two figures indicates that severe Class III patients are characterized by the presence of groups of strongly inter-correlated features, i.e. tend to act as a single whole system.

Once the pattern of a malocclusion has been identified, it becomes easier to analyze the force flow in the orofacial network, to define the local functional entities involved (in Graph theory, *motifs*) and localize signaling gates that provide among between modules, rather than taking solely into consideration the morphological characteristics of the system [8].

Table 1. The 21 cephalometric variables employed in our study.

SN	anteroposterior length of the cranial base
Wits	Wits appraisal
Co-A	midfacial length as distance from Co to A
Co-Gn	mandibular length as distance from Co to Gn
Ar-Go	mandibular ramus height
NS-GoGn	divergence of the mandibular plane relative to the anterior cranial base
NS-Ar	saddle angle
ArGoMe	gonial angle
SNA	anteroposterior maxillary position to the anterior cranial base
SNB	anterorposterior mandibular position to the anterior cranial base
IMPA	angle between the lower incisor with the mandibular plane
ANB	anteroposterior relation of the maxilla and the mandible
Interincisal	angle between the axis of the upper and the lower incisor
PP-SN	inclination of the palatal plane in relation to anterior cranial base
PP-PM	inclination of the palatal plane in relation to the mandible plane
NMe	anterior facial height
FMIA	angle between the axis of the lower incisor and the Frankfort plane
Overbite	Vertical distance between the incisal edges of the most protrusive maxillary and mandibular central incisors.
Overjet	Horizontal distance between the incisal edge of the most protrusive maxillary central incisors and the most facial aspect of the crown of the most protrusive mandibular central incisor
Go-Pg	distance between gonion and pogonion points
Co-Go	distance between condylion and gonion points

Most of the cephalometric variables are angles or distances derived from the cephalometric reference landmarks (Fig. 2).

The present study shows that during the growth process of Class III malocclusion the skeletal vertical and sagittal growth features (SN-GoGn, PP-PM) are central in the interacting network of the system components: these nodes can be considered the "driver nodes" for the growth of the orofacial system. The ability of the orofacial system to function as an integrate unit may arise from the balance of activities between the modules: this may be the core design principle revealed by orthodontic network analysis. Network analysis revealed that the patients with more unbalanced cephalometric features ("severe patients") present a network topology with a preponderance of the skeletal nodes and minor relevance of adaptive dentoalveolar nodes. In the "mild" patient group, the network topology showed a greater balance between skeletal and adaptive craniofacial features. In the patients with more pronounced radiographic Class III features, we have identified two subnetworks of strong functional interaction (cliques). As observed in several metabolic pathways, these subnetworks are recognized as critical elements of biological organization [7,8]; they work as feed-forward loops, with high capacity of anticipatory regulation as opposed to the homeostatis effects of feed-back loops. Such analysis confirms the importance of considering the co-occurrence of the interrelated morphologic features, reinforcing the hypothesis that these sites of co-occurrence of the overall interrelated morphologic features are more suitable to indicate the favorable or unfavorable progression of this type of disharmony respect to the individual orthodontic features. Presumably, the convergence of the orthodontic therapeutic approaches into these modules allows the clinician to maximize results and to shorten treatment times.

Computational technology has proved to be most useful in the handling of mass data (in the present case, a set of cephalometric measurements). As orthodontic studies shift from local description to system analysis, we need to identify the design principles of large craniofacial features networks. The limitations of viewing the head region in two dimensions only are well known. However, postnatal growth differences and the high incidence and magnitude of anteroposterior and vertical dentofacial abnormalities render this record useful for characterizing the overall morphology of the growing orofacial system.

The result of the present study indicate that, in their most basic abstraction level, the orofacial radiographic characteristics can be represented as networks using nodes to represent orthodontic characteristics, and edges to represent their various types of interactions. A substantial portion of the Class III issues during growth is driven by only a few nodes. By linking radiographic data and phenotypes to clinical characteristics in a causal or correlative manner, these observations may contribute to the construction of a model that provides a theoretical framework of the reciprocal interaction between organizing craniofacial pathways, growth, and malocclusion.

In conclusion, due to their generality, the application of network mathematical models could increase the interpretation of quantitative, patient-specific information and help to better targeting of therapy not only in orthodontics but also in other medical fields.

Acknowledgments

P. Auconi and M. Scazzocchio thank Matthias Reimann for help and support with the Power Graphs plugin.

Author Contributions

Conceived and designed the experiments: AS PA MS GC JAM LF. Performed the experiments: AS PA MS GC JAM LF. Analyzed the data: AS PA MS GC JAM LF. Contributed reagents/materials/analysis tools: AS PA MS GC JAM LF. Wrote the paper: AS PA MS GC JAM LF.

References

1. Albert R (2007) Network inference, analysis, and modelling in systems biology. The Plant Cell 19: 3327–3338.
2. Barabàsi A-L, Oltvai ZN (2004) Network biology: under standing the cell's functional organisation. Nat Rev Genet 5: 101–113.
3. Caldarelli G (2007) Scale-free networks. Complex webs in nature and technology. Oxford: Oxford Univ Press.
4. Newman MEJ (2006) Modularity and community structure in networks. Proc Natl Acad Sci USA 103: 8577–8582.
5. Barabasi A-L (2009) Scale-free networks: a decade and beyond. Science 325: 412–413.
6. Barrat A, Barthelemy M, Pastor-Satorras, Vespignani A (2004) The architecture of complex weighted networks. Proc Natl Acad Sci USA 101: 3747–3752.
7. Royer L, Reimann M, Andreopulos B, Schroeder M (2008) Unraveling protein networks with power graph analysis. PLoS Comput Biol 4: 1–8.
8. Ma'ayan A, Blitzer RD, Iyngegar R (2004) Toward predictive models of mammalian cells. Annu Rev Biophys Biomol Struct 34: 319–349.
9. Mesarovic MD, Sreenath SN, Keene JD (2004) Search for organising principles: understanding in system biology. Sys Biol 1: 19–27.
10. Janes KA, Yaffe MB (2006) Data-driven modelling of signal-transduction networks. Nat Mol Cell Biol 7: 820–828.
11. Kitano H (2002) Systems Biology: a brief overview. Science 295: 1662–1664
12. Auconi P,Caldarelli G, Scala A, Ierardo G, Polimeni A(2011) A network approach to orthodontic diagnosis. Orthod Craniofac Res 14: 189–197.
13. Staley RN (1995) Orthodontic diagnosis and treatment plan. In: Bishara SE Textbook of Orthodontics. Philadelphia: WB Saunders Co. pp. 98–113.
14. Baccetti T, Reyes BC, McNamara JA (2005) Gender differences in Class III malocclusion. Angle Orthod 75: 510–520.
15. Battagel JM (1994) The identification of Class III malocclusions by discriminand analysis. Eur J Orthod 16: 71–80.
16. Betzemberger D, Ruf S, Panchez H (1999) The compensatory mechanism in high angle malocclusions: a comparison of subjects in the mixed and permanent dentition. Angle Orthod. 69: 27–32.
17. Franchi L, Baccetti T, McNamara JA (1998) Cephalometric floating norms for north American adults. Angle Orthod 68: 497–502.
18. Solow B (1980) The dentoalveolar compensatory mechanism background and clinical implications. Br J Orthod 7: 145–151.
19. Stellzig-Eisenhauer A, Lux CJ, Schuster G (2002) Treatment decision in adult patients with Class III malocclusion: orthodontic therapy or orthognatic surgery? Am J Orthod Dentofacial Orthop 122: 27–38.
20. Freer T J (1973) Selection of predictor variables in assessing the severity of malocclusion. Am J Orthod 64: 155–161.
21. Bui C, King T, Proffit W, Frazier-Bowers S (2006) Phenotypic characterization of Class III patients. Angle orthod 76: 564–569.
22. Sanborn R T (1955) Differences between the facial skeletal pattern of Class III malocclusion and normal occlusion. Angle Orthod 24:208–219.
23. Reyes BC, Baccetti T, McNamara JA (2006) An estimate of craniofacial growth in Class II malocclusion. Angle orthod 76: 577–584.
24. Buchanan M, Caldarelli G (2010) A networked world. Phys. World 23: 22–23.
25. Zhu X, Gerstein M, Snyder M (2007) Getting connected: analysis and principles of biological networks. Gene Dev 21: 1010–1024.
26. Baccetti T, Reyes BC and McNamara JA Jr. (2007) Craniofacial changes in Class III malocclusion as related to skeletal and dental maturation. Am J Orthod Dentofacial Orthop. 132(2):171.e1–171.e12
27. Berthold M R, Cebron N, Dill F, Gabriel T R, Kotter T et al. (2007), "KNIME: The Konstanz Information Miner", in "Studies in Classification, Data Analysis, and Knowledge Organization", Springer ISBN = 978-3-540-78239-1, ISSN = 1431-8814 http://www.knime.org/ last accessed on 29 Aug 2012
28. Bonnanno G, Caldarelli G, Lillo F, and Mantegna R N (2003) Topology of correlation-based minimal spanning trees in real and model markets. Phys Rev E (68): 046103
29. Langfelder P, Horvath S (2008) WGCNA: an R package for weighted correlation network analysis, BMC Bioinformatics (9): 559. Published online 2008 December 29. doi: 10.1186/1471-2105-9-559
30. http://www.yworks.com/en/products_yed_about.html last accessed on 29 Aug 2012
31. http://wiki.cytoscape.org/CyOog last accessed on 29 Aug 2012
32. Smoot M, Ono K, Ruscheinski J, Wang PL, Ideker T (2011) Cytoscape 2.8: new features for data integration and network visualization. Bioinformatics (27): 431–432. Published online 2010 December 12.

5

Experimental Gingivitis Induces Systemic Inflammatory Markers in Young Healthy Individuals: A Single-Subject Interventional Study

Jörg Eberhard[1*], Karsten Grote[2], Maren Luchtefeld[2], Wieland Heuer[1], Harald Schuett[2], Dimitar Divchev[2], Ralph Scherer[3], Ruth Schmitz-Streit[5], Daniela Langfeldt[5], Nico Stumpp[1], Ingmar Staufenbiel[4], Bernhard Schieffer[2], Meike Stiesch[1]

1 Department of Prosthetic Dentistry and Biomaterials Science, Hannover Medical School, Hannover, Germany, **2** Department of Cardiology and Angiology, Hannover Medical School, Hannover, Germany, **3** Department of Medical Statistics, Hannover Medical School, Hannover, Germany, **4** Department of Operative Dentistry and Periodontology, Hannover Medical School, Hannover, Germany, **5** Institute for Microbiology, Christian-Albrechts-University Kiel, Kiel, Germany

Abstract

Objectives: We here investigated whether experimental gingivitis enhances systemic markers of inflammation which are also known as surrogate markers of atherosclerotic plaque development.

Background: Gingivitis is a low-level oral infection induced by bacterial deposits with a high prevalence within Western populations. A potential link between the more severe oral disease periodontitis and cardiovascular disease has already been shown.

Methods: 37 non-smoking young volunteers with no inflammatory disease or any cardiovascular risk factors participated in this single-subject interventional study with an intra-individual control. Intentionally experimental oral inflammation was induced by the interruption of oral hygiene for 21 days, followed by a 21-days resolving phase after reinitiation of oral hygiene. Primary outcome measures at baseline, day 21 and 42 were concentrations of hsCRP, IL-6, and MCP-1, as well as adhesion capacity and oxLDL uptake of isolated blood monocytes.

Results: The partial cessation of oral hygiene procedures was followed by the significant increase of gingival bleeding (34.0%, $P<0.0001$). This local inflammation was associated with a systemic increase in hsCRP (0.24 mg/L, $P=0.038$), IL-6 (12.52 ng/L, $P=0.0002$) and MCP-1 (9.10 ng/l, $P=0.124$) in peripheral blood samples between baseline and day 21, which decreased at day 42. Monocytes showed an enhanced adherence to endothelial cells and increased foam cell formation after oxLDL uptake ($P<0.050$) at day 21 of gingivitis.

Conclusions: Bacterial-induced gingival low-level inflammation induced a systemic increase in inflammatory markers. Dental hygiene almost completely reversed this experimental inflammatory process, suggesting that appropriate dental prophylaxis may also limit systemic markers of inflammation in subjects with natural gingivitis. International Clinical Trials Register Platform of the World Health Organization, registry number: DRKS00003366, URL: http://apps.who.int/trialsearch/Default.aspx.

Editor: Hugo ten Cate, Maastricht University Medical Center, The Netherlands

Funding: This study was in part supported by the Deutsche Forschungsgemeinschaft DFG, Bonn, Germany (Eb 223/5-1). The authors acknowledge funding of the publication costs by the Deutsche Forschungsgemeinschaft. The funders had no role in study design, data collection and analysis, decision to publish, or preparation of the manuscript.

Competing Interests: The authors have declared that no competing interests exist.

* E-mail: eberhard.joerg@mh-hannover.de

These authors contributed equally to this work.

Introduction

Gingivitis and periodontitis are two distinct chronic inflammatory processes belonging to the spectrum of periodontal diseases of the oral cavity affecting the tooth supporting tissues in response to bacterial accumulation. In contrast to periodontitis, gingivitis is initiated only after a few days of inadequate oral hygiene procedures by local plaque deposits adjacent to the highly vascularised gingival tissues. Gingivitis is a superficial inflammatory affection and is not destructive towards the surrounding connective and bone tissues and completely declines with the initiation of adequate oral hygiene procedures. In gingivitis bleeding of the gums may occur even after gentle mechanical stimulation in severe cases or following tooth brushing and chewing [1]. In contrast, in susceptible subjects periodontitis is characterized by the irreversible loss of bone and periodontal ligament that is if untreated followed by tooth loss [2]. In addition to various epidemiological studies demonstrating a potential link between periodontitis and cardiovascular diseases [3] it has been demonstrated that the treatment of patients suffering from periodontitis reduces acute parameters of atherosclerosis and improves endothelial function [4,5]. Equivalent data are not available for gingivitis, although the prevalence of moderate to severe periodontitis in western populations is 3% to 46% whereas gingivitis affects almost all individuals [6,7,8].

Inflammatory processes play a pivotal role in the pathogenesis of atherosclerosis and mediate the development of the disease, from initial leukocyte recruitment to sudden plaque rupture and subsequent myocardial infarction with often fatal outcome [9,10]. Several systemic inflammatory markers have been identified as independent risk factors for cardiovascular diseases. The ability to measure levels of these inflammatory markers in the systemic circulation has provoked interest in their development as biomarkers or surrogate markers for potential use in risk assessment [11,12]. In this regard, the acute phase reactant C-reactive protein (CRP) is a potential predictor of future atherosclerotic vascular disease, whereas cytokines and chemokines such as interleukin (IL)-6 or monocyte chemoattractant protein-1 (MCP-1, also known as CCL2) are established mediators of the chronic inflammatory process within the vascular wall in various experimental models (6–9). Activation of blood monocytes represents an early and crucial event in the development of atherosclerosis. Activated monocytes are prone to adhere more likely at inflamed sites of the endothelium to invade the arterial wall. Subsequently, they differentiate into foam cells in order to initiate atherosclerotic plaque growth. In this regard, chronic systemic inflammation has been shown to be linked to adverse cardiovascular outcomes [10]. Systemic or local infection may provide an additional inflammatory stimulus that could accelerate atherogenesis. However, the pathophysiological pathways between chronic extravascular infections and atherosclerosis remain unclear [3].

Although gingivitis is a highly prevalent chronic bacterial disease in susceptible children, adults and the elderly, persisting for decades in subjects, and is an essential precursor of periodontitis limited data are available today addressing detrimental systemic effects of gingivitis. Systemic effects of experimental or natural gingivitis have been rarely investigated and the existing studies did not show correlations between gingivitis and systemic levels of pro-inflammatory mediators or surrogate markers of atherosclerosis [13]. Recently, studies using broad-range frequency techniques using 454 pyrosequencing of 16S rRNA genes identified bacteria associated with gingivitis in atherosclerotic plaques and potentially highlight a mechanism by which low-level gingival inflammation may also affect cardiovascular diseases [14].

We now report the results of an intervention study using a single-subject design with an intra-individual control. Experimentally induced gingivitis in young, healthy volunteers was initiated by termination of oral hygiene and resolved after restart of oral hygiene to determine the effects and causal association of this highly prevalent chronic inflammatory oral disease on circulating inflammatory markers which in some studies have been suggested as surrogate markers of atherosclerotic plaque development.

Methods

Study Design

Over a period of 42 days, it was our goal to evaluate the effects of oral hygiene cessation and restart on surrogate markers of atherosclerotic plaque development and activation of blood monocytes in young healthy individuals (Fig. 1). Oral hygiene cessation was selected as the intervention for the present study because of the high reproducibility of the following inflammatory responses in the gingival tissues. This model was introduced by Löe et al. as the "Experimental Gingivitis Model" in 1965 [15]. The primary outcome was the in-group differences between baseline and day 21 in clinical, laboratory and experimental parameters of inflammation during the study. Participants were selected according to the following inclusion criteria: (1) 20–30 years of age, (2) non-smokers, (3) no clinical signs of gingival inflammation (redness, swelling, bleeding) at ≥90% sites observed, (4) no probing pocket depth >3 mm at any site and (5) no alveolar bone loss. Exclusion criteria were: (1) presence of systemic diseases (e.g., diabetes mellitus or cardiovascular, kidney, liver or lung disease) (2) pregnancy or breastfeeding, (3) history of drug abuse, (4) allergic diathesis, (5) medications, in particular currently ingestion of non-steroidal or steroidal anti-inflammatory drugs, analgesic or antibiotics within 3 months before entering the study, (6) untreated carious lesions and/or insufficient restorations, implants, crowns at teeth in the maxillary right quadrant and (7) mouth breathing. All participants gave written informed consent. The study was performed in accordance with the Helsinki Declaration, approved by the ethical Committee of Hannover Medical School and registered at the International Clinical Trials Register Platform of the World Health Organization (http://apps.who.int/trialsearch/Default.aspx, ID: DRKS00003366).

Volunteers, which were addressed by public announcement in the Hannover area, who met the inclusion criteria were scheduled for a dental and periodontal screening appointment and full medical and dental histories were collected. All participants had a college degree. After inclusion in the study, all participants received a professional scaling and polishing of all tooth surfaces to remove supra- and subgingival plaque, stain and calculus 14 days prior to the start of the experimental gingivitis phase. The intervention was initiated at baseline when all participants refrained from any oral hygiene at seven upper teeth of the right maxilla. This model of limited inflammation has been described previously and was used as a model for an inflammatory status in the oral cavity that may represent a inflammatory condition affecting the majority of cases in the general population [16]. The subjects were clinically examined and 20 ml peripheral venous blood was sampled at baseline as well as on day 21 (experimental gingivitis) and at the follow-up appointment 21 days after termination and 42 days after initiation of the experimental gingivitis phase. Professional tooth cleaning and topical fluoride application was applied at day 21 of the experimental gingivitis phase (Fig. 1). Hereby at day 21 the intervention was terminated and during the following 21 days rigorous oral hygiene procedures were applied in order that the subjects served as their own control.

Periodontal Clinical Examination

Periodontal data were recorded by three experienced and calibrated dentists at baseline and day 21. The data included the presence or absence of supragingival dental plaque using a modification of the Silness-Löe plaque index (PI) at the buccal and oral sites of the selected teeth and the observable inflammatory changes of the gingival tissues by the gingival index (GI) at four sites per tooth [17,18]. The volume of the gingival crevicular fluid (GCF) was determined after gentle drying of the tooth for ten seconds followed by insertion of a filter paper strip (Periopaper, Pro Flow Incorporated) for 30 seconds into the gingival sulcus at four sites of the upper right first premolar. The GCF was measured with a calibrated Periotron 6000 gingival fluid meter (Pro Flow Incorporated) and expressed in Periotron units (PU). Gingival bleeding on probing was also recorded (BOP) with a

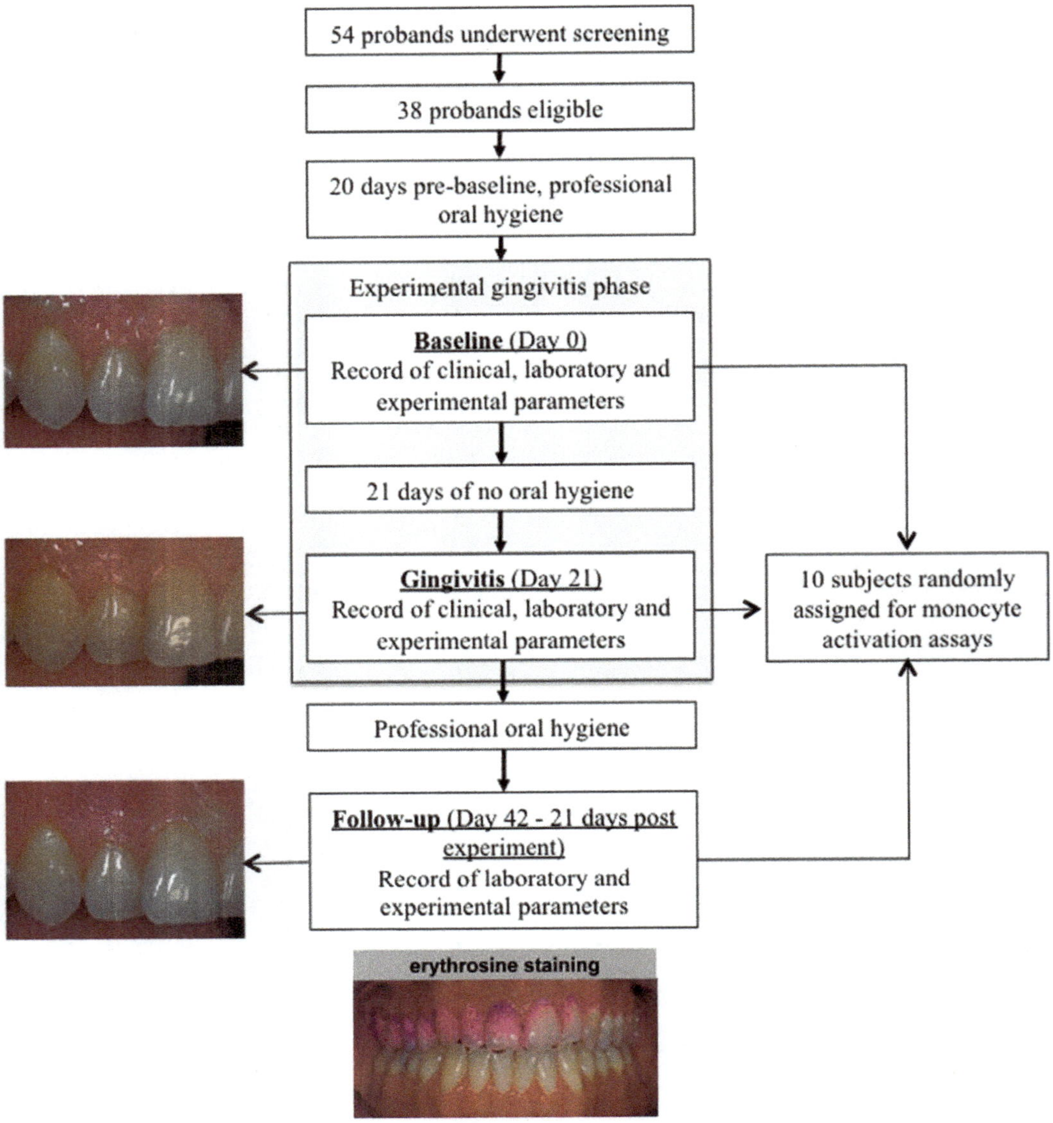

Figure 1. Flowchart of the study design from screening to follow-up. After a baseline visit, eligible volunteers were scheduled for intensive professional tooth cleaning and oral hygiene instructions to remove all biofilm deposits before starting the experimental gingivitis phase. After 21-days of cessation from any oral hygiene procedures in the upper right maxilla massive bacterial biofilms has been formed on the selected tooth hard substances, which are visible to the naked eye as yellowish plaques. Plaque covering of the tooth was routinely documented after erythrosine staining. The professional removal of all bacterial deposits and the restart of oral homecare terminated the experimental gingivitis phase. At baseline, day 21 (gingivitis) and 21 days after completion of the experimental gingivitis phase (follow-up) blood samples were obtained for serum parameters and monocyte activation assays.

pressure-calibrated probe (TPS probe, Vivacare) at four sites of all selected tooth sites: mesio-buccal, disto-buccal, mesio-oral and disto-oral. All measurements were recorded at four identical sites per tooth. The averaged scores for supragingival plaque and gingival inflammation (the sum of indexed scores divided by the total number of recorded sites), the amount of gingival crevicular fluid (the sum of the Periotron units per tooth divided by the number of sites) and the score for gingival bleeding on probing (the number of sites with gingival bleeding divided by the total number of sites, multiplied by 100) were calculated for each subject.

Species-specific Detection of Bacteria in Plaque Samples

Supragingival plaque was collected with sterile paper strips (VDW) at day 21 from all participants at the upper teeth of the right maxilla. Total genomic DNA was isolated using the QIAamp DNA Mini kit (Qiagen) according to the manufacturer's protocol for Gram-positive bacteria, but including a mechanical disruption step with a Precellys 24 bead mill (Bertin Technologies) prior to the first step of the protocol. Total genomic DNA was used as template for PCR-based detection of ten representative bacterial species commonly found in supragingival plaque samples belonging to different complexes according to Socransky et al. and Haffajee et al. [19,20]. The 'red complex', comprising of *Porphyromonas gingivalis*, *Tannerella forsythia*, and *Treponema denticola*, has been identified as the 'disease-related' complex. For supragingival plaque it has been shown that members of the red and orange complexes (e.g. *Fusobacterium nucleatum*) were most frequently associated with inflamed sites [19]. In the remaining clusters (purple, green and yellow) were moderately pathogenic species, including initial and early colonizers. The species-specific primers for the selected microorganisms are listed in table 1. All PCR reactions were performed on a TProfessional thermocycler (Biometra) in a total reaction volume of 20 µl. The reaction mix contained 2 µl of genomic DNA as template, 200 nM of each specific primer, 1x PCR buffer (including 1.5 mM magnesium chloride; Qiagen), 1.5 U HotStar Taq polymerase (Qiagen), 200 mM of each dNTP (Roth) and PCR-grade water (Roche). The thermal cycling protocol for each primer set was as follows: Initial denaturation at 95°C for 15 min; 40 amplification cycles consisting of denaturation at 94°C for 30 s, annealing at 55°–68°C for 45 s, elongation at 72°C for 1 min; final extension at 72°C for 10 min. 5 µl of each amplification reaction were analyzed by 1% agarose gel electrophoresis. A clear single band of expected size (table 1) was evaluated as positive detection signal and respective PCR products were subsequently sequenced.

Cardiovascular and Laboratory Assessment

Carotid intima-media thickness (IMT) was assessed at baseline and at day 42 by B-mode duplex sonography using a 10.5-MHz linear transducer. IMT was measured at the common carotid artery approximately 10 mm proximal to the bifurcation. The mean values from both sides are reported. Non-invasive blood pressure measurement was performed at baseline and at day 42 in seated position by Riva-Rocci/Korotkow's method. A standard 2D-Doppler transthoracic echocardiogram was performed at baseline and at day 21. Left ventricular function was assessed qualitatively. Valvular status was quantified by color and continuous-wave Doppler flow.

Serum and plasma samples were obtained at baseline, day 21 of the experimental gingivitis phase and at the follow-up re-evaluation at day 42. All samples were collected between 7.45 and 8.30 a.m. after a period of at least eight hours of fasting. Blood counts and measurements of lipid levels were done by standard laboratory testing. Serum concentrations of hsCRP were determined by immunonephelometry (detection limit 0.23 mg/L, Cardiophase hsCRP, Siemens). Serum levels of IL-6 (detection limit 0.70 pg/mL) and MCP-1 (detection limit 5.0 pg/mL) were measured by enzyme-linked immunosorbent assay (Quantikine HS, R&D Systems) with the help of a plate reader (µQuant; Bio-Tek Instruments).

Cell Culture

Human endothelial cells (human umbilical vein endothelial cells = HUVECs) were obtained from Lonza. Cells were cultured in endothelial cell growth medium (EGM-2; Lonza) supplemented with 2% FCS and growth factors and cultured on gelatin coated cell culture plates. Cells between passage 2 and 4 were used for experiments. Human leukocytes were isolated from the blood of the subjects. Erythrocytes were removed by hemolysis (155 mM NH_4Cl, 10 mM $KHCO_3$, 0.01% ethylenediaminetetraacetic acid; for 10 min) and cells were resuspended in X-vivo 15 medium (Lonza). Monocytic cells were enriched by plastic adherence over night, non-adherent cells were removed.

Table 1. Species-specific primers used to identify ten different bacterial species in plaque samples of experimental gingivitis at day 21 of the study.

Bacterial species	Primer	Annealing temperature	Expected amplicon size (bp)	Reference
Prevotella intermedia	F: 5′-CGTGGACCAAAGATTCATCGGTGGA-3′	64°C	259	[40]
	R: 5′-CCGCTTTACTCCCCAACAAA-3′			
Fusobacterium nucleatum	F: 5′-AGAGTTTGATCCTGGCTCAG-3′	60°C	360	[41]
	R: 5′-GTCATCGTGCACACAGAATTGCTG-3′			
Streptococcus oralis	F: 5′-TCCCGGTCAGCAAACTCCAGCC-3′	66°C	374	[42]
	R: 5′-GCAACCTTTGGATTTGCAAC-3′			
Streptococcus sanguinis	F: 5′-GGATAGTGGCTCAGGGCAGCCAGTT-3′	70°C	313	[42]
	R: 5′-GAACAGTTGCTGGACTTGCTTGTC-3′			
Capnocytophaga sputigena	F: 5′-AGAGTTTGATCCTGGCTCAG-3′	55°C	185	[43]
	R: 5′-GATGCCGCTCCTATATACCATTAGG-3′			
Eikenella corrodens	F: 5′-CTAATACCGCATACGTCCTAAG-3′	60°C	688	[44]
	R: 5′-CTACTAAGCAATCAAGTTGCCC-3′			
Tannerella forsythia	F: 5′-GCGTATGTAACCTGCCCGCA-3′	60°C	641	[44]
	R: 5′-TGCTTCAGTGTCAGTTATACCT-3′			
Porphyromonas gingivalis	F: 5′-AGGCAGCTTGCCATACTGCG-3′	60°C	404	[44]
	R: 5′-ACTGTTAGCAACTACCGATGT-3′			
Treponema denticola	F: 5′-TAATACCGAATGTGCTCATTTACAT-3′	60°C	316	[44]
	R: 5′-TCAAAGAAGCATTCCCTCTTCTTCTTA-3′			
Veillonella parvula	F: 5′-GAAGCATTGGAAGCGAAAGTTTCG-3′	57°C	623	[45]
	R: 5′-GTGTAACAAGGGAGTACGGACC-3′			
Aggregatibacter actinomycetemcomitans	F: 5′-TAGCCCTGGTGCCCGAAGC-3′	68°C	557	[46]
	R: 5′-CATCGCTGGTTGGTTACCCTCTG-3′			

Cell Adhesion

50,000 monocytes/well were seeded on a confluent monolayer of HUVECs in a 96-well plate in EGM-2 medium (Lonza). Adhesion was carried out for two hours at 37°C and 5% CO_2. Non-adherent cells were removed by 2 washing steps with PBS. Adherent cells were visualized per well in triplicates using a cell culture microscope (CKX31; Olympus) and captured with a digital camera (C-5060; Olympus). Adherent monocytes on a monolayer of endothelial cells were quantified using computer-assisted image analysis software (ImageJ 1.43 h, NIH).

Foam Cell Formation

50,000 monocytes/well were seeded in a 96-well plate in X-vivo 15 medium (Lonza) and monocyte-derived macrophages were obtained by plastic adherence for 4 days. Macrophages were stimulated for 4 hours with oxLDL (10 µg/ml). After treatment, cells were washed twice with PBS, fixed with formalin and dehydrated with 2-propandiol. Cellular lipids were stained with oil red O (Sigma) for 30 minutes. Oil red O-stained cells were visualized in three randomly chosen microscopic fields per well using a cell culture microscope (CKX31; Olympus) and captured with a digital camera (C-5060; Olympus). Percentage of Oil red O-positive cells was quantified using computer-assisted image analysis software (ImageJ 1.43 h, NIH).

Statistical Analysis

The statistical analysis was conducted with the statistical programming language R for the hypothesis testing and for the construction of graphs. The local two-sided Type-I-errors were set to 5% resulting in an explorative data analysis. In all comparisons of baseline values against gingivitis status and gingivitis status against follow-up, two-sided Wilcoxon signed-rank tests for paired samples were used. The exact *P*-values and exact confidence intervals were calculated for the monocytes adhesion assays and foam cell formations. Due to the exploratory character of the study all *P*-values were not adjusted for multiplicity. Results are presented as median differences with two-sided 95% confidence intervals as well as corresponding two-sided *P*-values. Post-hoc power calculations were based on the two-sample t test for paired data using a two-sided significance level of 0.05. The estimators for the mean differences and standard deviations were calculated from the present data.

Results

Subjects Characteristics

52 individuals were screened at the Hannover Medical School of Dentistry; of those 38 met the inclusion criteria and 37 subjects completed the clinical trial (Fig. 1). First subject in was 1st March 2010, last subject out was 28 July 2010. One volunteer showed clinical signs of congenital heart valve insufficiency and was withdrawn from the study. 37 non-smoking young and healthy volunteers (mean age 23.35±3.64 years) were enrolled in this study free of any traditional risk factor or inflammatory disease. The baseline characteristics of the subjects are presented in table 2.

As safety parameter and as marker of pre-existing atherosclerosis, the intima-media thickness of the left and right common carotid artery was determined. At baseline and after 42 days no differences were found (baseline: 0.55±0.16 mm, 21 days: 0.54±0.18 mm, $P=0.160$). Neither blood pressure nor serum cholesterol fraction showed significant differences when baseline was compared to day 21. Moreover, echocardiographical assessment of left ventricular function and valvular status was performed at baseline and at day 21 and showed no differences within the individuals.

Markers of Experimental Gingivitis

All volunteers developed experimental gingivitis as determined by all recorded parameters. The cessation of oral hygiene for 21 days in the upper right maxilla was followed by the accumulation of bacterial deposits on the tooth surfaces adjacent to the gingival tissues surrounding the teeth (absolute difference 2.04 PI, 95% CI, 1.91 to 2.17; $P<0.0001$) and is depicted in Figure 2A. This plaque formation was followed by the induction of inflammatory changes of the gingival tissues that became obvious by redness and swelling of the marginal gingiva categorized by the Gingival Index (absolute difference -1.29 GI, 95% CI, 1.11 to 1.40; $P<0.0001$, Fig. 2B). The accumulating inflammatory processes in the marginal gingival tissues between baseline and day 21 were associated with an increased volume of the gingival sulcus fluid (absolute difference 33.20 PU, 95% CI, 25.13 to 40.12; $P<0.0001$, Fig. 2C) and increased frequencies of bleeding on probing (absolute difference 34.00%, 95% CI, 28.00 to 39.00%; $P<0.0001$, Fig 2D).

Verification of Bacterial Plaque Composition

Aiming to identify ten bacterial species belonging to different clusters introduced by Haffajee et al. [19] and commonly found in sub- or supragingival plaque a species-specific PCR amplification was performed. We identified bacteria belonging to the red-complex in low detection frequencies within the study population of 37 subjects, *Porphyromonas gingivalis* (0.0%), *Tanerella forsythus* (13.5%) and *Treponema pallidum* (0.0%). Whereas *Fusobacterium nucleatum* (orange complex) was detected in every plaque sample from all test persons (100.0%). *Veilonella parvula* (purple complex) was observed in 97.3%, *C. sputigena* (green complex) in 94.1%, *E. corrodens* (green complex) in 88.6% and *S. sanguinis* (yellow complex) in 65.7% of all samples (Fig. 3). In summary, we could detect seven from ten representative bacterial species commonly found in plaque samples in high frequency across the whole group of participants. Whereas species from the red-complex associated with periodontitis, were absent or in low frequency.

Surrogate Markers of Atherosclerosis

Analysis of plasma samples revealed enhanced levels of circulating markers of inflammation when experimental gingivitis was induced. First of all, hsCRP mean difference was found to be significantly elevated under experimental gingivitis conditions 0.24 mg/L, 95% CI 0.01 to 1.20; $P=0.038$ (Fig. 4A). At follow-up, hsCRP levels tended to decline but were still slightly enhanced (median difference −0.02 mg/lL, 95% CI 0.28 to 0.71; $P=0.927$. Likewise, we observed enhanced circulating levels of the inflammatory mediators for IL-6 (Median difference 12.52 ng/l, 95% CI 1.25 to 43.85; $P=0.0002$) and MCP-1 (Median difference 9.10 ng/l, 95% CI −3.70 to 28.65; $P=0.124$) (Fig. 4B and C) between baseline and gingivitis, which both returned to baseline levels at the follow-up appointment (Median difference for IL-6 −12.51 ng/l, 95% CI −44.65 to −1.36; $P=0.001$ and median difference for MCP-1 −12.10 ng/l, 95% CI −27.00 to 0.50; $P=0.057$). Compared to baseline blood leukocyte and monocyte cell counts were increased upon experimental gingivitis (median differences 0.45×10^9/L, 95% CI −0.049 to 0.949, $P=0.0001$, respectively 0.010×10^9/L, 95% CI 0.099 to 0.150, $P=0.068$) and did not yet decline back to baseline levels at follow-up (mean differences for leukocytes 0.15×10^9/L, 95% CI −0.499 to 0.700,

Table 2. Baseline characteristics of the patients.

Characteristic	Study Group	Reference intervals*
	(N = 37)	(Male/Female)
Age - yr	23.4±3.6	
Male/Female sex - no. (%)	6/31 (16.2/83.8)	
Smoking status - no. (%)		
Never smoked	31 (83.8)	
Former Smoker¶	6 (16.2)	
Current smoker	0 (0)	
Family history of cardiovascular disease - no. (%)	3 (8.1)	
Race or ethnic group - no. (%)§		
White	31 (83.8)	
Asian	6 (16.2)	
Black	0 (0)	
Body-mass index§§	22.9±4.5	18.5–24.9
Blood pressure - mm Hg		
Systolic	124.0±12.0	<140
Diastolic	81.0±8.8	<90
Cholesterol fractions Male/Female (SD) - mmol/l		
S-cholesterol	5.9±1.8/6.2±2.1	3.3–6.2/3.3–6.2
S-HDL-cholesterol	1.8±0.3/2.4±0.8	>1.0/>1.2
S-LDL-cholesterol	4.0±1.4/4.0±1.4	1.8–4.5/1.7–4.2
Haemogram		
haemoglobin - g/dl	13.2±1.4	12.0–17.5
erythrocyte count - $\times 10^{12}$/liter	4.6±0.5	4.0–5.9
thrombocyte count - $\times 10^{9}$/liter	261.5±55.9	150.0–450.0
neutrophile count - $\times 10^{9}$/liter	5.8±0.8	1.1–8.8
eosinophile count - $\times 10^{9}$/liter	0.2±0.1	<0.5
basophile count - $\times 10^{9}$/liter	0.5±0.3	0.0–1.0
haematocrit - %	41.3±3.2	36.0–50.4

¶Smoking was terminated at least 12 months prior to the start of the study.
§Race was self-reported.
§§Body-mass index is defined as the weight in kilograms divided by the square of the hight in meters.
*All parameters fall within the reference intervals or are designated as "normal".

$P = 0.404$, and for monocytes 0.000×10^9/L, 95% CI −0.049 to 0.100, $P = 0.591$ (Fig. 4D, E).

Monycyte Activation Assays

Monocytes were isolated from the blood of ten randomly assigned study participants and subsequently subjected to ex vivo cell culture assays verifying monocyte activation. Of note, experimentally induced gingivitis led to significantly enhanced adherence of monocytes on endothelial cells (Fig. 5A) as well as to augmented oxLDL-uptake and foam cell formation (Fig. 5B). Both processes returned to baseline levels at day 42. Of note, monocyte activation is known to be crucially involved in the development of atherosclerosis and thereby fundamental to the etiology of coronary artery disease.

A post-hoc power analysis using observed mean differences and SDs demonstrated that this study had more than 80% power to detect differences between baseline and gingivitis for all parameters, except for MCP-1 (11% power), hsCRP (62% power) and Leucocyte counts (55% power).

Discussion

The present interventional study showed that even in healthy young individuals, experimentally induced gingivitis as low-level extravascular oral bacterial infection lead to an acute systemic inflammation with enhanced systemic levels of CRP, IL-6, MCP-1 and activated monocytes known as markers and mediators of vascular atherosclerotic disease. This inflammatory process seems to be almost completely reversible by appropriate dental hygiene.

Gingivitis is a chronic local infection affecting the tooth surrounding tissues, caused by bacteria of the dental plaque (e.g. *Streptococcus oralis*, *Veilonella ssp.* etc.) and is accompanied by a local inflammatory response of the host. The oral inflammatory response is, in contrast to periodontitis, limited to the soft gingival tissues not affecting the bone. Moreover, gingivitis differs from periodontitis with respect to its microbial composition and inflammatory responses [21]. In consequence, it was not expected at the beginning of the study to observe systemic effects from gingivitis, although they have already been shown for periodontitis [5]. Recently, Wahaidi et al. [13] was not able to show an

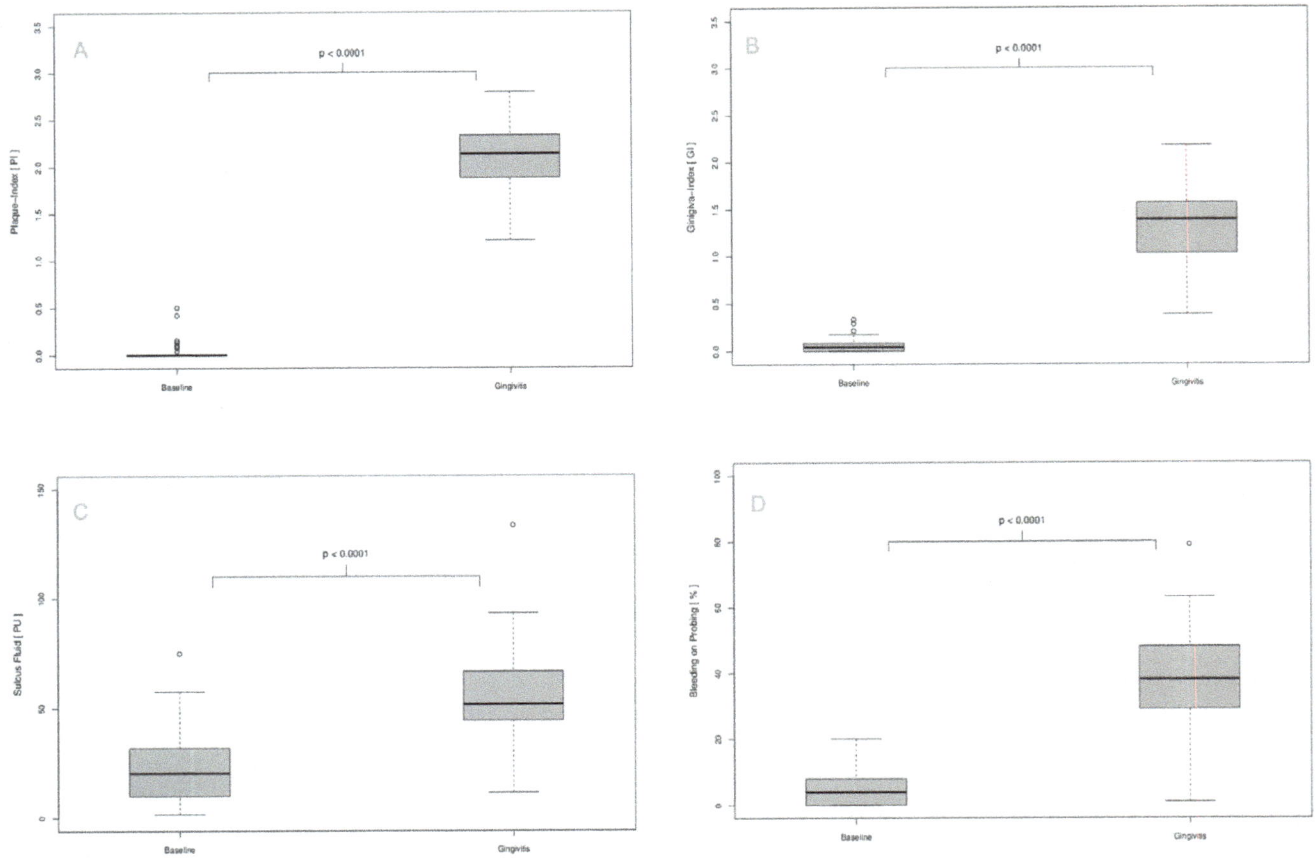

Figure 2. Characterization of oral clinical parameters at baseline and after 21 days of experimental gingivitis. The box-plots illustrate the plaque accumulation on tooth hard-substances during the 21-days non-brushing period followed by the progression of three selected clinical inflammatory parameters documenting the inflammatory status of the gingival tissues. The time interval and clinical observations are characteristic for an inflammatory lesion denoted as gingivitis.

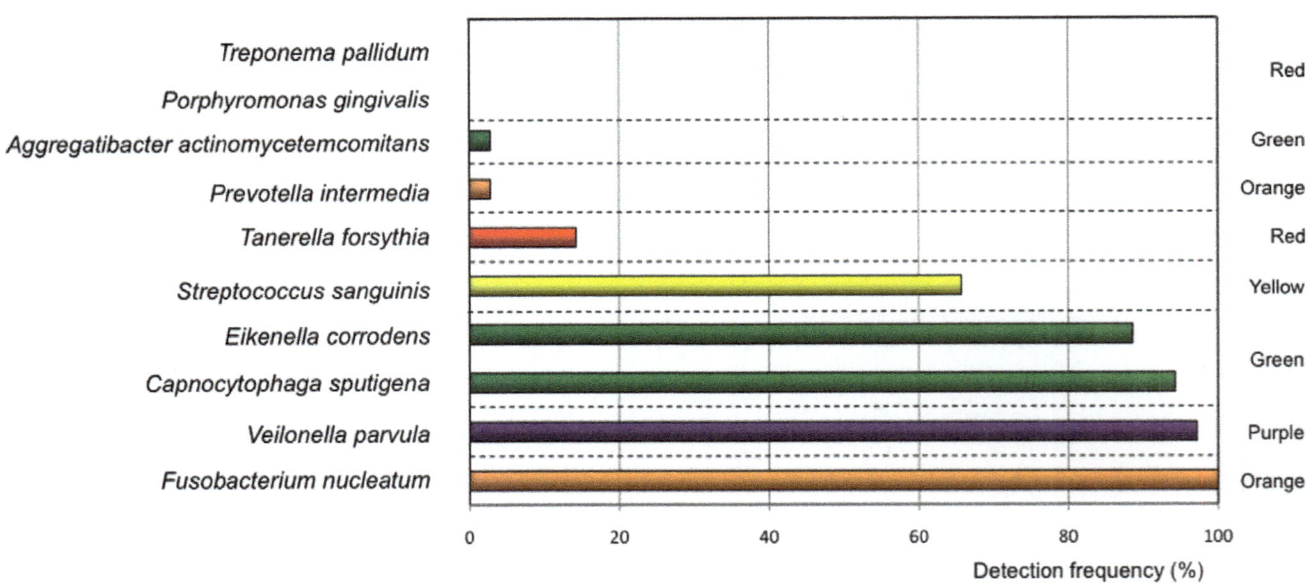

Figure 3. Species-specific detection of bacteria in 21-day old dental biofilms. The box-plots represent the PCR-based detection frequency of ten representative bacterial species within the study population of 37 subjects. The colors of the bars comply with the color codes of the bacterial complexes introduced by Socransky et al. [20].

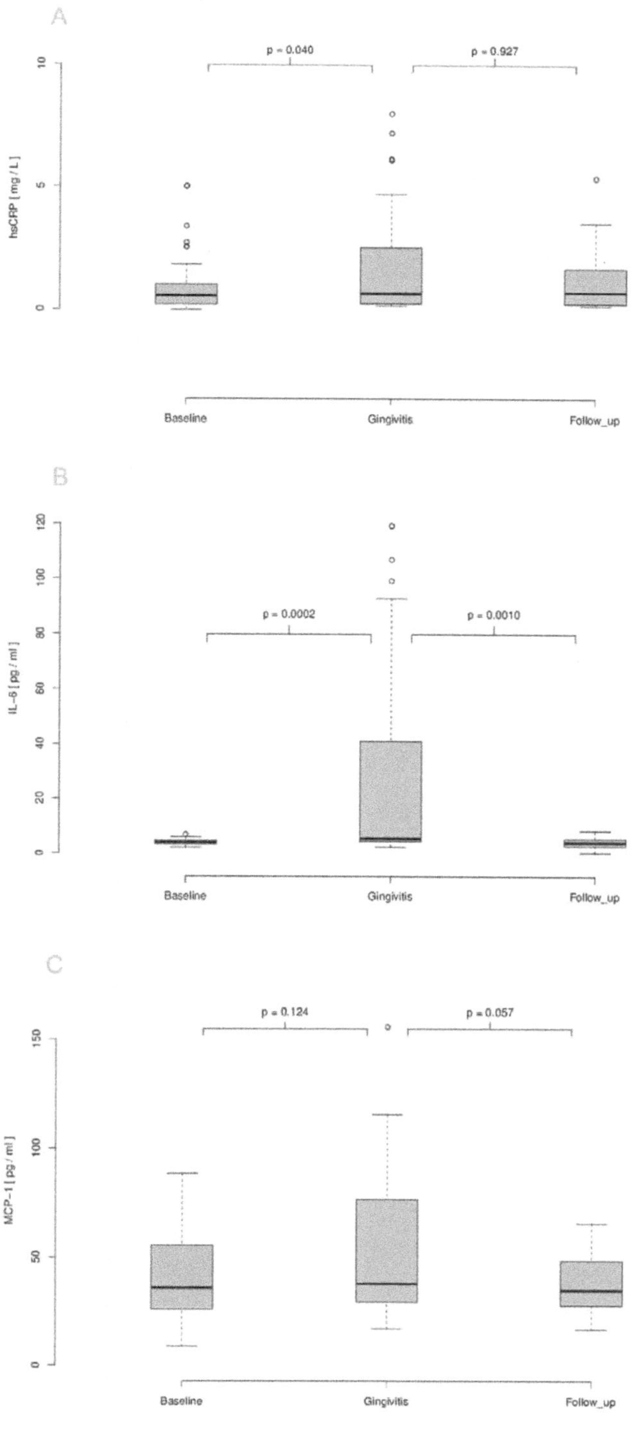

Figure 4. Characterization of serum parameters of inflammation at baseline, experimental gingivitis and follow-up. (A) Serum of participants was analyzed for hsCRP by immunonephelometrie. Plasma of participants was analyzed for IL-6 (B) and MCP-1 (C) by ELISA. Serums of participants were analyzed for leucocyte (D) and monocyte (E) cell counts by flow cytometry. *P*-values were calculated using two-sided Wilcoxon signed-rank tests for paired samples.

association of experimental gingivitis and systemic CRP and IL-6 levels in a population of healthy adults aged 18 to 30 years. These experiments were in accordance with a study of natural gingivitis by Wohlfeil et al. [22]. This group also showed no correlation between serum CRP levels and the degree of gingivitis. In contrast, elevated levels of serum IL-6 were found in patients suffering from type 2 diabetes and natural gingivitis compared to patients with diabetes and healthy gingival conditions [23]. The different observations between these studies and the present study may be explained at least in part by the young healthy participants of the present study, which do not have any traditional risk factors for cardiovascular diseases. In addition, a very sensitive method for the detection of CRP in serum was used.

Most likely, the observed gingival inflammatory processes, which was induced in the present study affect approximately 75% of Western populations [1]. In contrast to periodontitis, gingivitis affects children, adults and elderly in nearly equal ratios [8]. Clinically, this inflammatory process becomes obvious by bleeding during brushing the teeth, normally on a limited number of teeth. For the present study this clinical appearance was tried to mimick by inducing the inflammatory processes also just on a limited number of teeth, here seven, during a 21-days plaque accumulation phase. The inflammatory reactions of the gingival tissues are only mild and clinically nearly inconspicuous to the untrained eye. We studied well-characterized young healthy volunteers that yet did not show any traditional risk factor for cardiovascular diseases. Thus, we are assured that the observed systemic changes are a consequence of the local gingival inflammatory processes. However, the participants did not respond equally and showed inter-individual differences regarding the amount of dental plaque load, clinical signs of inflammation and serum markers of inflammation.

To further address the oral inflammatory status, we analyzed the presence of ten different species belonging to variable complexes according to Haffajee et al. [19], in which potential pathogens spread across different clusters. Bacterial species predominantly associated with subgingival lesions of destructive periodontitis were if at all in very low numbers present in the developing supragingival plaques of the present study [24,25]. Only *Fusobacterium nucleatum*, a so called 'bridge-bacterium' between health and disease, could be detected in high frequency in all plaque samples. Generally periopathogens, namely *Porphyromonas gingivalis*, are in the focus of research aimed to identify pathological mechanisms between periodontitis and systemic diseases [26]. The present study demonstrated that systemic effects could also be induced by low-level gingival inflammation and by bacterial plaques that do not harbour traditional periopathogens like *Porphyromonas gingivalis*. Hence, the present study is the first report that demonstrates adverse effects of local experimentally induced gingival inflammation on circulating serum levels of CRP, IL-6 and MCP-1 and activation of monocytes. These results demonstrated an enhanced systemic inflammatory status of the subjects during the course of the study. Future experiments are warranted to evaluate if natural gingivitis also enhances systemic inflammatory markers and the risk for atherosclerotic diseases. Elevated CRP, IL-6 and MCP-1 serum levels could serve as a direct marker of the inflammatory activity in the subjects' gingiva. The serum concentrations of hsCRP and IL-6 during the state of gingivitis reached levels, which were previously shown to be associated with high cardiovascular event rate i.e. myocardial infarction [27,28]. The broad concordance between clinical markers of gingival inflammation and systemic inflammatory markers and monocyte activation suggests a relationship between the local and systemic recations. Only one epidemiological study has been published aimed to identify associations between gingival inflammation and angina pectoris, however, the reported results are critical due to various confounding factors and unpredictable outcomes of self-reported data sampling [29]. For the present study the clinical parameters

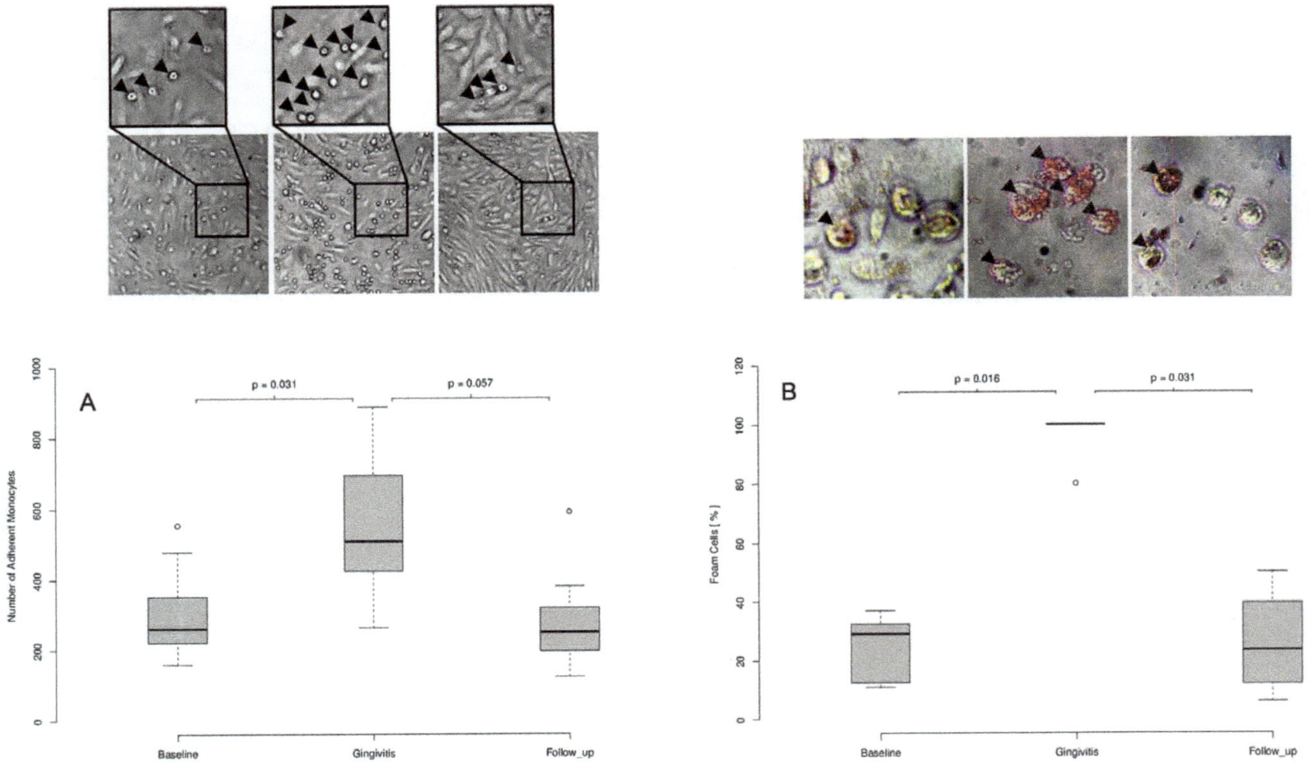

Figure 5. Monocyte adhesion assays and foam cell formation at baseline, gingivitis and follow-up. Blood monocytes were isolated from the blood of the volunteers at baseline (day 0), gingivitis (day 21) and follow-up (day 42) and subjected to ex vivo activation assays. (A) Number of adherent monocytes on cultured endothelial cells (HUVECs). Arrowheads in the enlarged picture detail indicate adherent monocytes. (B) Percentage foam cell formation after stimulation with oxLDL (10 μg/ml). Arrowheads indicate oil red O-positive foam cells. Representative pictures are shown. *P*-values were calculated using two-sided Wilcoxon signed-rank tests for paired samples.

of experimental gingivitis were not followed after day 21 of the experimental gingivitis phase, because multiple studies have shown that the clinical signs of gingivitis decline within seven days after the re-initiation of oral hygiene procedures in a group of subjects highly familiar with oral hygiene [30,31].

A potential limitation of this study is the sample size of 37 volunteers. However, the single-subject design with the subject as its own control is highly sensitive to detect individual differences. The here presented findings with young healthy individuals could not be generalized since elder subjects have an overall higher risk burden. Nevertheless, we especially have chosen young healthy subjects with no cardiovascular risk factors, to study systemic effects of experimental gingivitis. Thus, this approach offers the best prospect to uncover a potential relationship between local oral inflammation in gingivitis and systemic effects on surrogate markers of atherosclerosis. Definitely, larger randomised multi-center trials with elder subjects are necessary to investigate the hypothesis whether oral low-level gingivitis increases the risk for atherosclerosis or even enhances cardiovascular events.

The mechanisms by which local inflammatory processes of the oral cavity affect systemic conditions remain largely unknown and future experimental studies are warranted. Gingivitis involves bacterial infection with a range of Gram-positive and Gram-negative bacteria that invade the superficial gingival tissues [32]. During progression of the gingival disease, the epithelium becomes ulcerated to expose the underlying connective tissues and blood capillaries and facilitates entry of biofilm organisms or their products (e.g. bacterial heat-shock proteins) to the circulation during eating or tooth brushing [33]. Pathogens which have entered the bloodstream can directly invade blood vessel walls and atherosclerotic plaques [34,35,36]. Finally both, local oral infection and circulating infection products lead to an increase in the levels of circulating cytokines, chemokines and acute phase proteins, which are known to be associated with an increased cardiovascular event rate. The present study is the first report that demonstrated elevated serum levels of CRP, IL-6 and MCP-1 in the course of experimental gingivitis. Of interest, even gingival tissues were found to synthesize CRP [37]. Other inflammatory diseases, such as lupus erythematosus and rheumatoid arthritis are also associated with an increased cardiovascular risk supporting a mechanistic link between local extravascular inflammation and cardiovascular diseases [38,39].

It will be a task for future studies to identify the mechanisms that may account for the observed individual levels of local and systemic host responses. The potential confirmation that natural gingival inflammatory processes are an extravascular stimuli for systemic inflammation and atherogenesis will have great public health implications.

Supporting Information

Checklist S1.

Protocol S1.

Author Contributions

Conceived and designed the experiments: JE KG BS MS. Performed the experiments: JE ML WH DD HS RSS DL NS IS. Analyzed the data: JE KG RS BS MS. Contributed reagents/materials/analysis tools: JE KG ML RS RSS DL BS MS. Wrote the paper: JE KG ML BS MS.

References

1. Kebschull M, Demmer RT, Papapanou PN (2010) "Gum bug, leave my heart alone!"–epidemiologic and mechanistic evidence linking periodontal infections and atherosclerosis. J Dent Res 89: 879–902.
2. Pihlstrom BL, Michalowicz BS, Johnson NW (2005) Periodontal diseases. Lancet 366: 1809–1820.
3. Lockhart PB, Bolger AF, Papapanou PN, Osinbowale O, Trevisan M, et al. (2012) Periodontal disease and atherosclerotic vascular disease: does the evidence support an independent association?: a scientific statement from the American Heart Association. Circulation 125: 2520–2544.
4. Elter JR, Hinderliter AL, Offenbacher S, Beck JD, Caughey M, et al. (2006) The effects of periodontal therapy on vascular endothelial function: a pilot trial. Am Heart J 151: 47.
5. Tonetti MS, D'Aiuto F, Nibali L, Donald A, Storry C, et al. (2007) Treatment of periodontitis and endothelial function. N Engl J Med 356: 911–920.
6. Demmer RT, Papapanou PN (2010) Epidemiologic patterns of chronic and aggressive periodontitis. Periodontol 2000 53: 28–44.
7. Ericsson JS, Abrahamsson KH, Ostberg AL, Hellstrom MK, Jonsson K, et al. (2009) Periodontal health status in Swedish adolescents: an epidemiological, cross-sectional study. Swed Dent J 33: 131–139.
8. Li Y, Lee S, Hujoel P, Su M, Zhang W, et al. (2010) Prevalence and severity of gingivitis in American adults. Am J Dent 23: 9–13.
9. Hansson GK (2005) Inflammation, atherosclerosis, and coronary artery disease. N Engl J Med 352: 1685–1695.
10. Libby P, Ridker PM, Hansson GK (2011) Progress and challenges in translating the biology of atherosclerosis. Nature 473: 317–325.
11. Uno K, Nicholls SJ (2010) Biomarkers of inflammation and oxidative stress in atherosclerosis. Biomark Med 4: 361–373.
12. Drakopoulou M, Toutouzas K, Stefanadi E, Tsiamis E, Tousoulis D, et al. (2009) Association of inflammatory markers with angiographic severity and extent of coronary artery disease. Atherosclerosis 206: 335–339.
13. Wahaidi VY, Kowolik MJ, Eckert GJ, Galli DM (2011) Endotoxemia and the host systemic response during experimental gingivitis. J Clin Periodontol 38: 412–417.
14. Koren O, Spor A, Felin J, Fak F, Stombaugh J, et al. (2011) Human oral, gut, and plaque microbiota in patients with atherosclerosis. Proc Natl Acad Sci U S A 108 Suppl 1: 4592–4598.
15. Loe H, Theilade E, Jensen SB (1965) Experimental Gingivitis in Man. J Periodontol 36: 177–187.
16. Slawik S, Staufenbiel I, Schilke R, Nicksch S, Weinspach K, et al. (2011) Probiotics affect the clinical inflammatory parameters of experimental gingivitis in humans. Eur J Clin Nutr 65: 857–863.
17. Silness J, Löe H (1964) Periodontal Disease in Pregnancy. II. Correlation between Oral Hygiene and Periodontal Condition. Acta Odontol Scand 22: 121–135.
18. Löe H, Silness J (1963) Periodontal Disease in Pregnancy. I. Prevalence and Severity. Acta Odontol Scand 21: 533–551.
19. Haffajee AD, Socransky SS, Patel MR, Song X (2008) Microbial complexes in supragingival plaque. Oral Microbiol Immunol 23: 196–205.
20. Socransky SS, Haffajee AD, Cugini MA, Smith C, Kent RL Jr (1998) Microbial complexes in subgingival plaque. J Clin Periodontol 25: 134–144.
21. Honda T, Domon H, Okui T, Kajita K, Amanuma R, et al. (2006) Balance of inflammatory response in stable gingivitis and progressive periodontitis lesions. Clin Exp Immunol 144: 35–40.
22. Wohlfeil M, Wehner J, Schacher B, Oremek GM, Sauer-Eppel H, et al. (2009) Degree of gingivitis correlates to systemic inflammation parameters. Clin Chim Acta 401: 105–109.
23. Andriankaja OM, Barros SP, Moss K, Panagakos FS, DeVizio W, et al. (2009) Levels of serum interleukin (IL)-6 and gingival crevicular fluid of IL-1beta and prostaglandin E(2) among non-smoking subjects with gingivitis and type 2 diabetes. J Periodontol 80: 307–316.
24. Zee KY, Samaranayake LP, Attstrom R (1996) Predominant cultivable supragingival plaque in Chinese "rapid" and "slow" plaque formers. J Clin Periodontol 23: 1025–1031.
25. Haffajee AD, Teles RP, Patel MR, Song X, Veiga N, et al. (2009) Factors affecting human supragingival biofilm composition. I. Plaque mass. J Periodontal Res 44: 511–519.
26. Gaetti-Jardim E Jr, Marcelino SL, Feitosa AC, Romito GA, Avila-Campos MJ (2009) Quantitative detection of periodontopathic bacteria in atherosclerotic plaques from coronary arteries. J Med Microbiol 58: 1568–1575.
27. Ridker PM, Rifai N, Stampfer MJ, Hennekens CH (2000) Plasma concentration of interleukin-6 and the risk of future myocardial infarction among apparently healthy men. Circulation 101: 1767–1772.
28. Ridker PM, Hennekens CH, Buring JE, Rifai N (2000) C-reactive protein and other markers of inflammation in the prediction of cardiovascular disease in women. N Engl J Med 342: 836–843.
29. Ylostalo PV, Jarvelin MR, Laitinen J, Knuuttila ML (2006) Gingivitis, dental caries and tooth loss: risk factors for cardiovascular diseases or indicators of elevated health risks. J Clin Periodontol 33: 92–101.
30. Eberhard J, Reimers N, Dommisch H, Hacker J, Freitag S, et al. (2005) The effect of the topical administration of bioactive glass on inflammatory markers of human experimental gingivitis. Biomaterials 26: 1545–1551.
31. Eberhard J, Jepsen S, Albers HK, Acil Y (2000) Quantitation of arachidonic acid metabolites in small tissue biopsies by reversed-phase high-performance liquid chromatography. Anal Biochem 280: 258–263.
32. Saglie FR, Pertuiset JH, Rezende MT, Sabet MS, Raoufi D, et al. (1987) Bacterial invasion in experimental gingivitis in man. J Periodontol 58: 837–846.
33. Forner L, Larsen T, Kilian M, Holmstrup P (2006) Incidence of bacteremia after chewing, tooth brushing and scaling in individuals with periodontal inflammation. J Clin Periodontol 33: 401–407.
34. Elkaim R, Dahan M, Kocgozlu L, Werner S, Kanter D, et al. (2008) Prevalence of periodontal pathogens in subgingival lesions, atherosclerotic plaques and healthy blood vessels: a preliminary study. J Periodontal Res 43: 224–231.
35. Chiu B (1999) Multiple infections in carotid atherosclerotic plaques. Am Heart J 138: S534–536.
36. Libby P, Egan D, Skarlatos S (1997) Roles of infectious agents in atherosclerosis and restenosis: an assessment of the evidence and need for future research. Circulation 96: 4095–4103.
37. Lu Q, Jin L (2010) Human gingiva is another site of C-reactive protein formation. J Clin Periodontol 37: 789–796.
38. de Groot L, Posthumus MD, Kallenberg CG, Bijl M (2010) Risk factors and early detection of atherosclerosis in rheumatoid arthritis. Eur J Clin Invest 40: 835–842.
39. Boucelma M, Haddoum F, Chaudet H, Kaplanski G, Mazouni-Brahimi N, et al. (2011) Cardiovascular risk and lupus disease. Int Angiol 30: 18–24.
40. Baumgartner JC, Watkins BJ, Bae KS, Xia T (1999) Association of black-pigmented bacteria with endodontic infections. J Endod 25: 413–415.
41. Conrads G, Gharbia SE, Gulabivala K, Lampert F, Shah HN (1997) The use of a 16s rDNA directed PCR for the detection of endodontopathogenic bacteria. J Endod 23: 433–438.
42. Hoshino T, Kawaguchi M, Shimizu N, Hoshino N, Ooshima T, et al. (2004) PCR detection and identification of oral streptococci in saliva samples using gtf genes. Diagn Microbiol Infect Dis 48: 195–199.
43. Conrads G, Mutters R, Fischer J, Brauner A, Lütticken R, et al. (1996) PCR reaction and dot-blot hybridization to monitor the distribution of oral pathogens within plaque samples of periodontally healthy individuals. J Periodontol 67: 994–1003.
44. Ashimoto A, Chen C, Bakker I, Slots J (1996) Polymerase chain reaction detection of 8 putative periodontal pathogens in subgingival plaque of gingivitis and advanced periodontitis lesions. Oral Microbiol Immunol 11: 266–273.
45. Igarashi E, Kamaguchi A, Fujita M, Miyakawa H, Nakazawa F (2009) Identification of oral species of the genus Veillonella by polymerase chain reaction. Oral Microbiol Immunol 24: 310–313.
46. Kim SG, Kim SH, Kim MK, Kim HS, Kook JK (2005) Identification of Actinobacillus actinomycetemcomitans using species-specific 16S rDNA primers. J Microbiol 43: 209–212.

6

Multivariate Analysis of Factors Affecting Presence and/or Agenesis of Third Molar Tooth

Mohammad Khursheed Alam[1]*, Muhammad Asyraf Hamza[1], Muhammad Aizuddin Khafiz[1], Shaifulizan Abdul Rahman[2], Ramizu Shaari[2], Akram Hassan[3]

1 Orthodontic Unit, School of Dental Science, Universiti Sains Malaysia, Kota Bharu, Kelantan, Malaysia, **2** Oral and Maxillofacial Surgery Unit, School of Dental Science, Universiti Sains Malaysia, Kota Bharu, Kelantan, Malaysia, **3** Periodontology Unit, School of Dental Science, Universiti Sains Malaysia, Kota Bharu, Kelantan, Malaysia

Abstract

To investigate the presence and/or agenesis of third molar (M3) tooth germs in orthodontics patients in Malaysian Malay and Chinese population and evaluate the relationship between presence and/or agenesis of M3 with different skeletal malocclusion patterns and sagittal maxillomandibular jaw dimensions. Pretreatment records of 300 orthodontic patients (140 males and 160 females, 219 Malaysian Malay and 81 Chinese, average age was 16.27±4.59) were used. Third-molar agenesis was calculated with respect to race, genders, number of missing teeth, jaws, skeletal malocclusion patterns and sagittal maxillomandibular jaw dimensions. The Pearson chi-square test and ANOVA was performed to determine potential differences. Associations between various factors and M3 presence/agenesis groups were assessed using logistic regression analysis. The percentages of subjects with 1 or more M3 agenesis were 30%, 33% and 31% in the Malaysian Malay, Chinese and total population, respectively. Overall prevalence of M3 agenesis in male and female was equal ($P>0.05$). The frequency of the agenesis of M3s is greater in maxilla as well in the right side ($P>0.05$). The prevalence of M3 agenesis in those with a Class III and Class II malocclusion was relatively higher in Malaysian Malay and Malaysian Chinese population respectively. Using stepwise regression analyses, significant associations were found between Mx ($P<0.05$) and ANB ($P<0.05$) and M3 agenesis. This multivariate analysis suggested that Mx and ANB were significantly correlated with the M3 presence/agenesis.

Editor: Sompop Bencharit, University of North Carolina at Chapel Hill, United States of America

Funding: The authors have no support or funding to report.

Competing Interests: The authors have declared that no competing interests exist.

* Email: dralam@gmail.com

Introduction

Tooth agenesis is the congenital lack of one or more of the deciduous or permanent teeth – the one not erupted in the oral cavity, and also not visible in a radiograph, is one of the most frequent human dental anomales [1]. The third molar (M3) is a tooth characterized by the variability in the time of its formation, its widely varying crown and root morphology, and its varying presence or absence in the oral cavity [2]. Agenesis of one or more permanent teeth is a common anomaly in man and many reports on M3 agenesis have been published for different populations over the last 50 years [3–24].

The wide range of prevalence of this anomaly might be attributed to the differences in the methods of sampling and examination, age and sex distribution, and racial origin of the subjects. 7.

M3 agenesis has been associated with dental numeric and structured variations. Garn et al. [25] have suggested that when a M3 is absent, agenesis of the remaining teeth is 13 times more likely. M3 is undoubtedly the most common dental reduction with up to 50% of some groups affected [16].

Investigators and clinicians, especially orthodontists, believe that an increase in agenesis of permanent teeth is related to dentofacial development, and development of malocclusion. There have been many debates for years on whether there is a relationship between third molars and crowding [25,26], Clinicians, especially orthodontist should consider the entire dentition including the presence or absence of the third molars because it relates with posterior crowding. A limited number of studies have been carried out to evaluate the relationship between M3 agenesis and different skeletal malocclusion patterns [18,20,27], sagittal jaw dimensions [27,28] and craniofacial morphology [27].

We have, therefore, given particular attention to the subjects of presence and/or agenesis of M3. As per our concern no studies have been carried out to evaluate the relationship between presence and/or agenesis of M3 with different skeletal malocclusion patterns and sagittal maxillomandibular jaw dimensions in Malaysian Malay and Chinese polpulation. On the basis of these facts, the aim of this study was to -.

1) investigate the presence and/or agenesis of third molar tooth germs in orthodontics patients in Malaysian Malay and chinese population.
2) examine the relationship between presence and/or agenesis of M3 and different sagittal skeletal malocclusions.
3) examine the relationship between presence and/or agenesis of M3 and different vertical patterns of the skeletal malocclusions.
4) to determine the existence of any relation between the presence and/or agenesis of third molar tooth germs and sagittal maxillomandibular jaw dimensions.

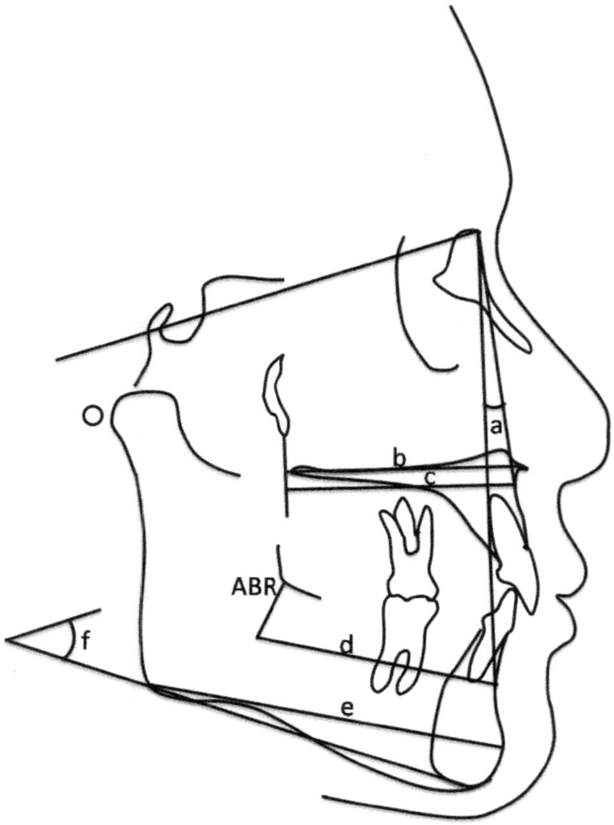

Figure 1. Angular cephalometric measurements relating to sagittal and vertical malocclusion and linear cephalometric measurements relating to sagittal jaw dimensions (descriptions are in Table 1).

Materials and Methods

All participants provide their written informed consent (One of the parents, either father and/or mother gave written consent for the adolescent subjects). This study was approved by the Ethical Committee of the Hospital Universiti Sains Malaysia (HUSM) [FWA Reg. No: 00007718; IRB Reg. No: 00004494], which complies with the Declaration of Helsinki. This study was designed and conducted according to the guidelines of Strengthening the Reporting of Observational studies in Epidemiology (STROBE), and we applied the STROBE checklist in the preparation of this manuscript [28].

Power and sample size software calculated the sample size with a power of 80%; the alpha was 0.05.

Sample size calculation:

$$n=\left(\frac{z}{\Delta}\right)^2(p(1-p))$$

n = number of sample.
z = z-score at 95% confidence interval = 1.96.
Δ = precision.
p = proportion taken from previous published study [18].

Considering the available resources, number of sample, n = 270.

Also, considering the missing data 10% of sample is added, so the sample size is 297.

Finally three hundred patients (140 males and 160 females, average age was 16.27±4.59) were selected for this study from the orthodontic unit of Hospital Universiti Sains Malaysia.

Inclusion criterion

1. the patients had not received any orthodontic treatment,
2. the patients had not undergone surgical removal or extraction of one or more M3s.

Exclusion criterion

1. subjects with congenital deformities,
2. radiographs of poor quality.

The digital images were investigated (Orthopantomogram [OPG]) measured (Lateral cephalograms) using Romexis software (Planmeca, Finland) operating with computer (DX2810 Microtower PC, HP Compaq, US) and 17-inch monitor screen (LE1711 LCD monitor, HP Compaq, US).

OPG investigation

Panoramic radiographs taken at the initial examination were used to determine the presence of M3 germs. In cases in which it was impossible to judge the presence of M3 germs from panoramic radiographs taken at the initial examination, were also excluded.

Cephalometric analysis

Lateral cephalograms also taken at the initial examination were used to measure linear and angular cephalometric variables (**Table 1 and Figure 1**). For the sagittal skeletal malocclusions, skeletal Class I (1° and 5°), Class II (>5°) and Class III (<1°) using the measurements of the ANB angle was used. SN-GoMe angle was used for classification of vertical patterns of the skeletal

Table 1. Cephalometrics angular and linear measurements.

Variable	Measuring unit	Description
(a) ANB	degree	Angle formed by a line joining NA and NB
(b) ANS-PNS	mm	Anteroposterior length of the nasal floor
(c) A-Ptm (Mx)	mm	Anteroposterior length of the maxillary basal bone
(d) ABR-B (Mn)	mm	anteroposterior length of the mandibular basal bone (ABR: cross point between occlusal plane and anterior edge of the ramus)
(e) Go-Pog	mm	anteroposterior length of the corpus
(f) SN-MP	degree	Angle formed by SN plane and mandibular plane.

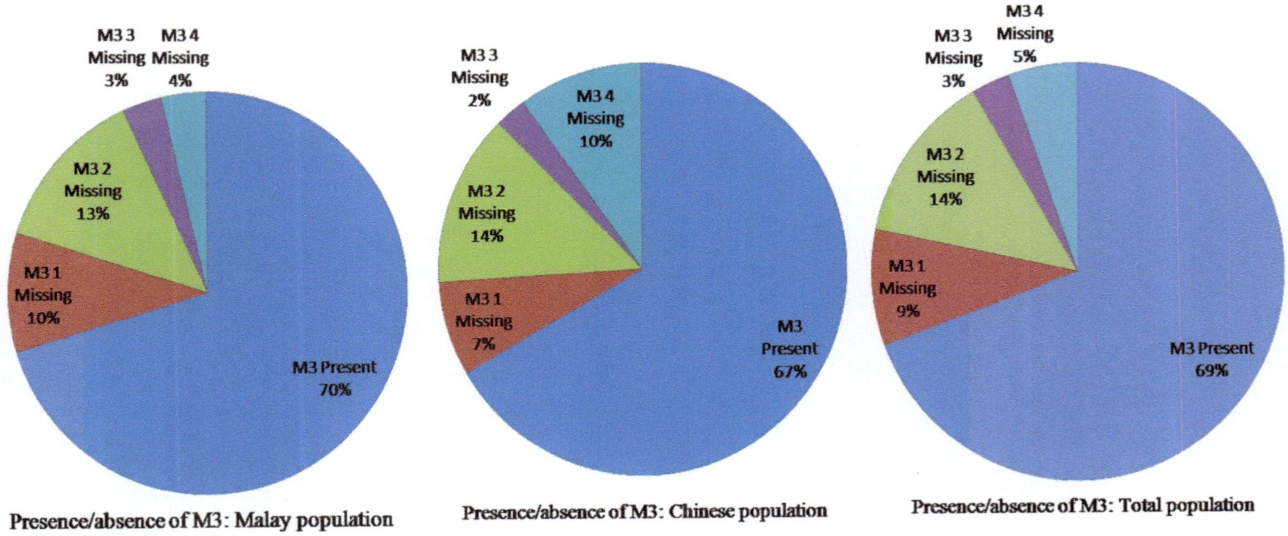

Figure 2. Distribution of Subjects with M3 Presence/Agenesis in Malysian Malay and Chinese.

malocclusions as being normal (27°–37°), hypo-divergent (<27°), and hyper-divergent (>37°).

Statistical Analysis

The data were verified and analysed statistically using IBM SPSS Statistics Version 20.0 with confidence level set at 5% ($P < 0.05$) to test for significance.

Randomly selected 50 OPG were evaluated by another researcher 4 weeks after the initial survey to determine the reliability of diagnosis of the M3 agenesis. The kappa statistics has been used to determine intra- and interexaminer agreements. There was 100% intra- and interexaminer agreement between the investigators. To determine the errors associated with digitizing and measurements, 50 radiographs were selected randomly. All procedures such as landmark identification, tracing, and measure-

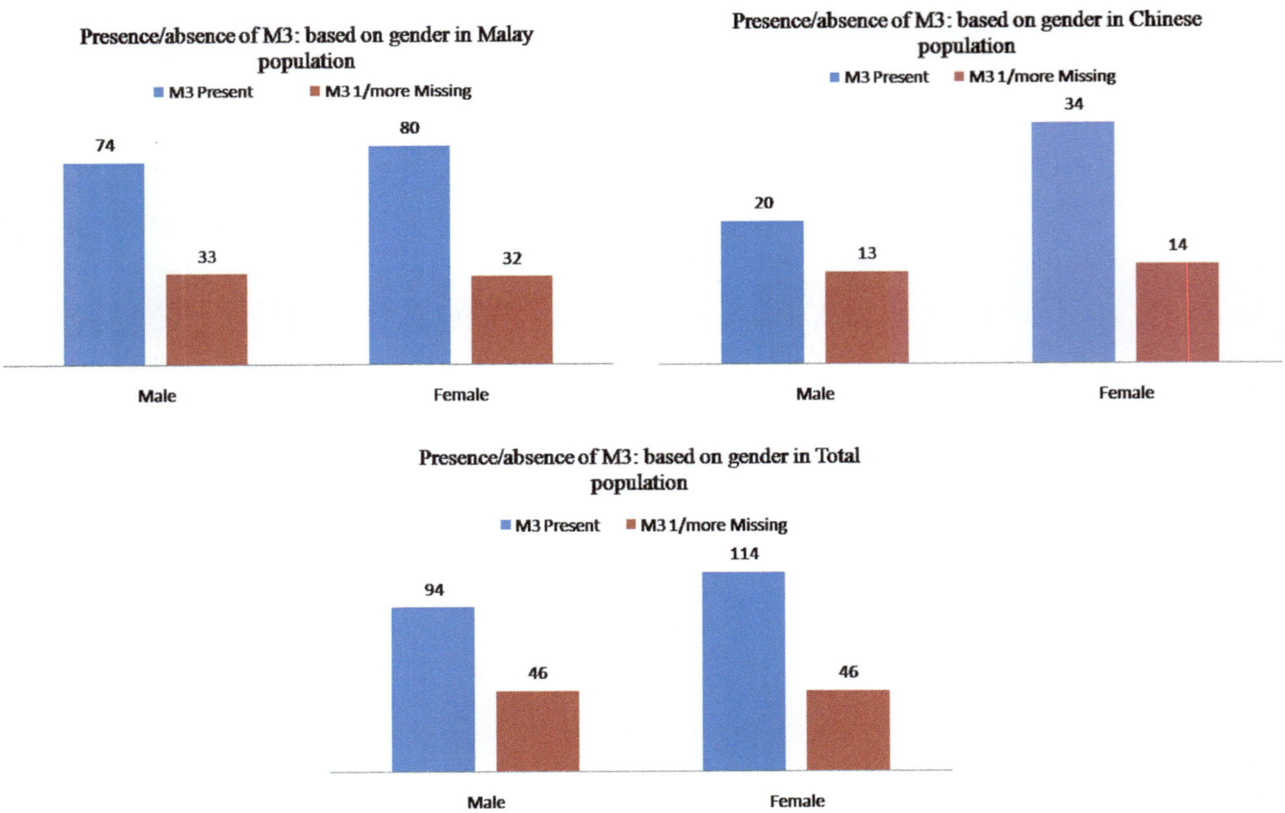

Figure 3. Distribution of Subjects with M3 Presence/Agenesis in male and female.

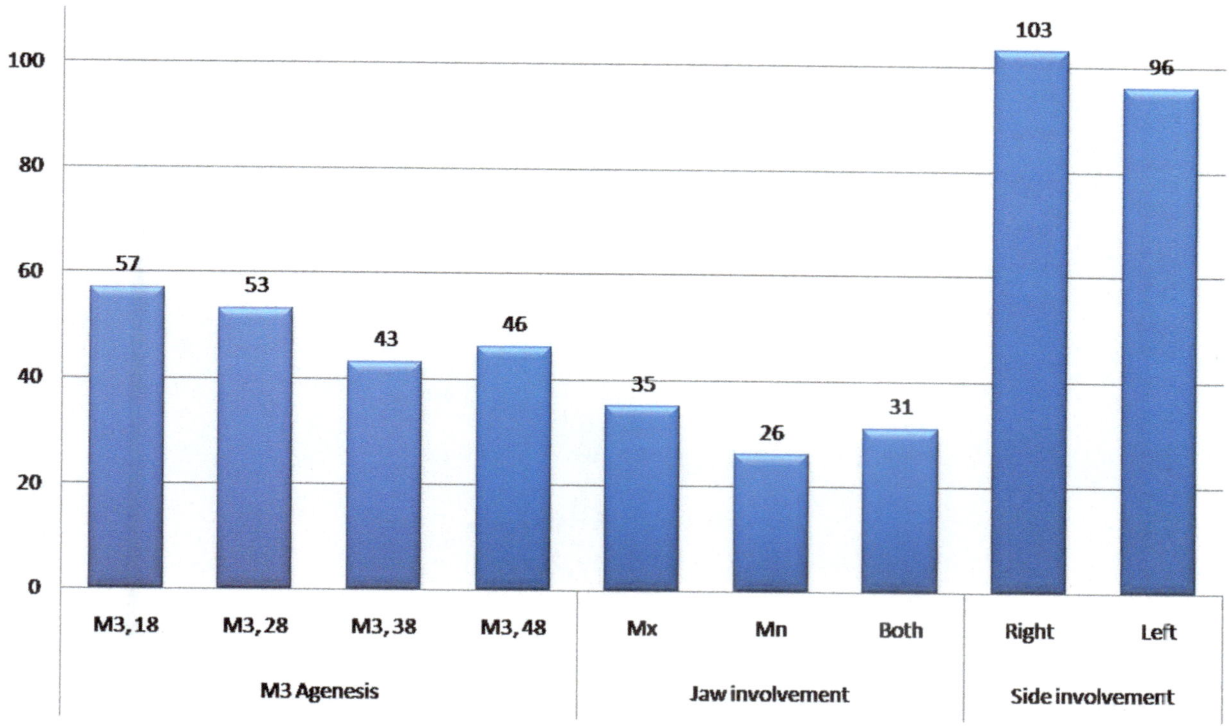

Figure 4. Distribution of Subjects in Total (Malaysian Malay and Chinese) population With M3 Agenesis, Jaw and side involvement.

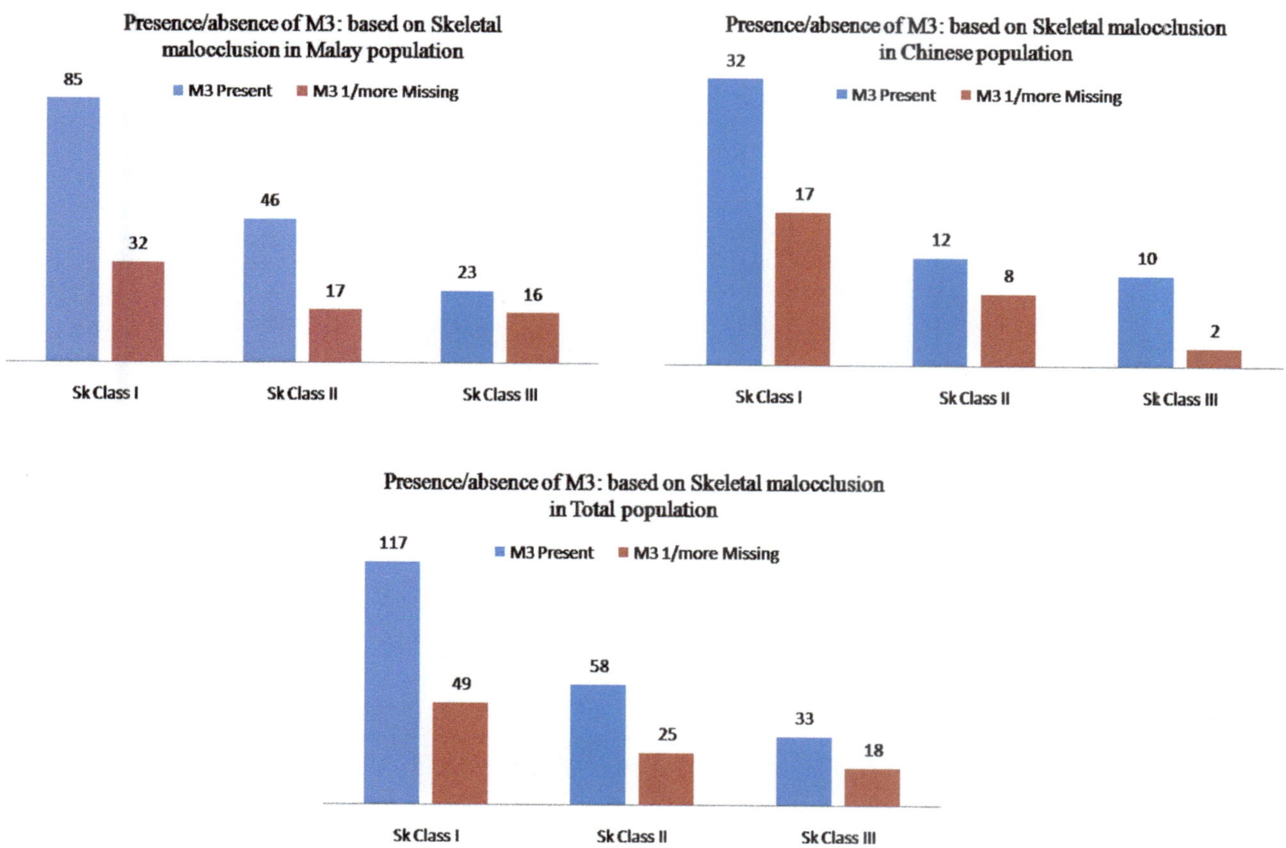

Figure 5. Distribution of Subjects with M3 Presence/Agenesis in Sagittal Skeletal Malocclusions.

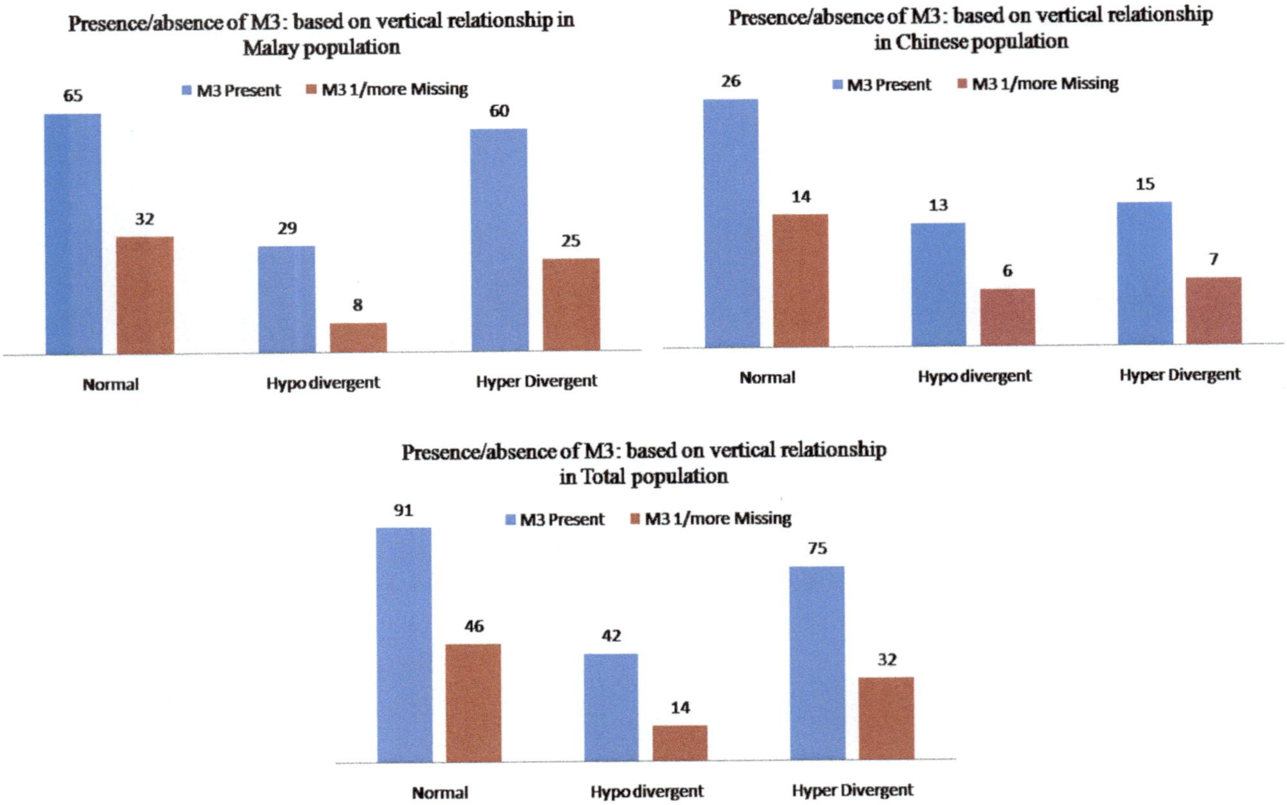

Figure 6. Distribution of Subjects with M3 Presence/Agenesis in Vertical Skeletal Malocclusions.

ments were repeated 4 weeks after the first examination by the same investigator. Intraclass correlation coefficients were performed to assess the reliability of the measurements and the coefficients of reliability of the measurements were between 0.93 and 0.99.

Dahlberg's formula was used to determine the method-error of cephalometric measurements, which did not exceed 0.38 mm for the linear variables, 0.63 degree for the angular variables. The combined error for any of the variable was small and considered to be within acceptable limit [29]. Dalhberg's formula: $\mathbf{ME = \sqrt{\Sigma(x1-x2)^2/2n}}$. Where x1 is the first measurement, x2 the second measurement and n the number of repeated records [29]. The M3 presence and/or agenesis were calculated with respect to race, genders, number of missing teeth, jaws, and skeletal malocclusion patterns. The Pearson chi-square test was performed to determine potential differences in the distribution of M3 agenesis when stratified according to the above parameters. The existence of significant differences between the presence and/or agenesis of third molar tooth germs and sagittal maxillomandibular jaw dimensions was analyzed by ANOVA for one factor and the Scheffe test for multiple comparisons.

Logistic regression analysis was performed using the dichotomous dependent variable, M3 presence vs agenesis groups. Both crude and backward stepwise logistic regression analyses were done to determine which factors associated with the M3 presence/agenesis [30].

Results

Presence and/or agenesis of third molar tooth germs in orthodontics patients in Malaysian Malay and Chinese population:

Inter races disparities

Figure 2 shows the percentages of subjects with all 4 M3 present and with 1 or more of the M3 missing. The percentages of subjects with all M3 were 70%, 67% and 69% in the Malaysian Malay, Chinese and total population, respectively. Therefore, the overall prevalence of M3 agenesis was 31% in this orthodontic population. The difference between the groups was not significant. Among the patients with M3 agenesis in Malaysian Malay population, the prevalence of patients with one, two, three, or four missing tooth/teeth were 10%, 13%, 3%, and 4%, respectively. In Malaysian Chinese population, the prevalence of patients with one, two, three, or four M3 missing tooth/teeth were 7%, 14%, 2%, and 10%, respectively. There is no significant difference in the occurrence of M3 agenesis between the numbers of M3s.

Inter sexes disparities

Figure 3 shows overall prevalence of M3 agenesis in male and female was equal. There was no significant gender difference.

Inter side (right and left) and jaw (maxilla, mandible and both)

The difference between the groups in relation to side and jaw involvement was not significant (data not shown). The distribution of M3s present in the maxilla and the mandible or both and on the right and the left side is depicted in **Figure 4**. Although the frequency of the agenesis of M3s is greater in maxilla as well in right side, the $\chi 2$ statistic revealed no significant relationship, indicating that there is no correlation between the frequencies of M3 existence.

Table 2. Linear and Angular Cephalometric Measurements in a Malay population With M3 Presence/Agenesis.

Variables	M3 Present		M3, 1 missing		M3, 2 missing		M3, 3 missing		M3, 4 missing	
	Mean	SD	Mean	SD	Mean	SD	Mean	SD	Mean	SD
ANS-PNS	51.18	5.06	50.38	3.74	52.59	5.30	50.04	4.82	50.83	4.13
Go-Pog	70.28	6.31	70.17	7.40	69.72	4.89	67.11	7.34	68.96	5.32
Mx	46.82	4.65	48.17	7.62	47.21	4.26	45.84	4.80	46.55	3.06
Mn	48.91	9.56	49.35	6.39	47.34	7.97	45.99	5.52	45.69	4.21
ANB	4.09	2.68	3.05	2.84	3.69	3.93	2.86	2.54	3.75	1.67
SN-MP	35.86	6.74	35.33	6.07	37.66	6.16	36.29	8.44	35.63	4.21

ANOVA applying Post Hoc Scheffe test * $P<0.05$. The groups did not show significant differences with any other.

Table 3. Linear and Angular Cephalometric Measurements in a Chinese population With M3 Presence/Agenesis.

Variables	M3 Present		M3, 1 missing		M3, 2 missing		M3, 3 missing		M3, 4 missing	
	Mean	SD	Mean	SD	Mean	SD	Mean	SD	Mean	SD
ANS-PNS	53.95	4.94	58.68	5.74	53.21	4.12	57.85	0.49	54.78	8.19
Go-Pog	73.83	7.02	77.27	7.92	75.05	4.67	78.25	3.04	73.99	10.97
Mx	48.48	4.12	52.88	5.20	48.07	3.17	50.85	1.77	50.24	7.11
Mn	48.30	7.61	50.20	7.11	46.03	7.42	50.05	1.34	45.28	7.24
ANB	3.83	2.41	5.67	1.37	3.55	1.69	3.50	2.12	3.88	2.36
SN-MP	34.59	6.85	32.33	4.63	34.64	5.97	34.50	2.12	34.25	5.70

ANOVA applying Post Hoc Scheffe test * $P<0.05$. The groups did not show significant differences with any other.

Table 4. Linear and Angular Cephalometric Measurements in Total (Malaysian Malay and Chinese) population With M3 Presence/Agenesis.

Variables	M3 Present		M3, 1 missing		M3, 2 missing		M3, 3 missing		M3, 4 missing	
	Mean	SD	Mean	SD	Mean	SD	Mean	SD	Mean	SD
ANS-PNS	51.90	5.17	52.22	5.43	52.76	4.96	51.78	5.41	52.80	6.59
Go-Pog	71.20	6.67	71.74	7.95	71.19	5.34	69.59	8.10	71.48	8.72
Mx	47.25	4.57	49.22	7.34	47.45	3.97	46.96	4.74	48.39	5.62
Mn	48.75	9.08	49.54	6.42	46.98	7.75	46.89	5.13	45.48	5.73
ANB	4.02	2.61	3.63	2.79	3.65	3.44	3.00	2.35	3.81	1.97
SN-MP	35.53	6.78	34.67	5.84	36.83	6.18	35.89	7.39	34.94	4.89

ANOVA applying Post Hoc Scheffe test * $P<0.05$. The groups did not show significant differences with any other.

Inter sagittal skeletal malocclusions disparities

Figure 5 shows the prevalence of M3 agenesis (total population) in those with a Class I, Class II, or Class III malocclusion was 29.5%, 30.1%, and 35.3%, respectively. The prevalence of M3 agenesis in those with a Class III malocclusion (41% in Malaysian Malay and 35% in total population) was relatively higher than in those with a Class I or a Class II. However in Malaysian Chinese population, the prevalence of M3 agenesis in those with a Class II malocclusion (40%) was relatively higher than in those with a Class I or a Class III. The difference between the groups was not significant.

Inter vertical patterns of the skeletal malocclusions disparities

Figure 6 shows the prevalence of M3 agenesis (total population) in those with a normal, hypo-divergent and hyper-divergent groups was 33.6%, 25%, and 29.9%, respectively. The difference between the groups was not significant.

Inter sagittal maxillomandibular jaw relationships disparities

Table 2, 3 and 4 shows the results obtained by linear and angular cephalometric measurement between 4 M3 present and with 1 or more of the M3 missing in Malaysian Malay, Chinese and total population. The frequency of M3 agenesis (4 M3s agenesis) increased with an increasing Mx (Table 3 and 4) and with a decreasing Mn (Table 2, 3 and 4). Significant differences between the groups were not detected.

Crude logistic regression analysis

Table 5 shows the results of the crude logistic regression analysis that estimated the associations between various factors (independent variable) and M3 presence/agenesis (dependent variable). Odds ratio, 95% confidence interval, and p value for the various factors are presented. No significant associations were found among various factors (age, sex, race, ANSPNS, GO-POG, Mx, Mn, ANB, SN-MP) with the M3 presence/agenesis.

Stepwise logistic regression analysis

Table 6 shows the results of the stepwise logistic regression analysis that estimated the associations between various factors and M3 presence/agenesis. Significant associations were found among various factors, Mx ($P<0.05$) and ANB ($P<0.05$) were significantly correlated with M3 presence/agenesis.

Discussion

In the present study based on panoramic radiographs, we attempted to determine the prevalence of M3 presence and/or agenesis in a sample of orthodontic patients from Malaysian Malay and Chinese. We found that 31% of the subjects had 1 or more M3s agenesis, These results indicate that about one third of the patients had 1 or more M3s agenesis, which is close to the frequency of 31.5% reported by Harris and Clark [16] for American white subjects, 32.4% reported by Rosario and Gonzalez [6] for Mexican subjects, 33.2% reported by Eloma and Eloma [13] for Finland subjects and 32% reported by Jacob et al. [24] for Malaysian Chinese subjects. Global distributions of the prevalence of M3 agenesis were shown in **Figure 7** [3–24]. These racial differences are interesting and suggest that some polygenetic inheritance on formation of M3 germs may differ among populations and races as well as may be due to differences in sample sizes.

Table 5. Crude logistic regression analysis: M3 presence vs. agenesis group.

	S.E.	Exp(B)	95% Confidence Interval		P - value
			Lower	Upper	
Age	0.029	1.030	0.973	1.089	0.310
Gender	0.251	0.825	0.504	1.348	0.442
Race	0.278	1.185	0.687	2.044	0.543
ANS-PNS	0.024	1.023	0.976	1.071	0.348
GO-POG	0.019	1.001	0.965	1.038	0.960
Mx	0.026	1.035	0.985	1.088	0.174
Mn	0.015	0.982	0.953	1.012	0.226
ANB	0.046	0.945	0.863	1.035	0.221
SN-MP	0.019	1.006	0.969	1.044	0.766

S.E. = Standard error, Exp(B = Odds ratio), * $P<0.05$.

In our study, the order of frequency for the M3 agenesis is two, one, four, and three M3s in Malaysian Malay subjects [24]. In Malaysian Chinese subjects, the order of frequency for the M3 agenesis is two, four, one, and three M3s. In total population, the order of frequency for the M3 agenesis is two, one, four, and three M3s [24]. The order of frequency for M3 agenesis in this study is incompatible with the reports published by those authors [16,18,22,23].

Intersexual comparisons revealed no significant differences in the incidence of M3 agenesis, despite the higher percentage noted for males than that for females (32.9% and 28.8%, respectively). The male predominance of M3 agenesis agrees with the results reported by Hattab et al. [19] but differs from data reported by Jacob et al. [24], Barka et al. [12] and Sandhu and Kaur [22]. On the other hand, all the above-mentioned authors concluded that intersexual differences were not statistically significant, which is in agreement with our results. No significance was also reported for the Turkish [18], Chinese [23] and Japanese [20] populations.

The order of frequency for the M3 agenesis is 18, 28, 48 and 38 is found in the present study. However Jacob et al. [24] found 18, 28, 38 and 48. Studies performed in different populations demonstrate that the majority of missing M3s were located in the maxilla, with the differences being statistically significant [20,23]. Hattab et al. [19], Sandhu and Kaur [22], Barka et al. [12] and Jacob et al. [24] also reported that congenitally missing M3s showed a greater predilection for the maxilla over the mandible. The reason there may be a disparity in M3 agenesis in the maxilla and mandible is also not clear [31]. Besides, in the present study, no significant difference was found between the frequencies of at least one M3 missing in the maxilla and the mandible.

In this study, crude logistic regression analysis was used to estimate associations between each factors (age, sex, race, ANSPNS, GO-POG, Mx, Mn, ANB, SN-MP) and M3 presence/agenesis. Stepwise logistic regression analysis was used to explore the associations between precise factors (among various factors) and M3 presence/agenesis. Stepwise logistic regression analysis is used in the exploratory phase of research [30]. Backward stepwise regression appears to be the preferred method of exploratory analyses, in which the analysis begins with a full model and variables are eliminated one by one using the largest p value [30]. The final model is the last step model, in which eliminating another variable would not improve the model significantly [30].

Sanchez et al. [27] hypothesized that agenesis of wisdom teeth is not related with any particular craniofacial morphology which is in agreement with the results of the present study except for the Mx. Present study revealed presence and/or agenesis of M3 depends significantly on sagittal skeletal malocclusions (ANB), and sagittal jaw dimensions (Mx) in the exploratory phase of analysis. Perhaps the difference in results could be linked to racial differences. Such differences are interesting; the reasons stated that some polygenetic inheritance on formation of M3 germs may be related to genes that control maxillary and/or mandibular dimensions. Present study also revealed presence and/or agenesis of M3 do not depends significantly on vertical patterns of the skeletal malocclusions. However, Sanchez et al. [27] concluded as maxillary M3 agenesis are related to reduced mandibular plane angles and mandibular M3 agenesis showed a diminished lower

Table 6. Adjusted logistic regression analysis (stepwise regression analysis: backward method): M3 presence vs. agenesis group.

	S.E.	Exp(B)	95% Confidence Interval		P - value
			Lower	Upper	
Mx	0.033	1.084	1.015	1.158	0.016*
Mn	0.021	0.964	0.924	1.005	0.082
ANB	0.054	0.887	0.798	0.985	0.025*

S.E. = Standard error, Exp(B) = Odds ratio), * $P<0.05$.
Variables entered on step 1: age, sex, race, ANSPNS, GO-POG, Mx, Mn, ANB and SN-MP.

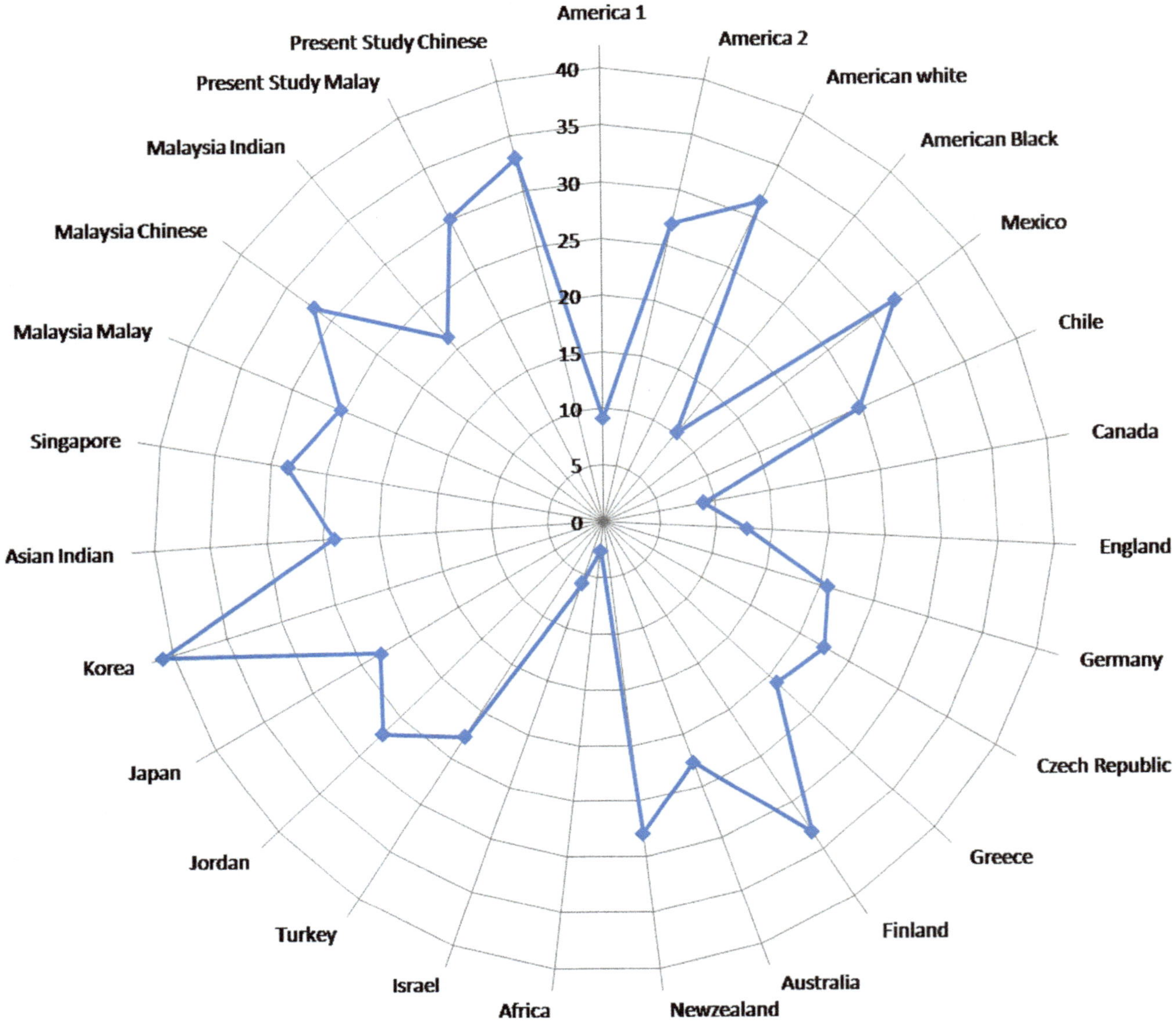

Figure 7. Global Distributions of prevalence of M3 Agenesis.

third and mandibular morphology characteristic of brachyfacial patterns.

Results of the present study are the evidence for the prevalence of M3 agenesis in those with a Class III malocclusion in Malaysian Malay population was relatively higher. However in Malaysian Chinese population, the prevalence of M3 agenesis in those with a Class II malocclusion was relatively higher. On the other hand Celikoglu and Kamak [18] and Kajii et al. [30] found that the prevalence of Class III subjects who had all four M3s was lower than that of subjects with Class II malocclusions. Celikoglu and Kamak [18] stated that the vertical patterns of the skeletal malocclusions for M3 agenesis patients showed with an order of prevalence in hyper-divergent, normal, and hypo-divergent groups. On the other hand, Sanchez et al. [27] found that agenesis of maxillary M3s was related to a reduced mandibular plane angle. In our study, we found that the order of prevalence is normal, hyper-divergent and hypo-divergent groups without any significant difference [18].

In a study of a group of Spanish, Sanchez et al. [27] evaluated the relationship of third molar agenesis to craniofacial morphology. They reported that subjects with bilateral maxillary agenesis, bilateral mandibular agenesis and control group (All M3 present) have no significant association with sagittal jaw dimensions which is in agreement with our finding. However, Kajii et al. [31] reported that subjects with bilateral maxillary agenesis of the M3 were significantly associated with maxilla and no significant association was shown between the sagittal dimension of the mandible and M3 agenesis.

In a prospect study, polygenetic inheritance on formation of M3 germs and the genes that control maxillary and/or mandibular dimensions and of craniofacial maturation need to be studied.

Conclusion

- The present results showed that in this orthodontic population from Malaysian Malay and Chinese, M3 agenesis accounted for 30% and 33% respectively.

- The frequency of M3 agenesis was found greater in the maxilla.
- These results revealed that Presence and/or agenesis of M3 do not depends significantly on age, sex, race, side, jaw involvement and vertical skeletal malocclusions.
- This multivariate analysis suggested that increasing Mx and ANB were significantly correlated with the M3 agenesis in this orthodontic population.

Author Contributions

Conceived and designed the experiments: MKA MAH MAK SAR RS AH. Performed the experiments: MKA MAH MAK. Analyzed the data: MKA MAH MAK SAR. Contributed reagents/materials/analysis tools: MKA MAH MAK SAR RS AH. Wrote the paper: MKA MAH MAK SAR RS AH. Critical review: MKA SAR RS AH.

References

1. Cameron J, Sampson WJ (1996) Hypodontia of the parmanent dentition. Case reports. Aust Dent J 41(1): 1–5.
2. Gravely JF (1965) A radiographic survey of third molar development. Br Dent J 119: 397–401.
3. Nanda RS (1954) Agenesis of the third molar in man. Am J Orthod 40: 698–706.
4. Harris EF, Clark LL (2008) Hypodontia: an epidemiologic study of American black and white people. Am J Orthod Dentofacial Orthop 134: 761–7.
5. Keene HJ (1965) The relationship between third molar agenesis and the morphologic variability of the molar teeth. Angle Orthod 35: 289–298.
6. Llarena del Rosario ME, Nuno Gonzalez MM (1990) Stages of formation and calcification of the third molar (Radiographic study of 500 Mexican children and adolescents). Rev ADM 47: 112–8. [In Spanish, English abstract].
7. Garcia-Hernandez F, Toro Yagui O, Vega Vidal M, Verdejo Meneses M (2008) Third Molar Agenesis in Young People Between 14 and 20 Years of Age, Antofagasta, Chile. Int J Morphol 26: 825–32. [In Spanish, English abstract].
8. Levesque GY, Demirijian A, Tanguay R (1981) Sexual dimorphism in the development, emergence, and agenesis of the mandibular third molar. J Dent Res 60: 1735–41.
9. Shinn DL (1976) Congenitally missing third molars in a British population. J Dent 4: 42–4.
10. Bredy E, Erbring C, Hubenthal B (1991) The incidence of hypodontia with the presence and absence of wisdom teeth. Dtsch Zahn Mund Kieferheilkd Zentralbl 79: 357–63. [In German, English abstract].
11. Rozkovcova E, Markova M, Lanik J, Zvarova J (2004) Agenesis of third molars in young Czech population. Prague Med Rep 105: 35–52.
12. Barka G, Tretiakov G, Theodosiou T, Ioannidou-Marathiotou I (2012) Presence of third molars in orthodontic patients from northern Greece Int J Gen Med 5: 441–7.
13. Elomaa M., Elomaa E (1973) Third molar aplasia and formation in orthodontic patients. Proc Finn Dent Soc 69: 141–146.
14. Lynham A (1990) Panoramic radiographic survey of hypodontia in Australian Defence Force recruits. Aust Dent J 35: 19–22.
15. Kruger E, Thomson WM, Konthasinghe P (2001) Third molar outcomes from age 18 to 26: findings from a population-based New Zealand longitudinal study. Oral Surg Oral Med Oral Pathol Oral Radiol Endod 92: 150–5.
16. Hellmann M (1936) Our third molar teeth: their eruption, presence and absence. Dent Cosmos 78: 750–762.
17. Goren S, Tsoizner R, Dinbar A, Levin L, Brezniak N (2005) Prevalence of congenitally missing teeth in Israeli recruits. Refuat Hapeh Vehashinayim 22: 49–5, 87. [In Hebrew, English abstract].
18. Celikoglu M, Kamak H (2012) Patterns of third-molar agenesis in an orthodontic patient population with different skeletal malocclusions Angle Orthod 82: 165–169.
19. Hattab FN, Rawashdeh MA, Fahmy MS (1995) Impaction status of third molars in Jordanian students. Oral Surg Oral Med Oral Pathol Oral Radiol Endod 79(1): 24–29.
20. Kajii T, Imai T, Kajii S, Iida J (2001) Presence of third molar germs in orthodontic patients in Japan. Am J Orthod Dentofacial Orthop 119(3): 245–250.
21. Lee SH, Lee JY, Park HK, Kim YK (2009) Development of third molars in Korean juveniles and adolescents. Forensic Sci Int 188: 107–11.
22. Sandhu S, Kaur T (2005) Radiographic evaluation of the status of third molars in the Asian–Indian students. J Oral Maxillofac Surg 63(5): 640–645.
23. Mok YY, Ho KK (1996) Congenitally absent third molars in 12 to 16 year old Singaporean Chinese patients: a retrospective radiographic study. Ann Acad Med Singapore 25: 828–30.
24. Jacob J, Phrabhakaran N, Shani AM, Nor Himazian M, Nur Fazwani A, Norain Azman M (2012) Third molar agenesis among children and youths from three major races of Malaysians. J Dent Sci 7(3): 211–217.
25. Garn SM, Lewis AB, Vicinus JH (1962) Third molar agenesis and reduction in the number of other teeth. J Dent Res 41: 717.
26. Bishara SE (1999) Third molars: a dilemma! Or is it? Am J Orthod Dentofacial Orthop 115: 628–633.
27. Sanchez MJ, Vicente A, Bravo LA (2009) Third molar agenesis and craniofacial morphology. Angle Orthod 79(3): 473–8.
28. Vandenbroucke JP, von Elm E, Altman DG, Gotzsche PC, Mulrow CD, Pocock SJ et al. (2007) Strengthening the reporting of observational studies in epidemiology (STROBE): Explanation and elaboration. Plos Med 4: e297.
29. Houston WJB (1983) The analysis of error in orthodontic measurements. Am J Orthod 83: 382–390.
30. Kleinbaum DG (1994) Logistic regression. Springer.
31. Kajii TS, Sato Y, Kajii S, Sugawara Y, Iida J (2004) Agenesis of third molar germs depends on sagittal maxillary jaw dimensions in orthodontic patients in Japan. Angle Orthod 74: 337–342.

7

Characterization of Novel MSX1 Mutations Identified in Japanese Patients with Nonsyndromic Tooth Agenesis

Seishi Yamaguchi[1,2,3], Junichiro Machida[1,7], Munefumi Kamamoto[1,5], Masashi Kimura[1,3], Akio Shibata[1,3], Tadashi Tatematsu[1,3], Hitoshi Miyachi[1], Yujiro Higashi[3], Peter Jezewski[6], Atsuo Nakayama[4], Kazuo Shimozato[1], Yoshihito Tokita[1,3]*

1 Department of Maxillofacial Surgery, School of Dentistry, Aichi-Gakuin University, Nagoya, Aichi, Japan, **2** Department of Dentistry and Oral Surgery, Aichi Children's Health and Medical Center, Obu, Aichi, Japan, **3** Department of Perinatology, Institute for Developmental Research, Aichi Human Service Center, Kasugai, Aichi, Japan, **4** Department of Embryology, Institute for Developmental Research, Aichi Human Service Center, Kasugai, Aichi, Japan, **5** Department of Oral and Maxillofacial Surgery, Japanese Red Cross Society Himeji Hospital, Himeji, Hyogo, Japan, **6** Department of Periodontology, University of Alabama at Birmingham School of Dentistry, Institute of Oral Health Research, Birmingham, Alabama, United States of America, **7** Department of Oral and Maxillofacial Surgery, Toyota Memorial Hospital, Toyota, Aichi, Japan

Abstract

Since *MSX1* and *PAX9* are linked to the pathogenesis of nonsyndromic tooth agenesis, we performed detailed mutational analysis of these two genes sampled from Japanese patients. We identified two novel *MSX1* variants with an amino acid substitution within the homeodomain; Thr174Ile (T174I) from a sporadic hypodontia case and Leu205Arg (L205R) from a familial oligodontia case. Both the Thr174 and Leu205 residues in the MSX1 homeodomain are highly conserved among different species. To define possible roles of mutations at these amino acids in the pathogenesis of nonsyndromic tooth agenesis, we performed several functional analyses. It has been demonstrated that MSX1 plays a pivotal role in hard tissue development as a suppressor for mesenchymal cell differentiation. To evaluate the suppression activity of the variants in mesenchymal cells, we used the *myoD*-promoter, which is one of convenient reporter assay system for MSX1. Although the gene products of these *MSX1* variants are stable and capable of normal nuclear localization, they do not suppress *myoD*-promoter activity in differentiated C2C12 cells. To clarify the molecular mechanisms underlying our results, we performed further analyses including electrophoretic mobility shift assays, and co-immunoprecipitation assays to survey the molecular interactions between the mutant MSX1 proteins and the oligonucleotide DNA with MSX1 consensus binding motif or EZH2 methyltransferase. Since EZH2 is reported to interact with MSX1 and regulate MSX1 mediated gene suppression, we hypothesized that the T174I and L205R substitutions would impair this interaction. We conclude from the results of our experiments that the DNA binding ability of MSX1 is abolished by these two amino acid substitutions. This illustrates a causative role of the T174I and L205R MSX1 homeodomain mutations in tooth agenesis, and suggests that they may influence cell proliferation and differentiation resulting in lesser tooth germ formation *in vivo*.

Editor: Ludmila Prokunina-Olsson, National Cancer Institute, National Institutes of Health, United States of America

Funding: This study was supported in part by grants from the Institute for Developmental Research, Aichi-Human Service Center (YT), and from the Aichi-Gakuin University, School of Dentistry (KS). The funders had no role in study design, data collection and analysis, decision to publish, or preparation of the manuscript.

Competing Interests: The authors have declared that no competing interests exist.

* Email: tokita@inst-hsc.jp

Introduction

Coding mutations within *MSX1* and *PAX9* have been identified in patients with either nonsyndromic or syndromic forms of tooth agenesis [1–9]. Based on the number of missing permanent teeth, excluding the third molars, tooth agenesis is classified into three categories. Hypodontia is generally defined as agenesis with the absence of less than six teeth, oligodontia is a condition in which six or more teeth are missing, and anodontia is the term used for complete tooth loss. Both in vivo and in vitro studies have revealed that Msx1 and Pax9 are essential for the induction of bone morphogenetic protein 4 (Bmp4), which is regarded as the pivotal step in mammalian tooth development [10]. Whilst the induction of BMP4 is considered to play the principal role in tooth germ development, repression of mesenchymal cell differentiation mediated by MSX1 has also been demonstrated to be a pivotal step for early development of hard tissues [12]. In addition, it is noteworthy that MSX1 by itself, unlike PAX9, cannot activate the Bmp4-promoter in vitro, but can potentiate PAX9 activity as a synergic cofactor. The molecular mechanism of human tooth agenesis mediated by MSX1 mutation is however independent of PAX9, since most MSX1 mutations related to oligodontia can potentiate PAX9-induced Bmp4-promoter activation [11]. Furthermore, it has been reported that MSX1 reduces the expression level of several genes that promote mesenchymal cell differentiation both in vitro [13], and in vivo [12]. Hence, to evaluate the ability of transcriptional gene repression of MSX1 mutation, we selected *MyoD*-promoter since it is a well-characterized system to assess the MSX1 mediated gene suppression activity [14–16]. In addition to this, it has been demonstrated previously that the molecular interaction between Msx1 and Enhancer of Zeste 2 (EZH2) histone H3 methyltransferase, one of the components of PRC2 (polycomb repressive complex 2), is required to suppress mesenchymal cell differentiation both in vitro and in vivo [12].

According to that report, EZH2 mediates gene suppression via the enrichment of tri-methylated histone H3 at lysine 27 on MSX1 genomic binding sites and ectopic myoblast cell differentiation is observed in the limb bones of MSX1-deficient mice [12]. The evidence to date thus suggests that the role of MSX1 is to prevent cell differentiation, and to maintain dental mesenchymal cells in a proliferative state to ensure robust tooth germ formation. We therefore hypothesize that EZH2 is the central player in the downstream cascade of MSX1 during the early development of human hard tissue, including permanent teeth.

In our current study, we describe two novel variants of the *MSX1* gene identified in two Japanese patients with isolated tooth agenesis. Since both of these variants involved amino acid substitutions in the MH4/homeodomain of MSX1, we performed functional analyses to confirm their pathogenicity. We conclude from our analysis that these amino acid substitutions are etiologic because they impair the transcriptional repression of MSX1 due to a loss of the DNA binding ability of the mutant proteins, whilst exhibiting no differences from wild-type MSX1 in terms of nuclear localization and molecular interactions with EZH2.

Subjects and Methods

Patients

This study was approved by the Committee on the Ethics of Human Experimentation, Aichi-Gakuin University, and the Institute for Developmental Research. A blood or hair sample was obtained from the participants with written informed consent. Well-characterized Japanese tooth agenesis patients were investigated in this study (four oligodontia cases involving the absence of six or more permanent teeth excluding the third molars; and 15 hypodontia cases with an absence of one to five permanent teeth excluding the third molars). The diagnoses of all patients were based on X-rays or study models. The control group comprised 100 Japanese samples from unrelated individuals who had no family history of tooth agenesis and/or facial malformation.

Sequencing and Mutation Analysis of Candidate Genes

All exons of the *MSX1* and *PAX9* genes including the splice sites were sequenced. The primers for *MSX1* and *PAX9* have been described previously [6,17,18]. The sizes of the amplified DNA fragments were as follows: *MSX1* exon1, 766 bp; exon2, 698 bp; *PAX9* exon1, 273 bp; exon2, 695 bp; exon3, 264 bp; exon4, 450 bp. The PCR products were sequenced using the BigDye Terminator v1.1 Cycle Sequencing Kit (Applied Biosystems, Foster City, CA) as previously described [19].

Plasmids

To construct the variant MSX1 expression vectors, *in vitro* site-directed mutagenesis was performed with FLAG-tagged human wild-type MSX1 [6] as a template. The amplified DNA fragments were subcloned into pcDNA3 (Invitrogen, San Diego, CA). The *myoD*-reporter plasmid (6.9 kb of DNA fragment of *myoD*-promoter region-driven firefly luciferase) [20] and myc-EZH2 plasmid [21] were kindly provided by Dr. Cory Abate-Shen (Columbia University) and Dr. Akiko Murayama (University of Tsukuba), respectively.

3D Models of MSX1 Variants

Since the MH4/homeodomain protein sequence in MSX1 is conserved between human and mouse, 3D structural data of the mouse Msx1-DNA molecular complex was retrieved from the NCBI Brookhaven Protein Data Bank (PDB) database (PDB ID, 1IG7) and used as a modeling template. The 3D models of the MSX1 variants were generated using Waals software ver. 1.1.2. (Altif Laboratories Inc., Tokyo, Japan) based on crystal structure.

Culture conditions for C2C12 Cell Differentiation

The mouse C2C12 cell line (ATCC CRL-1772; American Type Culture Collection, Manassas, VA) can differentiate into muscle, adipocyte, or osteoblastic lineages [22–24]. According to previous reports, these cells are maintained in Dulbecco's modified Eagle's medium (DMEM; Sigma) containing 20% fetal bovine serum. Differentiation was induced using differentiation medium containing DMEM and 2% horse serum.

DNA Transfection and Luciferase Reporter Assays

DNA transfections and luciferase assays were performed according to previously reported methods with minor modifications [6,25]. Briefly, transfection experiments were carried out in mouse C2C12 cells at 40–50% confluence using Lipofectamine 2000 (Invitrogen) in accordance with the manufacturer's instructions. Each transfection was done in triplicate in a gelatin coated 24-well plate (Iwaki glass, Tokyo, Japan) with 2.0 µg of *myoD*-firefly luciferase reporter vector, 3–20 ng of MSX1 expression vectors, and 2 ng of pRL-TK, an expression vector for sea pansy (*Renilla reniformis*) luciferase used as an internal control. Cells were incubated for 72 hours after transfection. Firefly luciferase and Renilla luciferase activities were measured in a luminometer using the Dual Luciferase Reporter assay system kit (Promega, Madison, WI). Cells were lysed in 100 µl of passive lysis buffer with agitation for 30 minutes at room temperature and 10 µl aliquots were used for measurements. Luciferase activity elicited by the *myoD*-promoter constructs was normalized for variations in transfection efficiency using Renilla luciferase as an internal standard.

Western Blotting

Western blotting was done as described previously [26] with minor modifications. Briefly, HEK293 transfectants were extracted with lysis buffer (1% Triton X-100, 1 mM EDTA in Tris-buffered saline; TBS) and these lysates were subjected to SDS-PAGE (12% gel), and transferred to Immobilon-P membranes (Millipore Corporation, Bedford, MA). The membranes were probed with an anti-FLAG M2 monoclonal antibody (1:2000; Sigma, St. Louis, MO), and signals on the blots were detected with a horseradish peroxidase-conjugated secondary antibody and ECL2 reagent (Amersham Life Science, Cleveland, OH).

Immunoprecipitation

HEK293 cells were cultured in DMEM supplemented with 10% FBS and transfected with FLAG-MSX1 and myc-EZH2 expression vectors. The cells were then treated with lysis buffer (10 mM Tris, pH 7.4, 150 mM NaCl, 1 mM EDTA, 0.1 mM dithiothreitol, 1% Triton X-100). MSX1 variants were immunoprecipitated from the lysates with anti-FLAG M2 monoclonal antibody and protein G sepharose beads (GE Healthcare Life Sciences, Piscataway, NJ). After washing of the beads, the samples were run on a 9% SDS-PAGE gel and analyzed by Western blotting with an anti-myc antibody.

Immunolocalization of Variant MSX1 Proteins in Mammalian Cells

To demonstrate the *in vivo* expression of wild-type and mutant MSX1, HEK293 cells were transfected with expression vectors for these products using Lipofectamine 2000 (Invitrogen, Grand Island, NY) as described previously [6]. Forty-eight hours post-

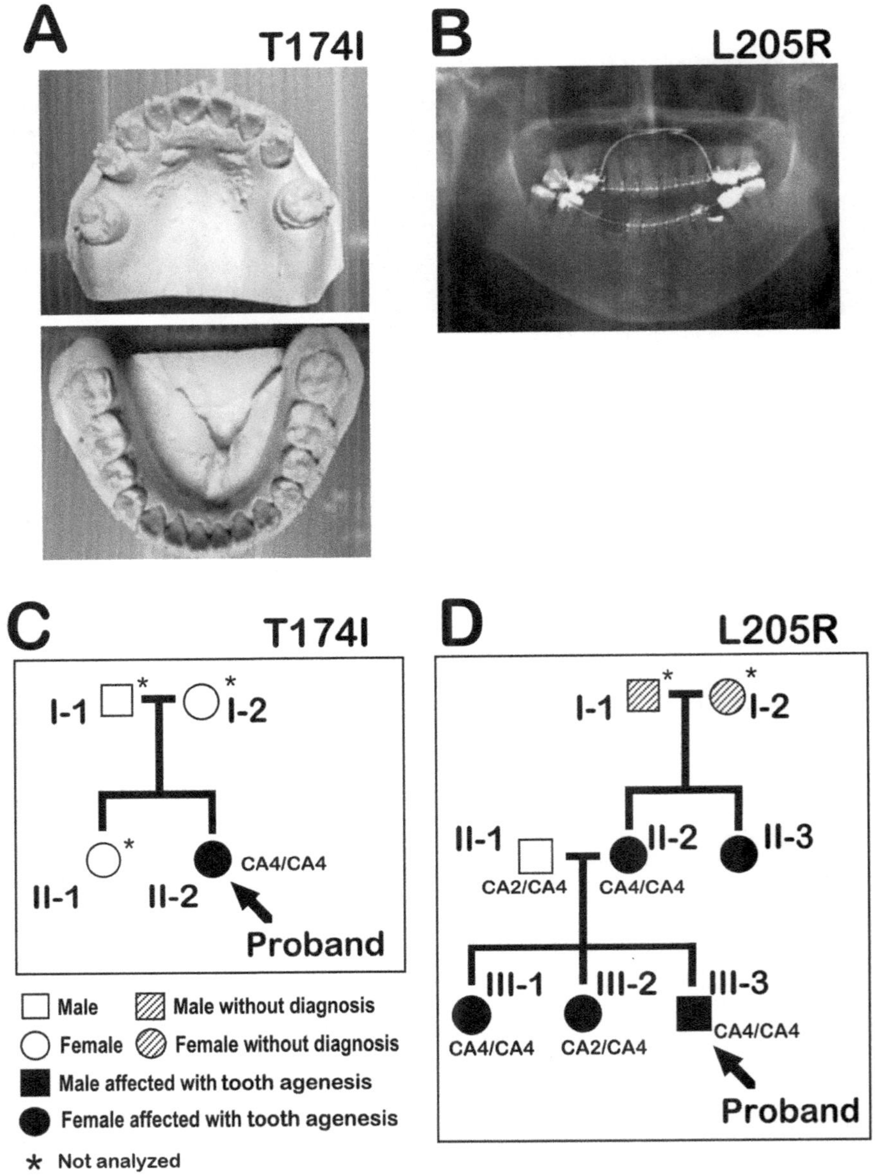

Figure 1. Pedigree analysis of tooth agenesis. A: Plaster cast of the maxillary (upper panel), and mandibular (lower panel) of the T174I proband exhibiting five missing teeth. **B:** Panoramic radiograph of the L205R proband with nine missing teeth. **C and D:** Pedigree for the tooth agenesis family of both the T174I (C), and L205R (D) probands. Darkened symbols represent affected, clear symbols indicate normal unaffected, hatched symbols indicate unable to diagnose caused by acquired tooth loss, squares indicate males, and circles indicate females. A type of CA-repeat polymorphism in the *MSX1* intron is indicated i.e. CA1 (12×CAs), CA2 (11×CAs), CA3 (10×CAs), CA4 (9×CAs), CA5 (8×CAs). Asterisks indicate family members that were not analyzed.

transfection, the cells were fixed with 4% paraformaldehyde/TBS and permeabilized with 1% Triton X-100/TBS prior to incubation with an anti-FLAG M2 monoclonal antibody (1:1000) for 60 minutes at 37°C. The cells were then incubated for 60 minutes at room temperature with DAPI (1 μg/ml), Alexa-488 phalloidin (2 U/ml), and Cy3-conjugated goat anti-mouse antibody (Jackson ImmunoResearch Laboratories Inc., West Grove, PA, 1:1000), respectively, in PBS. After washing of the cells with PBS three times, immunostaining signals were visualized under an Olympus BH-2 microscope.

Electrophoretic Mobility Shift Assay (EMSA)

EMSA was performed as described previously [21]. Briefly, complementary oligonucleotides harboring the MSX1 binding sequence (5′-CATGACCCCAATTAGTCCTGGCAG-3′ and 5′-gtgCTGCCAGGACTAATTGGGGTCATG-3′) were annealed and labeled with [α-^{32}P]dCTP [27]. The labeled probe at volumes corresponding to 10,000–20,000 cpm was incubated with 5 μl of cell lysates (prepared as described above) in a total volume of 15 μl (10 mM HEPES, 50 mM KCl, 0.1 mM EDTA, 1 mM dithiothreitol, 10 mM MgCl, and 10% glycerol), containing 1 μg of poly(dI-dC) for 15 minutes at room temperature. The reactions were analyzed by non-denaturing 4% polyacrylamide gel

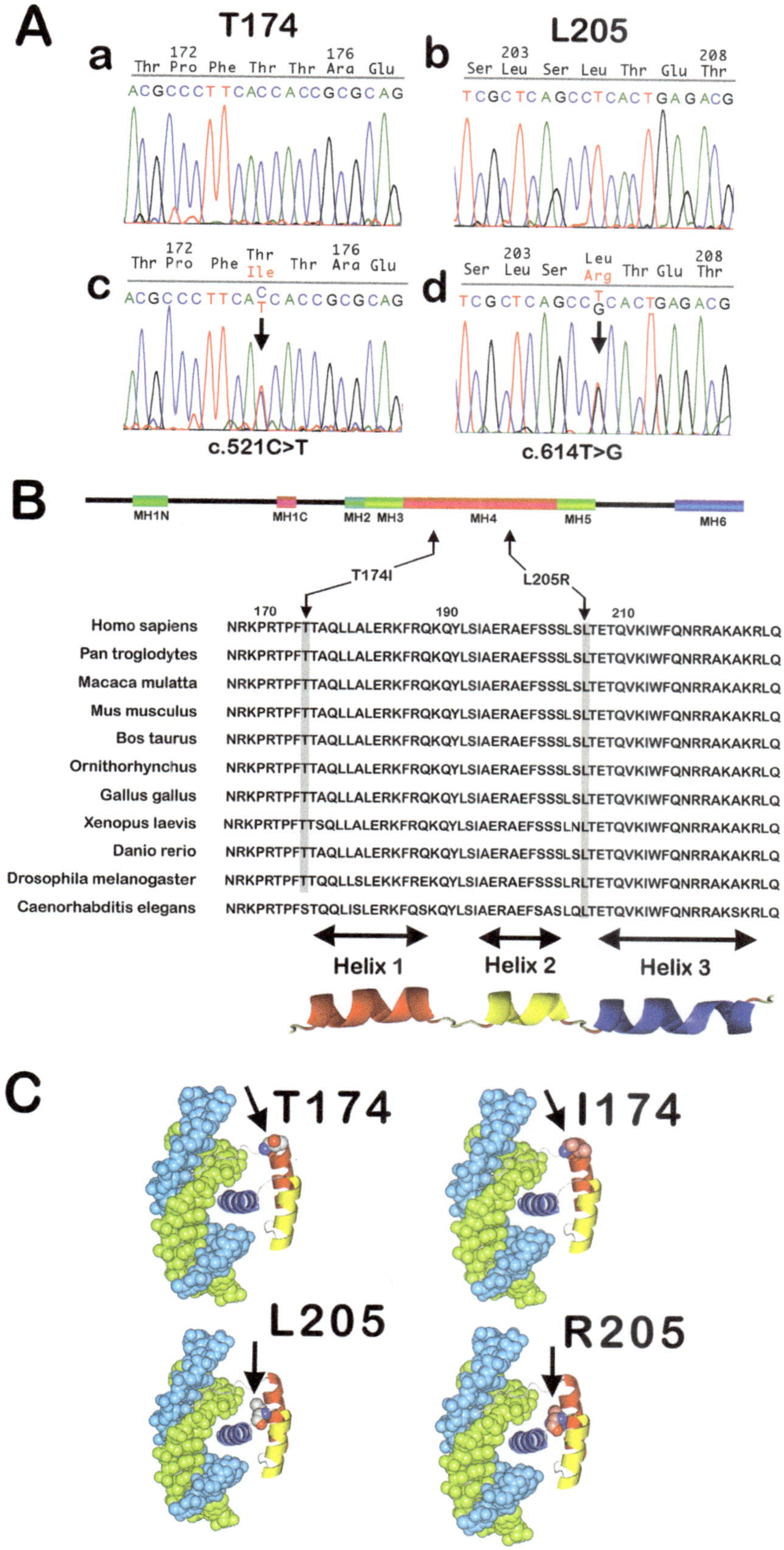

Figure 2. MSX1 variants isolated from tooth agenesis patients. A: DNA sequences of MSX1 exon 2 in unaffected (a and b) and affected (c and d) individuals. The C-T transition at position 521 (T174I), and T-G transition in position 614 (L205R) in the mutant sequences cause amino acid substitutions within the MH4/homeodomain of MSX1. **B:** Schematic representation of the human MSX1 protein. Multiple sequence alignments of the MSX1 MH4/homeodomain sequences sorted by species and homology are shown. Sequences were obtained from the SwissProt database and thereby aligned. Conservation of the key Thr174 and Leu205 amino acids (black arrows) across species is indicated by gray shading. The leucine at

position 205 is universally conserved at that position but the threonine at position 174 is replaced by serine, which has a similar polarity, in *C. elegans* Msx1 (See Additional file 1 in [43]). **C:** 3D models of mutant and wild-type MSX1 based on the crystal structures of the Msx1 MH4/homeodomain in complex with DNA (PDB ID 1IG7).

electrophoresis. For supershift assays, 2 μg of anti-FLAG M2 monoclonal antibody was added to the binding reaction.

Results

Pedigree and Diagnosis

We analyzed the *MSX1* and *PAX9* nucleotide sequences of 19 Japanese tooth agenesis patients, and thereby identified two novel mutations in the *MSX1* gene (Fig. 1, 2A, B). The first case harboring a novel *MSX1* variant was an apparent sporadic form of hypodontia in a 23-year-old female proband involving five missing teeth (plus the absence of an additional four third molars for a total of nine missing teeth; Fig. 1A, C). Unfortunately, we were forced to exclude the other members of her family from this study as we could not obtain informed consent. There was, however, no family history of congenitally missing teeth (assessed by medical interview). The second case was determined to be a familial case of oligodontia, wherein five of eight family members were affected in the pedigree through three generations (Fig. 1B, D). The proband (III-3) was a 26-year-old male missing 9 teeth (plus an additional four missing third molars for a total of 13 missing teeth). His two sisters (III-1 and III-2) also exhibited an oligodontia phenotype (Table 1). No orofacial cleft or other craniofacial abnormalities and no *PAX9* gene variations were present in any members of the families of these two cases.

In another pedigree investigated in this study, we identified one sporadic hypodontia case with a unilateral cleft lip and palate, but no *MSX1* or *PAX9* gene variations were detected. All the mothers of the probands had neither been smokers nor habitual drinkers. All of the primary teeth of these study participants were reported to be normal in size, shape, and number.

Mutation Search in Tooth Agenesis Patients

We analyzed the entire coding regions of the *MSX1* and *PAX9* genes. Two novel single-base substitutions were identified in the *MSX1* gene of two unrelated patients: a C to T transition at nucleotide 521 (C521T, T-allele: ACGCCCTTCA***C/T***CACCGCGCAG), and a T to G transition at nucleotide 614 (T614G, G-allele: TCGCTCAGCC***T/G***CACTGAGACG), and not in the unaffected members of the corresponding families (Fig. 2A). These variants had not been previously recorded in the 1000 Genomes Project database, dbSNP 137 database, or UCSC browser database. In addition, these variants were not evident in 200 normal Japanese control chromosomes (not shown), nor among 500 other population control individuals as described in our previous report [18], giving a global allele frequency estimation of <.001. The C to T transversion results in a replacement of threonine with isoleucine at position 174 (T174I), and the T to G transversion a substitution of the leucine residue at position 205 with arginine (L205R), within the MH4/homeodomain region of *MSX1* (Fig. 2B, C).

MyoD-Promoter Repression Activity of MSX1 Variants in vitro

It has been reported that MSX1 suppresses *myoD*-promoter activity and maintains cell proliferation during mesenchymal cell differentiation. Thus, the transcriptional regulation activities of the novel MSX1 variants in our current study were measured in a mesenchymal cell line, C2C12, transfected with a luciferase-reporter vector containing the *myoD*-promoter. A considerable level of luciferase activity was measured in differentiated C2C12 cells in this assay. In addition, whereas the reporter activity was remarkably reduced in the wild-type MSX1 transfected cells in a dose-dependent manner, no repression activity was detectable in the MSX1 variant-transfected cells (Fig. 3Aa, b). However, the stability of these variant proteins appeared to be unaffected by the amino acid substitutions since we could not detect any significant differences in the protein expression level between wild-type MSX1 and the T174I or L205R mutant proteins (Fig. 3B).

DNA Binding Ability of the MSX1 variants

Electrophoretic mobility shift assay (EMSA) analyses showed that the DNA-binding ability of the MSX1 protein was abolished by either the T174I or L205R mutations. Since there were two molecular complexes detected by a DNA probe containing the MSX1 consensus binding site (indicated by the small arrowhead and arrow in Fig. 3Ca, lane 1), we performed an additional supershift assay with an anti-FLAG antibody to confirm that these were FLAG-MSX1 containing complexes. The results showed that one of the molecular complexes indeed contained FLAG-MSX1, as previously reported [27], because the FLAG-MSX1/DNA complex (indicated by the arrow) was shifted to a higher molecular weight following incubation with an anti-FLAG antibody (Fig. 3Cb, lane 2, large arrowhead). The protein indicated by the small arrowhead is therefore an unknown endogenous protein in the HEK293 cells. In contrast to the wild-type MSX1 protein (Fig. 3Ca, lane 1, arrow), the mutant T174I or L205R MSX1 variants showed an absence of DNA binding activity (Fig. 3Ca, lanes 2–4).

Molecular Interactions between the MSX1 Variants and EZH2

Since the C-terminus incorporating the MH4/homeodomain of MSX1 is responsible for the interaction with EZH2 [12], we investigated whether the T174I or L205R substitutions could disrupt this complex formation. However, no significant differences were detected between wild-type and T174I or L205R variants with respect to molecular complex formation with the EZH2 protein (Fig. 3D).

Nuclear Localization of the T174I or L205R MSX1 proteins

The homeodomain of MSX1 is also responsible for the nuclear localization of this protein [11]. Thus, we investigated whether the T174I or L205R mutations had any effect on this process. HEK293 cells were transfected with plasmids encoding FLAG-tagged wild-type, T174I or L205R MSX1. By immunocytochemistry, FLAG signals were equally localized in the nucleus in all transfectants at 48 hours post-transfection (Fig. 4).

CA-repeat in the MSX1 Intron

It has been suggested that the tooth phenotypes may be a subphenotype of oral-facial clefting disorders [28]. The intronic CA-repeat (CA4) has been shown to be associated with oral-facial clefting [29,30], whereas the CA2 allele is known to be significantly undertransmitted in a biallelic model of oral facial clefting [31–33], and may be protective against that phenotype. Although it is conceivable that the complex disease alleles marked

Table 1. Summary of Tooth Agenesis Phenotypes in the L205R and T174I families.

Pedigree ID		*Congenitally Missing Permanent Teeth																
Dental Arch		**Right**								**Left**								
A	**T174I**	**8**	**7**	**6**	**5**	**4**	**3**	**2**	**1**	**1**	**2**	**3**	**4**	**5**	**6**	**7**	**8**	
	II-2:																	MSX1- c.521C>T T174I (heterozygous)
	Maxillary	*	*		*								*	*		*	*	
	Mandibular	*															*	
B	**L205R**	**8**	**7**	**6**	**5**	**4**	**3**	**2**	**1**	**1**	**2**	**3**	**4**	**5**	**6**	**7**	**8**	
	II-1																	no mutations in MSX1
	Maxillary	no congenitally missing teeth																
	Mandibular																	
	II-2				hypodontia, but it's unknown which teeth are congenitally missing													MSX1- c.614T>G L205R (heterozygous)
	Maxillary																	
	Mandibular																	
	III-1																	MSX1- c.614T>G L205R (heterozygous)
	Maxillary	?	*	*		*			*	*	*		*		*		?	
	Mandibular	?		*	*	*	*		*	*		*	*	*	*		?	
	III-2																	MSX1- c.614T>G L205R (heterozygous)
	Maxillary	*			*			*				*		*			*	
	Mandibular	*			*	*							*	*			*	
	III-3:																	MSX1- c.614T>G L205R (heterozygous)
	Maxillary	*			*	*							*	*			*	
	Mandibular	*			*	*		*					*	*			*	

1, central incisor; 2, lateral incisor; 3, canine; 4 and 5, first and second premolars, respectively; and 6–8, first, second, and third molars, respectively.

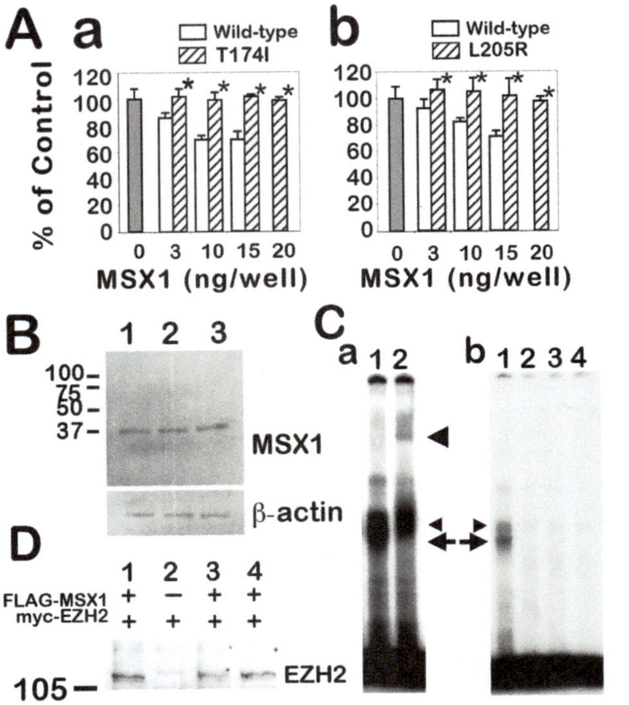

Figure 3. Functional analysis of tooth agenesis-causing MSX1 mutations. A: *myoD*-promoter repression activity of T174I and L205R variants in C2C12 cells. The C2C12 cells were cotransfected with an MSX1 expression vector, the firefly luciferase reporter gene driven by the *myoD*-promoter and sea pansy luciferase reporter gene driven by the thymidine kinase promoter. After differentiation treatments, firefly luciferase activity was measured and normalized with respect to the sea pansy luciferase activity. Open bars indicate human wild-type MSX1 transfectant data (3–15 ng/well); hatched bars denote data from experiments utilizing transfectants of the T174I (a) and L205R (b) variants of MSX1 (3–20 ng/well), respectively. The relative luciferase activity is expressed as a percentage of the negative control (gray bars). Each transfection point was carried out in triplicate in a gelatin-coated 24-well plate. The experiments were performed three times and representative data are shown. Error bars indicate standard deviation. Asterisks indicate no significant differences against the control (P-value >0.1). **B:** Stability and expression level of wild-type and mutant proteins. Western blot analysis was performed using extracts prepared from HEK293 cells transfected with FLAG-wild-type-MSX1 (lane 1), FLAG-T174I-MSX1 (lane 2) or FLAG-L205R-MSX1 (lane 3). These whole-cell extracts were immunoblotted with an anti-FLAG antibody (upper panel) and anti-beta actin antibody as an internal standard (lower panel). **C:** Electrophoretic mobility shift assay of MSX1. **a:** A double-stranded oligonucleotide probe containing a consensus binding-site for MSX1 interacts with proteins in the wild-type MSX1 transfectant cell lysate (lane 1, arrow and small arrowhead). The DNA binding ability of MSX1 is diminished by the T174I and L205R substitutions. Wild-type-MSX1 protein and oligo DNA complex observed in lane 1 (arrow) was not detected in the MSX1 variant transfectant lysates (lane 2, T174I-MSX1; lane 3, L205R-MSX1), or HEK293 parental cells (lane 4, negative control). **b:** Supershift experiments using an anti-FLAG antibody. The binding specificity was confirmed by a super-shift induction with anti-FLAG antibody (lane 2). A protein-DNA-antibody complex formed (large arrowhead), and the band indicated by the arrow disappeared. This indicates that this molecular complex denoted by the arrow contained FLAG-tagged wild-type MSX1 protein, and that the protein indicated by the small arrowhead is an unknown product that bound to the probe. **D:** Molecular interaction between MSX1 and EZH2 histone methyltransferase. Myc-EZH2 protein was coimmunoprecipitated with FLAG-MSX1 (lane 1). EZH2 protein was not detected in the MSX1-null EZH2 transfectant HEK293 cell lysate (lane 2). The MSX1-EZH2 interaction was observed in the FLAG-T174I-MSX1 sample (lane 3), and in the FLAG-L205R-MSX1 sample (lane 4).

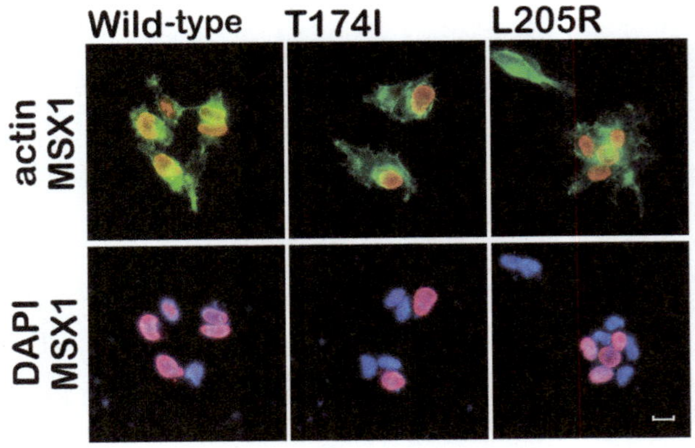

Figure 4. Nuclear localization of MSX1 variants. Immunolocalizations of FLAG-tagged wild-type, T174I, and L205R MSX1 products were similar when these variants were expressed in HEK293 cells. MSX1 (FLAG, red signal); nuclei (DAPI, blue signal). Cell morphologies were visualized by F-actin staining (Phalloidin, green signal). Neither the T174I nor L205R mutation affects the nuclear localization of MSX1 in vitro. Scale bar 20 μm.

by these CA-repeats could potentially influence the tooth phenotype, our DNA sequencing revealed that the CA-repeat genotype of the T174I proband was unexpectedly homozygous for the CA4 allele (9×CAs; Fig. 1C). Moreover, a heterozygous CA2 allele (11×CAs) was found in one of the affected family members in the L205R pedigree (Fig. 1D; III-2).

Discussion

We have found in our current study that MSX1 mutations in a familial-form of oligodontia (in a proband with a 13 tooth-loss including four third molars), and in an apparently sporadic-form of hypodontia (a proband with a nine tooth-loss including four third molars; Fig. 1). These mutations are contained within the beginning of the 1st helix of the MH4/homeodomain (T174I) and at the loop domain between the 2nd and 3rd helix in the MH4/homeodomain (L205R), which are highly conserved regions among various species (Fig. 2B, C). We show from reporter analysis using the *myoD*-promoter that both amino acid substitutions affect the transcriptional suppression activity of MSX1, which is one of key molecular mechanisms in mesenchymal cell differentiation (Fig. 3Aa, b). Our EMSA results indicate that the normal MSX1 DNA binding ability is impaired by the T174I and L205R mutations (Fig. 3C). Cory and colleagues have described in their previous report that the EZH2 protein binds to the C-terminus of MSX1 that incorporates its homeodomain [12]. We thus investigated whether these mutations affected the EZH2 binding ability of MSX1. Although we found that these variants can still interact with EZH2 (Fig. 3D) and show a normal subcellular-localization (Fig. 4), the loss of DNA binding ability in these mutant proteins would likely affect the recruitment of EZH2 to the MSX1 target genes that relate to mesenchymal cell differentiation, a process which needs to be suppressed for tooth germ formation.

The MH4/homeodomain of MSX1 is a DNA binding domain that assembles into a three-helical chain fold. The N-terminal arm of this domain is composed of nine amino acid residues, and the 2nd and 3rd helices are arranged in a helix-turn-helix motif (Fig. 2B). Crystallographic studies of the MSX1 homeodomain in complex with DNA have revealed a general model of DNA recognition by homeoproteins [34–36]. According to these studies, homeodomains contact their target DNA regions in the major and minor groove using their third helix and N-terminal arm, respectively. In the case of MSX1, the T174 residue contacts the minor groove of the DNA as a part of the N-terminal arm [37] (Fig. 2C). On the other hand, the polypeptide segment Ser204-Leu205-Ser206-Leu207 forms a type IV beta-bend in the predicted structure of the 2nd and 3rd helix of the MH4/homeodomain [38]. Thus, an amino acid substitution at this segment may affect the bend angle between the 2nd and 3rd helices. It is therefore plausible that the T174I and L205R substitutions directly impair DNA binding by MSX1. We were unable to observe any influence of the CA association markers within the families that we evaluated in our current analyses, since a significant correlation between the CA-repeat mutations and tooth phenotypes was not observed in these pedigrees (Fig. 1C, D).

Since our T174I proband was classified as a case of hypodontia based on well-established standards, we had expected that the T174I substitution would partially diminish the suppression activity of MSX1 against the *myoD*-promoter in a manner similar to another MSX1 variant that we previously described [6]. The *myoD*-promoter suppression activity was, however, found to be similar to that of the L205R variant (Fig. 3A), which causes a more severe phenotype (Table 1). There are two possible explanations for this finding. First, it has been reported that the R196P MSX1 mutant isolated from an oligodontia pedigree [1] loses its ability to suppress another MSX1 target, WIP-element [39], which is a regulatory element for restricted expression of Wnt-1 protein in the embryonic mouse forebrain [40]. In the R196P pedigree, the numbers of missing teeth range from 4 to 13. Therefore, it is possible that the T174I substitution may also relate to a more severe tooth agenesis phenotype, and such variable expressivity may result from varying genetic backgrounds associated with the risk of nonsyndromic tooth agenesis [41,42]. Second, there may be differences between the MSX1 transcriptional regulation that occurs at the *myoD*-promoter and at other promoters related to odontoblast differentiation such as bmp2, bmp4, and runx2, which have been previously shown to be suppressed by MSX1 [13].

Further studies are needed to evaluate MSX1 variants related to tooth agenesis including a deficiency in the regulatory activity of histone H3 tri-methylation. In any case, we show from our current analysis that Thr174 and Leu205 are both crucial for a properly functioning MSX1 MH4/homeodomain structure and robust odontogenesis.

Acknowledgments

We thank all of the family members and dentists who participated in this study. We are grateful also to Dr. Cory Abate-Shen (Columbia University) for kindly providing the *myoD*-reporter plasmid and to Dr. Akiko Murayama (University of Tsukuba) for donating the EZH2 expression vector. This study was supported in part by grants from the Institute for Developmental Research, Aichi-Human Service Center (YT), and from the Aichi-Gakuin University, School of Dentistry (KS). The authors declare no conflicts of interest.

Author Contributions

Conceived and designed the experiments: JM HM YH PJ KS YT. Performed the experiments: SY M. Kamamoto M. Kimura AS TT AN. Analyzed the data: SY YT. Contributed reagents/materials/analysis tools: SY JM HM KS. Wrote the paper: SY YT.

References

1. Vastardis H, Karimbux N, Guthua SW, Seidman JG, Seidman CE (1996) A human MSX1 homeodomain missense mutation causes selective tooth agenesis. Nat Genet: 417–421.
2. Stockton DW, Das P, Goldenberg M, D'Souza RN, Patel PI (2000) Mutation of PAX9 is associated with oligodontia. Nat Genet 24: 18–19.
3. van den Boogaard MJ, Dorland M, Beemer FA, van Amstel HK (2000) MSX1 mutation is associated with orofacial clefting and tooth agenesis in humans. Nat Genet 24: 342–343.
4. Jumlongras D, Bei M, Stimson JM, Wang WF, DePalma SR, et al. (2001) A nonsense mutation in MSX1 causes Witkop syndrome. Am J Hum Genet 69: 67–74.
5. Das P, Stockton DW, Bauer C, Shaffer LG, D'Souza RN, et al. (2002) Haploinsufficiency of PAX9 is associated with autosomal dominant hypodontia. Hum Genet 110: 371–376.
6. Kamamoto M, Machida J, Yamaguchi S, Kimura M, Ono T, et al. (2011) Clinical and functional data implicate the Arg(151)Ser variant of MSX1 in familial hypodontia. Eur J Hum Genet 19: 844–850.
7. Mostowska A, Biedziak B, Jagodzinski PP (2012) Novel MSX1 mutation in a family with autosomal-dominant hypodontia of second premolars and third molars. Arch Oral Biol 57: 790–795.
8. Liang J, Zhu L, Meng L, Chen D, Bian Z (2012) Novel nonsense mutation in MSX1 causes tooth agenesis with cleft lip in a Chinese family. Eur J Oral Sci 120: 278–282.
9. Kimura M, Machida J, Yamaguchi S, Shibata A, Tatematsu T, et al. (2013) Novel nonsense mutation in MSX1 in familial nonsyndromic oligodontia: subcellular localization and role of homeodomain/MH4. Eur J Oral Sci: in press.
10. Chen Y, Bei M, Woo I, Satokata I, Maas R (1996) Msx1 controls inductive signaling in mammalian tooth morphogenesis. Development 122: 3035–3044.
11. Wang Y, Kong H, Mues G, D'Souza R (2011) Msx1 mutations: how do they cause tooth agenesis? J Dent Res 90: 311–316.
12. Wang J, Kumar RM, Biggs VJ, Lee H, Chen Y, et al. (2011) The Msx1 Homeoprotein Recruits Polycomb to the Nuclear Periphery during Development. Dev Cell 21: 575–588.
13. Feng XY, Zhao YM, Wang WJ, Ge LH (2013) Msx1 regulates proliferation and differentiation of mouse dental mesenchymal cells in culture. Eur J Oral Sci 121: 412–420.
14. Woloshin P, Song K, Degnin C, Killary AM, Goldhamer DJ, et al. (1995) MSX1 inhibits MyoD expression in fibroblast×10T½ cell hybrids. Cell 82: 611–620.
15. Lee H, Habas R, Abate-Shen C (2004) Msx1 Cooperates with Histone H1b for Inhibition of Transcription and Myogenesis. Science 304: 1675–1678.
16. Lee H, Quinn JC, Prasanth KV, Swiss VA, Economides KD, et al. (2006) PIAS1 confers DNA-binding specificity on the Msx1 homeoprotein. Genes Dev 20: 784–794.
17. Frazier-Bowers SA, Guo DC, Cavender A, Xue L, Evans B, et al. (2002) A novel mutation in human PAX9 causes molar oligodontia. J Dent Res 81: 129–133.
18. Jezewski PA, Vieira AR, Nishimura C, Ludwig B, Johnson M, et al. (2003) Complete sequencing shows a role for MSX1 in non-syndromic cleft lip and palate. J Med Genet 40: 399–407.
19. Kamamoto M, Machida J, Miyachi H, Ono T, Nakayama A, et al. (2011) A novel mutation in the C-terminal region of RUNX2/CBFA1 distal to the DNA-binding runt domain in a Japanese patient with cleidocranial dysplasia. Int J Oral Maxillofac Surg 40: 434–437.
20. Zhang H, Hu G, Wang H, Sciavolino P, Iler N, et al. (1997) Heterodimerization of Msx and Dlx homeoproteins results in functional antagonism. Mol Cell Biol 17: 2920–2932.
21. Nakayama A, Murakami H, Maeyama N, Yamashiro N, Sakakibara A, et al. (2003) Role for RFX transcription factors in non-neuronal cell-specific inactivation of the microtubule-associated protein MAP1A promoter. J Biol Chem 278: 233–240.
22. Murayama A, Ohmori K, Fujimura A, Minami H, Yasuzawa-Tanaka K, et al. (2008) Epigenetic control of rDNA loci in response to intracellular energy status. Cell 133: 627–639.
23. Urist MR, Strates BS (2008) Bone morphogenetic protein. J Dent Res. 50: 1392–1406.
24. Honda T, Yamamoto H, Ishii A, Inui M (2010) PDZRN3 negatively regulates BMP-2-induced osteoblast differentiation through inhibition of Wnt signaling. Mol Biol Cell 21: 3269–3277.
25. Yumimoto K, Matsumoto M, Onoyama I, Imaizumi K, Nakayama KI (2013) F-box and WD repeat domain-containing-7 (Fbxw7) protein targets endoplasmic reticulum-anchored osteogenic and chondrogenic transcriptional factors for degradation. J Biol Chem 288: 28488–28502.
26. Tokita Y, Keino H, Matsui F, Aono S, Ishiguro H, et al. (2001) Regulation of neuregulin expression in the injured rat brain and cultured astrocytes. J Neurosci 21: 1257–1264.
27. Shi X, Yang X, Chen D, Chang Z, Cao X (1999) Smad1 interacts with homeobox DNA-binding proteins in bone morphogenetic protein signaling. J Biol Chem 274: 13711–13717.
28. Letra A, Menezes R, Granjeiro JM, Vieira AR (2007) Defining subphenotypes for oral clefts based on dental development. J Dent Res 86: 986–991.
29. Hewitt JE, Clark LN, Ivens A, Williamson R (1991) Structure and sequence of the human homeobox gene HOX7. Genomics 11: 670–678.

30. Padanilam BJ, Stadler HS, Mills KA, McLeod LB, Solursh M, et al. (1992) Characterization of the human HOX 7 cDNA and identification of polymorphic markers. Hum Mol Genet 1: 407–410.
31. Lidral AC, Romitti PA, Basart AM, Doetschman T, Leysens NJ, et al. (1998) Association of MSX1 and TGFB3 with nonsyndromic clefting in humans. Am J Hum Genet 63: 557–568.
32. Vieira AR, Orioli IM, Castilla EE, Cooper ME, Marazita ML, et al. (2003) MSX1 and TGFB3 contribute to clefting in South America. J Dent Res 82: 289–292.
33. Suzuki Y, Jezewski PA, Machida J, Watanabe Y, Shi M, et al. (2004) In a Vietnamese population, MSX1 variants contribute to cleft lip and palate. Genet Med 6: 117–125.
34. Qian YQ, Billeter M, Otting G, Muller M, Gehring WJ, et al. (1989) The structure of the Antennapedia homeodomain determined by NMR spectroscopy in solution: comparison with prokaryotic repressors. Cell 59: 573–580.
35. Wolberger C, Vershon AK, Liu B, Johnson AD, Pabo CO (1991) Crystal structure of a MAT alpha 2 homeodomain-operator complex suggests a general model for homeodomain-DNA interactions. Cell 67: 517–528.
36. Klemm JD, Rould MA, Aurora R, Herr W, Pabo CO (1994) Crystal structure of the Oct-1 POU domain bound to an octamer site: DNA recognition with tethered DNA-binding modules. Cell 77: 21–32.
37. Li H, Tejero R, Monleon D, Bassolino-Klimas D, Abate-Shen C, et al. (1997) Homology modeling using simulated annealing of restrained molecular dynamics and conformational search calculations with CONGEN: application in predicting the three-dimensional structure of murine homeodomain Msx-1. Protein Sci 6: 956–970.
38. Lewis PN, Momany FA, Scheraga HA (1973) Chain reversals in proteins. Biochim Biophys Acta 303: 211–229.
39. Hu G, Vastardis H, Bendall AJ, Wang Z, Logan M, et al. (1998) Haploinsufficiency of MSX1: a mechanism for selective tooth agenesis. Mol Cell Biol 18: 6044–6051.
40. Iler N, Rowitch DH, Echelard Y, McMahon AP, Abate-Shen C, et al. (1995) A single homeodomain binding site confers spatial restriction of Wnt-1 expression in the developing brain. Mech Dev 53: 87–96.
41. van den Boogaard MJ, Creton M, Bronkhorst Y, van der Hout A, Hennekam E, et al. (2012) Mutations in WNT10A are present in more than half of isolated hypodontia cases. J Med Genet 49: 327–331.
42. Mostowska A, Biedziak B, Zadurska M, Dunin-Wilczynska I, Lianeri M, et al. (2013) Nucleotide variants of genes encoding components of the Wnt signalling pathway and the risk of non-syndromic tooth agenesis. Clin Genet 84: 429–440.
43. Finnerty JR, Mazza ME, Jezewski PA (2009) Domain duplication, divergence, and loss events in vertebrate Msx paralogs reveal phylogenomically informed disease markers. BMC Evol Biol 9: 18.

8

A Phage Display Selected 7-mer Peptide Inhibitor of the *Tannerella forsythia* Metalloprotease-Like Enzyme Karilysin Can Be Truncated to Ser-Trp-Phe-Pro

Peter Durand Skottrup[1]*, Grete Sørensen[1], Miroslaw Ksiazek[2], Jan Potempa[2,3], Erik Riise[1]

1 Biomolecular Interaction Group, Department of Drug Design and Pharmacology, Faculty of Health and Medical Sciences, University of Copenhagen, Copenhagen, Denmark, **2** Department of Microbiology, Faculty of Biochemistry, Biophysics and Biotechnology, Jagiellonian University, Krakow, Poland, **3** Oral Health and Systemic Diseases Research Group, University of Louisville, School of Dentistry, Louisville, Kentucky, United States of America

Abstract

Tannerella forsythia is a gram-negative bacteria, which is strongly associated with the development of periodontal disease. Karilysin is a newly identified metalloprotease-like enzyme, that is secreted from *T. forsythia*. Karilysin modulates the host immune response and is therefore considered a likely drug target. In this study peptides were selected towards the catalytic domain from Karilysin (Kly18) by phage display. The peptides were linear with low micromolar binding affinities The two best binders (peptide14 and peptide15), shared the consensus sequence XWFPXXXGGG. A peptide15 fusion with Maltose Binding protein (MBP) was produced with peptide15 fused to the N-terminus of MBP. The peptide15-MBP was expressed in *E. coli* and the purified fusion-protein was used to verify Kly18 specific binding. Chemically synthesised peptide15 (SWFPLRSGGG) could inhibit the enzymatic activity of both Kly18 and intact Karilysin (Kly48). Furthermore, peptide15 could slow down the autoprocessing of intact Kly48 to Kly18. The WFP motif was important for inhibition and a truncation study further demonstrated that the N-terminal serine was also essential for Kly18 inhibition. The SWFP peptide had a Ki value in the low micromolar range, which was similar to the intact peptide15. In conclusion SWFP is the first reported inhibitor of Karilysin and can be used as a valuable tool in structure-function studies of Karilysin.

Editor: Richard C. Willson, University of Houston, United States of America

Funding: This work was supported by the Lundbeck Foundation [grant number R54-A5291 to PDS]; the National Institutes of Health [Grant number DE 09761, United States of America to JP); National Science Center [2011/01/B/NZ6/00268, Kraków, Poland to JP]; the European Community [FP7-HEALTH-2010-261460 "Gums&Joints" to JP]; the Foundation for Polish Science [TEAM project DPS/424–329/10 to JP]; the Faculty of Biochemistry, Biophysics and Biotechnology of the Jagiellonian University (FBB&B-UJ) [project no. K/DSC/000361 to MK); and structural funds from the European Union [POIG.02.01.00-12-064/08 to FBB&B-UJ]. The funders had no role in study design, data collection and analysis, decision to publish, or preparation of the manuscript.

Competing Interests: The authors have declared that no competing interests exist.

* E-mail: pds@farma.ku.dk

Introduction

Periodontitis is a serious bacterial infection-driven inflammatory disease affecting the periodontium, i.e., the tissues that surround and support the teeth. The 'red complex' is a term used for the three bacterial taxa that are considered the major periodontopathogens (*Treponema denticola*, *Porphyromonas gingivalis* and *Tannerella forsythia*) that lead to disease development [1]. These pathogens all produce high levels of extracellular proteolytic activity [2–8], which contributes to the periodontitis symptoms; loss of attachment between the tooth and the gingiva, which is due to bone degradation and weakening of the soft tissues surrounding the root of a tooth. This ultimately leads to formation of deep periodontal pockets and teeth loss [9]. Furthermore, accumulating evidence suggests that severe forms of periodontitis contribute to development of the systemic diseases, stroke, diabetes and rheumatoid arthritis [10–14]. Current periodontitis therapies are based upon mechanical removal of supra- and subgingival bacterial plaque from the tooth surface in conjunction with the use of antibiotics. Unfortunately, this treatment is not always fully effective, and focus was therefore directed towards development of protease inhibitors as an alternative weapon towards the periodontopathogen effects. In fact, a factor Xa inhibitor could inhibit the *P. gingivalis* gingipain proteases RgpA and RgpB and was bactericidal towards *P. gingivalis* [15]. Furthermore, chlorhexidine and benzamidine were used successfully to inhibit *P. gingivalis* gingipains [16,17]. Furthermore, doxycycline could inhibit protease activity from *P. gingivalis* and *T. denticola* [18].

T. forsythia is a gram-negative bacteria, which secrete proteases that act as virulence factors (PrtH, a cysteine protease and BspA, a trypsin-like protease). PrtH displays hemolysin activity and one study suggested that BspA mediates *T. forsythia* attachment to fibronectin and fibrinogen [19–21]. Karilysin, a newly identified metalloprotease isolated from *T. forsythia* [6] is secreted as a 472-residue protein and has the following composition; a 20-residue signal sequence, a 14-residue pro-peptide, an 18 kDa catalytic peptidase domain and a 30 kDa C-terminal domain of unknown function. The full length enzyme could be recombinantly expressed but the enzyme matured through sequential autolysis, by first generating a fully active 48 kDa variant, followed by formation of the catalytic domain (named Kly18) [6,22]. Kly18 structural analysis demonstrated a similarity to mammalian matrix metalloproteinases (MMPs) [22]. MMPs are a separate family within the 'metzincin' clan of MPs and participate in turnover of extracellular-matrix components and selective activation/inactivation of other proteins and enzymes. The MMP activity is tightly regulated, however uncontrolled MMP-proteolysis can occur, leading to tissue destruction, apoptosis and inflammation [23]. Metalloproteases derived from microbial pathogens were documented as important virulence factors contributing to evasion of antimicrobial mechanisms of the innate immune system [24].

Only limited information is available on the biology of Karilysin. Recent data demonstrated that Karilysin can inactivate the antimicrobial peptide LL-37 by proteolytic cleavage [7]. This suggests that Karilysin can contribute to evasion of the human immune response. This hypothesis has been further substantiated by recent findings that Karilysin-expressing *T. forsythia* isolates inhibits all pathways of the complement system by Karilysin-mediated degradation of complement system proteins (mannose-binding lectin, ficolin-2, ficolin-3, C4 and C5) [25]. For these reasons Karilysin is considered a potential target for therapeutic intervention but no Karilysin inhibitors currently exist.

In this study phage display was used to identify a peptide that specifically bound Karilysin and efficiently inhibited the proteolytic activity of Karilysin.

Materials and Methods

Miscellaneous Reagents

Karilysin catalytic domain (Kly18) and intact Kly48 were produced as previously described [6]. Active human MMP-3 catalytic domain, Bovine Serum Albumine (BSA), LB-medium and FITC-Casein were from Sigma-Aldrich. Maltose-binding protein (MBP) was from ProSpec-Tany TechnoGene Ltd. Peroxidase conjugated mouse anti-M13 phage monoclonal antibody, LMW (Low Molecular Weight)-SDS Marker and 1 ml MBPTrap HP columns were from GE-Healthcare. Peptide phage libraries (7-mer and 7-mer cysteine-constrained), pMAL-pIII vector, M13KE insert extension primer (NEB #E8101), −96 gIII sequencing primer (NEB #S1259), monoclonal anti-MBP HRP-conjugate, *EagI* and *Acc65I* were from New England Biolabs. Maxisorp microtiter plates and black fluorescence non-surface treated plates were both from NUNC. OPD-tablets (*o*-Phenylenediamine dihydrochloride) were from DAKO. All peptides were synthesised by Genscript. T4-DNA ligase was from Invitrogen. QIAquick gel extraction kit was from QIAgen. Ampicillin was from Calbiochem. Isopropyl β-D-thiogalactoside (IPTG) was from VWR.

Biopanning

Phage libraries displaying seven amino acids in random sequence order at the N-terminal end of protein III were used for affinity selection of peptide binders towards Kly18. Both a linear and a constrained version of the peptide library were used for the selection. Microtiter plates were coated at 4°C for 16 hours with purified Kly18 at 0.66 μM using 100 μl per well. These plates were subsequently washed in PBS (20 mM sodium phosphate, 150 mM NaCl, pH 7.4) supplemented with 0.05% Tween-20 (PBS-T) and then blocked with 4% BSA in PBS for 2 h at room temperature. Bacteriophage at 10^{11} pfu/100 μl were used for each panning round. The constrained and linear libraries were mixed and panned together as a mixture in PBS supplemented with 0.1% Tween20, pH = 7.4. After incubation for one hour at room temperature plates were washed ten times with PBS-T (0.1% Tween20) and bound peptide-phage were eluted with glycine/HCl, pH = 2.2 for 10 min. followed by neutralisation with Tris-base, pH = 9.0. Eluted phage were used to infect exponentially growing TG1 cells overnight at 37°C. The following day peptide-phage were precipitated from the cell supernatant with phage precipitation buffer (20% (w/v) PEG6000), 2.5 M NaCl) and re-dissolved in PBS as described [26]. After four rounds of panning, single clones were isolated and tested for Kly18 binding in phage ELISA (see below). Single stranded DNA was extracted from positive clones according to [27] and the DNA was sequenced in the region corresponding to the random peptide region.

Phage ELISA

Kly18 wells were coated and blocked as above. The following washes and incubations were performed at room temperature. After blocking, the plates were washed three times in PBS-T and one hundred μl solutions of the individual phage clones diluted 1:1 in 4% BSA/PBS were added in a concentration of 1×10^{10} pfu/ml and further incubated for one hour. Wells were washed ten times with PBS-T and next 100 μl of peroxidase conjugated mouse anti-M13 monoclonal antibody diluted 1/1000 in 2% BSA/PBS, pH = 7.4 was added and incubated for one hour. The plates were washed ten times and detection was carried out by adding 100 μl of an OPD solution (1 OPD-tablet dissolved in 3 ml H_2O and 5 μl 30% H_2O_2). The reaction was stopped by adding 100 μl of 1 M H_2SO_4 and absorbance values (*A*) were measured at 490 nm using an immunoreader (Emax).

Estimation of Peptide-phage Binding Affinity by the Use of Inhibition ELISA

Nunc Maxisorp plates were coated with Kly18 and blocked as described earlier. Titration curves of each clone revealed the phage concentration that gave half-maximum response, and this concentration was used for the individual inhibition assays. The inhibition assay was performed essentially as described previously [28]. Briefly, the individual phage clones were incubated with decreasing concentrations of Kly18 in 4% skimmed milk/PBS for 1 hour with extensive mixing. The mix was added to Kly18 coated and blocked wells and the unbound free phage were allowed to bind for 1 hour. Wells were washed with PBS-T five times and developed as above. The absorbance values were measured at 490 nm after 30 min of incubation at 22°C. Absorbance values determined at each Kly18 concentration (*A*) were divided by the absorbance measured in the presence of zero Kly18 (A_0), thereby yielding normalized values (A/A_0). These values were plotted against the Kly18 concentration to construct the inhibition curve. Curve fitting revealed the Kly18 concentration required for 50% inhibition (I_{50}) as described previously [28]. The assay was performed in triplicate.

Subcloning, Expression and Purification of the Maltose Binding Protein-peptide15 Fusion Protein

Peptide15 phage single stranded DNA was isolated as above and 25 ng of DNA was used as template for amplification of the peptide15 DNA by PCR using the M13KE insert extension primer and the −96 gIII sequencing primer. The programme used was 25 cycles of 95°C for 30 sec., 55°C for 30 sec. and 72°C for 30 sec. The PCR product was isolated as a single DNA band after agarose gel electrophoresis and digested with *Acc65I* and *EagI1*. The peptide15 DNA with flanking sequences was again purified after agarose gel electrophoresis. The peptide15 DNA was subcloned into *Acc65I/EagI* digested pMAL-pIII vector by T4-DNA ligase and transformed into chemocompetent TG1 cells. Clones were amplified, sequenced and preserved as glycerol stocks. A MBP-peptide15 clone was used for fusion-protein production by expansion in LB-medium (supplemented with 10 mM $MgCl_2$, 0.2% glucose and 1 mM ampicillin) and when $OD_{600} = 0.6$ was reached the culture was induced with 1 mM IPTG for 3 hours at

A

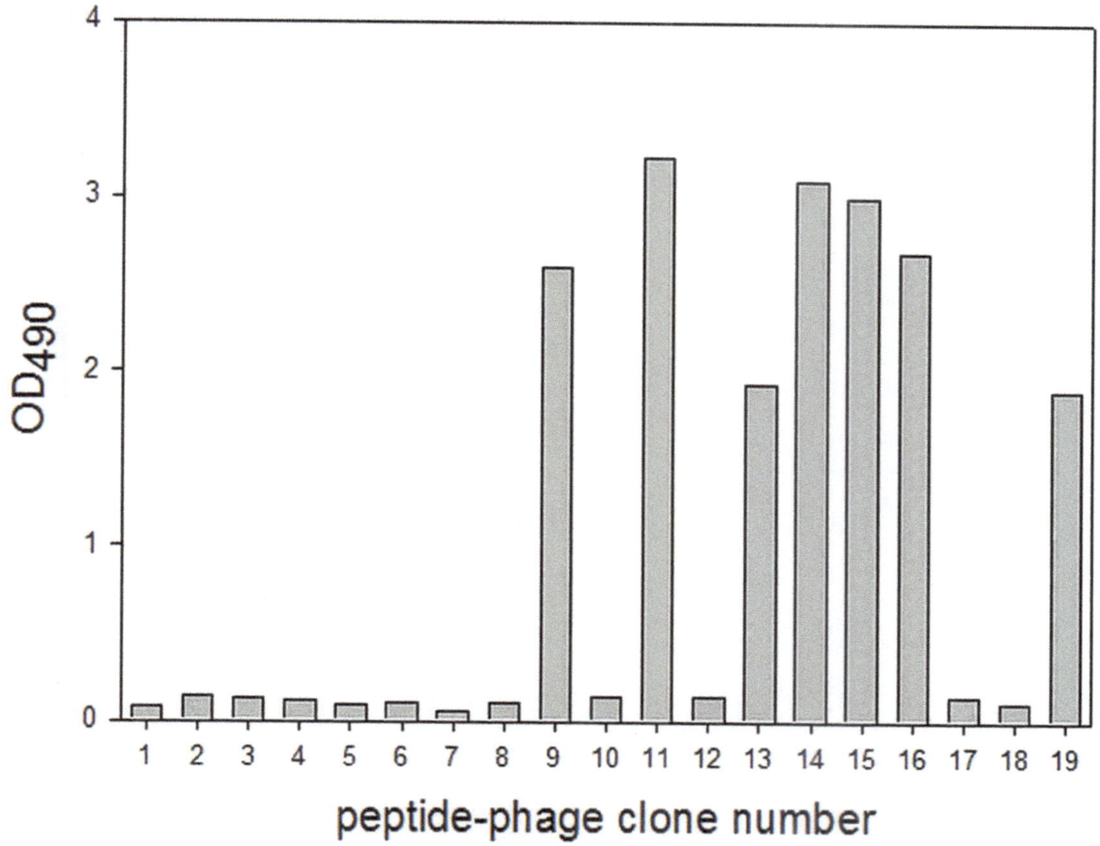

B

Phage clone	$I_{0.5}$ (µM Kly18)	Sequence
Peptide9	4.3	FWLPSPTGGG
Peptide11	3.1	WWRPPVLGGG
Peptide13	2.9	WWKYPPQGGG
Peptide14	1.5	YWFPAPPGGG
Peptide15	1.6	SWFPLRSGGG
Peptide16	4.2	YWLPYFSGGG
Peptide19	2.7	WWLPPGSGGG

Figure 1. Phage ELISA test of nineteen selected clones after four panning rounds, peptide sequences and estimated apparent afffinity. A) Optical density responses detected after the binding of peptide-phage to immobilized Kly18 are shown. Background binding to BSA has been subtracted for each clone. Clones with signals above 0.5 were deemed positive and further sequenced. B) Peptide-phage clones were tested in inhibition ELISA for estimation of affinity. All clones (except clone 13) shared the WXP motif.

30°C. The periplasmic fraction was isolated according to [29] and extensively dialysed into buffer A (20 mM Tris-HCl, 200 mM NaCl, 1 mM EDTA, pH 7.4). The dialysed fraction was applied to a 1 ml MBPTrap HP column at a flow rate of 1 ml/min and following extensive column wash with buffer A, MBP-peptide15 was eluted with 100% buffer B (20 mM Tris-HCl, 200 mM NaCl, 1 mM EDTA, 10 mM Maltose, pH 7.4). After dialysis into PBS, MBP-peptide15 purity was confirmed by SDS-PAGE.

Kly18 Detection by MBP-peptide15 ELISA

Kly18 and human MMP-3 catalytic domains were coated at the concentration of 0.66 µM. Blank wells were included for background determination. All wells were blocked in 4% BSA/PBS for 1 hour. After wash with PBS-T (5 times), MBP-peptide15 in 2% BSA/PBS diluted to 25 µg/ml was incubated for one hour with shaking. After wash with PBS-T (5 times), a monoclonal anti-MBP HRP-conjugate was added diluted 1:5000 in 2% BSA/PBS. Wells were washed ten times in PBS-T and developed with OPD substrate as above. To demonstrate that binding to Kly18 was mediated by peptide15 and not by MBP itself, control ELISA experiments were performed using MBP instead of MBP-peptide15.

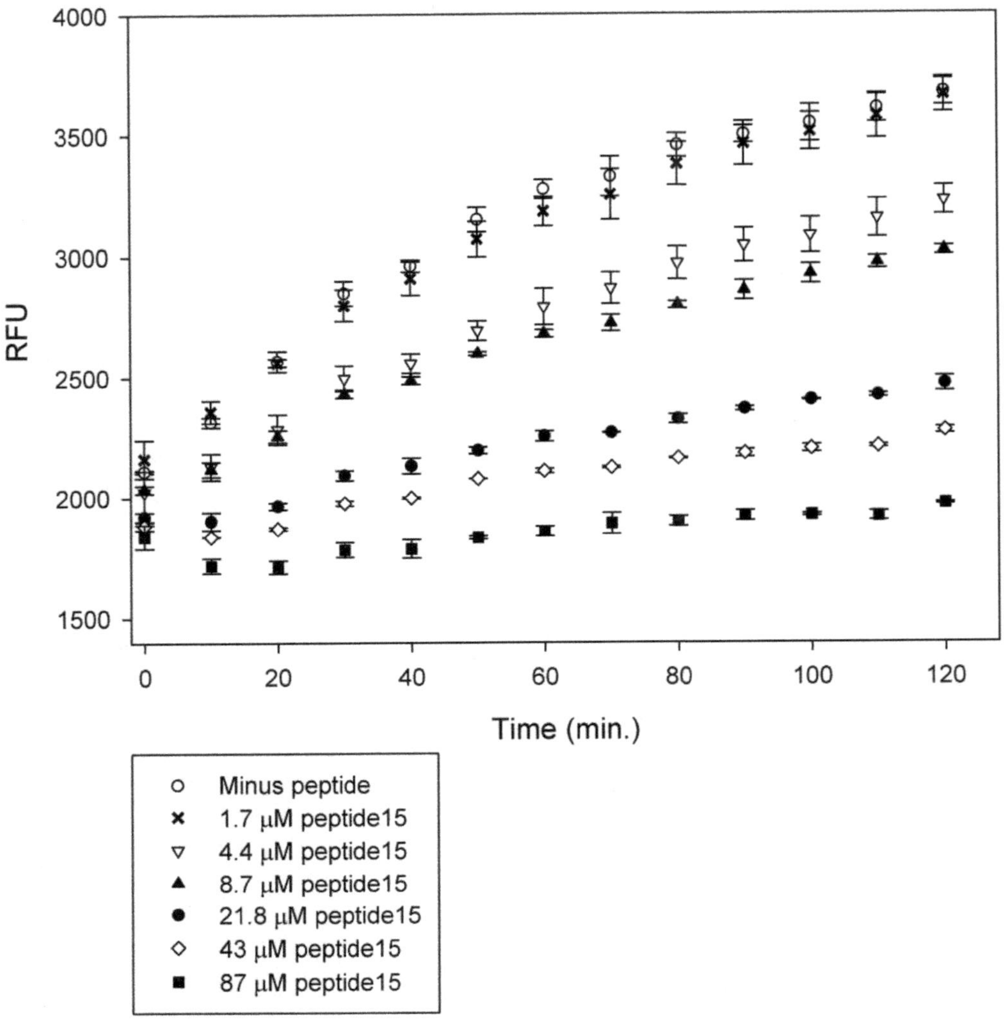

Figure 2. Peptide15 inhibits the proteolytic activity of Kly18. Peptide15 was pre-incubated with Kly18 in varying concentrations followed by addition of the substrate FITC-casein. The peptide15 inhibitory effect was seen as a decrease in Relative Fluorescence Units (RFU) in a dose-response manner. Error bars represent standard deviations between three experiments.

Assay for Monitoring Peptide15 Inhibitory Activity towards Kly18

Kly18 and Kly48 protease activities were monitored essentially as described [6]. One hundred μl working volumes were used in black untreated polypropylene microtitre plates and FITC-casein was used as the substrate. Assays were performed at 37°C using 500 nM of Kly18 (or Kly48) in assay buffer (100 mM Tris-HCl, 5mM $CaCl_2$, pH 8.0), at a FITC-casein concentration of 25 μg/ml. Released fluorescence was measured using a micro-titer plate reader at excitation/emission wavelengths of 485/538 nm. Peptides were dissolved in Milli Q water and added in varying molarities. The assay setup was as follows; Kly18 (or Kly48) was diluted in assay buffer together with peptide, followed by 30 minutes incubation on a vertical shaker at 22°C. Then FITC-casein was added and fluorescence formation was monitored at 37°C for 90 minutes with measurements every ten minutes. For estimation of inhibition constants (Ki) for peptide inhibition of Kly18, a fixed amount of Kly18 (500 nM as above) was incubated with varying concentrations of FITC-casein (5–25 μg/ml) in the presence of varying amounts of Kly18 peptide inhibitor (0–10 μM). Enzyme velocities were plotted, curves fitted and determination of Ki was performed using GraphPad Prism 5.04 using the macro for competitive inhibitor.

Assay for Monitoring the Effect of Peptide15 on the Auto-processing of Kly48

Karilysin (Kly48) at 13 μM was incubated at 37°C in 50 mM Tris-HCl, 2.5 mM $CaCl_2$, 0.02% NaN_3 pH 8.0 alone or in the presence of the peptide SWFPL at 455 μM. At different time points samples were withdrawn and the Kly48 autocatalytic processing was monitored by SDS-PAGE using 10% gels and the Tris-HCl/Tricine buffer system [30]. Gels were stained with 0.1% Coomassie Brilliant Blue R-250 in 10% acetic acid followed by destaining. Samples were run alongside a Low Molecular Weight SDS-PAGE Marker.

Results and Discussion

Isolation of Kly18 Binding Peptide-phage

Peptide phage display is an excellent tool for fast identification of lead structures that can be further modified as protease inhibitors [31]. In the present study 7-mer peptide libraries were

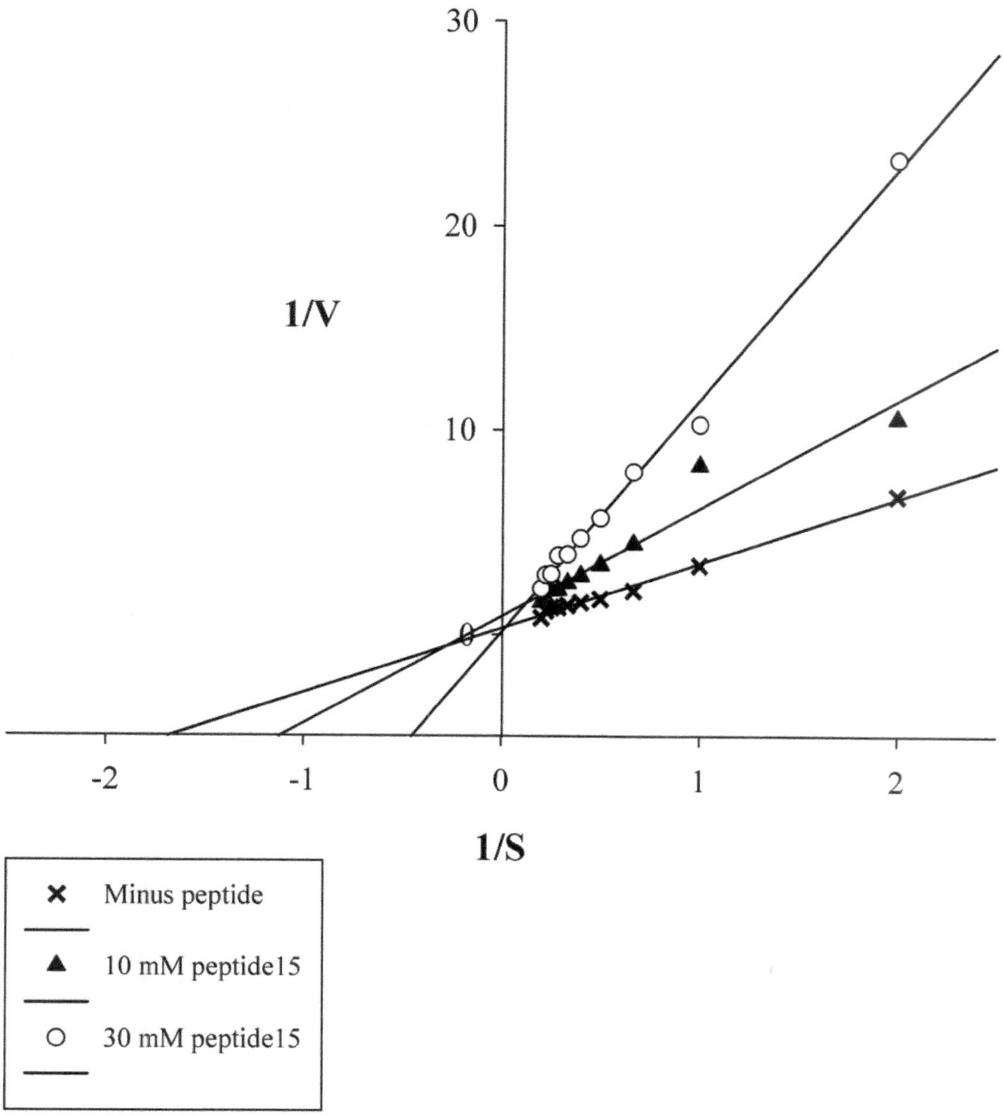

Figure 3. Peptide15 displays the characteristics of a competitive inhibitor. Shown are 1/V-1/S plot of peptide15 inhibition of Kly18. Kly18 was pre-incubated with fixed concentrations of peptide15 (10 μM and 30 μM) for 30 minutes, followed by incubation with varying concentrations of FITC-casein (5–50 μg/ml). As seen from the Lineweaver-Burke plot the Y-intercept is approximately the same for un-inhibited Kly18 as Kly18 inhibited with 10 μM and 30 μM, respectively. This suggested that peptide15 was a competitive inhibitor of Kly18. Linear regression lines were made using SigmaPlot 11.0. Data represent mean values from three experiments per substrate concentration.

used for bio-panning against the catalytic domain from Karilysin (Kly18). A cyclic 7-mer disulfide-constrained library (ACX_7CGGGS) and a linear 7-mer library (X_7GGGS) were mixed and used for selection on Kly18. Both libraries were fused to the N-terminal of protein III and displayed on phage. After four bio-panning rounds against surface-immobilized Kly18 a large enrichment in Kly18 binding phage was observed (>500 compared to the BSA control, data not shown). Nineteen clones were amplified and phage ELISA revealed seven Kly18-binders, peptide-phage 9,11,13,14,15,16,19 (Figure 1A). All seven peptide-phage displayed apparent affinities in the low micromolar range (Figure 1B). Only linear binders were isolated suggesting that the linear binders were of higher affinity than any potential cyclic peptides present in the library. In bio-panning experiments against other protein targets, we have used the same approach of mixing linear and cyclic libraries, but in these cases we isolated constrained peptides as well as linear peptides (unpublished). This suggested that we could exclude the possibility of a higher growth rate of the linear peptide library as the reason why we only isolated linear binders. All identified Kly18-binding peptide-phage (except peptide13) had the WXP motif, clearly demonstrating that these amino acids are important for Kly18 binding (Figure 1B). Interestingly, no peptides were found with the WXP motif in position 1–3 and all the peptides had the WXP peptide motif placed in position 2–4, thereby suggesting that an amino acid is essential in position one prior to the WXP motif for structural stability. Furthermore, it was evident that the X-position in the Kly18-binding motif was dependent upon basic amino acids (arginine/lysine) or bulky hydrophobic residues (leucine/phenylalanine) (Figure 1B). A decision was made to further focus on peptide15 (SWFPLRSGGGS).

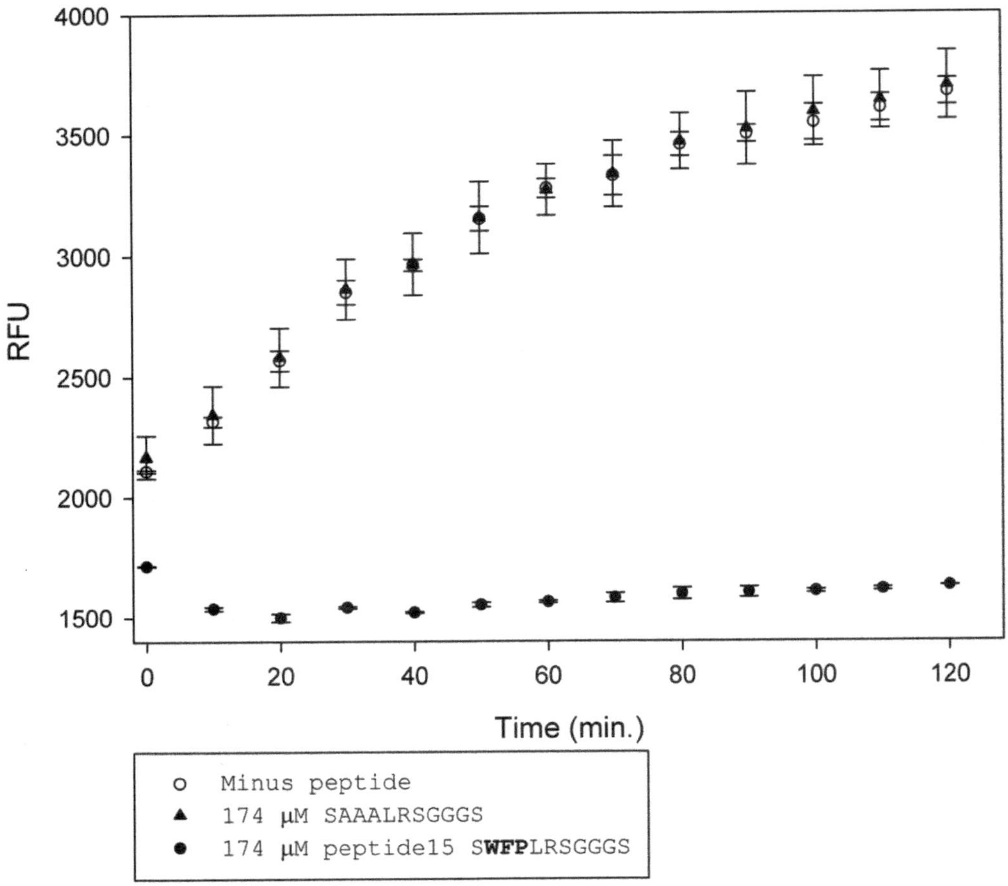

Figure 4. The WFP peptide motif is reponsible for Kly18 binding and inhibition. Pre-incubation of Kly18 with peptide15, (NH_2)-SWFPLRSGGGS-$(CONH_2)$, and a control peptide (NH_2)-SAAALRSGGGS-$(CONH_2)$, demonstrated that Kly18 inhibition could only be achieved with peptide15. Therefore, we concluded that the WFP motif was not only important for Kly18 binding but also for Kly18 inhibition. Error bars represent standard deviations between two experiments.

Free Soluble Peptide15 Inhibits Kly18 Proteolytic Activity

Peptide15 was chemically synthesised for activity testing. Initially, the peptide was synthesised in its entirety, mimicking all of the sequence displayed on phage. The peptide15 N-terminal was free during panning, however the C-terminal was fused to the phage. Consequently, peptide15 did not have a free negatively charged carboxylate at its C-terminal during panning. Therefore, in order to limit an effect of a C-terminal carboxylate, peptide15 was synthesised with a C-terminal amidation to block any unwanted C-terminal effects. The peptide15 synthesised was therefore (NH_2)-SWFPLRSGGGS-$(CONH_2)$. The Kly18 proteolytic activity was monitored with FITC-casein as the substrate and peptide15 inhibited Kly18-mediated FITC-casein cleavage in a dose-response manner (Figure 2). Furthermore, peptide15 displayed the characteristics of a competitive inhibitor as shown from a 1/V-1/S plot of peptide15 inhibition of Kly18. As seen from the Lineweaver-Burke plot the Y-intercept is approximately the same for un-inhibited Kly18 as Kly18 inhibited with 10 μM peptide15 and 30 μM peptide15, respectively (Figure 3). This suggested that peptide15 was a competitive inhibitor of Kly18.

To investigate the importance of the peptide15 WFP motif for Kly18 inhibition a control peptide was chemically synthesised with the WFP motif replaced by a triple alanine, (NH_2)-SAAALRSGGGS-$(CONH_2)$. Even in a very high dose (174 μM) the control peptide had a curve similar to that of Kly18 with no peptide present, thereby demonstrating that the WFP motif was crucial for inhibition of Kly18 (Figure 4).

Peptide15 Truncation Study and Comparative Kinetic Analysis

Peptide15 was synthesised in its entirety, including the linker sequence attached to the phage (GGGS) and the question arose if the amino acids flanking the WFP motif were necessary for Kly18 inhibition. To answer this, fifteen truncation variants of peptide15 were designed, termed 15-1 to 15–16 and the peptide15 lead structure was named 15-0 (Table 1). Peptide version 15-9 (WFPLRSGGGS) was too hydrophobic for synthesis but all others could be produced. Initially all peptide versions were screened in a relatively high single concentration (87 μM) to reveal if omission of single amino acid residues displayed dramatic effects on Kly18 inhibition. The peptide15 truncated version (NH_2)-SWFP-$(CONH_2)$ retained efficient inhibitory potency but the peptide (NH_2)-WFP-$(CONH_2)$ was completely inactive towards Kly18 (Figure 5). The data clearly demonstrated that the serine in position 1 was crucial for inhibition of Kly18 as all peptide versions lacking this serine (15-8,15-10,15-11,15-12,15-13,15-14,15-15) lost most or all of their Kly18 inhibition capacity (Figure 5). Therefore, the Kly18 inhibiting peptide motif was expanded to (NH_2)-SWFP-$(CONH_2)$. A possible explanation is that in absence of serine the presence of a charged amino group attached directly to the

Table 1. Peptides used in the truncation study.

Name	Sequence
15-0	(NH_2)-SWFPLRSGGGS-($CONH_2$)
15-1	(NH_2)-SWFPLRSGGG-($CONH_2$)
15-2	(NH_2)-SWFPLRSGG-($CONH_2$)
15-3	(NH_2)-SWFPLRSG-($CONH_2$)
15-4	(NH_2)-SWFPLRS-($CONH_2$)
15-5	(NH_2)-SWFPLR-($CONH_2$)
15-6	(NH_2)-SWFPL-($CONH_2$)
15-7	(NH_2)-SWFP-($CONH_2$)
15-8	(NH_2)-WFP-($CONH_2$)
15-9*	(NH_2)-WFPLRSGGGS-($CONH_2$)
15-10	(NH_2)-WFPLRSGGG-($CONH_2$)
15-11	(NH_2)-WFPLRSGG-($CONH_2$)
15-12	(NH_2)-WFPLRSG-($CONH_2$)
15-13	(NH_2)-WFPLRS-($CONH_2$)
15-14	(NH_2)-WFPLR-($CONH_2$)
15-15	(NH_2)-WFPL-($CONH_2$)
15-16	(NH_2)-SWAPLRSGGGS-($CONH_2$)

Shown are all possible truncation combinations of peptide15, while still retaining the WFP motif. Each structure is given a number. The peptide15 lead structure has the number 15-0. Structure 15-9 was too hydrophobic for synthesis.

tryptophan of the (NH_2)-WFP-($CONH_2$) motif could interfere with the binding and inhibitory mechanism of the peptide. Interestingly, full length peptide15 with an alanine substitution in position 3 (15-16), (NH_2)-SWAPLRSGGGS-($CONH_2$), was also inactive towards Kly18 (Figure 5). This demonstrated that the phenylalanine was also crucial for the inhibitory activity of peptide15.

Detailed kinetic analysis of peptides 15-0.,15-5., 15-6. and 15-7. revealed similar Ki values in the low micromolar area (Figure 6). This demonstrated that peptide15 can be truncated to the tetrapeptide (NH_2)-SWFP-($CONH_2$) without compromising inhibitory potency.

Peptide15 (SWFPL) Inhibits the Proteolytic Activity of Intact Karylysin (Kly48) and Delays the Auto-processing of Kly48 to Kly18

We next wanted to test if the inhibitory effect of peptide15 on Kly18 could be reproduced on intact Karilysin (Kly48). The experiment was performed essentially as described for Kly18 and the results demonstrated a clear dose-response inhibition of Kly48 by (NH_2)-SWFPL-($CONH_2$) (Figure 7A). Kly48 is unstable and auto-processes itself into Kly38 and Kly18 over time. Consequently, it was important to establish if SWFPL could modulate the Kly48 auto-processing. As seen from the SDS-PAGE gels in Figure 7B and 7C, (NH_2)-SWFPL-($CONH_2$) inhibited the auto-processesing efficiently and even after 48 hours there was still a considerable amount of Kly48 present. Taken together these two studies confirmed that peptide15 inhibited the proteolytic activity of Kly48 and this dataset strongly suggested that it may be possible to use peptide15 to lock Karilysin in the intact Kly48 form, and

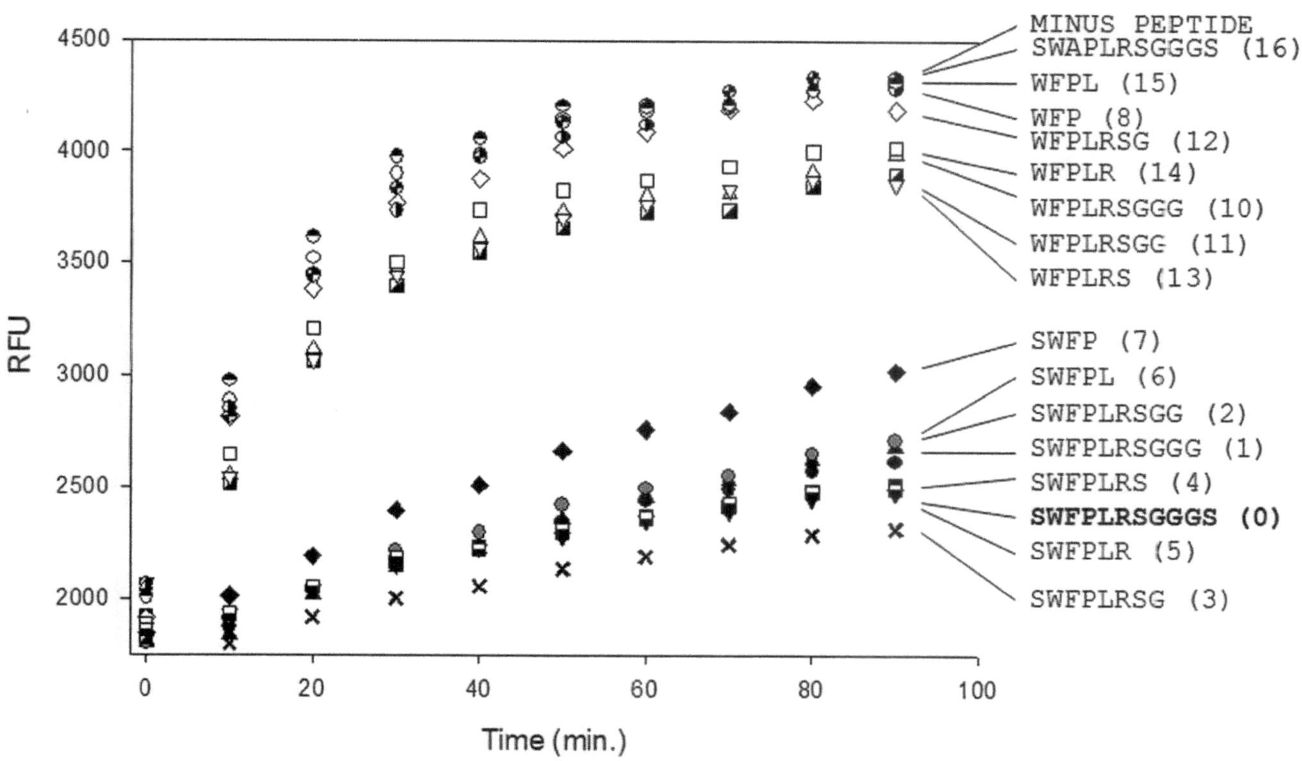

Figure 5. Screening of truncated peptides demonstrates that a tetra-peptide version of peptide15 can inhibit Kly18. Different length versions of peptide15 were tested for Kly18 inhibitory activity. All peptides were screened in a relatively high single concentration (87 μM) to reveal if omission of single amino acid residues displayed dramatic effects on Kly18 inhibition. The data demonstrated that peptide15 can be limited to (NH_2)-SWFP-($CONH_2$) (structure 15-7) and still inhibit Kly18.

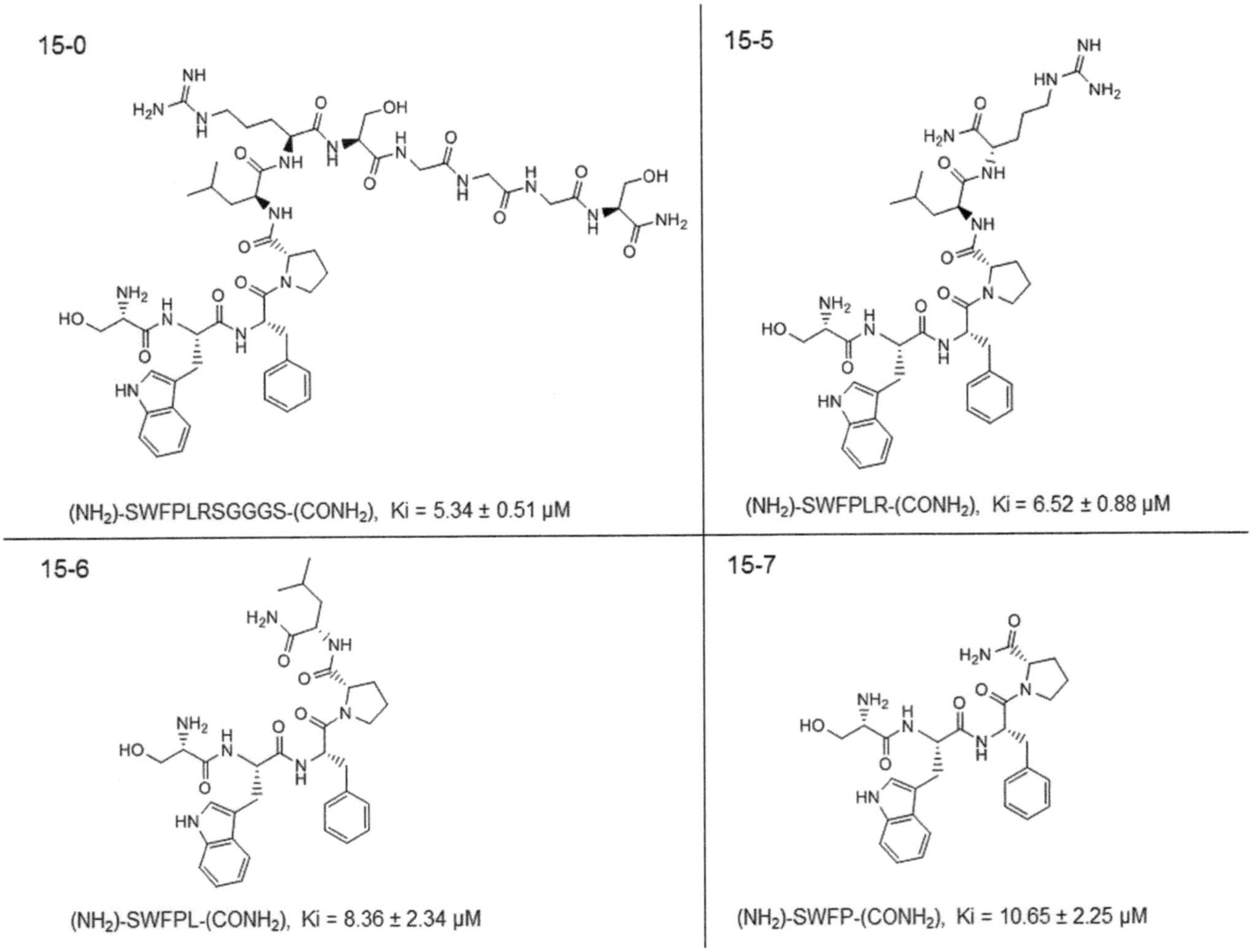

Figure 6. The tetrapeptide displays a Ki value similar to that of the peptide 15 lead structure. Shown are chemdraw structure models of the peptide versions 15-0, 15-5, 15-6 and 15-7. All truncated versions of peptide15 and intact peptide15 had low micromolar Ki values.

use that complex for crystallisation trials. This could reveal the structure of the intact enzyme.

Expression of MBP-peptide15 Fusion Construct and Specificity Test

In figure 8 a structural alignment of Kly18 and the catalytic domain of human MMP-3 is shown and as is the case with most human MMP's (MMP-1, MMP-7-14), Kly18 and human MMP-3 are structurally similar [22]. It was therefore important to establish if peptide15 was a general binder of MMP catalytic domains. To develop a probe for cross-reactivity tests, peptide15 was expressed as a MBP N-terminal fusion protein and purified in a simple one-step purification strategy. Purity was judged to be greater than 90% by SDS-PAGE (data not shown) and the MBP-peptide15 was used in ELISA to test cross-reactivity towards human MMP-3. MBP-peptide15 bound Kly18 but not MMP-3, thereby underlining peptide15 specificity (figure 9A). By performing a control ELISA experiment using MBP instead of MBP-peptide15, we could confirm that the binding observed was due to the specific interaction between peptide15 and Kly18 (Figure 9B).

As MMP catalytic domains are highly similar it is a challenge to find specific peptides. This was demonstrated in a recent study, which identified a cyclic MMP-9-binding peptide (CTTHWGFTLC) by phage display with high affinity. However, this peptide also had high affinity for MMP-2 [32]. Peptide phage display has also been used to identify substrate specificity of individual MMPs and by using a 15-mer peptide library Deng and co-workers demonstrated that collagenase 3/MMP-13 has a preference towards the peptide sequence GPLGMRGL. But three other MMPs (stromelysin-1/MMP-3, gelatinase B/MMP-9 and collagenase 1/MMP-1) had lower activity towards the isolated peptide substrate [33]. Furthermore, a recent study demonstrated that a unique MMP-11 substrate peptide could be isolated by phage display, which explained why MMP-11 does not have any activity towards substrates specific for other MMPs [34]. Consequently, one could argue that the peptide15 mode of action is that of a substrate competitive inhibitor. This is especially relevant due to the fact that the exact peptide sequence needed for Kly18 substrate cleavage is yet to be fully elucidated [6]. To explore this possibility peptide15 was incubated with or without a large excess of Kly18 and the mixture was analyzed by liquid chromatography mass spectrometry. The results demonstrated that peptide15 could not be cleaved by Kly18 as the mass peak m/z = 1149, corresponding to (NH_2)-SWFPLRSGGGS-$(CONH_2)$, was found in both preparations and no cleavage products were found (data not shown).

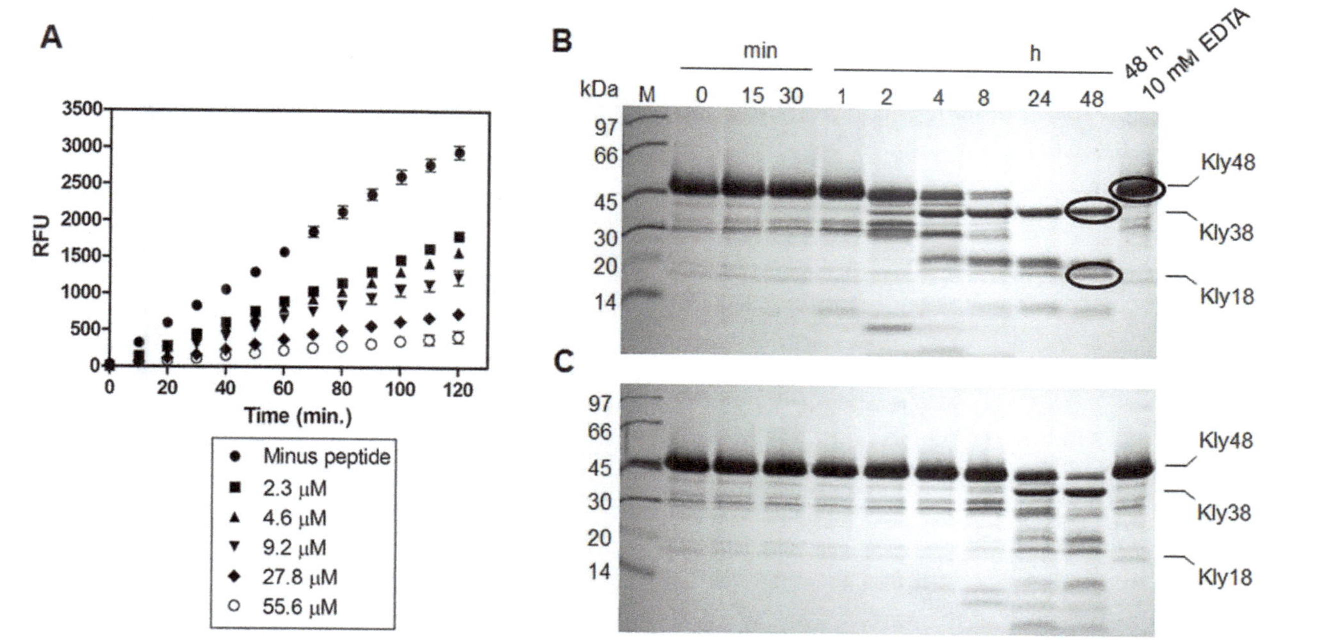

Figure 7. SWFPL inhibits the proteolytic activity of intact Karilysin (Kly48) and delays the auto-processing of Kly48 to Kly18. A) Kly48 was pre-incubated with SWFPL in varying concentrations (2.3 μM to 55.6 μM) followed by addition of the substrate FITC-casein. The SWFPL inhibitory effect was seen as a decrease in Relative Fluorescence Units (RFU) in a dose-response manner. Error bars represent standard deviations between three experiments. B+C) Intact Karilysin (Kly48) at 13 μM was incubated alone (B) or with the peptide inhibitor (C) at 455 μM. At indicated time points samples were withdrawn for SDS-PAGE analysis. It is clear that SWFPL inhibited the time-dependent autoprocessing of Kly48 to Kly38 and Kly18. Even after 48 hours a significant amount of Kly48 was still present.

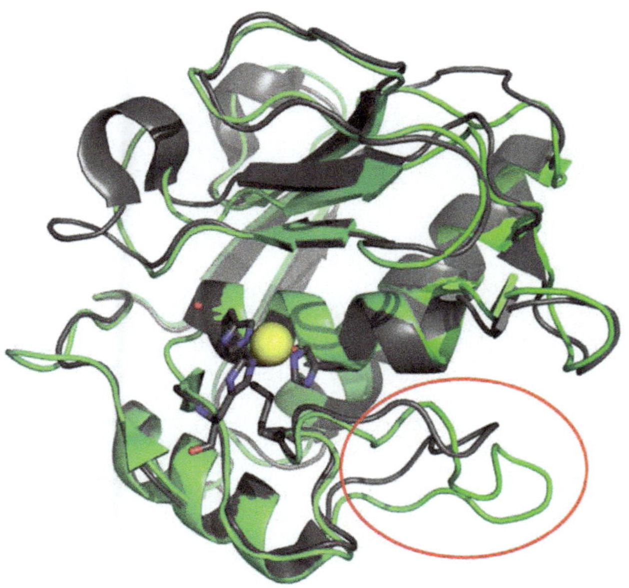

Figure 8. Structural alignment of the catalytic domains from Karilysin (Kly18) and human Matrix Metalloprotease-3 (MMP-3). MMP-3 is seen in green and Kly18 is seen in grey. The figure was prepared using Pymol (DeLano Scientific LLC) and the coordinate files 1CQR (MMP-3) and 2XS3 (Kly18). The structure alignment was performed using the 'align' function in PyMol. The Kly18 was structurally similar to MMP-3 as well as other mammalian MMP's (MMP-1 to 3, MMP-7 to MMP-14, MMP-16 and MMP-20) (Cerda-Costa *et al.* 2011). The figure displays the zinc (yellow sphere) that is coordinated by the three active site histidines (H155, H159 and H165). The specificity loop is indicated with a red circle.

The development of MMP inhibitors is highly relevant, due to the involvement of MMPs in several pathologies [23]. Some candidate molecules act by blocking the MMP-active sites via binding to the catalytic Zn^{2+} through chelators such as hydroxamate [23]. These approaches have been successful for MMP inhibition. However, the inhibitors have a broad specificity towards other MMPs due to very similar active site geometries of matrix metalloproteinases [23]. An alternative approach to specific MMP inhibitor design is to utilize larger molecules, such as peptides, that interact with the active site as well as exosites unique to individual MMPs [35]. Kly18 contains the metzincin MMP 3-histidine zinc-binding motif (HEXXHXXGXXH) and Kly18 was previously inhibited by small molecules chelators (EDTA, 1,10-phenanthroline) similar to mammalian MMPs [6]. Furthermore, the active site of the Kly18 structure had the classical MMP composition with small deviations in the specificity loop (seen as a red circle in Figure 8) [22]. As peptide15 binds exclusively to Kly18 and at the same time inhibits the enzyme, peptide15 may act by a combined effect of active site targeting and specificity loop exosite interaction. However, detailed structural analysis of Kly18-peptide15 co-crystals will provide final proof on the inhibition mechanism.

Conclusions

Periodontitis is a devastating disease of great discomfort to affected patients. Furthermore, recent findings link periodontitis to inflammatory diseases like rheumatoid arthritis, thereby further underlining the importance of disease treatment and containment [36]. Inhibitors of the periodontopathogen-derived proteases by small molecules, peptides or antibodies represent a rational approach to disease management. Inhibitors toward the most relevant proteases, of which Karilysin could be one, might be

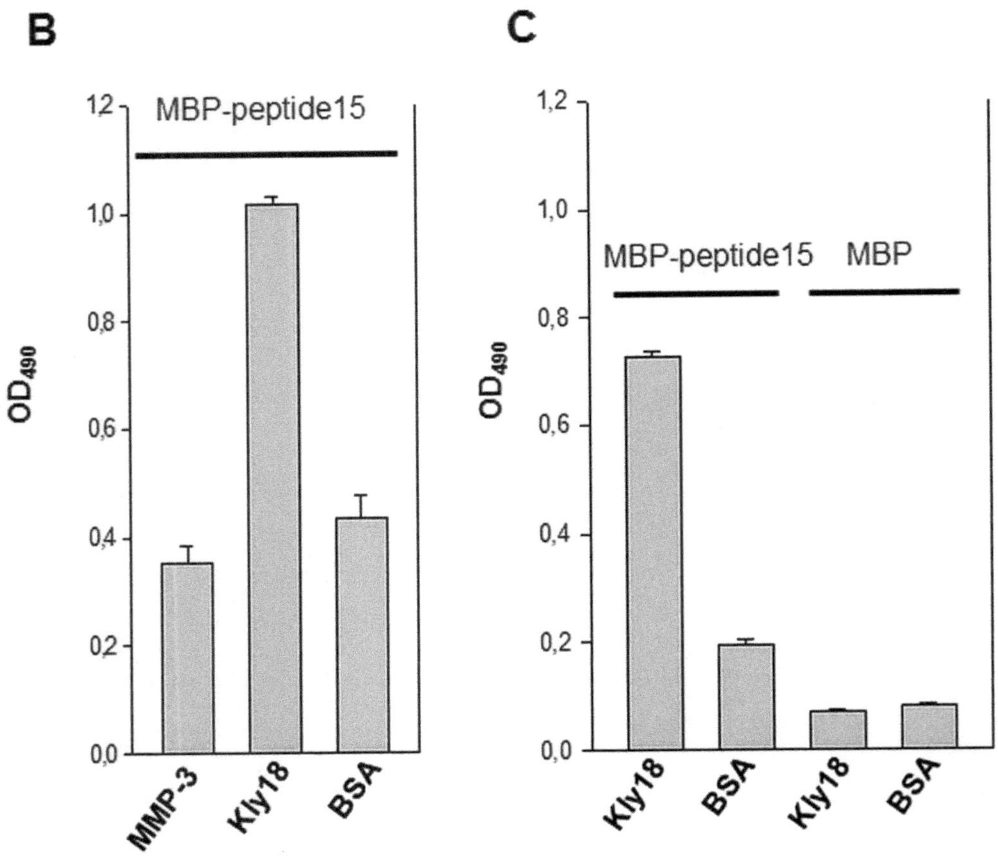

Figure 9. Peptide15-MBP is specific for Kly18. A) The peptide15-MBP fusion protein interacted exclusively with Kly18, thereby demonstrating that peptide15 was specific for Kly18. **B)** To demonstrate that binding to Kly18 was mediated by peptide15 and not by MBP itself, control experiments were performed using MBP instead of MBP-peptide15. Error bars represent standard deviations between three experiments.

applied as a combination therapy in the fight against the periodontopathogens of the 'red complex'. These inhibitors could be formulated in existing media, such as mouth wash, tooth paste or even chewing gum.

In this study, the first inhibitor of Karilysin was identified and characterized. The results supplied us with a detailed understanding of which amino acid residues were important for the inhibitory function of peptide15. The peptide will be a valuable probe in structure-function studies of Karilysin and detailed co-crystallisation studies can reveal the underlying molecular mechanism for the inhibition. From co-crystallisation structural data it may be possible to design peptidomimetics with improved Ki-values.

Author Contributions

Conceived and designed the experiments: PDS JP ER. Performed the experiments: PDS GS MK. Analyzed the data: PDS MK JP ER. Wrote the paper: PDS JP ER.

References

1. Socransky SS, Haffajee AD, Cugini MA, Smith C, Kent RL (1998) Microbial complexes in subgingival plaque. Journal of Clinical Periodontology 25: 134–144.
2. Byrne DP, Wawrzonek K, Jaworska A, Birss AJ, Potempa J, et al. (2009) Role of the cysteine protease interpain A of Prevotella intermedia in breakdown and release of haem from haemoglobin. Biochem J 425: 257–264.
3. Carlisle MD, Srikantha RN, Brogden KA (2009) Degradation of human alpha- and beta-defensins by culture supernatants of Porphyromonas gingivalis strain 381. J Innate Immun 1: 118–122.
4. Fitzpatrick RE, Aprico A, Wijeyewickrema LC, Pagel CN, Wong DM, et al. (2009) High molecular weight gingipains from Porphyromonas gingivalis induce cytokine responses from human macrophage-like cells via a nonproteolytic mechanism. J Innate Immun 1: 109–117.
5. Ishihara K, Wawrzonek K, Shaw LN, Inagaki S, Miyamoto M, et al. (2010) Dentipain, a Streptococcus pyogenes IdeS protease homolog, is a novel virulence factor of Treponema denticola. Biol Chem 391: 1047–1055.
6. Karim AY, Kulczycka M, Kantyka T, Dubin G, Jabaiah A, et al. (2010) A novel matrix metalloprotease-like enzyme (karilysin) of the periodontal pathogen Tannerella forsythia ATCC 43037. Biological Chemistry 391: 105–117.
7. Koziel J, Karim AY, Przybyszewska K, Ksiazek M, Rapala-Kozik M, et al. (2010) Proteolytic inactivation of LL-37 by karilysin, a novel virulence mechanism of Tannerella forsythia. J Innate Immun 2: 288–293.
8. Monteiro AC, Scovino A, Raposo S, Gaze VM, Cruz C, et al. (2009) Kinin danger signals proteolytically released by gingipain induce Fimbriae-specific IFN-gamma- and IL-17-producing T cells in mice infected intramucosally with Porphyromonas gingivalis. J Immunol 183: 3700–3711.
9. Imamura T (2003) the role of gingipains in the pathogenesis of periodontal disease. Journal of periodontology 74: 111–118.
10. Behle JH, Papapanou PN (2006) Periodontal infections and atherosclerotic vascular disease: an update. Int Dent J 56: 256–262.
11. Jordan RC (2004) Diagnosis of periodontal manifestations of systemic diseases. Periodontol 2000 34: 217–229.
12. Persson GR (2006) What has ageing to do with periodontal health and disease? International dental journal 56: 240–249.
13. Pihlstrom BL, Michalowicz BS, Johnson NW (2005) Periodontal diseases. Lancet 366: 1809–1820.
14. Wegner N, Wait R, Sroka A, Eick S, Nguyen KA, et al. (2010) Peptidylarginine deiminase from Porphyromonas gingivalis citrullinates human fibrinogen and

alpha-enolase: implications for autoimmunity in rheumatoid arthritis. Arthritis Rheum 62: 2662–2672.
15. Matsushita K, Imamura T, Tancharoen S, Tatsuyama S, Tomikawa M, et al. (2006) Selective inhibition of Porphyromonas gingivalis growth by a factor Xa inhibitor, DX-9065a. Journal of Periodontal Research 41: 171–176.
16. Cronan CA, Potempa J, Travis J, Mayo JA (2006) Inhibition of Porphyromonas gingivalis proteinases (gingipains) by chlorhexidine: synergistic effect of Zn(II). Oral Microbiol Immunol 21: 212–217.
17. Krauser JA, Potempa J, Travis J, Powers JC (2002) Inhibition of arginine gingipains (RgpB and HRgpA) with benzamidine inhibitors: zinc increases inhibitory potency. Biological Chemistry 383: 1193–1198.
18. Grenier D, Plamondon P, Sorsa T, Lee HM, McNamara T, et al. (2002) Inhibition of proteolytic, serpinolytic, and progelatinase-b activation activities of periodontopathogens by doxycycline and the non-antimicrobial chemically modified tetracycline derivatives. J Periodontol 73: 79–85.
19. Grenier D (1995) Characterization of the trypsin-like activity of Bacteroides forsythus. Microbiology 141: 921–926.
20. Saito T, Ishihara K, Kato T, Okuda K (1997) Cloning, expression, and sequencing of a protease gene from Bacteroides forsythus ATCC 43037 in Escherichia coli. Infect Immun 65: 4888–4891.
21. Sharma A, Sojar HT, Glurich I, Honma K, Kuramitsu HK, et al. (1998) Cloning, expression, and sequencing of a cell surface antigen containing a leucine-rich repeat motif from Bacteroides forsythus ATCC 43037. Infect Immun 66: 5703–5710.
22. Cerda-Costa N, Guevara T, Karim AY, Ksiazek M, Nguyen KA, et al. (2011) The structure of the catalytic domain of Tannerella forsythia karilysin reveals it is a bacterial xenologue of animal matrix metalloproteinases. Mol Microbiol 79: 119–132.
23. Overall CM, Lopez-Otin C (2002) Strategies for MMP inhibition in cancer: innovations for the post-trial era. Nat Rev Cancer 2: 657–672.
24. Potempa J, Pike RN (2009) Corruption of Innate Immunity by Bacterial Proteases. Journal of Innate Immunity 1: 70–87.
25. Jusko M, Potempa J, Karim AY, Ksiazek M, Riesbeck K, et al. (2012) A metalloproteinase karilysin present in the majority of *Tannerella forsythia* isolates inhibits all pathways of the complement system. Journal of immunology 188 in press.
26. Skottrup PD, Leonard P, Kaczmarek JZ, Veillard F, Enghild JJ, et al. (2011) Diagnostic evaluation of a nanobody with picomolar affinity toward the protease RgpB from Porphyromonas gingivalis. Anal Biochem 415: 158–167.
27. Sambrook J, Fritsch EF, Maniatis T (1989) Molecular Cloning: A Laboratory Manual.
28. Rath S, Stanley CM, Steward MW (1988) An inhibition enzyme-immunoassay for estimating relative antibody-affinity and affinity heterogeneity. Journal of Immunological Methods 106: 245–249.
29. Johansen LK, Albrechtsen B, Andersen HW, Engberg J (1995) pFab60: A new, efficient vector for expression of antibody Fab fragments displayed on phage. Protein Engineering 8: 1063–1067.
30. Schagger H, von Jagow G (1987) Tricine-sodium dodecyl sulfate-polyacrylamide gel electrophoresis for the separation of proteins in the range from 1 to 100 kDa. Anal Biochem 166: 368–379.
31. Nixon AE (2002) Phage display as a tool for protease ligand discovery. Curr Pharm Biotechnol 3: 1–12.
32. Koivunen E, Arap W, Valtanen H, Rainisalo A, Medina OP, et al. (1999) Tumor targeting with a selective gelatinase inhibitor. Nat Biotechnol 17: 768–774.
33. Deng SJ, Bickett DM, Mitchell JL, Lambert MH, Blackburn RK, et al. (2000) Substrate specificity of human collagenase 3 assessed using a phage-displayed peptide library. J Biol Chem 275: 31422–31427.
34. Pan W, Arnone M, Kendall M, Grafstrom RH, Seitz SP, et al. (2003) Identification of peptide substrates for human MMP-11 (stromelysin-3) using phage display. J Biol Chem 278: 27820–27827.
35. Jani M, Tordai H, Trexler M, Banyai L, Patthy L (2005) Hydroxamate-based peptide inhibitors of matrix metalloprotease 2. Biochimie 87: 385–392.
36. Detert J, Pischon N, Burmester GR, Buttgereit F (2010) The association between rheumatoid arthritis and periodontal disease. Arthritis Res Ther 12: 218.

9

Arterial Stiffness and Pulse Wave Reflection Are Increased in Patients Suffering from Severe Periodontitis

Yvonne Jockel-Schneider[1]*, Inga Harks[2], Imme Haubitz[1], Stefan Fickl[1], Martin Eigenthaler[1], Ulrich Schlagenhauf[1], Johannes Baulmann[3]

1 Department of Periodontology, University Hospital Wuerzburg, Wuerzburg, Germany, **2** Department of Periodontology, University Hospital Muenster, Muenster, Germany, **3** Clinic of Internal Medicine II, University Hospital Schleswig-Holstein, Luebeck, Germany

Abstract

Aim: This single blind cross-sectional study compared the vascular health of subjects suffering from severe chronic periodontitis, severe aggressive periodontitis and periodontal healthy controls by evaluating pulse wave velocity (PWV), augmentation index (AIx) and pulse pressure amplification (PPA).

Material and Methods: In a total of 158 subjects, 92 suffering from severe periodontitis and 66 matched periodontal healthy controls, PWV, AIx, central and peripheral blood pressure were recorded using an oscillometric device (Arteriograph).

Results: Subjects suffering from severe chronic or aggressive periodontitis exhibited significantly higher PWV ($p = 0.00004$), higher AIx ($p = 0.0049$) and lower PPA ($p = 0.028$) than matched periodontal healthy controls.

Conclusions: The results of this study confirm the association between periodontal inflammation and increased cardiovascular risk shown by impaired vascular health in case of severe periodontitis. As impaired vascular health is a common finding in patients suffering from severe periodontal disease a concomitant routine cardiovascular evaluation may be advised.

Editor: Giuseppe Schillaci, University of Perugia, Italy

Funding: This study was funded externally by a grant of the German Research Foundation (EH 365/1-1) and by the IZKF Wuerzburg (Z-2/34). The funders had no role in study design, data collection and analysis, decision to publish, or preparation of the manuscript.

Competing Interests: The authors have declared that no competing interests exist.

* Email: jockel_y@klinik.uni-wuerzburg.de

Introduction

The association between oral inflammation and the risk for myocardial infarction or stroke has been firstly described already more than two decades ago [1,2]. Ever since, a steadily increasing number of studies and reviews have firmly established a positive association between atherosclerosis and periodontal inflammation [3–5]. Preliminary intervention studies were able to prove the positive influence of various periodontal therapeutic measures on endothelial dysfunction, e.g. sub- and supragingival debridement [6,7], debridement supplemented by systemic antibiotics [8] or debridement in conjunction with local antibiotics [9]. For the evaluation of endothelial dysfunction, the first measurable stage of developing atherosclerosis, in these studies usually the flow-mediated dilatation FMD (endothelium-dependent) or the nitro-glycerin-mediated dilatation (endothelium-independent) of the brachial artery, have been recorded. While the validity of data obtained by FMD and nitro-glycerine-mediated dilatation has been verified by various trials, both methods require a very high level of examiner training to avoid faulty measurements and are time-consuming and expensive. Therefore the need for less expensive and clinically less demanding alternatives for routine vascular recording lead to the re-evaluation of the well-established principle of pulse wave velocity (PWV), augmentation index (AIx) and central pressures as clinically highly relevant indicators of vascular health.

The measurement of arterial stiffness by pulse wave reflection may be regarded as a prognostic significant extension of conventional vascular diagnosis. PWV is a direct marker of arterial stiffness [10,11]. Increased PWV is a strong predictor for future cardiovascular events and mortality in patients with and without diverse risk factors, as for example end-stage renal disease [12], patients with type 2 diabetes [13] hypertension [14], elderly people [15] or the general population [16–18].

An indirect measure of arterial stiffness and a direct measure of pulse wave reflection is the augmentation pressure and the augmentation index [19]. Augmentation can be described as the effect of wave reflection on the aortic systolic pressure peak. Accordingly, augmentation is a measure for the additional pressure caused by pulse wave reflection stressing the left ventricle [20]. AIx may be calculated by dividing the augmentation pressure by the pulse pressure. In principle, the AIx may be obtained by calculating the quotient of the pressure peak of the initial and the reflected wave (Fig. 1 [19]. All parameters influencing the AIx subsequently also have an impact on the central blood pressure. The measurement of the pulse wave reflection therefore allows an estimation of the central blood pressure, and may differ substantially from the recordable peripheral blood pressure [19]. It correlates well with left ventricular mass in hypertensive and in normotensive young men [21] and is an independent marker for premature coronary artery disease [22]. In different populations e.g. patients with end-stage renal failure, the AIx is also an independent predictor of mortality [23].

Both, PWV and AIx, provide essential information on the status of the arterial vascular system. The prognostic significance of arterial stiffness is very high. Measurements of PWV and AIx calculations allow stratifying patients with a high risk profile for cardiac and cerebral events who might benefit from more intensive cardiovascular treatment schemes [19].

Recently a new recording system for the assessment of vascular function on the basis of recorded pulse wave data has been developed, the so called Arteriograph. The Arteriograph was the very first validated device that allowed the measurement of PWV, AIx and central pressures by analysis of the oscillometric pressure curves registered on the upper arm with a single pressure cuff [24]. The principle of the oscillometric method is based on plethysmography and registers oscillometric pulsatile pressure changes in the brachial artery. Pressure fluctuations in the brachial artery are revealed by a pressure sensor in the cuff passing the recorded data to a computer for further analysis and computation of pulse pressure waves (Fig. 1). PWV is calculated in m/s for a given patient by relating the recorded time difference (ms) between the onset of the first pulse wave and the onset of the reflected pulse wave to the measured distance between the jugulum and the symphysis. The AIx corresponds to the pressure difference (amplitude difference; P1–P2, Fig. 1) between the first and second wave in relation to the pulse pressure (PP). The Arteriograph calculates the AIx based on a fixed formula and thus provides the aortic AIx without applying a transfer function [24].

Aim

The aim of this cross sectional study was to assess the cardiovascular status of patients suffering from severe aggressive or chronic periodontitis by recording pulse wave velocity, augmen-tation index and central blood pressure with the Arteriograph and compare it to data recorded from matched periodontal healthy controls.

Materials and Methods

Study design

This investigation was designed as a single blind cross-sectional trial. The study protocol, prepared in accordance with the declaration of Helsinki of 1973 and meeting the GCP criteria, was approved by the ethics committee of the University of Wuerzburg. All subjects included have signed the informed consent. A positive vote of the ethics committee of the University of Wuerzburg from 2009 (file #39-09) is easily available (e.g. on request via mail to the corresponding author).

Study setting

Study subjects were screened and recruited from individuals seeking dental care at the School of Dental Medicine of the University of Wuerzburg.

Inclusion criteria

Patients suffering from untreated severe generalised chronic or aggressive periodontitis were eligible for participation in test group. The diagnosis of generalised severe chronic or aggressive periodontitis was based on the classification criteria of the International Workshop for a Classification of Periodontal Diseases and Conditions [25].

The severity of disease expression was categorized according to the proposal of the working group of the Centers for Disease Control (CDC) and the American Academy of Periodontology (AAP) [26].

In order to restrict inclusion only to subjects with extensive periodontal lesions study patients additionally had to meet the following criteria: Patients with clinical detectable attachment loss ≥6 mm in a minimum of two different sextants and a minimum of

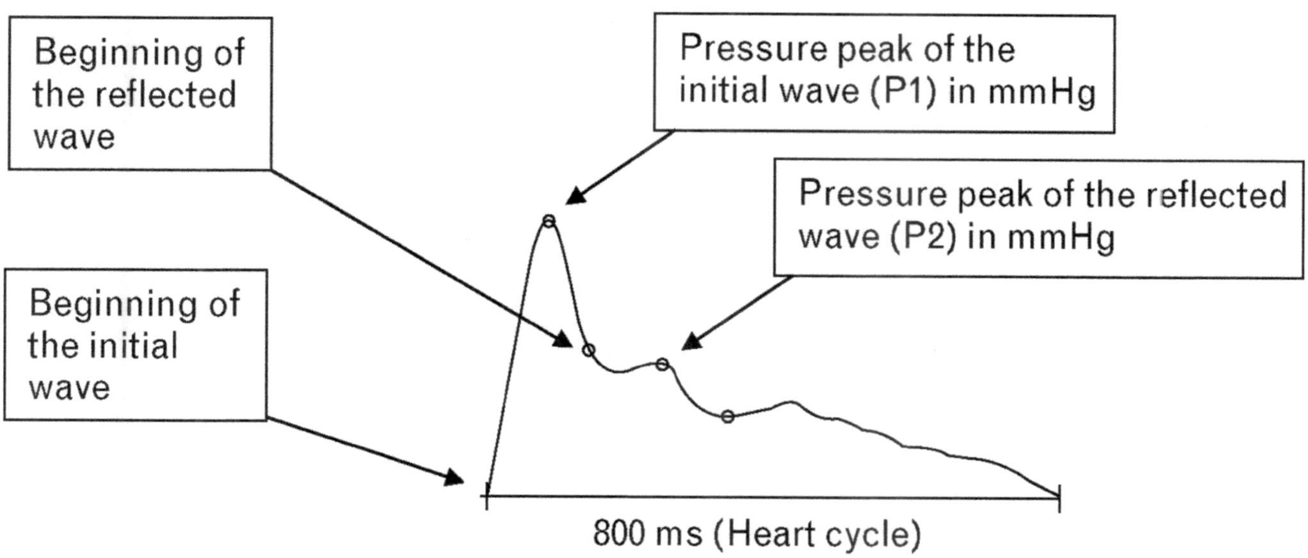

Figure 1. Original recording of an oscillometrically generated pulse wave (modified by Baulmann et al. 2008).

six interproximal sites on six different teeth were eligible for inclusion in the test group.

Individuals exhibiting minor periodontal pockets ≤3 mm were designated periodontal healthy and were eligible for inclusion in the control group.

Exclusion criteria

Individuals meeting the following criteria were not eligible for study participation: Less than ten natural teeth, age <18 years, pregnancy or breastfeeding, infectious disease, systematic periodontal therapy within the last five years, antibiotic medication within the last six months, intellectual inability to fully comprehend the aims of the study, severely decayed teeth, atrial fibrillation, or severe cardiac valve vitium.

Screening, recruitment and examination

A total of 724 subjects were screened, 256 met the inclusion criteria. Ultimately 158 subjects (75 male/83 female) were enrolled in the study. 92 patients were assigned to the test group (severe periodontitis). 74 received the diagnosis of severe chronic periodontitis and 18 suffered from aggressive periodontitis. 66 subjects served as periodontally healthy controls. Individuals meeting the inclusion criteria after the screening examination were informed about the aims of the study and asked for their participation. All patients who participated in the study signed informed consent and received an assessment of their periodontal health by recording a comprehensive periodontal status as well as an assessment of their cardiovascular status by using the Arteriograph within the next seven days. For matching purposes furthermore age, gender, weight, height, smoking habits and the presence of known systemic medical problems (e.g. diabetes) were recorded using a questionnaire.

Background factors

After setting the age of the evaluated subjects to older than 35 years it was not necessary to match the patients in the sense of pair wise assignment. The limit of 35 years was chosen because in the periodontitis group no one was younger than 36. After this exclusion, except the peripheral pulse pressure, there were no significant differences between the periodontally healthy controls and the test group suffering from severe periodontal diseases regarding the following parameters: gender, age, body mass index, height, weight, smoking habits, arterial hypertension, and presence of hypercholesterolemia. The same holds true for medication (tables 1 and 2).

Periodontal examination

The periodontal examination comprised the following parameters: Number of intraoral visible teeth, pocket probing depth (PPD) and clinical attachment level (CAL). Measurements were performed at six sites per tooth using a CP-12 Marquis periodontal probe (Hu Friedy Co., USA); Recorded measurements were rounded to the nearest millimeter. All periodontal examinations were executed by a single clinically experienced dentist. To ensure the reproducibility of the clinical test results, an intra-individual calibration was performed. For this, 4 phantom models with periodontal defects with each 27 teeth were measured at two points in time. The examiner was calibrated if the first measurement and the measurement 48 hours later was were equal at 75% of the measurements with total agreement and 95% within±1 mm [27].

Vascular examination

After the periodontal examination the recording of the cardiovascular parameters was performed during a subsequent appointment within the next seven days using the Arteriograph (TensioMed Ltd, Hungary) with the corresponding TensioMed analysis software (version 1.9.9.12).

In accordance with the international guidelines for the implementation of arterial stiffness measurements, all measurements were made in the same room under quiet conditions and dim illumination, unaffected by external environmental influences [28].

Firstly the distance between the sternal notch (jugulum) and the symphysis was recorded with a tape measure. Subsequently, in order to minimize sources of recording error each patient had a rest period of ten minutes before the onset of the cardiovascular measurements. All measurements were performed three times, with a predetermined free interval of two minutes between the individual measuring periods. During the examination the study subjects lay relaxed on an examination couch with eyes closed. All vascular data were recorded by the same trained medical technical assistant who was unaware of the assignment of the study subjects to the test or control group.

The analysis of the Arteriograph data was performed by an experienced cardiologist (JB) who also was unaware of the assignment of the data to the different groups.

Table 1. Clinical characteristics of the studied population.

	Unit	Group		P
		no/mild periodontitis	severe chronic/aggressive periodontitis	
		n = 66	n = 92	
Age	years	55±13	55±10	0.71
BMI	kg/m^2	25±4	26±3	0.60
Male gender	%	43,9	50,0	0.45
Smoker	%	30,3	21,7	0.22
Hypertension	%	17.2	22.5	0.44
Hypercholesteremia	%	10.0	10.9	1.0

Values are expressed as mean ± SD as a result of Mann-Whitney U-Test for age and BMI or in % as a result of Chi-squared for the others.

Table 2. Medication of the studied population.

	Unit	Group no/mild periodontitis n = 66	severe chronic/aggressive periodontitis n = 91	P
Diuretics (treated)	%	0	3.3	0.29
Statins (treated)	%	8.8	12.0	0.54
β-Blockers (treated)	%	7.0	16.3	0.086
Calcium channel blockers (treated)	%	3.5	3.3	1.0
NSAID (treated)	%	17.5	14.1	0.58
ACE-inhibitors (treated)	%	8.8	15.2	0.24

Values are expressed in % as result of Chi-squared test. NSAID = non-steroidal anti-inflammatory drugs; ACE = angiotensin converting enzyme.

Statistical analysis

Statistical data analysis was performed by a professional statistician using the WinMEDAS (C. Grund, Germany) statistical software package.

To calculate the differences between both groups the Mann-Whitney U-test was used for continuous variables. The Chi-square-test or Fishers test for expected values below 5 was used for nominal scale data. The level of significance was set to $p<0.05$.

Results

1. Pulse Wave Velocity (PWV)

The results of the PWV data analysis are depicted in figure 2. Data evaluation revealed significantly higher PWV values for patients suffering from severe chronic periodontitis or severe aggressive periodontitis when compared to the periodontal healthy controls ($p = 0.00004$).

2. Aortic Augmentation Index (AIx)

The results of the calculation of the AIx data for the test and control group are shown in figure 3. AIx scores calculated for the periodontally healthy individuals of the control group proved to be significantly lower ($p = 0.0049$) than the AIx scores calculated for those with severe aggressive periodontitis or severe chronic periodontitis.

3. Pulse pressure amplification (PPA) and central pressure

In the periodontally healthy controls the peripheral diastolic blood pressure was lower, peripheral systolic blood pressure higher and consequently the peripheral pulse pressure significantly higher ($p = 0.0024$) than the values recorded for the periodontitis group (see table 3). However when central pulse pressures were compared the differences disappeared, indicating that the pulse pressure and thus the central pressure is higher and pulse pressure amplification lower in the periodontitis group when compared to the healthy controls ($p = 0.028$ for PPA, table 4). The observed central augmentation pressure shows the tendency to be higher in the periodontitis group ($p = 0.064$, table 4).

Discussion

The main finding of this study is that in patients suffering from severe chronic or aggressive periodontitis arterial stiffness and pulse wave reflection are significantly increased.

It further supports the evidence for an association between periodontal and cardiovascular health and is in line with the data of several other studies [1,29–32].

The specific relationship between arterial stiffness and periodontitis was documented only once before in a subgroup of patients suffering from arterial hypertension [33]. The data of that study failed to prove a difference in PWV. They revealed a significantly higher left ventricular hypertrophy and significant differences in pulse wave reflection including increased central aortic pressures and increased augmentation in the periodontal disease group in the situation of arterial hypertension. A correlation between the pulse wave velocity and oral inflammation was, by contrast to our data, not confirmed. In terms of pulse wave reflection the results are in concordance with the findings of this study. We were able to identify higher AIx scores in the study subjects suffering from severe periodontal disease when compared to the periodontally healthy controls. Besides a higher sample rate in our study the main difference between Franek's and our study is patient selection. As in many other studies the study by Franek et al. 2009 evaluated a highly selected population. Only patients with hypertension were included in their trial. Other studies have shown that hypertensive patients themselves display higher pulse wave velocity scores than patients with normal blood pressure [14,34]. That may be one reason for the diverging study results. Differences induced by hypertension might have superimposed changes caused by periodontal inflammation. Whereas Franek focused on a subgroup of hypertension we included a wide range of cardiovascular compromised as well as cardiovascular healthy subjects. The higher number of evaluated individuals ($n = 724$) in the present study allowed for a meaningful statistical analysis.

Nevertheless, data analysis revealed that the mean peripheral blood pressure of both groups is within the normal range (≤140 systolic, and ≤90 diastolic). On the basis of a routine peripheral blood pressure control by the method of Riva-Rocci, the average individual in the test group would have been classified as patient with no risk factor for cardiovascular events. This illustrates the potential benefits of the oscillometric pulse wave analysis (e.g. Arteriograph) compared to ordinary blood pressure measurements for the detection of early or preclinical signs of cardiovascular dysfunction.

Another point to discuss is the diagnosis and thus the grouping of the patients. The use of the established Community Periodontal Index of Treatment Needs CPITN [35], for classifying the severity of periodontal disease as done in many previous investigations including the study by Franek et al. should be questioned critically. The scoring system of the CPITN tends to overestimate the

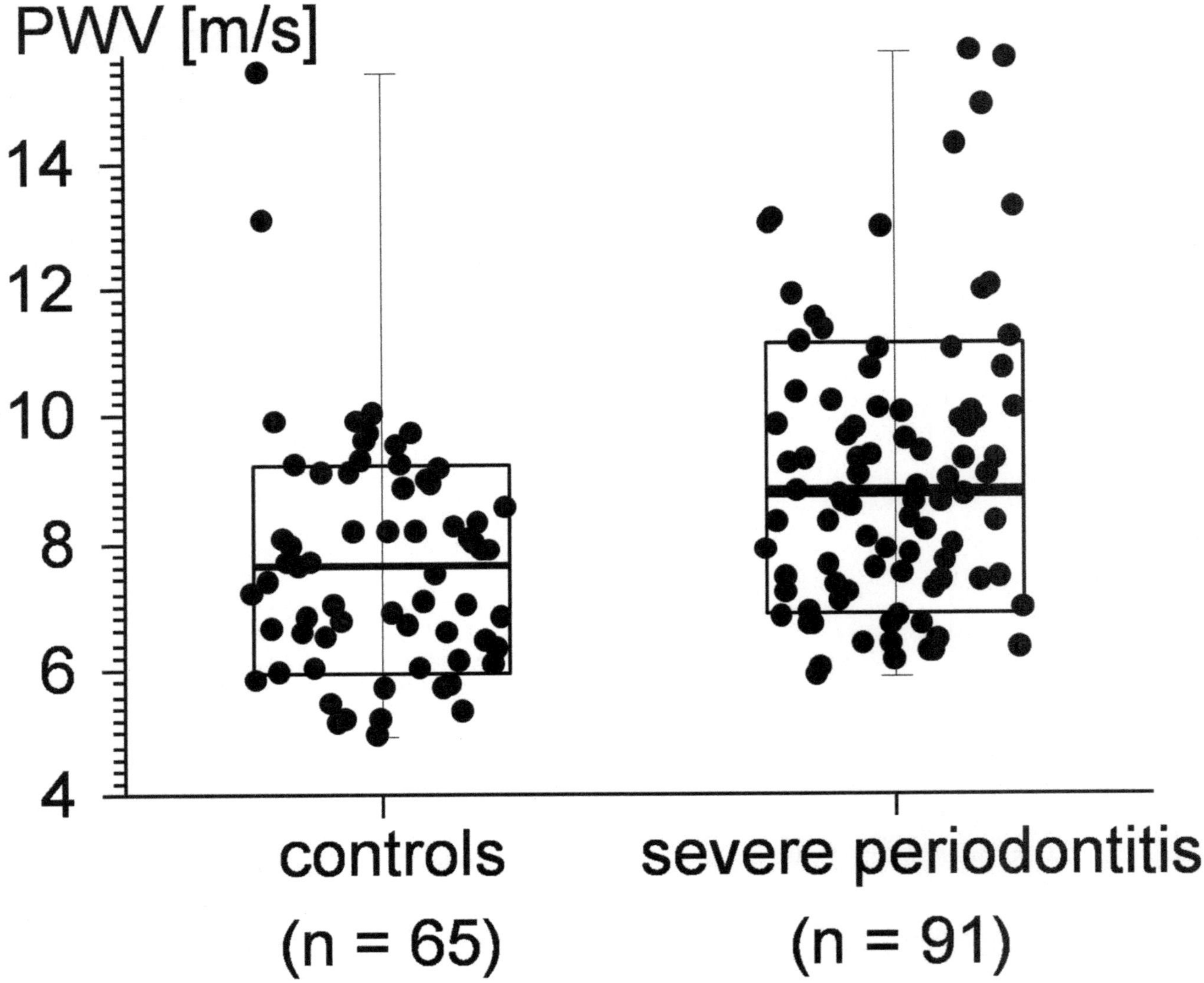

Figure 2. Pulse wave velocity (PWV) data recorded for the 2 experimental groups.

severity of periodontal disease expression [1,36]. For this reason, in all study participants we recorded a comprehensive periodontal status and the severity of disease expression was classified following the proposal of the working group of the Centers for Disease Control (CDC) and the American Academy of Periodontology (AAP) [26]. To ensure the inclusion of individuals with a substantial inflammatory burden in the periodontitis group, only subjects with a minimum of six teeth displaying pockets depth ≥ 6 mm were recruited, which is also in contrast to the disease severity of patients evaluated in other preceding investigations.

Particularly in young individuals with a diagnosis of aggressive periodontitis the recorded pulse wave velocity values were significantly higher than those found in the periodontally healthy controls (data not shown). This is consistent with findings from other studies documenting a much stronger association between periodontal infections and vascular endpoints in younger patients [37,38]. By which mechanisms the observed vascular changes are correlated with the manifestation of severe periodontal disease may not be answered by the present data.

"Translating" the arterial stiffness measurements observed in this study into a biological vascular age may serve as an illustration for the importance of the present findings [39]. For this purpose, the results of the present study are compared to standard values obtained from measurements made in the healthy general population. Patients with aggressive periodontitis or severe chronic periodontitis, displaying an average pulse wave velocity of 9.1 m/s their biological vascular age is about 20 years higher than that of the healthy age-corrected group and therefore pre-aged to a huge extent. Even more dramatic are is the interpretation of the results in terms of mortality and the incidence of cardiovascular events. An increase in pulse wave velocity of 1 m/s implies an estimated 14% increased risk for cardiovascular events, and a 15% increased risk for overall mortality rate accordingly to mortality rates of Vlachopoulos' review [17].

For the prediction of cardiovascular events the central pressure is more important than the peripheral [40]. Again, the present study revealed that periodontitis patients exhibit significantly higher central pressures (expressed as PPA) than periodontal healthy controls reflecting the higher cardiovascular risk of the periodontitis patients. Increased PWV as marker of stiffening of the large arteries suggest that periodontitis patients suffer from a broad range of subclinical vasculature dysfunction.

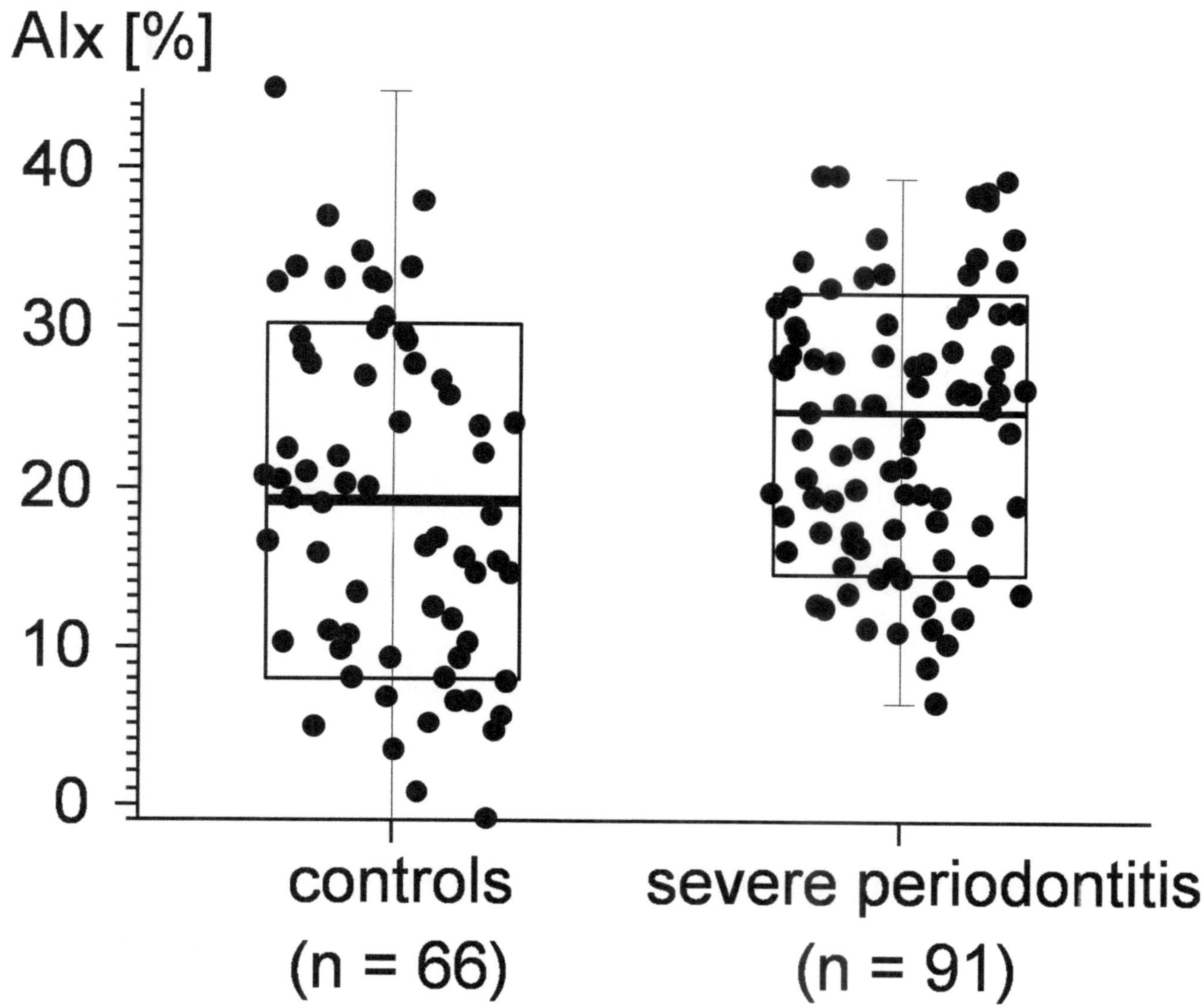

Figure 3. Aortic Augmentation Index (AIx) data calculated for the 2 experimental groups.

The most frequently cited reason for the intake of beta-blocker is the diagnosis "hypertension". Beta-blockers per se (possible exception nebivolol) affect arterial stiffness possibly indirectly by lowering of peripheral blood pressure and/or the initially ejected pressure wave without changing central hemodynamics. Though beta-blockers are known to lower PWV the group with the more frequent intake of β-blockers is showing higher PWV (the periodontitis group). One might speculate that if the intake of beta-blockers would be completely uniformly distributed, the difference in PWV of the groups could even be more pronounced.

Table 3. Hemodynamic characteristics of the studied population.

	Unit	Group: no/mild periodontitis n = 66	Group: severe chronic/aggressive periodontitis n = 92	P
Heart rate	bpm	69±10	67±10	0.089
Peripheral systolic blood pressure	mmHg	134±21	129±16	0.18
Peripheral diastolic blood pressure	mmHg	80±11	82±10	0.89
Peripheral pulse pressure	mmHg	54±14	47±10	0.0024**

Values are expressed as mean ± SD as a result of Mann-Whitney U-Test.

Table 4. Stiffness- and pulse wave reflection related hemodynamics of the studied population.

	Unit	Group no/mild periodontitis n = 66	severe chronic/aggressive periodontitis n = 91	P
Central systolic blood pressure	mmHg	125.9±22.9	124.3±17.8	0.87
Central pulse pressure	mmHg	46.2±16.3	42.1±11.3	0.15
Pulse pressure amplification		1.2±0.2	1.1±0.1	0.028*
Aortic augmentation index (AIx)	%	19.1±10.6	23.7±8.3	0.0049**
Augmentation pressure	mmHg	9.9±8.8	10.4±5.8	0.064
Pulse wave velocity (PWV)	m/s	7.7±1.9	9.1±2.2	0.00004***

Values are expressed as mean ± SD as a result of Mann-Whitney U-Test.

The same holds true for PPA. Nevertheless both, the intake of beta-blockers and the diagnosis hypertension, are not significantly different in both groups.

This cross-sectional study shows for the first time a pathophysiological and highly significant predictive risk marker of PWV in addition to the above described pulse wave reflection to be higher in patients suffering from severe periodontitis. Further intervention studies using these markers of vascular dysfunction and vascular structure as endpoints may be required to elucidate possible causal relationships between periodontal and cardiovascular disease.

Author Contributions

Conceived and designed the experiments: YJ I. Harks I. Haubitz SF ME US JB. Performed the experiments: YJ JB. Analyzed the data: YJ I. Harks I. Haubitz SF ME US JB. Contributed reagents/materials/analysis tools: YJ I. Harks ME US JB. Contributed to the writing of the manuscript: YJ I. Harks I. Haubitz ME US JB.

References

1. Mattila KJ, Nieminen MS, Valtonen VV, Rasi VP, Kesaniemi YA, et al. (1989) Association between dental health and acute myocardial infarction. BMJ 298: 779–781.
2. Syrjanen J, Peltola J, Valtonen V, Iivanainen M, Kaste M, et al. (1989) Dental infections in association with cerebral infarction in young and middle-aged men. J Intern Med 225: 179–184.
3. Humphrey LL, Fu R, Buckley DI, Freeman M, Helfand M (2008) Periodontal disease and coronary heart disease incidence: a systematic review and meta-analysis. J Gen Intern Med 23: 2079–2086. 10.1007/s11606-008-0787-6 [doi].
4. Janket SJ, Baird AE, Chuang SK, Jones JA (2003) Meta-analysis of periodontal disease and risk of coronary heart disease and stroke. Oral Surg Oral Med Oral Pathol Oral Radiol Endod 95: 559–569. 10.1067/moe.2003.107 [doi];S1079210402917075 [pii].
5. Kebschull M, Demmer RT, Papapanou PN (2010) "Gum bug, leave my heart alone!"–epidemiologic and mechanistic evidence linking periodontal infections and atherosclerosis. J Dent Res 89: 879–902. 0022034510375281 [pii];10.1177/0022034510375281 [doi].
6. Elter JR, Hinderliter AL, Offenbacher S, Beck JD, Caughey M, et al. (2006) The effects of periodontal therapy on vascular endothelial function: a pilot trial. Am Heart J 151: 47. S0002-8703(05)00901-4 [pii];10.1016/j.ahj.2005.10.002 [doi].
7. Mercanoglu F, Oflaz H, Oz O, Gokbuget AY, Genchellac H, et al. (2004) Endothelial dysfunction in patients with chronic periodontitis and its improvement after initial periodontal therapy. J Periodontol 75: 1694–1700. 10.1902/jop.2004.75.12.1694 [doi].
8. Seinost G, Wimmer G, Skerget M, Thaller E, Brodmann M, et al. (2005) Periodontal treatment improves endothelial dysfunction in patients with severe periodontitis. Am Heart J 149: 1050–1054. S0002870305000669 [pii];10.1016/j.ahj.2004.09.059 [doi].
9. Tonetti MS, D'Aiuto F, Nibali L, Donald A, Storry C, et al. (2007) Treatment of periodontitis and endothelial function. N Engl J Med 356: 911–920. 356/9/911 [pii];10.1056/NEJMoa063186 [doi].
10. Ferrari AU, Radaelli A, Centola M (2003) Invited review: aging and the cardiovascular system. J Appl Physiol 95: 2591–2597. 10.1152/japplphysiol.00601.2003 [doi];95/6/2591 [pii].
11. Safar H, Mourad JJ, Safar M, Blacher J (2002) Aortic pulse wave velocity, an independent marker of cardiovascular risk. Arch Mal Coeur Vaiss 95: 1215–1218.
12. Blacher J, Guerin AP, Pannier B, Marchais SJ, Safar ME, et al. (1999) Impact of aortic stiffness on survival in end-stage renal disease. Circulation 99: 2434–2439.
13. Cruickshank K, Riste L, Anderson SG, Wright JS, Dunn G, et al. (2002) Aortic pulse-wave velocity and its relationship to mortality in diabetes and glucose intolerance: an integrated index of vascular function? Circulation 106: 2085–2090.
14. Boutouyrie P, Tropeano AI, Asmar R, Gautier I, Benetos A, et al. (2002) Aortic stiffness is an independent predictor of primary coronary events in hypertensive patients: a longitudinal study. Hypertension 39: 10–15.
15. Meaume S, Benetos A, Henry OF, Rudnichi A, Safar ME (2001) Aortic pulse wave velocity predicts cardiovascular mortality in subjects >70 years of age. Arterioscler Thromb Vasc Biol 21: 2046–2050.
16. Mitchell GF, Hwang SJ, Vasan RS, Larson MG, Pencina MJ, et al. (2010) Arterial stiffness and cardiovascular events: the Framingham Heart Study. Circulation 121: 505–511. CIRCULATIONAHA.109.886655 [pii];10.1161/CIRCULATIONAHA.109.886655 [doi].
17. Vlachopoulos C, Aznaouridis K, Stefanadis C (2010) Prediction of cardiovascular events and all-cause mortality with arterial stiffness: a systematic review and meta-analysis. J Am Coll Cardiol 55: 1318–1327. S0735-1097(10)00280-9 [pii];10.1016/j.jacc.2009.10.061 [doi].
18. Willum-Hansen T, Staessen JA, Torp-Pedersen C, Rasmussen S, Thijs L, et al. (2006) Prognostic value of aortic pulse wave velocity as index of arterial stiffness in the general population. Circulation 113: 664–670. 113/5/664 [pii];10.1161/CIRCULATIONAHA.105.579342 [doi].
19. Baulmann J, Nurnberger J, Slany J, Schmieder R, Schmidt-Trucksass A, et al. (2010) [Arterial stiffness and pulse wave analysis]. Dtsch Med Wochenschr 135 Suppl 1: S4–14. 10.1055/s-0030-1249183 [doi].
20. O'Rourke MF (1999) Wave travel and reflection in the arterial system. J Hypertens Suppl 17: S45–S47.
21. Marchais SJ, Guerin AP, Pannier BM, Levy BI, Safar ME, et al. (1993) Wave reflections and cardiac hypertrophy in chronic uremia. Influence of body size. Hypertension 22: 876–883.
22. Weber T, Auer J, O'Rourke MF, Kvas E, Lassnig E, et al. (2004) Arterial stiffness, wave reflections, and the risk of coronary artery disease. Circulation 109: 184–189. 10.1161/01.CIR.0000105767.94169.E3 [doi];01.-CIR.0000105767.94169.E3 [pii].
23. London GM, Blacher J, Pannier B, Guerin AP, Marchais SJ, et al. (2001) Arterial wave reflections and survival in end-stage renal failure. Hypertension 38: 434–438.
24. Baulmann J, Schillings U, Rickert S, Uen S, Dusing R, et al. (2008) A new oscillometric method for assessment of arterial stiffness: comparison with tonometric and piezo-electronic methods. J Hypertens 26: 523–528. 10.1097/HJH.0b013e3282f314f7 [doi];00004872-200803000-00022 [pii].
25. Armitage GC (1999) Development of a classification system for periodontal diseases and conditions. Ann Periodontol 4: 1–6. 10.1902/annals.1999.4.1.1 [doi].
26. Page RC, Eke PI (2007) Case definitions for use in population-based surveillance of periodontitis. J Periodontol 78: 1387–1399. 10.1902/jop.2007.060264 [doi].
27. Grossi SG, Dunford RG, Ho A, Koch G, Machtei EE, et al. (1996) Sources of error for periodontal probing measurements. J Periodontal Res 31: 330–336.

28. Van Bortel LM, Duprez D, Starmans-Kool MJ, Safar ME, Giannattasio C, et al. (2002) Clinical applications of arterial stiffness, Task Force III: recommendations for user procedures. Am J Hypertens 15: 445–452. S0895706101023263 [pii].
29. Briggs JE, McKeown PP, Crawford VL, Woodside JV, Stout RW, et al. (2006) Angiographically confirmed coronary heart disease and periodontal disease in middle-aged males. J Periodontol 77: 95–102. 10.1902/jop.2006.77.1.95 [doi].
30. Hujoel PP, Drangsholt M, Spiekerman C, DeRouen TA (2000) Periodontal disease and coronary heart disease risk. JAMA 284: 1406–1410. joc00373 [pii].
31. Morrison HI, Ellison LF, Taylor GW (1999) Periodontal disease and risk of fatal coronary heart and cerebrovascular diseases. J Cardiovasc Risk 6: 7–11.
32. Tonetti MS (2009) Periodontitis and risk for atherosclerosis: an update on intervention trials. J Clin Periodontol 36 Suppl 10: 15–19. CPE1417 [pii];10.1111/j.1600-051X.2009.01417.x [doi].
33. Franek E, Klamczynska E, Ganowicz E, Blach A, Budlewski T, et al. (2009) Association of chronic periodontitis with left ventricular mass and central blood pressure in treated patients with essential hypertension. Am J Hypertens 22: 203–207. ajh2008330 [pii];10.1038/ajh.2008.330 [doi].
34. Sigurdsson E, Sigfusson N, Sigvaldason H, Thorgeirsson G, Silent S (1996) The changes in an epidemiologic cohort study – a marker of hypertension or coronary heart disease, or both: the Reykjavik study. 27: 1140–1147.
35. Ainamo J, Barmes D, Beagrie G, Cutress T, Martin J, et al. (1982) Development of the World Health Organization (WHO) community periodontal index of treatment needs (CPITN). Int Dent J 32: 281–291.
36. Micheelis W, Hoffmann T, Holtfreter B, Schroeder E (2008) Zur epidemiologischen Einschätzung der Parodontitislast in Deutschland - Versuch einer Bilanzierung. 7: 464–472.
37. Dietrich T, Jimenez M, Krall Kaye EA, Vokonas PS, Garcia RI (2008) Age-dependent associations between chronic periodontitis/edentulism and risk of coronary heart disease. Circulation 117: 1668–1674. CIRCULATIONAHA.107.711507 [pii];10.1161/CIRCULATIONAHA.107.711507 [doi].
38. Jimenez M, Krall EA, Garcia RI, Vokonas PS, Dietrich T (2009) Periodontitis and incidence of cerebrovascular disease in men. Ann Neurol 66: 505–512. 10.1002/ana.21742 [doi].
39. McEniery CM, Yasmin, Hall IR, Qasem A, Wilkinson IB, et al. (2005) Normal vascular aging: differential effects on wave reflection and aortic pulse wave velocity: the Anglo-Cardiff Collaborative Trial (ACCT). J Am Coll Cardiol 46: 1753–1760. S0735-1097(05)01781-X [pii];10.1016/j.jacc.2005.07.037 [doi].
40. Roman MJ, Devereux RB, Kizer JR, Okin PM, Lee ET, et al. (2009) High central pulse pressure is independently associated with adverse cardiovascular outcome the strong heart study. J Am Coll Cardiol 54: 1730–1734. S0735-1097(09)02607-2 [pii];10.1016/j.jacc.2009.05.070 [doi].

10

Education as a Predictor of Chronic Periodontitis: A Systematic Review with Meta-Analysis Population-Based Studies

Adrien Boillot[1], Bechara El Halabi[1], George David Batty[4], Hélène Rangé[1], Sébastien Czernichow[2,3], Philippe Bouchard[1]*

1 Department of Periodontology, Service of Odontology, Rothschild Hospital, AP-HP, Paris 7 - Denis Diderot University, U.F.R. of Odontology, Paris, France, 2 Department of Nutrition, Ambroise Paré Hospital, University Versailles St-Quentin, Boulogne-Billancourt, France, 3 INSERM, U1018, Centre for Research in Epidemiology and Population Health, Villejuif, France, 4 Department of Epidemiology and Public Health, University College London, London, United Kingdom

Abstract

Background: The impact of socioeconomic inequalities on health is well-documented. Despite the links of periodontal disease with cardiovascular diseases, adverse pregnancy outcomes and diabetes, no meta-analysis of socioeconomic variations in periodontal disease exists. This meta-analytic review was conducted to determine the extent to which education attainment influences risk of periodontitis in adults aged 35+ years in the general population.

Methods: The authors searched studies published until November 2010 using EMBASE and MEDLINE databases. References listed were then scrutinised, our own files were checked, and, finally, we contacted experts in the field. The authors included only general population-based studies conducted in adults aged 35 years and more. All articles were blind reviewed by two investigators. In the case of disagreement, a third investigator arbitrated. Using PRISMA statement, two reviewers independently extracted papers of interest.

Results: Relative to the higher education group, people with low education attainment experience a greater risk of periodontitis (OR: 1.86 [1.66–2.10]; $p<0.00001$). The association was partially attenuated after adjustment for covariates (OR: 1.55 [1.30–1.86]; $p<0.00001$). Sensitivity analyses showed that methods used to assess periodontitis, definition of cases, study country and categorization of education are largely responsible for the heterogeneity between studies. No significant bias of publication was shown using both the Egger ($p=0.16$) and rank correlation tests ($p=0.35$).

Conclusions: In the studies reviewed, low educational attainment was associated with an increased risk of periodontitis. Although this evidence should be cautiously interpreted due to methodological problems in selected studies, efforts to eliminate educational inequalities in periodontitis should focus on early life interventions.

Editor: Yiqing Song, Brigham & Women's Hospital, Harvard Medical School, United States of America

Funding: The authors have no support or funding to report.

Competing Interests: The authors have declared that no competing interests exist.

* E-mail: phbouch@noos.fr

Introduction

Chronic periodontitis is a bacterially induced inflammatory disease of the soft and hard tissues which support the tooth root [1]. It is caused by an accumulation of dental plaque, organized as a biofilm on the surface of the tooth crown and root [2], which lead to the destruction of periodontal connective tissue and alveolar bone; without treatment this results in tooth loss. Periodontitis may have long term consequences for health by increasing the risk of type 2 diabetes (T2D) [3], obesity [4], metabolic syndrome [5], cardiovascular diseases (CVD) and pulmonary diseases [6–8], adverse pregnancy outcomes [9], and premature mortality [8]. The condition is common, affecting up to 20% of the adult population in industrialised countries [10].

Chronic periodontitis is a multifactorial disease. However, the contribution of the different risk factors/indicators associated with the disease remains unclear. In addition to a role for oral hygiene, age, cigarette smoking [11] and T2D [3] in the aetiology of this disorder, a further risk factor may be poor social circumstances. There are good *prima facie* reasons to anticipate a relationship between low socio-economic status and chronic periodontitis, not least the strong link between socio-economic status and various health behaviours including smoking and diet [12]. Socio-economic adversity is also related to higher rates of a range of other important chronic diseases, including CVD [13] selected cancers [14], and mental illness [15].

Socio-economic status is typically characterised by income, occupational prestige, and educational achievement. Of these, educational attainment is stable across the adult life course [16] and, because it is usually peaks earlier in life than the other socio-economic indicators, it precedes the onset of most major chronic diseases so allowing investigators to separate cause from effect (reverse causality). Identifying socioeconomic at-risk subgroups for chronic periodontitis has the potential to enhance the effectiveness of preventative campaigns by focusing interventions, adopting specific strategies, reducing costs of public health decisions and obtaining active participation of target populations [17]. Given the strong associations described in the literature between chronic periodontitis and various systemic conditions (e.g, cardiovascular disease), such preventive programmes have also a global public health importance.

The most recent systematic review on socioeconomic variations in chronic periodontitis was published five six ago [18]. Accordingly, we undertook an updated systematic review of studies examining the association of educational attainment and chronic periodontitis in adults in the general population. Additionally, we aggregated the results from identified studies by conducting a meta-analysis.

Methods

Identification of Studies

Following the PRISMA statement [19], we performed a systematic review of all published observational studies conducted in individuals aged 35 and older, which investigated the association between level of education and risk of periodontitis. (Table S1)

Two independent reviewers trained in online article searches (AB and BEH) searched English language papers published before November 2010. We used a four-pronged approach to identifying papers. First, the MEDLINE and EMBASE searches were conducted using the MeSH and EMTREE. For MEDLINE, we used the following strategy: ("Periodontal diseases" [MeSH] OR "periodontitis" [MeSH] OR "chronic periodontitis" [MeSH] OR "periodontal attachment loss" [MeSH] OR "periodontal pocket" [MeSH] OR "alveolar bone loss" [MeSH]) AND ("education" [MeSH] OR "educational status" [MeSH] OR "marital status" [MeSH] OR "occupations" [MeSH] OR "income" [MeSH] OR "socioeconomic factors" [MeSH] OR "social class" [MeSH]). Limits: Human, English.. For EMBASE, search strategy was: ("periodontal disease" [EMTREE] OR "periodontitis" [EMTREE] OR "chronic periodontitis" [EMTREE] OR "periodontal pocket" [EMTREE] OR "alveolar bone loss" [EMTREE]) AND ("education" [EMTREE] OR "educational status" [EMTREE] OR "marital status" [EMTREE] OR "occupation" [EMTREE] OR "income" [EMTREE] OR "socioeconomics" [EMTREE] OR "social status" [EMTREE]). Limits: Human, English. Second, references listed in articles of interest were scrutinised. Third, we checked our own files. Fourth, we contacted selected experts in the field.

Inclusion Criteria

We included all observational studies conducted in adults aged 35+ years in the general population with 1) case definition of periodontitis (probing or radiographic assessment, self-reported data) (Text S1), 2) a variable describing the level of education, 3) a quantitative assessment of the relationship between these two variables. Studies conducted in non-representative populations (e.g. samples of attendees in dental settings) were excluded to maximise external validity. When more than one report used the same data, studies resulting in lowest power were excluded except when prospective data were available. In the case of disagreement, the two investigators discussed the article and tried to find agreement. When consensus was not reached, a third investigator (P.B.) was involved until agreement was found.

Data Abstraction

Two investigators (AB, BEH) independently extracted and tabulated basic information on each study: design, country where the study was conducted, sample size, number of cases, age range, definition of chronic periodontitis, partial or full-mouth recording, categories of level of education. Crude odds ratios (OR), or the data to compute them when crude estimates were unavailable, were also identified and extracted. Adjusted effect measures, including the covariates features in the multivariable model, were tabulated.

Data Analysis

We transformed OR by taking their natural logarithms and calculating standard errors and corresponding confidence intervals [20]. Effects measures and their standard errors were pooled using an inverse variance method with random effects to account for statistical heterogeneity between studies. We calculated pooled OR and accompanying 95% confidence interval (95% CI) for the lowest versus the highest categories of education. Heterogeneity was assessed with the I^2 statistic [21]. We carried out sensitivity analyses based on study design (longitudinal versus cross-sectional studies), year of publication (≤2000 versus >2000), region where the study was conducted (US versus non-US countries), sample size (≤1000 versus >1000), age (≥35 versus olders (≥65)), periodontal assessment method (partial-mouth versus full-mouth recording), definition of cases (combined clinical attachment loss (CAL) and periodontal probing depth (PPD) versus single probing measurement), number of categories of education (2 versus >2). Significance was set at $p<0.05$ and 95% CI were quoted throughout [18]. The Kappa statistic was used to assess interrater reliability between the two independent reviewers [22]. Publication bias was assessed by visually examining a funnel plot with asymmetry being formally assessed with both the Egger test [23] and the rank correlation test [24]. The data were analysed using Review Manager (RevMan, version 5.0, The Cochrane Collaboration, 2008). Bias of publication was measured using CMA (Comprehensive Meta Analysis, version 2.2.055, Biostat, 2010).

Results

Study characteristics

The electronic search yielded 6048 publications, including 1288 duplicates. From the 4760 potentially relevant articles identified, 4528 were excluded. Among the 232 remaining papers, hand-searching of references was performed, resulting in 35 additional papers. From the 267 eligible articles, 249 were excluded resulting in 18 studies, which met all the inclusion criteria and were included in the analyses (Figure 1) [25–42]. The kappa coefficient between examiners was 0.78 (0.75–0.80) demonstrating a substantial agreement [43]. Characteristics of the included studies are presented in Table 1–3. The combined population resulted in 40783 participants. Only two studies were longitudinal [31–32]. The included studies were reformed in the following countries (n = 10): Australia, Brazil, Canada, Denmark, Iran, Norway, Sweden, USA, Taiwan, and Thailand. Crude effect estimates were computed in ten studies [27,29–31,33,34,37,39,41–42]. Eight studies met criteria of inclusion, but were excluded because they were conducted in duplicate surveys [44–51].

Four out of 18 studies did not use full-mouth clinical examination [29,35,37,41]. Only six studies, exhibiting a quite different level of adjustment, gave adjusted effect measures [26,29,32,35,38,40]. Two studies were performed on samples of male [28,41]; whereas two other studies were performed on samples of female [30,38]. One study has separated the outcomes

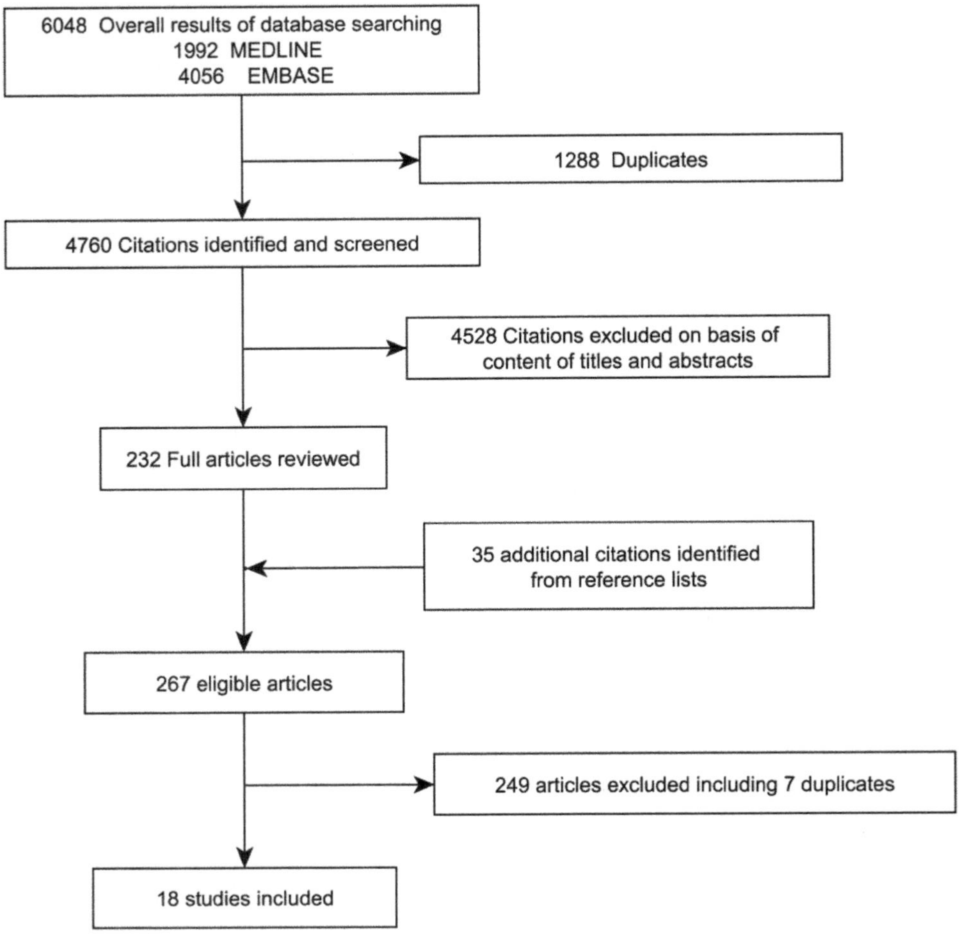

Figure 1. Flow chart for identifying eligible studies.

Table 1. Characteristics of selected US cross-sectional studies in a meta-analysis of education level and chronic periodontitis.

Study name	Study size (of interest/original)	Age (yrs)	Study design	Outcome (No of cases in education groups of interest/Total No of cases)	Comparison groups for education	Variables in multiple adjustment
Beck et al. 1990, USA [25].	689/689	≥65	CS	At least 4 sites with CAL≥5 mm with at least one of those sites with PPD≥4 mm. n = 224/224.	< versus ≥12 years of education.	None.
Borrell et al. 2006, USA [26].	3,240/5,677	≥52	CS	At least two sites with CAL≥6 mm and at least 1 site with PPD≥5 mm. n = 545/963.	<High School versus ≥college.	Age, gender, center, neighbourhood socio-economic score, income.
Dietrich et al. 2006, USA [28].	462/469	47–92	CS	At least one tooth with CAL and PPD≥5 mm. n = 86/86.	≤versus >High School.	None.
Dye et al . 2009, USA [29].	4,014/5,747	≥40	CS	At least one tooth with CAL≥3 mm and PPD≥4 mm. n = 843/1,063.	<High School versus ≥College.	Age, gender, smoking, race, diabetes, periodontal pathogens.
Famili et al. 2005, USA [30].	188/202	≥65	CS	More than 12 teeth with CAL>4 mm. n = 151/163.	≤versus >16 years of education.	None.
Phipps et al. 2009, USA [41].	672/1210	≥65	CS	30% or more of teeth examined with CAL≥5 mm. n = 248/463.	≤High School versus ≥Graduate School	None.

CAL: Clinical Attachment Loss; CPITN: Community Periodontal Index of Treatment Needs; CS: Cross-Sectional; L: Longitudinal; PPD: Periodontal Pocket Depth; t0: Baseline data; Un: Unknown.

Table 2. Characteristics of selected non-US cross-sectional studies in a meta-analysis of education level and chronic periodontitis.

Study name	Study size (of interest/ original)	Age (yrs)	Study design	Outcome (No of cases in education groups of interest/Total No of cases)	Comparison groups for education	Variables in multiple adjustment
Brennan et al. 2007, Australia [27].	709/709	45–54	CS	2 or more sites with CAL≥5 mm and one or more sites with PPD≥4 mm. n = 139/139.	Primary, Secondary, Certificate versus Diploma or degree	None.
Hessari et al. 2007, Iran [33].	2,764/7,949	35–44	CS	At least one sextant with CPITN score 4 (PPD>5.50 mm). Men: n = 136/457. Women: n = 158/360.	Illiterate versus any university education.	None.
Krustrup et al. 2006, Denmark [34].	386/1052	35–44; 65–74	CS	At least one tooth with CAL≥6 mm. n = 22/50.	≤10 versus ≥15 years of education.	None.
Lai et al. 2007, Taiwan [35].	4,347/8,462	35–44	CS	CPITN score 4 (PPD>5,5 mm). n = Un/414.	≤ Junior High School versus ≥ College.	Age, gender, occupation.
Locker et al. 1993, Canada [36].	624/624	≥50	CS	Mean CAL≥3.83. n = Un.	≤ versus >High School.	None.
Mucci et al. 2004, Sweden [37].	14,736/26,690	≥42	CS	Self-reported. Diagnosed by a dentist to have periodontal disease or ever had tooth mobility. n = 2,956/5,527.	Elementary versus University	None.
Nicolau et al. 2007, Brazil [38].	224/224	39,01 (4.70)	CS	More than 42% of teeth with loss of attachment. n = 90/90.	≤ versus >4 years of education.	Age, smoking, plaque, emotional support, conditions during childhood.
Paulander et al. 2004, Sweden [39].	549/549	50 ; 55	CS	Highest 20% of the CAL distribution (mean CAL: 2.4–7.1). n = 110/110.	≤ versus >7 years of education.	None.
Peres et al. 2007, Brazil [40].	6,086/11,342	35–44	CS	At least one site with PPD≥4 mm and at least one site with CAL≥4 mm. n = 542/1,018.	≤4 versus ≥12 years of education.	Age, gender, race, income.
Torrungruang et al. 2009, Thailand [42].	453/453	39–59	CS	3 or more sites with PPD≥5 mm. n = 164/164.	≤ versus >High School.	None.

CAL: Clinical Attachment Loss; CPITN: Community Periodontal Index of Treatment Needs; CS: Cross-Sectional; L: Longitudinal; PPD: Periodontal Pocket Depth; t0: Baseline data; Un: unknown.

for each gender [33]. Cases were defined by a combination of CAL and PPD conditions in six studies [25–29,40]; by a single CAL criteria in seven studies [30,31,34,36,38,39,41]; by CPITN score (Community Periodontal Index of Treatment Needs) in two studies [33,35]; and by self-reported assessment in one study (for more informations about periodontal indices, see supplemental material) [36]. No study with radiographic assessment met criteria of inclusion.

Summary estimates

The summary estimates of OR for each study were pooled to give a total estimate of risk (Figure 2). The overall OR (95% CI) for chronic periodontitis was 1.86 (1.66 to 2.10), indicating an increased risk of periodontitis associated with a low level of education when compared with the highest level of education. The effect size among studies showed a moderate to substantial heterogeneity ($I^2 = 55\%$).

Table 3. Characteristics of selected longitudinal studies in a meta-analysis of education level and chronic periodontitis.

Study name	Study size (of interest/ original)	Age (yrs)	Study design	Outcome (No of cases in education groups of interest/Total No of cases)	Comparison groups for education	Variables in multiple adjustment
Gilbert et al. 2005, USA [31].	559/560	≥45	L	At least one site with a 48-month worst attachment level 3 mm or more than the baseline worst attachment level on that same tooth. n = 123/123.	< versus ≥High School.	None.
Hansen et al. 1995, Norway [32].	81/81	35 (t0)	L	Increased in the number of C-scored quadrants (PTNS) from 1973 to 1988 (at least one site with PPD>5 mm). N = 16/16.	≤ versus >10 years of education.	Missing teeth, last dental visit, oral preventive behaviours, socioeconomic proxies, social class.

CAL: Clinical Attachment Loss; CPITN: Community Periodontal Index of Treatment Needs; CS: Cross-Sectional; L: Longitudinal; PPD: Periodontal Pocket Depth; t0: Baseline data; Un: unknown.

Study or Subgroup	log[Odds Ratio]	SE	Weight	Odds Ratio IV, Random, 95% CI
Beck JD 1990 Blacks	1.131	0.332	2.6%	3.10 [1.62, 5.94]
Beck JD 1990 Whites	0.956	0.36	2.3%	2.60 [1.28, 5.27]
Borrell LN 2006 Blacks	0.693	0.186	5.6%	2.00 [1.39, 2.88]
Borrell LN 2006 Whites	0.47	0.122	7.9%	1.60 [1.26, 2.03]
Brennan DS 2007	0.293	0.196	5.3%	1.34 [0.91, 1.97]
Dietrich T 2006	0.086	0.246	4.0%	1.09 [0.67, 1.77]
Dye BA 2009	0.982	0.087	9.5%	2.67 [2.25, 3.17]
Famili P 2005	0.315	0.372	2.2%	1.37 [0.66, 2.84]
Gilbert GH 2005	0.604	0.241	4.1%	1.83 [1.14, 2.93]
Hansen BF 1995	1.29	0.578	1.0%	3.63 [1.17, 11.28]
Hessari H 2007 Females	0.718	0.372	2.2%	2.05 [0.99, 4.25]
Hessari H 2007 Males	0.5	0.206	5.0%	1.65 [1.10, 2.47]
Krustrup 2006	0.531	0.439	1.6%	1.70 [0.72, 4.02]
Lai H 2007	0.315	0.14	7.2%	1.37 [1.04, 1.80]
Locker D 1992	0.788	0.234	4.2%	2.20 [1.39, 3.48]
Mucci LA 2004	0.723	0.043	11.1%	2.06 [1.89, 2.24]
Nicolau B 2007	0.207	0.267	3.6%	1.23 [0.73, 2.08]
Paulander J 2004	0.604	0.22	4.6%	1.83 [1.19, 2.82]
Peres MA 2007	0.788	0.16	6.4%	2.20 [1.61, 3.01]
Phipps KR 2008	0.513	0.176	5.9%	1.67 [1.18, 2.36]
Torrungruand K 2009	0.978	0.248	3.9%	2.66 [1.64, 4.32]
Total (95% CI)			**100.0%**	**1.86 [1.66, 2.10]**

Heterogeneity: $Tau^2 = 0.03$; $Chi^2 = 44.26$, df = 20 (P = 0.001); $I^2 = 55\%$
Test for overall effect: Z = 10.32 (P < 0.00001)

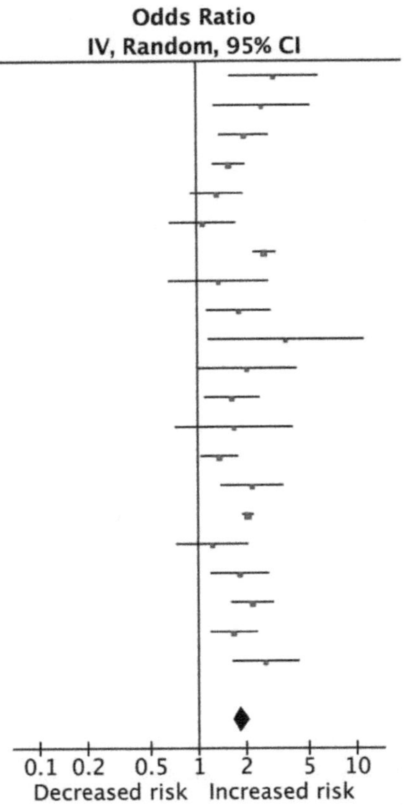

Figure 2. Results of primary meta-analysis: crude risk of periodontitis for individuals with lower education. Legend: Higher level of education as reference. Weights for individual studies calculated with random effects models and inverse variance method. The centre of each black square is placed at the point estimate, the area of the square is proportional to the sample size, and each horizontal line shows the 95% confidence interval for the estimate for each study. Pooled OR (95% CI): 1.86 (1.66–2.10). p<0.00001.

Secondary analyses

Results of the primary analysis were not changed in the sensitivity analysis (Table 4). Two exceptions were the alternative meta-analysis including longitudinal studies and those conducted before year 2000, which enhanced the overall odds ratio (respectively 2.11 (1.22 to 3.63) and 2.57 (1.87 to 3.53)). Within the sensitivity analyses, we examined also various variables as potential sources of heterogeneity. There was evidence of significant heterogeneity across studies that may be explained by geographical differences (Non US: $I^2 = 42\%$ versus US: $I^2 = 68\%$), the extent of the clinical assessment [partial-mouth ($I^2 = 89\%$) versus full-mouth ($I^2 = 22\%$)], and the definition of cases [clinical attachment loss and periodontal probing pocket combined ($I^2 = 74\%$) versus probing pocket depth solely ($I^2 = 0\%$)]. Other sources of heterogeneity have to be interpreted with caution because of the differences in the number of studies in each category. The sensitivity analyses with one by one exclusions showed that one study had a significantly effect on heterogeneity (Data not shown) [29]. When excluded, heterogeneity between studies was nearly non significant ($p = 0.04$, $I^2 = 39\%$).

When pooling studies with adjusted estimates, results were unchanged (OR = 1.55 (1.30 to 1.86); p<0.00001) but low heterogeneity between studies was found ($I^2 = 38\%$) (Figure 3). On the contrary, pooling crude estimates for same studies conducted to both an higher heterogeneity ($I^2 = 77\%$) and an higher risk estimate (OR = 1.88 (1.46 to 2.42)) (Data not shown). Funnel plot showed no asymmetry. No significant bias was shown using both the Egger (p = 0.16) and rank correlation tests (p = 0.35).

Discussion

Principal finding

The present analysis of studies conducted in the general population of adults reveals that individuals with a low level of education have an excess risk of chronic periodontitis when compared with adults with high level of education.

A number of mechanisms may explain this effect. Indirect mechanisms include the link between education and the two main risk factors for chronic periodontitis: smoking [52] and diabetes type 2 [53]. Lower educational attainment, which is a close correlate of IQ, may also directly lead to poorer coping strategies [54], higher BMI [55], lower levels of dental services use [56], low degree of periodontal health awareness [57], and irregular oral self-care practices [58], that in themselves are linked to poor oral hygiene habits may lead to higher levels of dental plaque [59]. Only one study which met our criteria of inclusion showed a significant decrease of the risk to develop chronic periodontitis in the low educated subgroup after adjustment for oral health behaviors [32].

Theories in social epidemiology could also explain such an association. The "pathway model" suggests circumstances in early-life influence social trajectories into and through adulthood, so increasing chronic disease risk [60]. Moreover, low education level is likely to lead to low prestige and low pay occupations, and residing in deprived area. The impact of environmental conditions on periodontal health has been widely described such that individuals living in a neighborhood in the most socially

Table 4. Results of sensitivity analyses to investigate differences between studies included in the meta-analysis (random-effects model).

Included studies	No of studies	OR	95% CI	Residual heterogeneity (I^2)
Study design				
Longitudinal [31,32]	2	2.11*	1.22, 3.63	17%
Cross-sectional [25–30,33–42]	16	1.85***	1.64, 2.09	58%
Baseline data				
≤2000 [25,32,36]	3	2.57***	1.87, 3.53	0%
>2000 [26–31,33–35,37–42]	15	1.79***	1.58, 2.03	61%
Study region				
US [25,26,28–30,41]	6	1.89***	1.51, 2.37	68%
Non US [27,31–40,42]	12	1.83***	1.58, 2.11	42%
Sample size				
≤1000 [25,27,28,30–32,34,36,38,39,41,42]	12	1.78***	1.49, 2.12	31%
>1000 [26,29,33,35,37,40]	6	1.94***	1.65, 2.27	70%
Age (years)				
No limitation [26–29,31–40,42]	15	1.85***	1.62, 2.10	60%
Olders only (≥65) [25,30,41]	3	1.98**	1.41, 2.78	29%
Oral examination				
Partial-mouth [29,35,41]	3	1.85*	1.18, 2.91	89%
Full-mouth [25–28,30–34,36,38–40,42]	14	1.81***	1.59, 2.06	22%
Periodontal assessment				
CAL and PPD [25–29,40]	6	1.93***	1.52, 2.46	74%
CAL or PPD [30–36,38,39,41,42]	11	1.70***	1.49, 1.94	0%
N° of classes for education				
2 [25,27,28,30–32,36,38,39,42]	10	1.81***	1.46, 2.24	42%
2 [26,29,33–35,37,40,41]	8	1.91***	1.66, 2.20	63%

*$P<0.01$.
**$P<0.001$.
***$P<0.0001$.
Higher level of education as reference. Random-effects model and inverse variance method.

Study or Subgroup	log[Odds Ratio]	SE	Weight	Odds Ratio IV, Random, 95% CI
Borrell LN 2006 Blacks	0.693	0.186	14.8%	2.00 [1.39, 2.88]
Borrell LN 2006 Whites	0.182	0.13	21.7%	1.20 [0.93, 1.55]
Dye BA 2009	0.713	0.188	14.6%	2.04 [1.41, 2.95]
Hansen BF 1995	0.723	0.306	7.2%	2.06 [1.13, 3.75]
Lai H 2007	0.336	0.156	18.1%	1.40 [1.03, 1.90]
Nicolau B 2007	0.182	0.327	6.5%	1.20 [0.63, 2.28]
Peres MA 2007	0.405	0.165	17.1%	1.50 [1.09, 2.07]
Total (95% CI)			**100.0%**	**1.55 [1.30, 1.86]**

Heterogeneity: $Tau^2 = 0.02$; $Chi^2 = 9.74$, df = 6 (P = 0.14); $I^2 = 38\%$
Test for overall effect: Z = 4.84 (P < 0.00001)

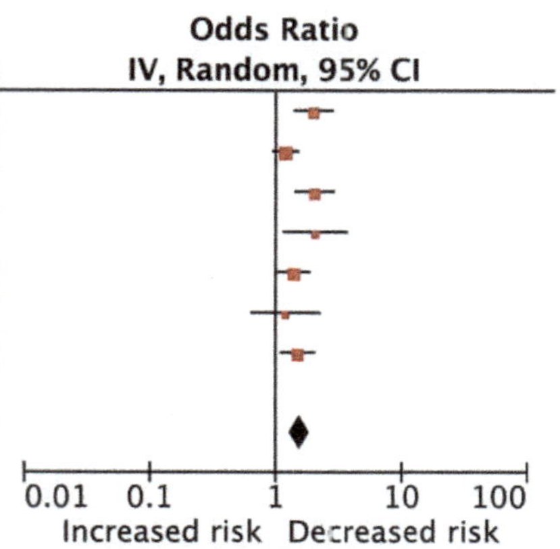

Figure 3. Results of primary meta-analysis: adjusted risk of periodontal diseases for individuals with low education. Legend: Higher level of education as reference. Weights for individual studies calculated with random effects models and inverse variance method. The centre of each black square is placed at the point estimate, the area of the square is proportional to the sample size, and each horizontal line shows the 95% confidence interval for the estimate for each study. Pooled OR (95% CI): 1.55 (1.30–1.86). p<0.00001.

marginalised areas experience twice the risk of periodontitis relative to those in the most affluent [61].

Exploration for heterogeneity

The pooled OR should be interpreted with caution, given the substantial heterogeneity detected between studies. Sensitivity analyses showed that several factors seem to account for this heterogeneity, including the region where the study was conducted, the extent of oral examination, the definition of cases and the number of categories for education level assessment. Taken together these factors might help us to improve our understanding of circumstances under which education interacts with periodontal health. In addition, the heterogeneity indicates that efforts should be made to adopt a standardised methodological approach when studying the association between periodontal diseases and socioeconomic factors.

Partial-mouth examinations may underestimate the prevalence of periodontal diseases [62,63]. Additionally, methods used in partial-mouth examination are numerous. Both result in a lower heterogeneity between studies when excluding studies with partial-mouth examination. For same reasons, exclusion of studies using both CAL and PPD to define periodontitis results in a low heterogeneity between studies. As an illustration, heterogeneity between studies became non-significant when we conducted a one-study removed sensitivity analysis excluding Dye study ($I^2 = 39\%$) [29]. In this cross-sectional study using data from NHANES III survey, cases of periodontitis were defined as a combination of clinical attachment loss and probing pocket depth criteria after a full-mouth examination.

The impact of education on periodontal status does not seem the same according to the geographic area. Heterogeneity was higher for US studies than for studies conducted in other countries. One explanation might be that the US studies were not focused on same spatial units, several using census data, whereas others were conducted in counties or neighbourhoods.

Heterogeneity could also be due to differences in the classification of education attainment. In the sensitivity analyses, we compared studies with two classes of education with other studies. When only studies separating education level into two classes were included in the analysis, a lower heterogeneity was found. This may be due to the method we used. We compared individuals from extreme categories of education attainment. Including studies with more than two classes of education; we excluded all individuals with an intermediate level of education. Further, the classification of education attainment differs between studies. Some authors use corresponding diploma; other authors use years of schooling to categorize the level of education. Both resulted in a higher heterogeneity between studies with more than two classes of education.

Pooling of studies with adjusted estimates showed a decrease in heterogeneity between studies. Confounders such as race, diabetes or smoking are a source of heterogeneity between studies, and no adjustment result in an overestimated association between education and chronic periodontitis [18].

Strengths and limitations

The present study has limitations inherent to meta-analyses. First, the results should be interpreted with caution and should not be considered as causal evidence because all studies were observational and most cross-sectional. Only two prospective studies met our criteria of inclusion [31–32]. Thus, associations are suggestive at best.

Secondly, there was significant heterogeneity between the included studies so overall conclusions must be regarded with caution. When we carried out sensitivity analyses to investigate possible sources of heterogeneity the results highlight a call for standardisation when studying social epidemiology in periodontal health, in particular concerning definition of cases. However, exclusion of only one study [29] resulted in a decrease of heterogeneity between studies, which became non significant ($p = 0.04$). Then, only six studies gave adjusted results for confounders [26,29,32,35,38,40], and two studies were adjusted for smoking [29,38], whereas it was described as a confounding factor [18].

Finally, because the physiopathology mechanisms for aggressive periodontitis differ from those involved in the development of chronic periodontitis [64] *a priori*, we elected not to include studies which captured the former outcome. This may have caused us to misclassify as unaffected some individuals with localized periodontitis. This is likely to have diluted the overall strength of the education-periodontal disease association.

However, our study has several strengths. It is the first, to our knowledge, including such a number of individuals (more than 40000), which quantifies the association between education attainment and periodontal diseases. The analysis is centred on chronic periodontitis, which is the most common form of periodontitis in adults. A previous systematic review has already shown a higher prevalence of periodontitis in a low socioeconomic group but the effect was not quantified [18]. The reason why no meta-analysis was performed in the above study maybe due (1) to the wide range of age (>19 year-old) that may include different diagnosis such as aggressive and chronic periodontitis, (2) to the difficulty to evaluate the socio-economic level in younger populations, and (3) to the low number of studies available when this review was conducted (our Medline search identified a nearly 60% increase in the number of studies from April 2004 to November 2010). Our search was conducted on multiple databases, and references listed in retrieved articles were adequately scrutinised according to the standards guidelines for systematic reviews. Finally, both Egger and rank correlation tests showed no significant bias of publication.

Conclusions and implications

Results from our meta-analysis support the growing body of evidence of a socioeconomic gradient in oral health. The impact is first clinical to identify at-risk patients and adopt preventive attitudes for them, such as motivation to institute healthy behaviours (smoking cessation, oral hygiene instruction, regular dental visits…). This socioeconomic gradient in periodontal health may also have several implications for public health. The association between periodontal disease and other diseases that may compromise health condition emphasises the need to identify at-risk populations. This would permit to target public health actions aiming to prevent periodontal diseases. Identifying socioeconomic at-risk populations for oral diseases enhances the effectiveness of preventive campaigns by focusing interventions, adopting specific strategies and obtaining active participation of target populations. Moreover, because of the associations between education level and various risk factors/indicators for chronic periodontitis, educational attainment appears as a main target in preventing the development of chronic periodontitis. Finally, because of the relationships between chronic periodontitis and numerous systemic conditions, such approaches may lead to the reduction of the morbidity for other chronic diseases and, as a consequence, to decrease the overall healthcare costs.

To conclude, the effect of low education attainment on higher risk of periodontal diseases has a series of potential mechanisms.

This notwithstanding, education may plausibly represent a main target for preventive programmes for periodontal diseases.

Supporting Information

Table S1 PRISMA checklist.

Text S1 Description of periodontal measurements.

Acknowledgments

The authors thank Marco Aurélio Peres, Departamento de Saúde Pública, Universidade Federal de Santa Catarina, Campus Universitário Trindade, Florianópolis, SC 88010-970, Brazil, and Annette Leclerc, Inserm U1018, Epidemiology of occupational and social determinants of health, Center for Research in Epidemiology and Population Health, Inserm, Villejuif, France, for giving additional information, which were necessary to write, respectively, the results and discussion sections.

Author Contributions

Conceived and designed the experiments: AB SC PB. Analyzed the data: AB SC. Wrote the paper: AB BEH GDB HR SC PB. ICMJE criteria for authorship read and met: AB BEH GDB HR SC PB. Agreed with the manuscript's results and conclusions: AB BEH GDB HR SC PB. Collected data: AB BEH HR. Wrote the first draft of the paper: AB GDB SC PB.

References

1. Darveau RP (2010) Periodontitis: a polymicrobial disruption of host homeostasis. Nat Rev Microbiol 8(7): 481–90.
2. Kolenbrander PE, Palmer RJ, Jr., Periasamy S, Jakubovics NS (2010) Oral multispecies biofilm development and the key role of cell-cell distance. Nat Rev Microbiol 8(7): 471–80.
3. Taylor GW (2010) Bidirectional interrelationships between diabetes and periodontal diseases: an epidemiologic perspective. Ann Periodontol 6(1): 99–112.
4. Chaffee B, Weston S (2010) Association Between Chronic Periodontal Disease and Obesity: A Systematic Review and Meta-Analysis. J Periodontol 81(12): 1708–24.
5. D'Aiuto F, Sabbah W, Netuveli G, Donos N, Hingorani AD, et al. (2008) Association of the metabolic syndrome with severe periodontitis in a large U.S. population-based survey. J Clin Endocrinol Metab 93(10): 3989–94.
6. Tonetti MS, D'Aiuto F, Nibali L, Donald A, Storry C, et al. (2007) Treatment of periodontitis and endothelial function. N Engl J Med 356(9): 911–20.
7. Garcia RI, Nunn ME, Vokonas PS (2001) Epidemiologic associations between periodontal disease and chronic obstructive pulmonary disease. Ann Periodontol 6(1): 71–7.
8. Li Q, Chalmers J, Czernichow S, Neal B, Taylor BA, et al. (2010) Oral disease and subsequent cardiovascular disease in people with type 2 diabetes: a prospective cohort study based on the Action in Diabetes and Vascular Disease: Preterax and Diamicron Modified-Release Controlled Evaluation (ADVANCE) trial. Diabetologia 53(11): 2320–7.
9. Wimmer G, Pihlstrom BL (2008) A critical assessment of adverse pregnancy outcome and periodontal disease. J Clin Periodontol 35(8 Suppl): 380–97.
10. Pihlstrom BL, Michalowicz BS, Johnson NW (2005) Periodontal diseases. Lancet 366(9499): 1809–20.
11. Bergstrom J (2006) Periodontitis and smoking: an evidence-based appraisal. J Evid Based Dent Pract 6(1): 33–41.
12. Shankar A, McMunn A, Steptoe A (2010) Health-related behaviors in older adults relationships with socioeconomic status. Am J Prev Med 38(1): 39–46.
13. Kerr GD, Slavin H, Clark D, Coupar F, Langhorne P, et al. (2010) Do Vascular Risk Factors Explain the Association between Socioeconomic Status and Stroke Incidence: A Meta-Analysis. Cerebrovasc Dis 31(1): 57–63.
14. Conway DI, Petticrew M, Marlborough H, Berthiller J, Hashibe M, et al. (2008) Socioeconomic inequalities and oral cancer risk: a systematic review and meta-analysis of case-control studies. Int J Cancer 122(12): 2811–9.
15. Chang-Quan H, Zheng-Rong W, Yong-Hong L, Yi-Zhou X, Qing-Xiu L (2010) Education and risk for late life depression: a meta-analysis of published literature. Int J Psychiatry Med 40(1): 109–24.
16. Ribet C, Melchior M, Lang T, Zins M, Goldberg M, et al. (2007) [Characterisation and measurement of social position in epidemiologic studies]. Rev Epidemiol Sante Publique 55(4): 285–95.
17. Watt RG (2002) Emerging theories into the social determinants of health: implications for oral health promotion. Community Dent Oral Epidemiol 30: 241–47.
18. Klinge B, Norlund (2005) A socio-economic perspective on periodontal diseases: a systematic review. J Clin Periodontol 32 Suppl 6: 314–25.
19. Moher D, Liberati A, Tetzlaff J, Altman DG, The PRISMA Group (2009) Preferred Reporting Items for Systematic Reviews and Meta-Analyses: The PRISMA Statement. PloS Med 6(7).
20. Altman DG, Bland JM (2003) Interaction revisited: the difference between two estimates. BMJ 326(7382): 219.
21. Higgins JP, Thompson SG, Deeks JJ, Altman DG (2003) Measuring inconsistency in meta-analyses. BMJ 327(7414): 557–60.
22. Cohen J (1960) A coefficient of agreement for nominal scales. Educ Psychol Meas 20: 37–46.
23. Egger M, Davey Smith G, Schneider M, Minder C (1997) Bias in meta-analysis detected by a simple, graphical test. BMJ 315(7109): 629–34.
24. Begg CB, Mazumdar M (1994) Operating characteristics of a rank correlation test for publication bias. Biometrics 50(4): 1088–101.
25. Beck JD, Koch GG, Rozier RG, Tudor GE (1990) Prevalence and risk indicators for periodontal attachment loss in a population of older community-dwelling blacks and whites. J Periodontol 61(8): 521–8.
26. Borrell LN, Beck JD, Heiss G (2006) Socioeconomic disadvantage and periodontal disease: The dental atherosclerosis risk in communities study. Am J Public Health 96(2): 332–9.
27. Brennan DS, Spencer AJ, Roberts-Thomson KF (2007) Periodontal disease among 45–54 year olds in Adelaide, South Australia. Aust Dent J 52(1): 55–60.
28. Dietrich T, Krall Kaye E, Nunn ME, Van Dyke T, Garcia RI (2006) Gingivitis susceptibility and its relation to periodontitis in men. J Dent Res 85(12): 1134–7.
29. Dye BA, Herrera-Abreu M, Lerche-Sehm J, Vlachojannis C, Pikdoken L, et al. (2009) Serum antibodies to periodontal bacteria as diagnostic markers of periodontitis. J Periodontol 80(4): 634–47.
30. Famili P, Cauley J, Suzuki JB, Weyant R (2005) Longitudinal study of periodontal disease and edentulism with rates of bone loss in older women. J Periodontol 76(1): 11–5.
31. Gilbert GH, Shelton BJ, Fisher MA (2005) Forty-eight-month periodontal attachment loss incidence in a population-based cohort study: Role of baseline status, incident tooth loss, and specific behavioral factors. J Periodontol 76(7): 1161–70.
32. Hansen BF, Bjertness E, Gronnesby JK, Eriksen HM (1995) Changes in periodontal treatment needs. A follow-up study of Oslo citizens from the ages of 35 to 50 years. J Periodontal Res 30(6): 410–7.
33. Hessari H, Vehkalahti MM, Eghbal MJ, Murtomaa HT (2007) Oral health among 35- to 44-year-old Iranians. Med Princ Pract 16(4): 280–5.
34. Krustrup U, Erik Petersen P (2006) Periodontal conditions in 35–44 and 65–74-year-old adults in Denmark. Acta Odontol Scand 64(2): 65–73.
35. Lai H, Lo MT, Wang PE, Wang TT, Chen TH, et al. (2007) A community-based epidemiological study of periodontal disease in Keelung, Taiwan: a model from Keelung community-based integrated screening programme (KCIS No. 18). J Clin Periodontol 34(10): 851–9.
36. Locker D, Leake JL (1993) Risk indicators and risk markers for periodontal disease experience in older adults living independently in Ontario, Canada. J Dent Res 72(1): 9–17.
37. Mucci LA, Hsieh CC, Williams PL, Dickman PW, Bjorkman L, et al. (2004) Birth order, sibship size, and housing density in relation to tooth loss and periodontal disease: a cohort study among Swedish twins. Am J Epidemiol 159(5): 499–506.
38. Nicolau B, Netuveli G, Kim JW, Sheiham A, Marcenes W (2007) A life-course approach to assess psychosocial factors and periodontal disease. J Clin Periodontol 34(10): 844–50.
39. Paulander J, Axelsson P, Lindhe J, Wennstrom JL (2004) Some characteristics of 50/55-year-old individuals with various experience of destructive periodontal disease: A cross-sectional study. Acta Odontol Scand 62(4): 199–206.
40. Peres MA, Antunes JLF, Boing AF, Peres KG, Bastos JLD (2007) Skin colour is associated with periodontal disease in Brazilian adults: A population-based oral health survey. J Clin Periodontol 34(3): 196–201.
41. Phipps KR, Chan BK, Jennings-Holt M, Geurs NC, Reddy MS, et al. (2009) Periodontal health of older men: the MrOS dental study. Gerodontology 26(2): 122–29.
42. Torrungruang K, Bandhaya P, Likittanasombat K, Grittayaphong C, Torrungruang K, et al. (2009) Relationship between the presence of certain bacterial pathogens and periodontal status of urban Thai adults. J Periodontol 80: 122–29.
43. Landis JR, Koch GG (1977) The measurement of observer agreement for categorical data. Biometrics 33(1): 159–74.
44. Brown LF, Beck JD, Rozier RG (1994) Incidence of attachment loss in community-dwelling older adults. J Periodontol 65(4): 316–23.
45. Cascaes AM, Peres KG, Peres MA (2009) Periodontal disease is associated with poor self-rated oral health among Brazilian adults. J Clin Periodontol 36(1): 25–33.
46. Dolan TA, Gilbert GH, Ringelberg ML, Legler DW, Antonson DE, et al. (1997) Behavioral risk indicators of attachment loss in adult Floridians. J Clin Periodontol 24(4): 223–32.

47. Hansen BF, Bjertness E, Gjermo P (1990) Changes in periodontal disease indicators in 35-year-old Oslo citizens from 1973 to 1984. J Clin Periodontol 17(4): 249–54.
48. Hansen BF, Bjertness E, Gronnesby JK (1993) A socio-ecologic model for periodontal diseases. J Clin Periodontol 20(8): 584–90.
49. Hessari H, Vehkalahti M, Eghbal M, Murtomaa H, Hessari H, et al. (2009) Lifelong exposure to smoking and oral health among 35- to 44-year-old Iranians. Oral Health Prev Dent 7(1): 61–8.
50. Torrungruang K, Tamsailom S, Rojanasomsith K, Sutdhibhisal S, Nisapakultorn K, et al. (2005) Risk indicators of periodontal disease in older Thai adults. J Periodontol 76(4): 558–65.
51. Tsai C, Hayes C, Taylor GW (2002) Glycemic control of type 2 diabetes and severe periodontal disease in the US adult population. Community Dent Oral Epidemiol 30(3): 182–92.
52. Huisman M, Van Lenthe FJ, Giskes K, Kamphuis CB, Brug J, et al. (2011) Explaining socio-economic inequalities in daily smoking: a social-ecological approach. Eur J Public Health. In press.
53. Kavanagh A, Bentley RJ, Turrell G, Shaw J, Dunstan D, et al. (2010) Socioeconomic position, gender, health behaviours and biomarkers of cardiovascular disease and diabetes. Soc sci Med 71: 1150–60.
54. Christensen U, Schmidt L, Kriegbaum M, Hougaard CO, Holstein BE (2006) Coping with unemployment: does educational attainment make any difference? Scand J Public Health 34: 363–70.
55. Molarius A, Seidell JC, Sans S, Tuomilehto J, Kuulasmaa K (2000) Educational level, relative body weight, and changes in their association over 10 years: an international perspective from the WHO MONICA Project. Am J Public Health 90: 1260–68.
56. Lang IA, Gibbs SJ, Steel N, Melzer D (2008) Neighbourhood deprivation and dental service use: a cross-sectional analysis of older people in England. J Public Health 30: 472–78.
57. Alwaeli HA, Al-Jundi SH (2005) Periodontal disease awareness among pregnant women and its relationship with socio-demographic variables. Int J Dent Hyg 3: 74–82.
58. Petersen PE, Aleksejuniene J, Christensen LB, Eriksen HM, Kalo I (2000) Oral health behavior and attitudes of adults in Lithuania. Acta Odontol Scand 58: 243–48.
59. Zini A, Sgan-Cohen HD, Marcenes W (2011) Socio-economic position, smoking, and plaque: a pathway to severe chronic periodontitis. J Clin Periodontol 38: 229–35.
60. Graham H (2002) Building an inter-disciplinary science of health inequalities: the example of lifecourse research. Soc Sci Med 55: 2005–16.
61. Borrell LN, Burt BA, Warren RC, Neighbors HW (2006) The role of individual and neighborhood social factors on periodontitis: the third National Health and Nutrition Examination Survey. J Periodontol 77: 444–53.
62. Eaton KA, Duffy S, Griffiths GS, Gilthorpe MS, Johnson NW (2001) The influence of partial and full-mouth recordings on estimates of prevalence and extent of lifetime cumulative attachment loss: a study in a population of young male military recruits. J Periodontol 72(2): 140–5.
63. Borges-Yanez SA, Maupome G, Jimenez-Garcia G (2004) Validity and reliability of partial examination to assess severe periodontitis. J Clin Periodontol 31(2): 112–8.
64. Lang N, Bartold PM, Cullinan M, Jeffcoat M, Mombelli A, et al. (1999) Consensus Report: Aggressive Periodontitis. Ann Periodontol 4: 53.

11

Differences in Functional Outcomes for Adult Patients with Prosthodontically-Treated and -Untreated *Shortened Dental Arches*: A Systematic Review

Saadika Khan[1]*, Alfred Musekiwa[2], Usuf M. E. Chikte[3], Ridwaan Omar[4]

1 Department of Restorative Dentistry, University of the Western Cape, Cape Town, South Africa, **2** Centre for Evidence-Based Health Care, Faculty of Medicine and Health Sciences, Stellenbosch University, Cape Town, South Africa, **3** Department of Interdisciplinary Health Sciences, Stellenbosch University, Cape Town, South Africa, **4** Head of Prosthodontics, Faculty of Dentistry, Kuwait University, Safat, Kuwait

Abstract

This review examined differences in functional outcomes and patient satisfaction when shortened dental arches are left untreated compared to their restoration to complete arch lengths with different prosthodontic interventions.

Methods: A protocol was developed according to the criteria for a systematic review. All relevant databases were searched to identify appropriate clinical trials regardless of language or publication status. Predetermined eligibility criteria were applied, trial quality assessed and data extracted for each study. Relevant outcomes assessed were: functioning ability, patient satisfaction and harmful effects on oral structures.

Results: Searches yielded 101 articles: 81 from electronic databases and 20 from reference lists of retrieved articles (PEARLing searches). Sixty-nine citations were assessed for eligibility after removing 32 duplicate records. After reading titles and abstracts, a total of 41 records were excluded and the full-texts of the remaining 28 records were read. Only 21 records were included for the SR because 7 records were excluded after reading the full-text reports. These 21 records report the outcomes of four randomized controlled trials (RCTs) and one non-randomized clinical trial (CT) which were pre-specified and used for this review. No on-going studies were found and no eligible studies were excluded for failure to report the reviewer's pre-specified outcomes. Outcomes were reported in the retrieved 21 articles. A narrative explanation of the pre-specified outcomes is reported for the 3 comparison groups (which were based on the different interventions used for the individual clinical trials). The shortened dental arch as a treatment option is encouraging in terms of functioning, patient satisfaction and cost-effectiveness. By using only high quality studies it was expected that the results would be more reliable when making conclusions and recommendations, but some of the included studies had to be downgraded due to methodological errors.

Editor: Kimon Divaris, UNC School of Dentistry, University of North Carolina-Chapel Hill, United States of America

Funding: University of the Western Cape funded the services of a statistician for this review. The funders had no role in study design, data collection and analysis, decision to publish, or preparation of the manuscript.

Competing Interests: The authors have declared that no competing interests exist.

* Email: skhan@uwc.ac.za

Introduction

Prosthodontic treatment planning customarily includes the replacement of all missing teeth with the intention of achieving complete dental arches (CDAs) comprising 28 teeth [1–3]. The rationale for this approach includes impaired oral function with a perceived detrimental impact on chewing ability, occlusal stability and temporomandibular joint (TMJ) function due to the loss of the molar teeth [4]. On the other hand, several studies and reviews have indicated that twenty occluding teeth provide sufficient oral functional ability and the need to replace all missing posterior teeth has been questioned [3–11].

The classic shortened dental arch (SDA) is defined as ten pairs of occluding anterior and premolar teeth [5,8]. Many patients present with SDAs since molars are the teeth more commonly lost due to caries, resulting in patients having a posteriorly reduced dental arch [12–13]. Variations of the SDA include a partially dentate arch described as an interrupted or discontinuous dental arch where individual anterior, premolar or even molar teeth are lost [7]. A considerable number of studies have been conducted, though mostly in industrialized countries, that confirm a range of benefits and adequate oral functioning with a SDA [4–12,14–20]. These studies also propose that the aesthetic features of such partially dentate patients are acceptable [5,8]. Research related to the SDA concept has also been conducted and promoted in some developing countries such as Tanzania and Nigeria [3,5–12]. The 1982 WHO oral health goal for developing countries was set as the retention of twenty functional, aesthetic natural teeth without resorting to a prosthesis which is in line with the findings of the SDA research [4–12,21].

When dentists extend or reconstitute reduced, shortened or discontinuous dental arches and replace missing teeth in either anterior or posterior regions to create a CDA, the following interventions are usually recommended: removable partial denture prosthesis (RPDP) or fixed denture prosthesis (FDP), including resin-bonded bridges and implant-retained prostheses [9,22–33]. Anecdotal evidence suggests that the choice is largely intuitively based upon the number of missing teeth, their location in the arch, and economic considerations. Currently, RPDPs, FDPs and implant procedures evidently operate on the premise of optimal occlusion encompassing the aesthetics, oral function, oral health and comfort created by the occluding teeth [4–5,33]. This practice appears to have evolved empirically, with no scientific or clinical evidence to support its widespread acceptance by clinicians [3,22–33].

Several research reports tend to support the view that the underlying objective of the SDA to preserve a functional dental arch can be realized through a functionally-oriented treatment approach [5,15–17,22,24,26]. This entails directing the limited resources towards that part of the dentition that can be successfully preserved and in the most cost-effective manner, rather than on the remaining molar teeth that often have a poorer prognosis [5,7,31–58]. The minimum number of teeth or shortness of the arch will also depend on the periodontal condition of the remaining teeth, the age of the patient, occlusal activity, food types and adaptive capacity of the patients' temporomandibular joints [3,7,9].

Research suggests that this seemingly beneficial SDA concept and its variations can be utilized to improve accessibility and affordability to treatment for socially- and economically-deprived middle-aged and elderly communities [5,16,22,24,26]. Other associated benefits of the SDA have been enumerated by several researchers [5–8,10–20,31–58]. A number of studies have been conducted in Tanzania where the evidence obtained was used to advise the government, medical and dental personnel to include the SDA concept within the prosthodontic management protocols for the country [12,16,50–52]. The consequence of the research was that dental institutions reviewed the dental curricula accordingly [12,16,50–52].

Following the large body of published research data related to the SDA conducted in different parts of the world, several efforts at collating these data have been made. Thus a number of systematic reviews (SR) focusing on the SDA have been completed [8,56–58]. A SR conducted by Gotfredsen and Walls (2007) focused on studies that reported on the assessment of normative needs only, although it did not include quality of life studies that considered the perceived oral health needs of partially dentate patients [8]. In the SR by Fueki et al (2011), different types of study designs were included, in addition to the randomised controlled trials (RCT) [56]. The quality of evidence from longitudinal studies related to restorative and non-restorative approaches to adult patients with SDAs were assessed by Faggion (2011) using GRADE (Grading of Recommendations Assessment, Development and Evaluation) approach [58]. With this study, even though all the results from the included studies were not reported, it demonstrated how important methodological rigor is and that these need to be reported [58]. In a recent electronic search in the Cochrane database for systematic reviews, Abt, Carr and Worthington (2012) focused on a broad research question to include all different types of interventions for partially dentate patients, including the SDA [57]. No conclusive evidence was found to indicate that any intervention was better for partially dentate patients, irrespective of particular interventions, procedures or materials used [57].

Given that so few RCTs have been conducted and are available, researchers conducting SRs are faced with the ineluctable option of including different types of study designs and systematic reviews [8,56–58]. This results in the inclusion of lesser strength studies which could affect the quality of the evidence presented [8,14,31–37,40–48,53–55].

The aim of this systematic review was to identify and analyse existing clinical trials which compare the functional outcomes of prosthodontic interventions used for treating shortened arches versus un-restored shortened arches in partially dentate adult patients.

The following research question addresses the aim and objectives of the study: In adult patients with shortened dental arches, what is the effect of prosthodontics interventions on the functional outcomes compared to having no treatment?

Methods

Protocol Development

A protocol (Registration No: 11/4/39) was developed (not published) to include all aspects of a SR namely: selection criteria, search strategy, selection methods using predetermined eligibility criteria, data collection, data extraction, assessment of risk of bias using the Cochrane tool, the GRADE tool to grade the evidence of each clinical trial and statistical analysis by calculating risk ratios (RR) for dichotomous outcomes and presented at 95% confidence intervals [59–60].

Criteria for considering studies for this review

Types of studies. Only RCTs and Clinical trials (CTs) are included in the systematic review (SR).

Types of interventions. Interventions included in this study are described as any prosthodontic intervention used to restore and treat the SDA such as RPDPs and FDPs. The control group for this study included patients with the classic SDA.

Types of participants. Participants included in the SR were:

1. Adult male and female participants aged 18 years and older.
2. Study population included patients with posteriorly reduced or shortened dental arches.

Types of outcome measures. Primary and secondary outcomes were pre-specified for the SR and these include:

Primary outcomes

1) Functional outcomes (patient- or investigator-reported) as measured by masticatory function, chewing ability, occlusal effects, nutrient intake (using nutritional assessments and haematological markers) and subjective functioning ability.
2) Survival of the interventions (fixed or removable partial denture prostheses) used for the extension of SDAs.

Secondary outcomes

1) Patient satisfaction and oral health-related quality of life (social interaction; aesthetics and effectiveness) using oral health indicators for example Oral Health Indicator Profile (OHIP) or the Oral Impacts of Daily Performance (OIDP).
2) Harmful effects (caries; tooth loss; periodontal status, plaque index (PI), gingival index (GI), temporomandibular joint (TMJ) problems, interdental spacing and overbite).

Inclusion criteria. Studies that included above interventions and outcomes and addressed the pre-specified outcomes were eligible for this SR.

Exclusion criteria. The following study designs: case-control, cross-sectional and cohort studies; case-series and case reports; other SRs; analytical and narrative reviews and different types of animal studies that were not eligible for inclusion, were excluded.

Search strategy. All relevant databases were searched: Medline, Cochrane Central Register of Controlled Trials, EMBASE, CINAHL, Science Direct, ProQuest, Science Journals, Scopus, PsycINFO, ClinicalTrials.gov, WHO ICTRP, TRIP and PACTR. Further hand-searching was conducted including citations from reference lists of retrieved studies (PEARLing searches) for additional references [59]. Where data were missing and full texts unavailable, these unclear reports were clarified by contacting authors or research institutes. Efforts were made to obtain English versions of studies reported in other languages either by requesting English versions from authors or using language experts to translate key findings. Authors were also contacted for unpublished reports or conference proceedings, where it was needed. Where registries were available for on-going studies, these were included as well and experts in the field of research related to the SDA were contacted.

Key terms were combined using Boolean operators and search strategies for each database were developed using the database specific functions [59]. Medical subject headings were applied in databases which allowed this function [59]. A wide search strategy was developed and modified according to the requirements of the different databases to ensure no eligible studies were excluded and an example includes the following:

(shortened dental arch OR shortened dental arches) AND (Clinical Trial OR Comparative Study OR Evaluation Studies OR Randomized Controlled Trial OR clinical trial) AND 1980/01/01-2014/12/31).

Search limits. Databases were searched for articles of over a period of three decades from 1980 to April 2014. The limits included in the search strategy were: human studies, adult patients and randomized and non-randomized controlled clinical trials.

Selection methods. Two review authors (SK and AM) independently screened titles and abstracts from the electronic searches to select potentially relevant studies using a predetermined eligibility form based on the inclusion criteria [59]. Full text articles of potential studies were then retrieved and re-assessed for eligibility. Each article was scrutinized to ensure that multiple publications from the same study were included only once. Where eligibility was unclear, clarification was sought from the trial authors and the corresponding articles were re-assessed. Differences between the eligibility results were resolved by consulting the other review authors (UMEC and RO). Studies that did not meet the inclusion criteria were excluded and the reasons for exclusion were reported. Data extraction for the selected studies was completed by the principal researcher (SK) using a specially designed pre-piloted data extraction form for this SR [59]. All disagreements regarding this process were resolved through discussion with the other review authors (AM, UMEC and RO).

Qualitative analysis. The quality of the studies included for this SR were evaluated for any risk of bias by researchers (SK and AM) using the Cochrane Risk of Bias tool and as described in the Cochrane Handbook for Systematic Reviews of Interventions [59]. The assessment was done across the following six components: random sequence generation, allocation concealment, blinding, incomplete outcome data, selective reporting, and other bias. Each of these were judged as 'yes', 'no', or 'unclear' corresponding to low, high, or unclear risk of bias respectively. Where information in the articles was insufficient for making the judgements, trial authors were contacted for clarification. Disagreements were resolved through discussion with other review authors. Results of risk of bias were summarised in a risk of bias table. In addition, GRADE assessments were completed by the researchers (SK and AM) for each clinical trial and these were used to grade the evidence and strength of recommendations for clinical intervention (where possible) using the GRADE Profiler system [60]. These are reported in the summary of findings tables.

Data synthesis and management. Results were reported separately for the following three comparisons: 1) FDP versus RPDP; 2) RPDP versus no treatment (SDA); 3) SDA versus CDA. No imputation of missing data was carried out and study authors were requested to provide any missing data. Available case analysis was applied where data were missing. Risk ratios with corresponding 95% confidence intervals were calculated for dichotomous outcomes using Review Manager 5 software. Although a meta-analysis of outcomes across study results had been anticipated, the included studies reported outcomes in different forms that could not be pooled in a meta-analysis. Consequently, results for individual studies were reported separately.

Results

The search strategy identified a total of 101 citations (Figure 1): electronic databases yielded 81 and 20 were from reference lists of retrieved articles (that is, through PEARLing searches). A total of 32 duplicate records were removed, leaving 69 citations which were assessed for eligibility. After reading titles and abstracts, a total of 41 records were excluded and the full-text of the remaining 28 records was retrieved. A further 7 records were excluded after reading the full-text reports, leaving the remaining 21 records as included studies for the SR (Figure 1). Only four RCTs and one CT were used for this review, but outcomes were reported in the retrieved 21 records [14,31–38,40–48,53–55]. No on-going studies were found and no eligible studies were excluded for failure to report the reviewer's pre-specified outcomes.

Study characteristics

The studies were grouped according to types of interventions into the following comparisons:

Comparison 1: FDPs versus RPDPs for SDAs in the lower jaw.

Two included studies from the UK and Denmark assessed comparison 1 [31–38].

Comparison 2: RPDPs versus no treatment (SDA).

Two studies from Germany and Ireland assessed comparison 2 [40–48].

Comparison 3: SDA versus CDA.

Only one study from the Netherlands assessed comparison 3 [14,53–55].

Characteristics of included studies. The study characteristics of the four RCTs and 1 CT included in this SR are summarized according to types of study, population characteristics, types of interventions and the follow-up periods and these are specified on Table 1 [14,31–38,40–48,53–55].

Qualitative analysis. Table 2 specifies the quality assessment of the included studies and these are summarized in the 'risk of bias table' and 'risk of bias graph' where judgements are categorized to indicate a low, high, or unclear risk of bias (Figure 2) following the Cochrane guidelines [59]. Below we give a detailed explanation of these results:

Sequence Generation: Three of the five trials were reported as having been randomised. For sequence generation, two clinical trials used computer-generated numbers and a third trial used randomly permuted block randomisation for generating the allocation sequence, which we judged as having a low risk of bias [34–38,40–48]. The Witter et al (2001) clinical trial invited subjects to join the department for a study, and no attempt was made to randomise patients, thus it is judged as having a high risk of bias [14,53–55]. The Budtz-Jorgensen and Isidor (1987) trial did not mention how the sequence was generated and provided

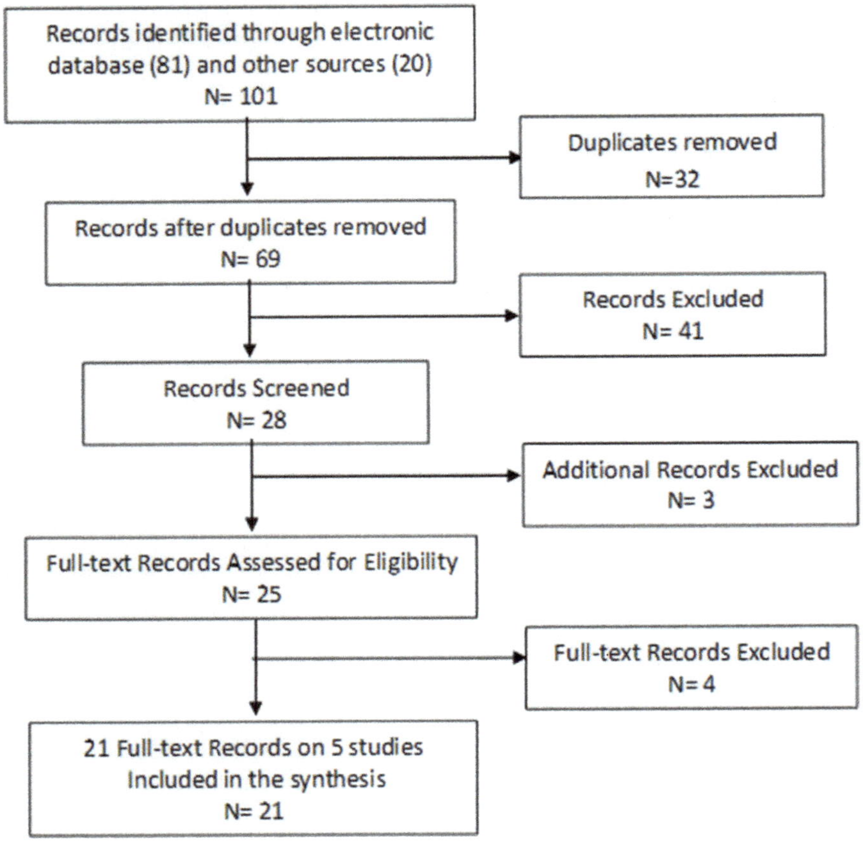

Figure 1. Prisma Flow Chart of Study Selection.

insufficient information to enable us to judge whether there was a high or low risk of bias, and we thus rated it as having an unclear risk of bias [31–33].

Allocation Concealment: The Moynihan et al (2000), Wolfart et al (2005) and Mc Kenna (2012) studies are described as having a low risk of bias for allocation concealment, as they indicated that the clinician was not involved in the allocation and that concealment was warranted following a central randomisation process after patient enrolment [34–38,40–48]. For the Budtz-Jorgensen and Isidor (1987) and Witter et al (2001) studies, there is no indication as to how intervention allocation was concealed and these were judged as having an unclear risk of bias [14,31–33,53–55].

Blinding: The Moynihan et al (2000) study was referred to as a double blinded study with the clinician blinded to allocation of intervention and statistician being blinded to treatment and thus it is judged as having a low risk of bias [34–38]. The Witter et al (2001) study can be considered as a single blinded study because evaluation of outcomes was completed by a calibrated observer at all intervals, but it was not stated as such, thus it is judged as having an unclear risk of bias [14,53–55]. Mc Kenna (2012) indicated that the researcher was not involved in the intervention allocation, making it a single-blinded study, thus it is judged as having a low risk of bias [47–48]. The Wolfart et al (2005) study indicated that it was impossible to blind the dentist and patient due to discrepancies of the treatments; thus it was judged as having a high risk of bias, whereas Budtz-Jorgensen and Isidor (1987) provided insufficient information related to blinding and it was regarded as having an unclear risk of bias [31–33,40–46].

Incomplete Outcome Data: Analyses for the Moynihan et al (2000), Wolfart et al (2005) and Mc Kenna (2012) studies were conducted on the "intention-to-treat" (ITT) principle; and the studies reported proportionate numbers of losses to follow-up (which were small) and some having no losses between the intervention and control [34–38,40–48]. Witter et al (2001) indicated that regression models accounted for the subjects lost during the study [53]. Thus, all 4 studies above were judged as having a low risk of bias [34–38,40–46,53–55]. On the other hand, Budtz-Jorgensen and Isidor (1987) did not indicate and specify how the analysis was completed, but all pre-specified outcomes were reported, and the number of losses to follow-up was small, thus it was judged as having a low risk of bias [31–33].

Selective Reporting: All studies were registered and approved with their respective Review boards [14,31–38,40–48,48,53–55]. The protocol for the Wolfart et al (2005) study was published (41). In the Budtz-Jorgensen and Isidor (1987) and Witter et al (2001) studies all outcomes were reported but outcomes were not pre-specified as primary or secondary outcomes [14,31–33,53–55]. Both these studies were thus judged as having a high risk of bias. The three remaining RCTs specified the outcomes as primary and secondary and reported these as such, thus these were judged as having a low risk of bias [34–38,40–46]. All the included studies except the Wolfart et al (2005) study reported all their pre-specified outcomes in subsequent publications [14,31–38,40–48,53–55].

Other potential sources of bias: No other sources of bias were detected with four of the five included studies. The Budtz-Jorgensen and Isidor (1987) study was judged as having high risk of bias because there were six patients who did not wear the RPDP at all during the study [32–33].

Table 1. Table of Included Studies.

Study Details	Methods	Participants	Interventions	Outcomes	Notes
Author: Budtz-Jorgensen and Isidor (31–33)	*Duration of trial*: 5 years	*Sample*: Total N = 53	*Intervention*: FDP (N = 27)	*Outcomes*: Caries; Prosthetic condition; periodontal conditions (PI/GI) and	Study approval by Ethics Board was not recorded
Country: Denmark	*Assessment periods*: 1 and 2 months; 2 and 5 years	*Age*: 61–83 yrs. (Mean age: 69) *Gender*: 28 Females; 25 Males	*Control*: RPDP (N = 26)	Masticatory system (TMJ) and patient opinion.	No verif cation
Study Design: CT		*Country and Setting*: Denmark, University Hospital		Outcomes were not divided into primary or secondary	
Author: Witter et al (14, 53–55)	*Duration of trial*: 9 years	*Sample*: Total N = 146	*Intervention*: SDA (N = 74)	*Outcomes*: Interdental spacing; periodontal support and	Study approved by University Nijmegen Ethics Board.
Country: Netherlands	*Assessment periods*: Baseline and 3, 6 and 9 years	*Age*: Mean −36.2 yrs. for CDA; Mean -40.5 yrs. for SDA *Gender*: 82 Females; 64 Males	*Control*: CDA (N = 72)	Occlusal contact; Overbite; occlusal wear and TMJ problems	Informed Consent from patients was obtained.
Study Design: CT		*Country and Setting*: Netherlands, Nijmegen Clinic		Outcomes were not divided into primary or secondary	
Author: Jepson et al (34–37)	*Duration of trial*: 2 and 5 years	*Sample*: Total N = 60	*Intervention*: FDP (N = 30)	*Primary*: Survival of prosthesis; Influence of diet and nutrient intake	Study approval received from Ethics Board.
Country: United Kingdom (UK)	*Assessment periods*: 3 months; 1, 2 and 5 years	*Age*: 39–81 yrs. (Mean age: 67) *Gender*: 35 Females; 25 Males	*Control*: RPDP (N = 30)	*Secondary*: Caries; Periodontal status; patient satisfaction	Informed Consent from patients obtained.
Study Design: RCT		*Country and Setting*: UK, Newcastle Dental Hospital			Power calculations were completed
Author: Walters et al (40–46)	*Duration of trial*: 3 year	*Sample*: Total N = 215 (pilot sample incl. in main study)	*Intervention*: SDA (N = 106)	*Primary*: First tooth loss	Study approved by Institutional Ethics Review Board
Country: Germany	*Assessment periods*: 4–8 wks.; 6 months and 1, 2, 3, 4 and 5 years	*Age*: 35 yrs. + (Mean age: 59) *Gender*: 107 Females and 108 Males	*Control*: RPDP (N = 109)	*Secondary*: 2nd tooth loss; caries; survival of treatment; oral health related quality of life; tooth mobility; PI; GI and TMJ Problems	Power calculations were completed
		Country and Setting: Germany, University Hospitals			
Author: McKenna et al (47–48)	*Duration of trial*: 1 year	*Sample*: Total N = 44	*Intervention*: RPDP (N = 21)	*Primary*: Oral health related quality of Life; Nutritional status	Study approved by Cork University's Ethics Review Board
Country: Ireland	*Assessment periods*: Baseline and 1 month	*Age*: 65–82 yrs. (Mean age: 68) *Gender*: 28 Females; 16 Males	*Control*: RBB/FDP (N = 23)	*Secondary*: cost-effectiveness of two treatments	Power calculations completed: Estimated that one treatment was not worse than the other
Study Design: RCT		*Country and Setting*: Ireland, University Hospitals			

KEY:
RCT–randomized controlled trial.
CT–Clinical Trial.
SDA–shortened dental arch.
CDA–complete dental arch.
FDP–fixed dental prosthesis.
RBB–resin-bonded bridge.

RPDP–removable partial denture/dental prosthesis.
PI–plaque index.
GI–gingival index.
TMJ–temporomandibular joint.

Effects of interventions

See: Summary of findings for the main comparisons of functional outcomes and patient satisfaction with FDPs compared to RPDPs in treating patients with SDAs (Table 3); Summary of findings for SDA patients treated with RPDPs compared to no treatment (Table 4) [59].

Comparison 1: Fixed Denture Prosthesis vs Removable Partial Denture Prosthesis. Primary Outcomes: 1. Functional Outcomes: *Occlusion:* Budtz-Jorgensen and Isidor (1987) showed no significant difference in the number of patients with satisfactory occlusion during the 2-year period after treatment between the FDP and RPDP groups (RR 1.16, 95%CI: 0.90 to 1.48, 53 participants) [31].

2. Survival: Thomason et al (2007) reported time to survival for the restoration of the shortened dental arch but there was no significant difference between the FDP and RPDP groups (Hazard Ratio 0.59, 95%CI: 0.27 to 1.29, 60 participants) [37].

Secondary Outcomes: 1. Patient Satisfaction: This outcome was only reported by Jepson et al (2003) but there was no significant difference in median satisfaction scores at 1 year after treatment between the FDP and RPDP groups (p = 0.092 as reported by authors, 52 participants: Table 5) [36].

2. Harmful Effects: (caries; tooth loss; periodontal status, plaque index, gingival index; TMJ problems; interdental spacing; overbite).

Caries: Both studies are in agreement regarding the development of caries lesions with FDPs and RPDPs where: Jepson et al (2001) found that treatment with FDPs showed a significant increase in number of patients with no caries experience compared to the RPDP patients (RR 1.89, 95% CI: 1.09 to 3.30, 50 participants) [35]. Similarly, Isidor and Budtz-Jorgensen (1990) observed 22 dental carious lesions in the RPDP group compared with only two lesions in the FDP group; however we could not calculate a treatment effect since the respective number of patients was not reported. Our unit of analysis was individual patients and not individual teeth [33].

The following effects were only reported for the Budtz-Jorgensen and Isidor study (33):

TMJ dysfunction: Isidor and Budtz-Jorgensen (1990) found no significant difference in the number of patients showing TMJ dysfunction between the FDP and RPDP groups (RR 0.64, 95%CI: 0.36 to 1.16, 53 participants) [33].

Tooth Loss: In the Isidor and Budtz-Jorgensen (1990) study, 11 teeth were extracted in the RPDP group compared with only one tooth in the FDP group during the five years of observation. However, no treatment effect could be calculated because the respective numbers of patients were not reported [33].

Plaque Index: Isidor and Budtz-Jorgensen (1990) reported the mean plaque index ranging from 0.4 to 0.7 in the FDP group and from 0.7 to 1.0 in the RPDP group; the difference between the two groups was significant ($p<0.05$) during the first two years of examination as reported by study authors [33].

Gingival Index: Isidor and Budtz-Jorgensen (1990) indicated that the mean gingival index was always higher in the RPDP than in the FDP group, the difference being significant ($p<0.05$) at the 12-, 18-, 36-, and 48-month examinations [33].

Comparison 2: Removable Partial Denture Prosthesis versus no treatment (SDA). Primary Outcomes: 1. Functional outcomes: *Mini Nutritional Assessment (MNA):* Mc Kenna (2012) reported the change in MNA scores from baseline to final (month 1) for the two treatment groups and these results are summarised in Table 6 [47]. The values in the table were used to calculate a treatment effect which showed no significant difference in the change in MNA score between the RPDP and SDA treatment groups (MD −0.03, 95%CI: −1.35 to 1.29, 42 participants: Table 6). A higher MNA score indicates better nutrition effect.

2. Survival: This outcome was not reported in the two studies assessing this comparison.

Secondary Outcomes: 1. Patient satisfaction: This outcome was measured using different tools for both the Mc Kenna (2012) and Wolfart studies (2012), but the time periods from baseline to the end of studies were significantly different, thus indicating differences in final outcomes.

Oral Health Related Quality of Life (OHRQoL): Mc Kenna (2012) reported a non-significant difference in the OHRQoL scores from baseline to the end of treatment (month 1) for the two treatment

Table 2. Risk of Bias Table.

Study	Budtz-Jorgensen (31–33)	Witter et al (14, 51–53)	Jepson et al (34–38)	Walter et al (40–46)	Mc Kenna et al (47–48)
Random Sequence Generation (Selection bias)	Unclear	Unclear	Yes	Yes	Yes
Allocation Concealment (Selection bias)	Unclear	Unclear	Yes	Yes	Yes
Blinding (Detection and Performance bias)	No	Unclear	Yes	No	Yes
Incomplete Outcome Assessment (Attrition bias)	Yes	Yes	Yes	Yes	Yes
Free of Selective Reporting (Reporting bias)	No	No	Yes	No	Yes
Free of Other Bias	No	Yes	Yes	Yes	Yes

"Yes" indicates a low risk of bias, "No" indicates a high risk of bias, and "Unclear" indicates either a lack of information or uncertainty over the potential for bias.

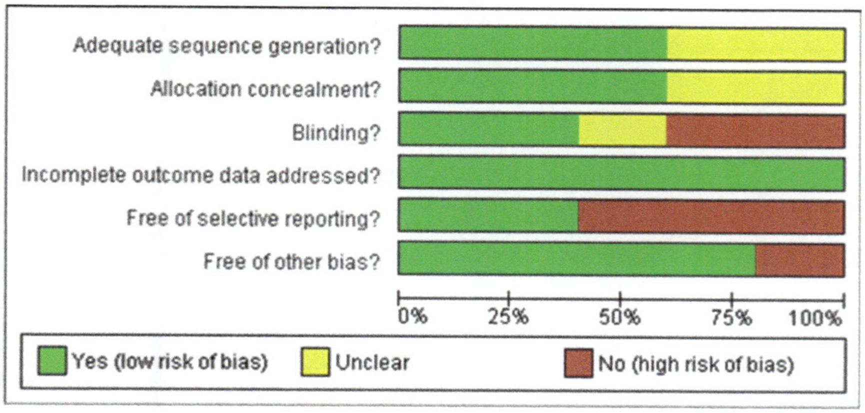

Figure 2. Risk of bias graph: review authors' judgements about each risk of bias item presented as percentages across all included studies.

groups (Table 7) [47]. The author used the oral health impact profile (OHIP-14) to give a score ranging from 0 (minimum) to 56 (maximum). A high score indicated a poor OHRQoL with low scales indicating good OHRQoL. However, no treatment effect could be calculated to compare the change in the OHIP-14 scores between the two treatment groups because standard deviations of change were not given and also because exact p-values were not reported.

For the Wolfart et al study (2012), the median OHIP-49 scores for pre-treatment, baseline, 1 and 5 years follow-up showed significant reduction of impacts ($p<0.05$). Before treatment, the median OHIP-49 total score was 38.0 for the RPDP group and 40.0 for the SDA group. Most significant reductions occurred at baseline (27.0; $p<0.0001$) and 1 year on (13.0; $p<0.0002$) for the RPDP group (compared to the Mc Kenna study after 1 month). For the SDA group, a significant change in impacts (19.0; $p<0.05$) were observed only at baseline, no further significant changes were reported [45].

2. Harmful Effects: (caries; tooth loss; periodontal status, plaque index, gingival index; TMJ problems; interdental spacing; overbite).

Tooth loss: The Walter et al study (2012) showed no significant difference in the number of patients experiencing first tooth loss within 38 months of observation after treatment between the RPDP and SDA groups (RR 1.23, 95%CI: 0.56 to 2.70, 150 participants) [44]. The respective Kaplan-Meier survival rates at 38 months were 0.83 (95%CI: 0.74 to 0.91) in the RPDP group and 0.86 (95%CI: 0.78 to 0.95) in the SDA group, the difference is not significant (as reported by study authors) [44].

Comparison 3: Shortened Dental Arches (SDA) versus Complete Dental Arches (CDA). Primary Outcomes: 1. Functional outcomes:

Occlusal contact: Witter et al, (2001) reported that a significantly higher percent (73%, 95%CI: 67–80%) of teeth in the anterior region had occlusal contact in intercuspal position of the SDA group compared with the CDA group (62%, 95%CI: 55–69%) ($p<0.05$) [53]. No treatment effect could be calculated because the number of patients per group was not specified [53].

Occlusal tooth wear: Witter et al (1994) reported the mean occlusal tooth wear scores using transformed values for subjects of 40 years of age [55]. However, no significant differences between the SDA subgroups [means (SD) ranging from 1.1(0.1) to 1.6(0.1)] and the CDA group [means (SD) of 1.4(0.0) and 1.5(0.0)] were found when comparing the means of the scores for the upper and for the lower anterior regions. Similarly for the premolar regions, no significant differences were found between the SDA subgroups [mean (SD) scores 0.7(0.1) to 1.0(0.1)] and the CDA group [mean (SD) score 0.9(0.1)]. No treatment effect could be calculated because the respective number of patients was not reported.

2. Survival: This outcome was not reported in the one study assessing this comparison.

Secondary Outcomes: 1. Patient satisfaction: This outcome was not reported in the one study assessing this comparison.

2. Harmful Effects: (caries; tooth loss; periodontal status, plaque index, gingival index; TMJ problems; interdental spacing; overbite).

Interdental spacing: Witter et al (1994) described a comparison of the mean scores of interdental spacing per region [55]. According to the authors, the premolar regions of the SDA subgroups had significantly higher means [mean (SD): 0.4(0.1) and 0.5(0.1)] than the CDA group [mean (SD): 0.1(0), $p<0.01$ as reported by authors]. For the anterior regions, the spacing was not significantly different for SDA [mean (SD) range from 0.2(0.1) to 0.5(0.1)]; CDA group [mean (SD) range from 0.1(0.0) to 0.3(0.1)]. They also reported that spacing remained the same in all regions over time in the SDA group [55]. No treatment effect could be calculated because the results were given per region and also because the respective number of patients were not specified in the results.

Overbite: Witter et al (1994) stated this outcome only for some subgroups but did not compare their results between the SDA and CDA groups [55]. Therefore we could not calculate a treatment effect.

Periodontal support: Witter et al (1994) described the mean relative bone heights using transformed values for subjects of 40 years of age [55]. The authors reported that maxillary premolars and mandibular second premolars in the SDA subgroups showed significantly lower mean bone height scores than those in the CDA group, whereas mandibular first premolars did not differ. The values reported were not sufficient for the calculation of a treatment effect.

TMJ problems: The Witter et al study (2007) indicated that patients with SDAs (65–79%) had similar prevalence, severity and changes in signs and symptoms related to the TMJ as patients with CDAs (70–75%) [54].

Excluded study characteristics: All non-RCTs and reviews were excluded from this SR. Other SRs and summary articles were viewed as potentially included studies, but these were however later not considered for inclusion (Table 8).

Table 3. COMPARISON 1: FDP versus RPDP for Treated and untreated Shortened Dental Arches (31–38).

Patient or population: patients with Treated and untreated Shortened Dental Arches
Settings: Hospital Setting
Intervention: FDP versus RPDP

Outcomes	Illustrative comparative risks* (95% CI)		Relative effect	No of Participants (studies)	Quality of the evidence	Comments
	Assumed risk	Corresponding risk	(95% CI)		(GRADE)	
	Control	FDP versus RPDP				
Number of patients with satisfactory occlusion	Study population		RR 1.16 (0.9 to 1.48)	53 (1 study)	⊕⊖⊖⊖ very low[1,2]	
	769 per 1000	892 per 1000 (692 to 1000)				
	Moderate					
	769 per 1000	892 per 1000 (692 to 1000)				
Number of patients with no caries experience	Study population		RR 1.89 (1.09 to 3.3)	50 (1 study)	⊕⊕⊕⊖ moderate[2]	
	391 per 1000	740 per 1000 (427 to 1000)				
	Moderate					
	391 per 1000	739 per 1000 (426 to 1000)				
Number of patients showing TMJ dysfunction	Study population		RR 0.64 (0.36 to 1.16)	53 (1 study)	⊕⊖⊖⊖ very low[1,2]	
	577 per 1000	369 per 1000 (208 to 669)				
	Moderate					
	577 per 1000	369 per 1000 (208 to 669)				
Survival of Intervention	Study population		HR 0.59 (0.27 to 1.29)	60 (1 study)	⊕⊕⊕⊖ moderate[2]	
	See comment	See comment				
	Moderate					
Patient Satisfaction	Study population		Not estimable[3]	52 (1 study)	⊕⊕⊕⊖ moderate[2]	
	See comment	See comment				
	Moderate					

EXPLANATION OF TABLE ABOVE: *The basis for the **assumed risk** (e.g. the median control group risk across studies) is provided in footnotes. The **corresponding risk** (and its 95% confidence interval) is based on the assumed risk in the comparison group and the **relative effect** of the intervention (and its 95% CI). **KEY: CI:** Confidence interval; **RR:** Risk ratio; **HR:** Hazard ratio.

Explanation for the GRADE Working Group QUALITY of evidence: *High quality*: Further research is very unlikely to change our confidence in the estimate of effect. **Moderate quality:** Further research is likely to have an important impact on our confidence in the estimate of effect and may change the estimate. *Low quality*: Further research is very likely to have an important impact on our confidence in the estimate of effect and is likely to change the estimate. **Very low quality:** We are very uncertain about the estimate.

REASONS for the QUALITY of the Evidence: [1]High risk of bias for blinding, selective reporting bias and other bias; [2]Small sample size; [3]No significant difference ($p = 0.092$).

Discussion

The focus of this review was the classic SDA, irrespective of whether it occurred naturally or was created by means of a FDP. An exhaustive and comprehensive search yielded four RCTs and 1 CT that were included [14,31–38,40–48,53–55]:

Jepson et al (2001) is in agreement with the research conducted by Isidor and Budtz-Jorgensen (1987, 1990) regarding an increase in caries incidence as reported 2 and 5 years post treatment [33,35,38]. In addition, the increase in caries incidence for the RPDP group also concurred with the research of Bergman et al, (1964), cited in Budtz-Jorgensen (1990) [32].

Survival of fixed bridges 5 years post study was similar to other trials [30–32,37–38]. RPDP patients chose not to wear RPDPs which was similar to other studies [31–32,37–38]. For patient satisfaction, the small sample size does not allow us to generalize our results to other settings, thus it is advised to conduct these studies amongst different populations.

For the Wolfart et al study (2010): Post hoc power calculations implied that the pilot sample size was too small to generalize results and for comparison to other studies [40–43]. The larger study results are free of bias with a large enough sample due to it being a multi-centre study. While it reduced the bias, it still could not be generalized to patients that are different to the study

Table 4. COMPARISON 2: RPD versus SDA for Treated and untreated Shortened Dental Arches (40–48).

Patient or population: patients with Treated and untreated Shortened Dental Arches						
Settings: Hospital setting						
Intervention: RPD versus SDA						
Outcomes	**Illustrative comparative risks* (95% CI)**		**Relative effect (95% CI)**	**No of Participants (studies)**	**Quality of the evidence (GRADE)**	**Comments**
	Assumed risk	Corresponding risk				
	Control	**RPD versus SDA**				
Change in MNA scores		The mean change in MNA scores in the intervention groups was **0.03 lower** (1.35 lower to 1.29 higher)		42 (1 study)	⊕⊕⊕⊖ **moderate**[1]	
Number of patients with first tooth loss in 38 months	**Study population**		**0.83** (0.74 to 0.91)	150 (1 study)	⊕⊕⊖⊖ **low**[2,3]	
	130 per 1000	**108 per 1000** (97 to 119)				
	Moderate					
	130 per 1000	**108 per 1000** (96 to 118)				
Patient Satisfaction	**Study population**		Not estimable[4]	215 (1 study)	See comment	
	See comment	See comment				
	Moderate					

EXPLANATION OF TABLE ABOVE: *The basis for the **assumed risk** (e.g. the median control group risk across studies) is provided in footnotes. The **corresponding risk** (and its 95% confidence interval) is based on the assumed risk in the comparison group and the **relative effect** of the intervention (and its 95% CI). **KEY: CI:** Confidence interval; **RR:** Risk ratio;

Explanation for the GRADE Working Group QUALITY of evidence: High quality: Further research is very unlikely to change our confidence in the estimate of effect. **Moderate quality:** Further research is likely to have an important impact on our confidence in the estimate of effect and may change the estimate. **Low quality:** Further research is very likely to have an important impact on our confidence in the estimate of effect and is likely to change the estimate. *Very low quality*: We are very uncertain about the estimate.

REASONS for the QUALITY of the Evidence: [1]Small sample size; [2]High risk of bias for blinding and selective reporting bias; [3]Wide confidence interval- the 95% CI includes both null effect and appreciable harm and [4]No significant changes were reported for the Irish study. For the German study: Significant differences were seen at baseline (27.0; $p<0.0001$) and 1 year on (13.0; $p<0.0002$) for the RPDP group and a significant change in impacts (19.0; $p<0.05$) were observed only at baseline for the SDA group.

Table 5. Summary satisfaction scores for the UK-based study at 1 year (a lower score indicates more satisfaction).

Group	N	Median (baseline)	Median (1 year)	p-value per group	p-value between groups
FDP (Intervention)	26	18	11	<0.001	0.092
RPDP (Control)	26	16.5	13	0.009	

FDP = Fixed dental prosthesis; RPDP = Removable partial denture/dental prosthesis (34–38).

sample. For the patient satisfaction outcome, the summary scores of the pilot study were similar to another German study (John and Micheelis, 2003, cited in Walter et al (2012) [45]. For temporomandibular disease (TMD) pain scores, the instrument used in other studies was more reliable (Dworkin, 2002, cited in Walter et al (2012) [44]. Tooth loss as a primary outcome is questioned due to extended time periods, thus it was advised to use caries and periodontal attachment loss as outcomes instead [44].

The Mc Kenna study (2012), which is the most recently conducted RCT; the results are similar to other RCTs completed in the past, where small sample sizes would not necessarily show a significant difference between interventions given the follow-up period [47–48]. In this case, follow-up after only one month of treatment was too short to show any difference between interventions [47–48]. But the cost-effectiveness reported with this RCT has been noted as researchers and clinicians are under the impression that the cost for FDPs far outweighs that of RPDP treatment [22,39,48]. And this has been in line with the findings of the Danish study published some years ago [32–33].

For the Witter et al study (2001), results were similar to other studies with regards to outcomes reported and the effect of outcomes on the dentition in the SDA group (tooth wear, TMJ effects) (Aukes, 1988; Mohl, 1988; Eliasson, 1997, cited in Witter et al (2001) [53].

The quality of the evidence is indicative of the integrity of the study and the research conducted. With reference to the quality assessment of the included studies, this has been described in detail above. More importantly, this quality is determined by the study designs. Study designs are graded according to the quality of evidence that they provide. Systematic reviews and RCTs are considered to be designs of the highest quality [59–60]. Within the different design groups, certain concessions can be made for those designs that do not follow the exact guidelines [59–60]. For instance RCTs can be downgraded if their risk of bias is high [59–60].

Only RCTs and CTs were however included in this systematic review which provides stronger evidence and increases the strength of the recommendations [59–60]. After completing the quality assessment (using the GRADE approach) of the included studies, it clearly showed that some of the studies had not followed the exact guidelines for RCTs, but nevertheless had the features thereof [59–60]. These can be regarded as downgraded RCTs (Tables 3–4). These downgraded RCTs did not use randomization, allocation concealment or blinding, and failed to specify the outcomes as primary or secondary. These downgraded RCTs could thus affect the quality of evidence only slightly [59–60]. For example, the Budtz-Jorgensen (1987, 1990) and Witter et al (2001) studies could be regarded as downgraded CTs [14,31–33,53–55,60].

A meta-analysis could not be completed for this SR for the following reasons: Some of the outcomes for the SR (for example survival of intervention) were not reported by all the included studies; sufficient RCTs were not found related to SDAs; the outcomes were reported in so many different ways for each of the studies that a narrative approach for this review had to be adopted and not all outcomes are reported for the Wolfart et al (2005) study (and no correspondence was received when the authors were contacted). In addition, there was insufficient information reported by studies to allow us to combine continuous data using the mean difference (MD). The outcomes from the studies were thus grouped for this review.

For this SR, a systematic approach to the evaluation of the evidence obtained from the studies was adopted by the researchers and disagreements were resolved by discussion. The researchers highlighted the areas where bias could have been expected (Table 2). Study samples, settings, age categories, interventions and outcomes for the included studies were mostly similar, creating strong evidence (Table 1). Comparison between the groups of the different studies could be systematically recorded in the stipulated groups. And again, for this SR all potential sources were searched and reported. Most studies followed guidelines to protect against bias (some without making reference to the method followed) [14,31–33,53–55]. And this was assessed using the Cochrane's risk of bias tool [59]. Since all the included studies in this SR were conducted in developed countries, our findings cannot be generalized to patients in all countries because cultural and socio-economic differences that exist between countries and within communities can influence patients' reactions.

Other SRs were also conducted in the past ten years [8,56–58], where researchers included studies with different study designs and not only RCTs. For the most current SR [57], the research question was so broad that the focus on the SDA was minimal, thus many of the data related specifically to SDAs were not even included in the analysis [57]. For this SR, only the British and

Table 6. Change in MNA scores for the Irish study.

Group	n	Baseline MNA score average	Final MNA score average	p-value per group	Calculated SD of change
RPDP	21	23.65	24.75	0.03	2.15
SDA	21	23.24	24.37	0.03	2.21

MNA = Mini nutritional assessment; SD = Standard Deviation; RPDP = Removable partial denture/dental prosthesis; SDA = Shortened dental arch (47–48).

Table 7. Change in OHIP-14 scores for the Irish study.

Group	n	Baseline OHIP-14 score average	Final OHIP-14 score average	p-value per group
RPDP	21	12.4	3.3	<0.001
SDA	21	11.4	1.8	<0.001

OHIP = Oral health impact Profile; RPDP = Removable partial denture/dental prosthesis; SDA = Shortened dental arch (47–48).

German RCTs were mentioned and only the results of the pilot study for the German RCT was reported [57]. The authors concluded citing insufficient evidence to report a difference between RPDP and FDPs in the treatment of SDAs [57]. In addition, when evaluating the quality of the evidence of a systematic review, it is recommended that the GRADE approach should be used [60]. It is a method of evaluating the quality of evidence and strength of recommendations in healthcare, and thus provides the needed rigor and transparency when making specific recommendations [60].

Quality of evidence

As stated above, the quality of evidence was assessed using the GRADE methodology for this SR (Tables 3 and 4). With the assessment, the small sample sizes seriously affected the imprecision, and the risk of bias was very serious with studies where no blinding and selective reporting was observed (Tables 3 and 4). From the combined effects, the overall quality of the assessment is regarded as being low (Tables 3 and 4). This implies that further research (as in conducting more RCTs) is likely to have an important impact on our confidence in the estimate of effect, and may change the estimate.

Implications for practice

The SDA concept has been researched and used in industrialized countries and this review aimed to highlight its appropriateness and relevance for a developing country such as South Africa. A change in paradigm or thinking should be encouraged, even though results of clinical trials conducted in other countries may not necessarily be generalizable to South African populations. By regarding the research related to SDAs in a positive light (patient satisfaction, caries incidence, TMJ effects and tooth loss), this SR specifies that policy-makers and/or institutions should be encouraged and recommend its teaching and clinical implemen-

Table 8. Excluded studies, with reasons for exclusion.

Study	Reasons for exclusion
Abt, Carr and Worthington (57)	A systematic review
	Focused on treatment options for all types of partially dentate patients
	Did not specifically focus on the interventions for SDAs
	SDA was considered as only one treatment option
Fueki et al (56)	A systematic review completed in Japan
	Included different study designs
	All the RCTs included in this review were used for the present review as well. But other RCTs were included for the present SR
	The analysis for this SR is different to that of the present SR
Faggion (58)	A systematic review
	Intention was to include RCTs and CTs, but a prospective study was included
	All RCTs used for this SR was included in the present review with the inclusion of other RCTs
	Outcomes that were not reported in this SR has been included in the present review
	Focus of this paper was the GRADE assessment completed
Emami and Feine: 2010 (62)	Is a summary of a clinical trial completed on this SDA subject. Above RCT has been included in this review
Gotfredsen and Walls (8)	Is a SR of the literature related to the SDA topic
	Similar outcomes as addressed in this SR
	Different study design types were included
	SR concluded the acceptable level of oral function obtained with 20 natural teeth (which is line with the WHO goal for the year 2000)

KEY:
SDA: shortened dental arch.
RCT: randomized controlled trial.
CT: clinical trial.
SR: systematic review.
GRADE: Grading of Recommendations Assessment, Development and Evaluation.
WHO: World Health Organization.

tation by students and clinicians. These are considered as instances where low-quality evidence can still make a strong recommendation due to the body of available evidence on SDAs.

Implications for research

Sufficient RCTs related to SDAs were not found, and thus it would be advisable to conduct more randomized clinical trials. The RCTs were also conducted in European and Nordic countries and these results may not be generalizable to other context, due to substantial cross-cultural and socio-economic differences between countries. External validity or generalizability of studies conducted in other countries depends on: settings where studies were conducted; participants' characteristics; interventions researched across studies; relevance of the endpoints achieved with each study; results obtained and their comparison to one another and the indirect/direct costs when conducting each study.

Conclusions

The results from this SR related to SDAs as a treatment option were encouraging in terms of functioning, patient satisfaction and cost-effectiveness. However, only the Moynihan et al (2000) study reported on the primary outcome of survival of the SDA, and had this been determined by the other studies, it would have strengthened the recommendation of the SDA as a treatment option even further [34].

Recommendations

The stronger the evidence, the stronger the recommendation for the implementation of the SDA as a treatment option for partially dentate patients. By using only high quality studies such as RCTs and CTs for this SR, it was expected that the results would be more reliable when making conclusions and recommendations. Nevertheless, any conclusion/s from such a SR can still be regarded in a positive light, even though the included studies had to be downgraded due to methodological errors [60]. It is also recommended that when conducting clinical trials, strict protocols need to be prepared and the reporting of the RCT should follow the CONSORT guidelines [61]. This could then be of great benefit to other researchers when critically appraising these clinical trials. More importantly, outcomes for the RCT have to be pre-specified and all should be reported so that future systematic reviews may be conducted with the inclusion of a meta-analysis, instead of a narrative report as needed to be done for this SR. Thus further research (as in conducting clinical trials) should be encouraged and for the different settings and contexts (for example developing countries) to create a comprehensive database related to SDAs.

Supporting Information

Checklist S1 PRISMA 2009 Checklist.

Author Contributions

Conceived and designed the experiments: SK AM UMEC RO. Performed the experiments: SK. Analyzed the data: SK AM. Contributed reagents/materials/analysis tools: SK AM UMEC RO. Wrote the paper: SK. Checked Drafts: AM UMEC RO.

References

1. Zarb GA, Bolender CL, Carlsson GE (1997) Boucher's Prosthodontics Treatment for edentulous Patients, 11th ed. Missouri, USA: Mosby.
2. Müller F, Naharro M, Carlsson GE (2007) What are the prevalence and incidence of tooth loss in the adult and elderly population in Europe? Clin Oral Impl Res 18(Sup 3): 2–14.
3. Carlsson GE (2010) Some dogmas related to prosthodontics, temporomandibular disorders an occlusion. Acta Odon Scand 68: 313–322.
4. Witter DJ, van Elteren P, Käyser AF, Van Rossum MJM (1989) The effect of removable partial dentures on oral function in shortened dental arches. J Oral Rehabil 16: 27–33.
5. Käyser AF (1981). Shortened dental arches and oral function. J Oral Rehabil 8: 457–462.
6. Witter DJ, van Elteren P, Käyser AF (1988) Signs and symptoms of mandibular dysfunction in shortened dental arches. J Oral Rehabil 15: 413–420.
7. Käyser AF (1989) The shortened Dental Arch: A Therapeutic concept in reduced dentitions and certain high risk groups. Int J Perio Rest Dent 9(6): 426–449.
8. Gotfredsen K, Walls AWG (2007) What dentition assures oral function? Clin Oral Impl Res (Suppl. 3): 34–45.
9. Creugers NHJ, Witter DJ, Van't Spijker A, Gerritsen AE, Kreulen CM (2010) Occlusion and temporomandibular function among subjects with Mandibular Distal Extension Removable Partial Dentures. Int J Dent 1–7. [DOI:10.115/2010/807850].
10. Gerritsen AE, Witter DJ, Bronkhorst EW, Creugers NHJ (2012) An observational cohort study on shortened dental arches- clinical course during a period of 27–35 years. Clin Oral Invest 1–8 [DOI:10.1007/s00784-012-0765-6].
11. Zhang Q, Witter DJ, Bronkhorst EM, Creugers NHJ (2012) Chewing ability in an urban and rural population over 40 years in Shandong Province, China. Clin Oral Invest 1–11.
12. Sarita PT, Witter DJ, Kreulen CM, Matee MI, Van't Hof MA, et al. (2007) Oral health status related to the shortened dental arch concept in Tanzania. Eur J Sci 115(4): 265–274.
13. Elias EC, Sheiham A (1998) The relationship between satisfaction with mouth and number and position of teeth. J Oral Rehabil 25: 649–661.
14. Witter DJ, de Haan AF, Kayser AF, van Rossum GM (1994) A 6-year follow-up study of oral function in shortened dental arches. Part I: Occlusal stability. J Oral Rehabil 21(2): 113–25.
15. Allen PF, Witter DF, Wilson NHF, Käyser AF (1996) Shortened dental arch therapy: views of consultants in restorative dentistry in the United Kingdom. J Oral Rehabil 23: 481–485.
16. Sarita PT, Witter DJ, Kreulen CM, Creugers NHJ (2003) The shortened dental arch concept and attitudes of dentists in Tanzania. Comm Dent Oral Epidimiol 31: 111–115.
17. Armellini DB, Von Fraunhofer JA (2004) The shortened dental arch: A review of the literature. J Prosthet Dent 92(6): 531–535.
18. Ueno M, Yanagisawa T, Shinada K, Ohara S, Kawaguchi Y (2008) Masticatory ability and functional tooth units in Japanese adults. J Oral Rehabil 35: 337–344.
19. Zeng X, Sheiham A, Tsakos G (2008) Relationship between clinical dental status and eating difficulty in an old Chinese population. J Oral Rehabil 35: 37–44.
20. Baba K, Igarashi Y, Nishiyama A, John MT, Akagawa Y, et al. (2008) Patterns of missing occlusal units and oral health-related quality of life in SDA patients. J Oral Rehabil 35: 621–628.
21. World Health Organization (1992) A review of current recommendations for the organization and administration of Community Oral Health services in Northern and Western Europe. Geneva: WHO regional office for Europe. WHO Technical Report Series No. 826: 16–17.
22. Khan S, Omar R, Chikte UME (2012) Perceptions of practitioners regarding shortened dental arch. SADJ 67(2): 60–68.
23. Ivanhoe JR, Cibirka RM, Parr GR (2002) Treating the modern complete denture patient: A review of the literature. J Prosthet Dent 88: 631–635.
24. Omar R (2004) Reappraising prosthodontic treatment goals for older, partially dentate people: Part I. Traditional management strategy. SADJ 59(5): 198–202.
25. Carlsson GE, Omar R (2010) The future of complete dentures in oral rehabilitation. A critical review. J Oral Rehabil 37: 143–156.
26. Khan S, Chikte UME, Omar R (2013) From classroom teaching to clinical practice: Experiences of senior dental students regarding the shortened dental arch concept. J Dent Educ (In press).
27. Creugers NHJ, Käyser AF, vant Hof MA (1992) A seven-and-half-year survival study of resin-bonded bridges. J Dent Res 71: 1822–1825.
28. Creugers NHJ, De Kanter RJ, vant Hof MA (1997) Long-term survival data from a clinical trial on resin bonded bridges. J Dent 25: 239–242.
29. De Kanter RJ, Creugers NHJ, Verzijden CW, vant Hof MA (1998) A five year multi-practice clinical study on posterior resin-bonded bridges. J Dent Res 77: 609–614.
30. Frank RP, Brudvik JS, Le roux B, Milgrom P, Hawkins N (2000) Relationship between the standards of removable partial denture construction, clinical acceptability and patient satisfaction. J Prosthet Dent 83: 521–7.
31. Budtz-Jorgensen E, Isidor F (1987) Cantilever bridges or removable partial dentures in geriatric patients: a two-year study. J Oral Rehabil 14: 239–249.

32. Budtz-Jorgensen E, Isidor F (1990) A 5-year longitudinal study of cantilever fixed partial dentures compared with removable partial dentures in a geriatric population. J Prosthet Dent 64: 42–47.
33. Isidor F, Budtz-Jorgensen E (1990) Periodontal conditions following treatment with distally extending cantilever bridges or removable partial dentures in the elderly patients. A 5-year study. J Periodont 61: 21–26.
34. Moynihan PJ, Butler TJ, Thomason JM, Jepson NJA (2000) Nutrient intake in partially dentate patients: the effect of prosthetic rehabilitation. J Dent 28: 557–563.
35. Jepson NJA, Moynihan PJ, Kelly P, Watson GW, Thomason JM (2001) Caries incidence following restoration of shortened lower dental arches in a randomized controlled trial. BDJ 191(3): 140–144.
36. Jepson NJA, Allen F, Moynihan PJ, Kelly P, Thomason JM (2003) Patient satisfaction following restoration of shortened mandibular dental arches in a randomized controlled trial. Int J Prosthodont 16(4): 409–414.
37. Thomason JM, Moynihan PJ, Steen N, Jepson NJA (2007) Time to Survival for the restoration of the Shortened lower Dental Arch. J Dent Res 86(7): 646–650.
38. Balevi B (2008) No difference in the 5-year survival rates between the resin-bonded cantilever bridge and removable partial denture for the restoration of the shortened dental arch. Evid Based Dent 9(4): 105–106.
39. Abu-Saleh T, Marnewick J (2008) Implant-supported crowns for a shortened dental arch: A Case Report. J Contemp Dent Prac 9(5): 114–121.
40. Wolfart S, Heydecke G, Luthardt RG, Marre B, Freesmeyer WB, et al. (2005) Effects of prosthetic treatment for SDAs on OHRQoL, self-reports of pain and jaw disability: results from pilot-phase of a randomized multicentre trial. J Oral Rehabil 32: 815–822.
41. Luthardt RG, Marré B, Heineck A, Gerss J, Aggstaller H, et al. (2010) The randomized shortened dental arch study (RaSDA): design and protocol. Trials 11(15): 1–9.
42. Walter MH, Weber A, Marré B, Gitt I, Gerβ J, et al. (2010) The randomized Shortened dental arch study: Tooth Loss. J Dent Res 89: 818–822.
43. Walter MH, Weber A, Marré B, Gitt I, Gerβ J, et al. (2012) The randomized shortened dental arch study: 5 year results of the pilot phase. Deutsch Zahnärzt Zeits 67: 360–363.
44. Walter MH, Hannak W, Kern M, Mundt T, Gernet W, et al. (2012) The randomized shortened dental arch study: tooth loss over five years. Clin Oral Invest 1–10 [DOI:10.1007/s00784-01-0761-x].
45. Wolfart S, Muller F, Gerβ J, Heydecke G, Marré B, et al. (2012) The randomized shortened dental arch study: oral-health-related quality of life. Clin Oral Invest, DOI:10.1007/s00784-013-0991-6.
46. Wolfart S, Marré B, Wöstmann B, Kern M, Mundt T, et al. (2012) The randomized shortened dental arch study: 5-year Maintenance. J Dent Res 91(1): 65–71.
47. McKenna G, Allen PF, Flynn A, O'Mahony D, DaMata C, et al. (2012) Impact of tooth replacement strategies on the nutritional status of partially-dentate elders. Gerodont 29: e883–e890. [DOI:10.1111/j.1741-2358.2011.00579.x].
48. McKenna G, Allen PF, Flynn A, O'Mahony D, DaMata C, et al. (2012) A preliminary report of the cost-effectiveness of tooth replacement strategies for partially-dentate elders. Gerodont 1–7.
49. De Sa e Frias V, Toothaker R, Wright RF (2004) Shortened Dental Arch: A review of current treatment concepts. J Prosthodont 13(2): 104–110.
50. Sarita PT, Kreulen CM, Witter DJ, Creugers NHJ (2003) Signs and symptoms associated with TMD in adults with shortened dental arches. Int J Prosthodont 16(3): 265–270.
51. Sarita PT, Witter DJ, Kreulen CM, Van't Hof MA, et al. (2003) A study on occlusal stability in shortened dental arches. Int J Prosthodont 16(4): 375–380.
52. Sarita PT, Witter DJ, Kreulen CM, Van't Hof MA, et al. (2003) Chewing ability of subjects with shortened dental arches. Comm Dent Oral Epidimiol 31(5): 328–334.
53. Witter DJ, Creugers NHJ, Kreulen CM, de Haan AF (2001) Occlusal stability in Shortened Dental Arches. J Dent Res 80(2): 432–436.
54. Witter DJ, Kreulen CM, Mulder J, Creugers NHJ (2007) Signs and symptoms related to temporomandibular disorders- Follow-up of subjects with shortened and complete dental arches. J Dent 35: 521–527.
55. Witter DJ, de Haan AF, Käyser AF, van Rossum GM (1994) A 6-year follow-up study of oral function in shortened dental arches. Part II: Craniomandibular dysfunction and oral comfort. J Oral Rehabil 21(4): 353–66.
56. Fueki K, Yoshida E, Igarashi Y (2011) A systematic review of prosthetic restoration in patients with shortened dental arches. Jap Dent Sci Rev 47: 167–174.
57. Abt E, Carr AB, Worthington HV (2012) Interventions for replacing missing teeth: partially absent dentition. Cochrane Database of Systematic Reviews Issue 2. Art. No: CD003814. DOI:10.1002/14651858.CD003814.pub2.
58. Faggion CM (2011) The shortened dental arch revisited: from evidence to recommendations by the use of the GRADE approach. J Oral Rehabil 38: 940–949.
59. Higgins JPT, Green S (2009) Cochrane Handbook for systematic reviews of interventions. 1st Edition. West Sussex, UK: Wiley-Blackwell.
60. Guyatt GH, Oxman AD, Vist GE, Kunz R, Falck-Ytter Y, et al. (2008) GRADE: an emerging consensus on rating quality of evidence and strength of recommendations. BMJ, 336: 924–926.
61. CONSORT Guidelines. Available: http://www.consort-statement.org.

12

Tooth Loss in the United Kingdom – Trends in Social Inequalities: An Age-Period-and-Cohort Analysis

Eduardo Bernabé[1], Aubrey Sheiham[2]*

1 King's College London Dental Institute at Guy's, King's College and St. Thomas' Hospitals, Division of Population and Patient Health, London, United Kingdom,
2 Department of Epidemiology and Public Health, University College London, London, United Kingdom

Abstract

This study assessed trends in social inequalities in tooth loss in the United Kingdom between 1988 and 2009. Data from 20,126 adults who participated in the latest three national Adult Dental Health Surveys in England, Wales and Northern Ireland were used. Social class was determined using the 6-point Registrar General's Social Class. Three indicators of tooth loss were analysed; the proportion of edentate people among all adults and the number of teeth and the proportion with functional dentition (defined as having 20+ teeth) among dentate adults. Trends were modelled within an age, period and cohort framework using partial least squares regression (PLSR). Confidence intervals for PLSR estimates were obtained using non-parametric bootstrapping. The Slope and Relative Index of Inequality (SII and RII) were used to quantify social inequalities in tooth loss. Between 1988 and 2009, absolute inequalities in total tooth loss narrowed (SII changed from −28.4% to −15.3%) while relative inequalities widened (RII from 6.21 to 20.9) in the whole population. On the other hand, absolute and relative social inequality in tooth loss remained fairly stable over time among dentate adults. There was an absolute difference of 2.5–2.9 in number of teeth and 22–26% in the proportion with functional dentition between the lowest and highest social classes. In relative terms, the highest social class had 10–11% more teeth and 25–28% higher probability of having functional dentition than the lowest social class. The findings show pervasive inequalities in tooth loss by social class among British adults despite marked improvements in tooth retention in recent years and generations. In the whole adult population, absolute inequalities in tooth loss have narrowed while relative inequalities have increased steadily. Among dentate adults, absolute and relative inequalities in number of teeth and proportion of people with functional dentition have remained significant but unchanged over time.

Editor: Kimon Divaris, UNC School of Dentistry, University of North Carolina-Chapel Hill, United States of America

Funding: The authors have no support or funding to report.

Competing Interests: The authors have declared that no competing interests exist.

* Email: a.sheiham@ucl.ac.uk

Introduction

Tooth loss is an outcome that reflects not only the individuals' history of dental diseases but also patients' and dentists' attitudes and behaviours, the availability and accessibility of dental services and the prevailing philosophies of dental care [1,2]. It is considered an effective marker of population oral health and is therefore monitored in many countries. Despite large declines in the prevalence and incidence of tooth loss at global, regional and country levels in the past two decades [3], socioeconomic inequalities in tooth loss persist even in developed countries [4–8]. There is a social gradient in tooth loss, regardless of how the latter is measured, either as the prevalence of total tooth loss, the number of teeth or the proportion of adults with functional dentition, commonly assessed as having 20 or more natural teeth.

Monitoring social inequalities in health over time is important to improve understanding of the social determinants of health and evaluate policies to promote health and reduce health inequalities [9,10]. Some recent studies have explored the trends in social inequality in tooth loss [8,11–14]. Cunha-Cruz et al. [11] showed that for 25–74 year-old Americans, absolute differences in total tooth loss between high and low socioeconomic groups remained stable from 1972 to 2001. Dye and Thornton-Evans [12] also reported little change in the absolute difference of no tooth loss between poor and non-poor groups from 1988/94 to 1999/04 for 35–44 year-old Americans, but the absolute difference in total tooth loss between poor and non-poor groups increased from 19% to 23% for 65–74 year-olds. Elani et al. [8] showed that for adults aged 20 years and older, absolute differences in total tooth loss by income remained wider in Canada (7.5% in 1970/72 to 4.0% in 2007/09) compared to the US (3.7% in 1971/74 to 3.1% in 2007/08), while absolute differences by education narrowed (13.8% to 2.8% in Canada and 9.0% to 3.6% in the US). Celeste et al. [14] found that the absolute difference in total tooth loss between the poorer and the richer groups decreased in Brazil from 1986 to 2002, and in Sweden, from 1968 to 2000, while relative differences remained the same (prevalence ratios of 2.58 and 2.70 for Sweden and 1.67 and 1.12 for Brazil, with no significant trends over time). Holst [13] reported that the absolute difference in total tooth loss between the highest and lowest income quintiles decreased by 10.5% from 1975 to 2002 in Norwegian adults, with changes of −0.1%, 9.8% and 5.4% for 20–34-, 35–59- and 60+ year-olds respectively, whereas relatively inequality increased from a prevalence ratio of 2.1 in 1975 to 14.2 in 2002, with decreases from 3.5 to 0 in 20–34 year-olds and 2.1 to 1.0 in 35–59- year-olds but an increase from 2.0 to 7.5 in 60+ year-olds. However, the absolute difference in the proportion of people with functional dentition between the highest and lowest income quintiles increased by 25% from 1985 to 2002, with increases of 3.9% and 10.3% in the two youngest groups but a decrease of 9.3% in the oldest group, whereas relative inequality in functional dentition remained stable; from 0.5 in 1985 to 0.9 in 2002, with even smaller changes in the three age groups [13].

All the aforementioned studies used the range, either absolute or relative, to describe inequalities in tooth loss over time, in spite of the fact that such measures overlook changes in the intermediate socioeconomic groups, do not take into account the sizes of the groups being compared and tell little about how these inequalities are affected by the distribution of disease [15,16]. Alternative measures of health inequalities are thus recommended [17,18]. More importantly, all previous studies assume that observed changes over survey years are due to period effects, after accounting for age effects. Since age, period and cohort effects are linearly dependent (cohort = period-age), they implicitly assume that cohort effects do not exist. Age, period and cohort effects refer to some type of time-related variation in the outcome of interest, but they have distinct meanings [19,20]. Age effects refer to variation associated with different age groups. Thus, age effects reflect the biological and social processes of aging internal to individuals and represent developmental changes across the life course. Period effects refer to variation over time periods or calendar years that affect all age groups simultaneously. Lastly, cohort effects refer to variation among groups born in different years [19]. Thus, not taking into account cohort effects may mask trends of social inequalities in health [21–23].

As large inequalities in oral health in adults have been reported in the United Kingdom (UK) [7,24] and improvements in oral health have occurred in children [25] and adults [26], we hypothesised that the pervasive social inequalities in tooth loss in adults have persisted, despite marked improvements in oral health in recent surveys and generations. Within an age, period and cohort framework, this study assessed the trend of social inequalities in tooth loss in the UK between 1988 and 2009.

Materials and Methods

Data source

The Adult Dental Health Survey (ADHS) is a national cross-sectional survey in the UK, first carried out in 1968 and repeated each decade thereafter. We used individual-level data from the latest three surveys (1988, 1998 and 2009) in England, Wales and Northern Ireland because Scotland did not participate in 2009 and data from earlier surveys are only available at aggregate level. Each survey is based on a nationally representative sample of adults aged 16 years and over, with participants selected using stratified multi-stage random sampling methods. The survey has two main components; an interview followed by a clinical examination for dentate adults only. Participation rates in the ADHS have varied between 74% and 94% for the interview and between 61% and 82% for the clinical examination, across surveys [27–29].

We used two analytical samples in this study (Table 1). The first included 20,126 adults who completed the interview and had no missing data in the variables selected for analysis, whereas the second included 12,206 dentate adults who were clinically examined and had no missing data (93% and 94% of the total number of adults and dentate adults that participated in the three surveys in England, Wales and Northern Ireland, respectively).

Socioeconomic classification

The 1988 and 1998 ADHS measured social class on the basis of occupation of the household reference person (HRP), formerly Registrar General's Social Class (RGSC), and grouped individuals with similar levels of occupational skill using an ordinal scale with six categories: professional (I); managerial and technical (II); skilled non-manual (IIINM); skilled manual (IIIM); partly skilled (IV); and unskilled (V). For RGSC, the HRP is defined as the head of household: the oldest householder, with men taking precedence over women in the case of couples or non-related joint householders. In 2009, the ADHS adopted the National Statistics Socioeconomic Classification (NS-SEC) which is derived from HRP's occupational unit group, employment status and size of establishment, and includes 14 operational categories that can be collapsed into eight analytical classes: higher managerial and professional (1), lower managerial and professional (2), intermediate (3), small employers and own account workers (4), lower supervisory and technical (5), semi-routine (6), routine (7) and never worked and long-term unemployed (8). For NS-SEC, the HRP is defined as the person responsible for owning or renting or who is otherwise responsible for the accommodation. In the case of joint householders, the person with the highest income takes precedence and becomes the HRP. Where incomes are equal, the oldest person is taken as the HRP. The operational categories of NS-SEC can be aggregated to produce an approximated version of RGSC and these approximations have been shown to achieve an overall continuity level of 87% [30].

Outcome measures

During interviews, participants were asked whether they still have some natural teeth or have lost them all. Dentate participants who completed the interview were invited to a subsequent clinical examination where the condition of all teeth, including third molars, was recorded [27–29]. Three indicators of tooth loss were selected for this study. They were the proportion of edentate people among all adults; second, the number of teeth and third, the proportion of people with functional dentition (i.e. defined as having 20 or more teeth) among dentate adults.

Covariates

During interviews, participants provided information on country of residence, sex and age. Age was grouped into eight 10-year brackets (16–24, 25–34, 35–44, 45–54, 55–64, 65–74 and 75+ years). Period was defined as survey year and coded as 0 for 1988, 1 for 1998 and 2 for 2009. Individuals were grouped into eight 10-year cohort bands by their year of birth. These cohorts were defined by their mid-point; for example, the cohort 1948 included individuals born between 1944 and 1953. The eight cohort groups were 1908, 1918, 1928, 1938, 1948, 1958, 1968 and 1978.

Measures of social inequalities in tooth loss

We used the Slope Index of Inequality (SII) and the Relative Index of Inequality (RII) to measure, respectively, absolute and relative social inequality in tooth loss in 1988, 1998 and 2009. The SII is the linear regression coefficient that shows the relation between the level of health (i.e. number of teeth) or the frequency of a health problem (i.e. proportion of edentate people or having 20+ teeth) in each socioeconomic category and the hierarchical ranking of each socioeconomic category on the social scale [16]. SII can be interpreted as the absolute change in health level or in

Table 1. Participation rates in the Adult Dental Health Surveys in England, Wales and Northern Ireland, by survey year.

Unweighted sample	1988	1998	2009	All
Eligible adults	5670	5560	13509	24739
No interview obtained	427	560	2129	3116
Interviewed adults	5243	5000	11380	21623
Edentate adults	1108	672	813	2593
Dentate adults	4135	4328	10567	19030
Examined adults with teeth	3405	3149	6469	13023
Analytical sample				
Adults with complete data	5048	4770	10308	20126
% of interviewed adults	96%	95%	91%	93%
Dentate adults with complete data	3307	2963	5936	12206
% of examined adults	97%	94%	92%	94%

the frequency of a health problem when moving from the lowest through the highest socioeconomic level [15,17]. Two versions of the RII are often used in the literature. The RII for the mean or $RII_{(mean)}$ is calculated dividing the SII by the mean level of population health or by the frequency of the health problem in the population whereas RII for the ratio or $RII_{(ratio)}$ is calculated diving the regression model's predicted value at the highest point by the regression model's predicted value at the lowest point [16,18]. Confidence intervals for SII and RII were obtained as described elsewhere [18,31].

Table 2. Characteristics of the analytical samples, by survey year.

Explanatory	All adults			Dentate adults only		
variables	**1988**	**1998**	**2009**	**1988**	**1998**	**2009**
Sample size[a]	5048	4770	10308	3307	2963	5936
Sex						
Male	49%	51%	49%	52%	53%	49%
Female	51%	49%	51%	48%	47%	51%
Age groups						
16–24 years	18%	13%	11%	23%	15%	11%
25–34 years	18%	19%	17%	23%	22%	17%
35–44 years	18%	18%	20%	21%	20%	21%
45–54 years	14%	17%	18%	14%	18%	18%
55–64 years	14%	13%	16%	11%	12%	16%
65–74 years	11%	11%	11%	6%	9%	10%
75+ years	8%	9%	9%	2%	4%	7%
Country						
England	92%	92%	92%	92%	92%	92%
Wales	5%	6%	5%	6%	5%	5%
Ireland	3%	3%	3%	3%	3%	3%
Social class[b]						
I (highest)	8%	7%	5%	10%	8%	6%
II	27%	29%	30%	31%	31%	31%
IIINM	13%	14%	22%	13%	14%	23%
IIIM	33%	30%	22%	31%	30%	21%
IV	14%	15%	16%	12%	14%	15%
V (lowest)	5%	5%	5%	4%	4%	4%

[a]Counts are unweighted.
[b]Social class groups are professional (I); managerial and technical (II); skilled non-manual (IIINM); skilled manual (IIIM); partly skilled (IV); and unskilled (V).

Table 3. Association of social class with three indicators of tooth loss from partial least squares regression (PLSR) for 20126 adults and 12206 dentate adults in the UK.

Explanatory variables	All adults		Dentate adults only			
	Edentulous		Number of teeth		Having 20+ teeth	
	OR[a]	(95% CI)	Coef.[b]	(95% CI)	OR[a]	(95% CI)
Social class[c]						
I (highest)	0.27	(0.20, 0.37)	1.53	(1.37, 1.68)	2.61	(2.54, 2.69)
II	0.46	(0.42, 0.51)	0.64	(0.57, 0.70)	1.46	(1.44, 1.47)
IIINM	0.71	(0.69, 0.73)	0.22	(0.18, 0.27)	1.17	(1.16, 1.17)
IIIM	1.43	(1.35, 1.50)	−0.58	(−0.63, −0.53)	0.78	(0.77, 0.78)
IV	1.71	(1.62, 1.81)	−0.79	(−0.89, −0.70)	0.61	(0.6, 0.62)
V (lowest)	2.37	(2.10, 2.67)	−1.78	(−1.97, −1.58)	0.37	(0.36, 0.39)
Sex						
Men	0.88	(0.87, 0.89)	0.16	(0.12, 0.19)	0.99	(0.99, 1.00)
Women	1.14	(1.13, 1.15)	−0.16	(−0.19, −0.12)	1.01	(1.00, 1.01)
Age groups						
16–24 years	0.00	(0.00, 0.00)	1.83	(1.76, 1.90)	14.54	(14.17, 14.9[illegible])
25–34 years	0.17	(0.16, 0.19)	1.95	(1.84, 2.05)	3.78	(3.74, 3.83)
35–44 years	0.25	(0.24, 0.27)	0.90	(0.84, 0.96)	1.77	(1.75, 1.78)
45–54 years	0.76	(0.75, 0.77)	−0.30	(−0.4, −0.19)	1.08	(1.07, 1.08)
55–64 years	1.25	(1.04, 1.50)	−2.33	(−2.49, −2.17)	0.54	(0.54, 0.54)
65–74 years	1.91	(1.86, 1.95)	−2.85	(−3.00, −2.70)	0.46	(0.45, 0.46)
75+ years	3.20	(3.06, 3.34)	−4.67	(−4.93, −4.41)	0.28	(0.27, 0.28)
Country						
England	0.89	(0.89, 0.90)	0.56	(0.53, 0.59)	1.31	(1.3, 1.33)
Wales	1.17	(1.16, 1.18)	−0.40	(−0.45, −0.35)	0.86	(0.85, 0.86)
Northern Ireland	1.03	(1.03, 1.03)	−0.80	(−0.89, −0.70)	0.69	(0.68, 0.7)
Period						
1988	1.65	(1.62, 1.68)	−0.42	(−0.44, −0.41)	0.82	(0.82, 0.83)
1998	1.09	(1.09, 1.10)	−0.05	(−0.09, −0.01)	1.04	(1.03, 1.04)
2009	0.59	(0.58, 0.60)	0.46	(0.43, 0.49)	1.14	(1.13, 1.15)
Cohort						
1908	7.20	(6.70, 7.75)	−7.01	(−7.30, −6.71)	0.17	(0.16, 0.17)
1918	3.20	(3.06, 3.35)	−5.67	(−5.96, −5.38)	0.19	(0.19, 0.19)
1928	2.27	(2.20, 2.35)	−3.45	(−3.57, −3.33)	0.35	(0.35, 0.36)
1938	1.35	(1.33, 1.37)	−1.80	(−1.86, −1.75)	0.54	(0.54, 0.55)
1948	0.68	(0.67, 0.69)	0.01	(−0.10, 0.12)	0.92	(0.91, 0.92)
1958	0.24	(0.23, 0.25)	1.11	(1.05, 1.17)	1.88	(1.86, 1.89)
1968	0.23	(0.22, 0.25)	1.62	(1.57, 1.67)	3.44	(3.39, 3.49)
1978	0.06	(0.05, 0.07)	1.55	(1.45, 1.65)	10.19	(9.99, 10.39)
1988	0.01	(0.00, 0.06)	2.24	(2.12, 2.35)	8.35	(7.99, 8.73)

[a]Odds ratios (OR) from logistic PLSR.
[b]Regression coefficients from linear PLSR.
[c]Social class groups are professional (I); managerial and technical (II); skilled non-manual (IIINM); skilled manual (IIIM); partly skilled (IV); and unskilled (V).

Statistical analysis

Each outcome was modelled separately, including social class, sex, age groups, country of residence, period and cohort as explanatory variables. As age, period and cohort are mathematically related (period-age = cohort), they cannot be entered into the same regression model due to perfect co-linearity [19,32]. To address this problem, we used partial least squares regression (PLSR) to separate and account for age, period and cohort effects [33]. PLSR does not use the original collinear covariates in the estimation process but extracts weighted components that maximise the covariance between the outcome and successively extracted components. The outcome is then regressed onto these components, and corresponding regression coefficients are calculated using linear algebra [34]. The first few components usually

Table 4. Predicted probabilities of being edentate for adults and predicted number of teeth and probability of having 20+ teeth for dentate adults in the UK, by survey year.

Survey year	Social class[a]	All adults		Dentate adults only			
		% edentate		Number of teeth		% with 20+ teeth	
		%	(95% CI)	Mean	(95% CI)	%	(95% CI)
1988	I (highest)	7%	(7%, 8%)	25.3	(25.2, 26.2)	89%	(86%, 91%)
	II	11%	(10%, 11%)	24.2	(24.1, 24.1)	80%	(79%, 81%)
	IIINM	17%	(16%, 18%)	23.9	(23.8, 24.1)	77%	(75%, 79%)
	IIIM	25%	(24%, 27%)	23.2	(23.1, 23.3)	73%	(73%, 74%)
	IV	28%	(27%, 30%)	23.2	(23.0, 23.3)	68%	(63%, 72%)
	V (lowest)	34%	(32%, 36%)	22.5	(22.4, 22.6)	62%	(46%, 76%)
1998	I (highest)	4%	(3%, 4%)	25.4	(25.3, 25.5)	89%	(80%, 94%)
	II	6%	(6%, 7%)	25.0	(24.9, 25.0)	87%	(86%, 87%)
	IIINM	11%	(11%, 11%)	24.4	(24.2, 24.6)	84%	(84%, 85%)
	IIIM	20%	(20%, 21%)	23.5	(23.5, 23.6)	75%	(24%, 97%)
	IV	21%	(20%, 22%)	23.1	(23,0, 23.2)	70%	(65%, 75%)
	V (lowest)	26%	(26%, 27%)	22.6	(22.5, 22.8)	64%	(58%, 70%)
2009	I (highest)	1%	(1%, 2%)	26.2	(26.1, 26.3)	95%	(93%, 97%)
	II	4%	(3%, 4%)	25.3	(25.2, 25.5)	87%	(86%, 87%)
	IIINM	5%	(4%, 5%)	24.8	(24.6, 25.0)	84%	(73%, 92%)
	IIIM	11%	(10%, 11%)	24.1	(24.0, 24.2)	78%	(77%, 79%)
	IV	13%	(12%, 14%)	24.1	(23.9, 24.2)	74%	(70%, 77%)
	V (lowest)	18%	(16%, 20%)	22.6	(22.4, 22.8)	55%	(51%, 59%)

Predicted probabilities and predicted means were estimated from logistic and linear PLSR models (adjusted for country of residence, sex and age, period and cohort effects), respectively.

[a]Social class groups are professional (I); managerial and technical (II); skilled non-manual (IIINM); skilled manual (IIIM); partly skilled (IV); and unskilled (V).

Table 5. Health inequality measures (with 95% confidence intervals) for the association of social class with three indicators of tooth loss for 20126 adults and 12206 dentate adults in the UK, by period.

Period	Measure[a]	All adults		Dentate adults only			
		% edentate		Number of teeth		% with 20+ teeth	
1988	SII	−28.4	(−35.0, −21.7)	2.5	(1.4, 3.6)	21.8	(14.4, 29.2)
	$RII_{(mean)}$	1.65	(1.38, 1.92)	0.10	(0.07, 0.14)	0.28	(0.22, 0.35)
	$RII_{(ratio)}$	6.21	(5.07, 7.61)	0.90	(0.87, 0.93)	0.75	(0.70, 0.80)
1998	SII	−24.9	(−33.8, −16.2)	2.9	(2.5, 3.4)	25.5	(16.9, 34.0)
	$RII_{(mean)}$	2.07	(1.55, 2.58)	0.12	(0.11, 0.14)	0.32	(0.24, 0.39)
	$RII_{(ratio)}$	14.89	(10.82, 20.49)	0.89	(0.87, 0.90)	0.72	(0.68, 0.78)
2009	SII	−15.3	(−22.7, −8.0)	2.6	(1.4, 3.8)	25.8	(7.5, 44.1)
	$RII_{(mean)}$	1.55	(1.03, 2.07)	0.10	(0.07, 0.14)	0.32	(0.16, 0.47)
	$RII_{(ratio)}$	20.94	(15.10, 29.05)	0.90	(0.87, 0.93)	0.73	(0.63, 0.83)

[a]SII: Slope Index of Inequality; $RII_{(mean)}$: Relative Index of Inequality for the mean; and $RII_{(ratio)}$: Relative Index of Inequality for the ratio.

explain most of the covariance with the outcome. Hence, increments in the explained variation in the outcome (R^2) were used as a criterion for selecting the number of PLSR components. Small changes in R^2 resulting from the inclusion of an additional component indicated the model without such component was preferred [33,34].

PLSR modelling was undertaken using R-3.1.0 for Windows. We modelled the proportion of edentate people and those having 20+ teeth, using logistic PLSR and number of teeth using linear PLSR. To improve stability in the iteration process for PLSR, all explanatory variables were centred at the mid-point of their respective scales and each converted to a set of indicator (dummy) variables before analysis [33]. As there is no distribution assumption for PLSR coefficients, 1000 non-parametric bootstraps were drawn to obtain 95% confidence intervals (CI) for estimates from PLSR. All analyses were weighted to take account of the survey design and possible non-response bias.

For each outcome, we first present PLSR estimates (adjusted odds ratios and regression coefficients for dichotomous and continuous outcomes respectively), followed by stratified results by survey year (period) to inspect for trends in social inequalities in tooth loss. In the stratified analysis by period, predicted probabilities for dichotomous outcomes and predicted means for continuous outcomes were reported along with the corresponding SII, $RII_{(mean)}$ and $RII_{(ratio)}$.

Results

The socio-demographic composition of the two analytical samples is shown, by periods, in Table 2. The proportion of edentate adults decreased over the last two decades, from 20% (95% CI: 19–21%) in 1988 to 12% (11–13%) in 1998 to 6% (5–6%) in 2009. These changes were accompanied by increases in the mean number of teeth among dentate adults, from 24.3 (24.0–24.5) in 1988 to 24.8 (24.6–25.0) in 1998 to 25.5 (25.4–25.7) in 2009, as well as in the proportion of dentate adults with 20+ teeth, from 83% (81–84%) in 1988 to 85% (84–86%) in 1998 to 87% (86–88%) in 2009.

Table 3 shows the results of the PLSR carried out with each outcome. The 95% CI revealed that all estimates (for the comparison of code 1 to code 0 used with each dummy variable) were statistically significant at the 5% level. Marked improvements in tooth retention were observed by periods and cohorts, independent of the negative effect of aging. Social gradients were found in the three outcomes after accounting for country of residence, sex and age, period and cohort effects. In the full sample of adults, the odds of being edentate increased gradually from the highest (I-NM) to the lowest (V-M) social class. Similarly, the number of teeth and odds of having 20+ teeth among dentate adults increased progressively from the lowest to the highest social class.

Table 4 reports the predicted probability of being edentate for all adults as well as the predicted number of teeth and probability of having 20+ teeth (with 95% CI) for dentate adults, by social class and period, calculated from their respective PLSR models. Monotonic gradients in the three outcomes were found by social class in every survey despite overall improvements over time. These findings were used to calculate measures of social inequalities in tooth loss, which were thus adjusted for all covariates (Table 5). Among all adults, absolute inequality in total tooth loss diminished over the two decades, as indicated by the change in SII from −28.4 in 1998 to −15.3 in 2009. The SII indicated that the probability of being edentate decreased by 15.3% from the lowest through the highest social class in 2009.

The $RII_{(mean)}$ varied from 1.65 in 1988, suggesting that the SII was 1.65 times the overall probability of being edentate, to 1.55 in 2009. And the $RII_{(ratio)}$ increased from 6.21 in 1998, implying that the probability of being edentate in the lowest social class was 6.21 times the probability in the highest social class, to 20.9 in 2009. On the other hand, measures of social inequality in tooth loss among dentate adults remained fairly stable over time. SII was positive and varied between 2.5 and 2.9 for the predicted number of teeth (indicating that the highest social class had 2.5–2.9 more teeth than the lowest social class) and between 21.8 and 25.8 for the probability of having 20+ teeth. The $RII_{(mean)}$ varied from 0.10 to 0.12 for the predicted number of teeth and from 0.28 to 0.32 for the probability of having 20+ teeth; and the $RII_{(ratio)}$ varied between 0.89 and 0.90 for the predicted number of teeth and between 0.72 and 0.75 for the probability of having 20+ teeth.

Discussion

There were pervasive inequalities in tooth loss by social class in the UK adult population. The findings on inequality are consistent with other UK reports on tooth loss [7,24]. However, we found that social gradients in tooth loss persisted through the two decades studied, regardless of the outcome used (total tooth loss, number of teeth or functional dentition) and despite marked improvements in tooth retention in recent years and generations.

Different trends in social inequality in tooth loss were observed for dentate adults and the whole population. For dentate adults, the SII and RII indicated that social inequalities in number of teeth and proportion with functional dentition have remained significant over the last two decades. There was an absolute difference of 2.5–2.9 in number of teeth and 22–26% in the proportion with functional dentition between the lowest and highest social classes. In relative terms, the top social class had 10–11% more teeth and 25–28% higher probability of having functional dentition than the bottom social class. On the other hand, the SII and RII showed opposite trends for the full population. While the SII implied that absolute inequality in total tooth loss between the highest and lowest social classes decreased over the past two decades (from −28.4% to −15.3%), the $RII_{(ratio)}$ indicated that relative inequality in total tooth loss increased steadily over the same period (from 6 to almost 21 times). Dramatic changes in the epidemiology of total tooth loss could explain the above findings. It has been previously suggested that relative differences may increase while absolute differences decrease if the frequency of the health problem declines [16,18]. Kassebaum et al. [3] speculate that massive declines in the global prevalence and incidence of total tooth loss between 1990 and 2010 are due to changes in societal and cultural norms as well as coordinated efforts in treating oral diseases and preventing tooth loss throughout life. More importantly, the situation of increasing relative but decreasing absolute inequality also occurs when the rate of improvement is smaller for the group with the worst initial health [35]. In our case, total tooth loss declined by 80% for the highest social class and 48% for the lowest social class. Taken together, our findings indicate that the significant decline in total tooth loss in the UK over the past two decades has not benefited all social classes evenly.

The magnitude of social inequalities in tooth loss is unlikely to change quickly [7]. Tooth loss reflects both the individuals' history of dental diseases and treatment by dental services over the life course. As such, it captures a lifetime cumulative experience. To eliminate social inequalities in tooth loss, the determinants of inequalities must be identified and avoidable determinants modified. More attention should be directed at preventing dental diseases at all stages of the life course and at addressing the common determinants of chronic diseases, including oral diseases.

Tracking social inequalities in oral health over time is important to inform social and oral health-related policy. This is the first study to quantify and provide time comparative analysis of social inequalities in tooth loss using rigorous measures of social inequalities in oral health. As all previous trend analyses on social inequalities in tooth loss have relied on the range measure of inequality, their results are difficult to compare with ours. In line with previous recommendations [15,17,18,36], future studies should report both absolute and relative measures of social inequalities in oral health.

Our findings should be interpreted in the light of some potential limitations. First, our findings were based on participants with complete data, which may raise concerns about representativeness of the data. However, the two analytical samples represented 93% and 94% of the adults and dentate adults that participated in the three surveys in England, Wales and Northern Ireland, respectively. In addition, the two samples were comparable with the general adult population in the three British countries in terms of demographic characteristics and social classes, which provides support for its representativeness and the generalization of the findings. Second, we used occupation-based social class to measure socioeconomic circumstances, ignoring other socioeconomic indicators relevant to oral health, such as education or income. A key strength of RGSC is its past official status in the UK, and hence, its widespread use in vital statistics and censuses over a long period of time. More importantly, it has been widely used to describe the socioeconomic gradient in health [37,38]. Third, in 2001 NS-SEC replaced RGSC as the official socioeconomic classification in the UK, which may raise concerns about the validity of comparisons between the old and new socioeconomic classifications. However, Rose and Pevalin [30] constructed derivation matrices for RGSC from NS-SEC to assist with maintaining comparability across surveys and showed that 87 per cent of cases in NS-SEC can be allocated to the correct RGSC category. Further studies should explore whether similar trends of social inequalities in oral health are observed using alternative socioeconomic measures and oral health outcomes over longer periods of evaluation.

Conclusions

There were pervasive inequalities in tooth loss by social class among British adults despite marked improvements in tooth retention in recent years and generations. In the whole population, absolute inequalities in total tooth loss have narrowed while relative inequalities have increased steadily. Among dentate adults, absolute and relative inequalities in number of teeth and proportion of people with functional dentition have remained significant, but unchanged over time.

Acknowledgments

The 2009 Adult Dental Health Survey was commissioned by the NHS Information Centre for Health and Social Care and was conducted on behalf of the Department of Health in England, the Welsh Assembly Health Department and the Department of Health, Social Services and Public Safety in Northern Ireland. The Survey was managed by the Office for National Statistics with a major contribution from The National Centre for Social Research.

Author Contributions

Conceived and designed the experiments: EB AS. Analyzed the data: EB. Contributed to the writing of the manuscript: EB AS.

References

1. Baelum V, van Palenstein Helderman W, Hugoson A, Yee R, Fejerskov O (2007) A global perspective on changes in the burden of caries and periodontitis: implications for dentistry. J Oral Rehabil 34: 872–906; discussion 940.
2. Fejerskov O, Escobar G, Jossing M, Baelum V (2013) A functional natural dentition for all - and for life? The oral healthcare system needs revision. J Oral Rehabil 40: 707–722.
3. Kassebaum NJ, Bernabé E, Dahiya M, Bhandari B, Murray CJ, et al. (2014) Global Burden of Severe Tooth Loss: A Systematic Review and Meta-analysis. J Dent Res 93: 20S–28S.
4. Sanders AE, Slade GD, Turrell G, John Spencer A, Marcenes W (2006) The shape of the socioeconomic-oral health gradient: implications for theoretical explanations. Community Dent Oral Epidemiol 34: 310–319.
5. Thomson WM (2012) Social inequality in oral health. Community Dent Oral Epidemiol 40 Suppl 2: 28–32.
6. Guarnizo-Herreno CC, Watt RG, Pikhart H, Sheiham A, Tsakos G (2013) Socioeconomic inequalities in oral health in different European welfare state regimes. J Epidemiol Community Health 67: 728–735.
7. Shen J, Wildman J, Steele J (2013) Measuring and decomposing oral health inequalities in an UK population. Community Dent Oral Epidemiol 41: 481–489.
8. Elani HW, Harper S, Allison PJ, Bedos C, Kaufman JS (2012) Socio-economic inequalities and oral health in Canada and the United States. J Dent Res 91: 865–870.
9. CSDH (2008) Closing the gap in a generation: health equity through action on the social determinants of health. Final Report of the Commission on Social Determinants of Health. Geneva: World Health Organization.
10. WHO (2013) Handbook on health inequality monitoring: with a special focus on low- and middle-income countries. Geneva: World Health Organization.
11. Cunha-Cruz J, Hujoel PP, Nadanovsky P (2007) Secular trends in socio-economic disparities in edentulism: USA, 1972–2001. J Dent Res 86: 131–136.
12. Dye BA, Thornton-Evans G (2010) Trends in oral health by poverty status as measured by Healthy People 2010 objectives. Public Health Rep 125: 817–830.
13. Holst D (2008) Oral health equality during 30 years in Norway. Community Dent Oral Epidemiol 36: 326–334.
14. Celeste RK, Nadanovsky P, Fritzell J (2011) Trends in socioeconomic disparities in oral health in Brazil and Sweden. Community Dent Oral Epidemiol 39: 204–212.
15. Wagstaff A, Paci P, van Doorslaer E (1991) On the measurement of inequalities in health. Soc Sci Med 33: 545–557.
16. Regidor E (2004) Measures of health inequalities: part 2. J Epidemiol Community Health 58: 900–903.
17. Mackenbach JP, Kunst AE (1997) Measuring the magnitude of socio-economic inequalities in health: an overview of available measures illustrated with two examples from Europe. Soc Sci Med 44: 757–771.
18. Cheng NF, Han PZ, Gansky SA (2008) Methods and software for estimating health disparities: the case of children's oral health. Am J Epidemiol 168: 906–914.
19. Yang Y, Land KC (2013) Age-Period-Cohort Analysis: New Models, Methods, and Empirical Applications. London: CRC Press.
20. Glenn ND (1977) Cohort analysis. Beverly Hills, California: Sage Publications.
21. Lynch SM (2003) Cohort and life-course patterns in the relationship between education and health: a hierarchical approach. Demography 40: 309–331.
22. Chen F, Yang Y, Liu G (2010) Social Change and Socioeconomic Disparities in Health over the Life Course in China: A Cohort Analysis. Am Sociol Rev 75: 126–150.
23. Beck AN, Finch BK, Lin SF, Hummer RA, Masters RK (2014) Racial disparities in self-rated health: trends, explanatory factors, and the changing role of socio-demographics. Soc Sci Med 104: 163–177.
24. Tsakos G, Demakakos P, Breeze E, Watt RG (2011) Social gradients in oral health in older adults: findings from the English longitudinal survey of aging. Am J Public Health 101: 1892–1899.
25. Pitts NB, Chestnutt IG, Evans D, White D, Chadwick B, et al. (2006) The dentinal caries experience of children in the United Kingdom, 2003. Br Dent J 200: 313–320.
26. Steele JG, Treasure ET, O'Sullivan I, Morris J, Murray JJ (2012) Adult Dental Health Survey 2009: transformations in British oral health 1968–2009. Br Dent J 213: 523–527.
27. Kelly M, Steele J, Nuttall N, Bradnock G, Morris J, et al. (2001) Adult Dental Health Survey: Oral Health in the United Kingdom in 1998. London: The Stationery Office.
28. O'Sullivan I, Lader D, Seymour-Beavean C, Chenery V, Fuller E, et al. (2011) Foundation Report: Adult Dental Health Survey 2009 London: The Health and Social Care Information Centre, Dental and Eye Care Team.
29. Todd JE, Lader D (1991) Adult Dental Health 1988 United Kingdom. London: Her Majesty's Stationery Office (HMSO).
30. Rose D, Pevalin D (2005) The National Statistics socio-economic classification: origins, development and use. London: Palgrave Macmillian. 1–120 p.
31. Hayes LJ, Berry G (2002) Sampling variability of the Kunst-Mackenbach relative index of inequality. J Epidemiol Community Health 56: 762–765.
32. Mason KO, Mason WM, Winsborough HH, Poole WK (1973) Some Methodological Issues in Cohort Analysis of Archival Data. Am Sociol Rev 38: 242–258.
33. Tu YK, Kramer N, Lee WC (2012) Addressing the identification problem in age-period-cohort analysis: a tutorial on the use of partial least squares and principal components analysis. Epidemiology 23: 583–593.
34. Vinzi VE, Chin WW, Henseler J, Wang H, editors (2010) Handbook of partial least squares: Concepts, methods and applications. Berlin, Germany: Springer Handbooks of Computational Statistics.
35. Harper S, King NB, Meersman SC, Reichman ME, Breen N, et al. (2010) Implicit value judgments in the measurement of health inequalities. Milbank Q 88: 4–29.
36. Kelly MP, Morgan A, Bonnefoy J, Butt J, Bergmann V (2007) The social determinants of health: developing an evidence based for action. WHO Commision on Social Determinants of Health.
37. Galobardes B, Shaw M, Lawlor DA, Lynch JW, Davey Smith G (2006) Indicators of socioeconomic position (part 2). J Epidemiol Community Health 60: 95–101.
38. Krieger N, Williams DR, Moss NE (1997) Measuring social class in US public health research: concepts, methodologies, and guidelines. Annu Rev Public Health 18: 341–378.

13

Application of Intra-Oral Dental Scanners in the Digital Workflow of Implantology

Wicher J. van der Meer[1]*, Frank S. Andriessen[2], Daniel Wismeijer[3], Yijin Ren[4]

1 Assistant professor, Department of Orthodontics, University Medical Centre Groningen, University of Groningen, Groningen, The Netherlands, **2** Postgraduate, Section of Oral Implantology, Academic Centre for Dentistry Amsterdam, Amsterdam, The Netherlands, **3** Professor and chair, Department of Oral Function and Restorative Dentistry, Head of the Section of Oral Implantology and Prosthodontics, Academic Centre for Dentistry Amsterdam, Amsterdam, The Netherlands, **4** Professor and chair, Department of Orthodontics, University Medical Centre Groningen, University of Groningen, Groningen, The Netherlands

Abstract

Intra-oral scanners will play a central role in digital dentistry in the near future. In this study the accuracy of three intra-oral scanners was compared. Materials and methods: A master model made of stone was fitted with three high precision manufactured PEEK cylinders and scanned with three intra-oral scanners: the CEREC (Sirona), the iTero (Cadent) and the Lava COS (3M). In software the digital files were imported and the distance between the centres of the cylinders and the angulation between the cylinders was assessed. These values were compared to the measurements made on a high accuracy 3D scan of the master model. Results: The distance errors were the smallest and most consistent for the Lava COS. The distance errors for the Cerec were the largest and least consistent. All the angulation errors were small. Conclusions: The Lava COS in combination with a high accuracy scanning protocol resulted in the smallest and most consistent errors of all three scanners tested when considering mean distance errors in full arch impressions both in absolute values and in consistency for both measured distances. For the mean angulation errors, the Lava COS had the smallest errors between cylinders 1–2 and the largest errors between cylinders 1–3, although the absolute difference with the smallest mean value (iTero) was very small (0,0529°). An expected increase in distance and/or angular errors over the length of the arch due to an accumulation of registration errors of the patched 3D surfaces could be observed in this study design, but the effects were statistically not significant.

Clinical relevance: For making impressions of implant cases for digital workflows, the most accurate scanner with the scanning protocol that will ensure the most accurate digital impression should be used. In our study model that was the Lava COS with the high accuracy scanning protocol.

Editor: Michael Glogauer, University of Toronto, Canada

Funding: These authors have no support or funding to report.

Competing Interests: The authors have declared that no competing interests exist.

* E-mail: w.j.van.der.meer@umcg.nl

Introduction

The basis for prosthetic work in dentistry has traditionally been an intra-oral impression that was subsequently poured in dental stone. The stone model forms the basis for the dental lab to manufacture crowns, fixed partial dentures and frames attached to natural teeth. Stone models are also used for producing frameworks for implant cases. This traditional workflow has proven itself in clinical practice, even though impression materials are prone to dimensional changes due to on-going chemical reactions [1] and stone will show expansion due to secondary reactions whilst setting [2]. Aforementioned dimensional changes may very wellresult in a misfit of the cast restorations. The misfit of fixed partial dentures on natural teeth will result in forces on the underlying teeth. Natural teeth however can move 25–100 μm in axial direction and 56–108 μm in lateral direction [3], [4] and adapt to a slightly different position in the bone due to the periodontal ligament should there be a slight misfit of the prosthetic work. Implants on the other hand will only show a range of motion of 3–5 μm in axial direction and 10–50 μm in lateral direction after osseointegration due to compression of the bone [4]. Ill-fitting framework will generate stress on the implants which may have a biological effect on the bone-implant interface [5], [6]. Also prosthetic complications as screw loosening or fracture may be related to ill-fitting framework fit [7]. A finite element analysis (FEA) study has also shown that passive fit will distribute masticatory forces more evenly over the implants [8]. The aforementioned factors have resulted in the paradigm that passive fit of the framework is one of the key factors for long-term success in implant dentistry [9], [10] stressing the importance of a reliable and precise impression procedure. Several strategies have been developed to ascertain passive fit [3], [11]. Even though none of the techniques has proven to be a panacea, the application of industrial-based digital production workflows is a solution that seems to gain popularity. As the impression procedure is at the origin of the workflow, the data collected during this phase is important as errors introduced in this phase will reverberate in the rest of the workflow. An intra-oral scanner could overcome some of the errors associated with traditional impression taking [12] and cast production [13], as digital output data can be fed directly into a digital workflow. The assessment of the accuracy of traditional impression materials has primarily been performed using linear or

3D measurements. The accuracy deviations that were found in those studies have been expressed in µm or percentages [14], [15], [16].

When considering accuracy one is inclined to consider only what we can refer to as "local accuracy" where the scan of a small geometrical form is compared to the original form and the difference between the two forms can be considered as the accuracy of the scanner. This would hold true for accuracy needed for single crown units in dentistry. This accuracy has been determined for intra-oral scanners by several authors [17], [18], [19]. Another form of accuracy would be the accuracy over more units across the dental arch, which could be referred to as "general accuracy", resembling the accuracy necessary for the production of multi-unit fixed partial denture on natural teeth or implants. This form of accuracy is especially interesting if one considers full arch impressions for implant framework. In those cases the accuracy of the full-arch impression and the distance between the implants leaves less room for errors due to the rigidity of the bone-implant interface [11]. Although the dichotomy between "local" and "general" accuracy may seem immaterial at first, the rationale behind it is that all the intra-oral scanners build their 3D models by combining several 3D images made of the same section of the model but from different angles. The composition of the different 3D patches inevitably leads to registration errors that may vary in magnitude depending on the scanning technology and the registration algorithms used [20] [21], [22]. *Even though other studies* have tried to establish the accuracy of some of the intra-oral digitizers [17], [18], [19], no consensus exists on how to assess the accuracy of intra-oral scanners. Some have looked at single teeth [18], several teeth in a row [17] or at quadrants [18]. One study has looked at full arch scans [19]. In order to simplify the comparison, the dataset comparison was always reduced to a single number depicting the difference between the dataset of the scanner and the golden standard. In our study we wanted to consider the accuracy necessary for multi-unit framework on implants and a single number does not indicate possible error fluctuations over a longer span in those cases. We have therefore chosen to measure the distance and angular changes over a longer span between simulated implants generating multiple numbers that can be compared.

The objective of this study was to assess the "general accuracy" of three commercially available intra-oral scanners, that employ different scanning technologies to obtain the 3D images, for the application in the digital workflow in implant prosthetics.

Materials and Methods

The model

Three high precision PEEK (polyether ether ketone) cylinders were manufactured by Createch Medical (Createch Medical, Mendaro, Spain) with an accuracy of 2 µm. PEEK was chosen for its excellent mechanical and chemical properties and to avoid a reflective surface that a metal cylinder would provide, as all intra-oral scanners have problems scanning reflective, shiny surfaces.

On a full arch stone model of a volunteer, the teeth 36, 46 and 41 were ground to gingival level. Subsequently a hole was drilled in the stone and implant analogues were placed in the prepared cavities and embedded in stone. The high precision cylinders were then screwed on the implant analogues.

The intra-oral scanners

The intra-oral scanners used in the study were the CEREC AC with the CEREC bluecam (Sirona Dental Systems Gmbh, Bensheim, Germany) with software version 3.85, the Cadent iTero (Cadent Inc, Carlstadt, USA) with software version 3.5.0 and the Lava COS (3M Espe, St. Paul, USA) with software version 2.1). All 3D scanners measure the distance from the scanner's sensor-tip to the object with different technologies to convert the optical data to a 3D model. The CEREC AC system employs light stripe projection and active triangulation (Figure 1) to generate 3D images [23]. The Cadent iTero scanner employs a parallel confocal imaging technique [24] for capturing 3D images (Figure 2). The Lava COS uses active wavefront sampling [25] to obtain a 3D model of the dentition (Figure 3). Both the CEREC AC and the Cadent iTero capture single 3D frames that are stitched with other frames to compose a complete 3D model in a short registration cycle. After each cycle the user can proceed to scan the next part of the model. After the scanning procedure the model can be uploaded to respectively CEREC or iTero for post processing. The Lava COS is a 3D video system that captures 20 3D frames per second, which are registered real-time. After the scanning procedure a post processing cycle is necessary to recalculate the registration and compensate for potential errors, resulting in a high resolution model that is uploaded to 3M.

Dusting or powdering

The iTero scanner does not need special preparation of teeth to be scanned. Before scanning with the Lava COS, teeth need to be dusted with Lava Powder (3M Espe, St. Paul, USA), a titanium-oxide powder. The latter has to do with the technology the scanner employs. The dust particles on the teeth are used for registration of the 3D patches obtained during scanning. When employing the CEREC AC, a matte finishing needs to be applied to the surface to be scanned to prevent reflections. For this purpose the surface is covered with a thin layer of Optispray (Sirona Dental Systems GmbH, Bensheim, Germany). To correctly mimic the clinical situation, the models were prepared according to the manufacturer's instructions with the appropriate powder before scanning the model. To avoid possible errors due to powder contamination, the order of scanning was decided to be

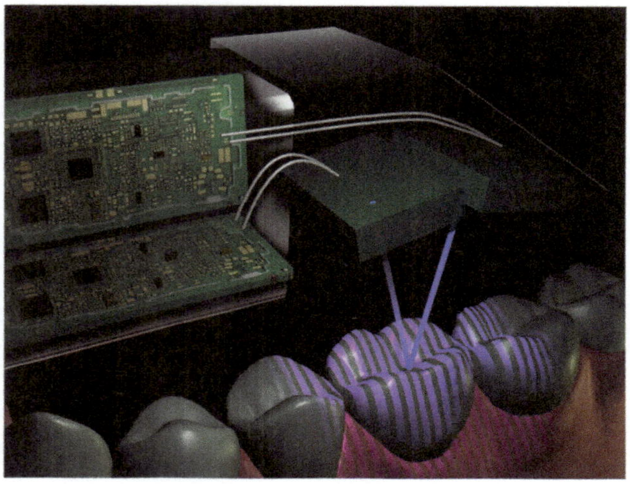

Figure 1. The technical principle of the CEREC scanner. The Cerec projects a light stripe pattern on the object. As each light ray is reflected back on the sensor, the distance between the projected ray and reflected ray is measured. Because the fixed angle between the projector and sensor is known, the distance to the object can be calculated through Pythagoras theorem, as one side and one angle (the fixed angle) of the triangle are now known. Hence the name "triangulation".

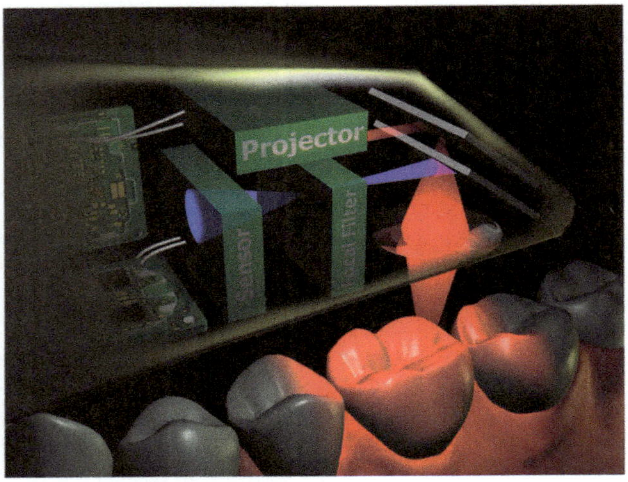

Figure 2. The technical principle of the iTero scanner. The iTero scanner uses confocal laser scanning in which a laser beam (red) is projected on an object. Via a beam splitter, the reflected beam (purple) is led through a focal filter so that only the image that lies in the focal point of the lens can project on the sensor. As the focal distance is known, the distance of the scanned part of the object to the lens is known (the focal distance). To scan the whole object, the lens is moved up and down, each time projecting a part of the object onto the sensor.

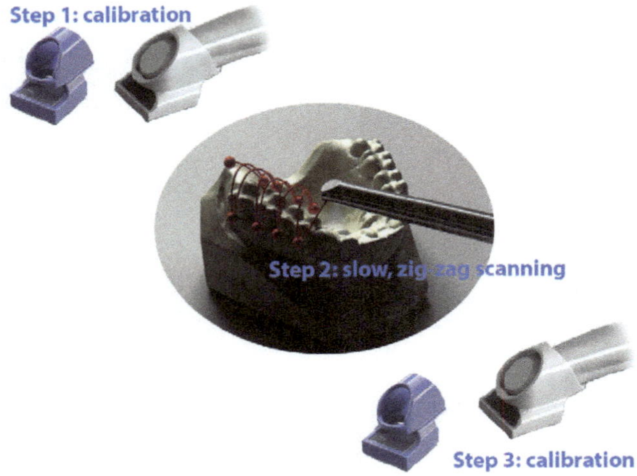

Figure 4. The hi-res scanning protocol for the Lava COS scans. The scanning protocol for the scans for the Lava COS is the normal scanning protocol, except that the scan-path is a slow zigzag scan and that at the end of the scan a second calibration is performed.

1. the iTero, as it required no powder
2. the Lava COS, as it required only light dusting
3. the CEREC, as it required the complete surface to be covered with a thin layer of Optispray.

3D scanning

The model was attached to a table and scanned 10 times with three different intra-oral scanners: the iTero (Cadent Inc, Carlstadt, USA), the Lava COS (3M Espe, St. Paul, USA) and the CEREC (Sirona Dental Systems GmbH, Bensheim, Germany). The manufacturers were asked for the protocol for high accuracy scanning as would be used for scanning implant locators and for special considerations for this type of scanning, e.g. calibration of the scanning unit or modification of the scanning protocol. The iTero and the CEREC had only one scanning protocol for all cases and did not distinguish between normal scanning and high accuracy scanning. The Lava COS had a high accuracy scanning protocol and subsequent calibration protocol. The normal Lava scanning protocol consists of a calibration with small calibration block before the intra-oral scan starts followed by scanning of the teeth according to a non-prescribed scan path. The

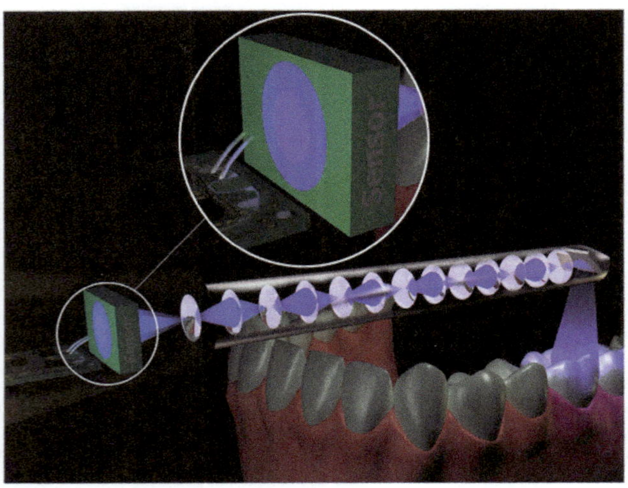

Figure 3. The technical principle of the Lava COS scanner. The Lava COS uses "active wavefront sampling" to calculate the 3D model of the teeth. For this the image reflected from the teeth is led through a lens system and eventually projected onto a sensor. If the image is in focus, the distance of the object coincides with the focal length of the lens. If the image is out of focus, the distance from the lens to the object can be calculated from the size of the blurred image through a simple mathematical formula.

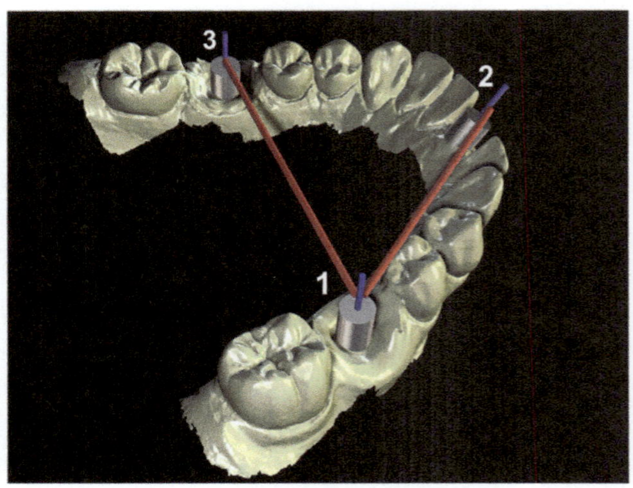

Figure 5. The measurements were made between the centers of the high-precision cylinders. Three 3D CAD models of the cylinders in the model were imported and registered with each of the scanned equivalents. The distance between the centre-lines was measured in the software using a linear measurement tool. The angular deflection of the cylinders was measured with an angular measurement tool, using the cylinder at the location of the lower right molar as the baseline.

Table 1. Absolute errors in the distance between the cylinders in micrometers.

	CEREC		iTero		Lava COS	
	ABS Error 1-2	ABS Error 1-3	ABS Error 1-2	ABS Error 1-3	ABS Error 1-2	ABS Error 1-3
MEAN	79,6	81,6	70,5	61,1	14,6	23,5
SD	77,1	52,5	56,3	53,9	12,7	14,2
CI (95%)	31,8–127,4	49,1–114,2	35,5–105,4	27,7–94,5	6,7–22,4	14,7–32,3

high accuracy scanning protocol for scanning implant abutments consists of a calibration with the aforementioned calibration block followed by a slow zig-zag scanning of the dentition. After the scan the calibration with the calibration block is performed for a second time (Figure 4). The calibration measurements are used to calculate and compensate for errors that have occurred during scanning.

All the scans were performed according to the instructions of the manufacturer by a dentist proficient with the specific intra-oral scanner. As only the iTero scanner does not require dusting or powdering of the model, the iTero scanner was used first to scan the model 10 times with a 10 minute interval between the scans. After this the model was dusted according to the instructions for the Lava COS with Lava Powder (3M Espe, St. Paul, USA) and the model was scanned 10 times with this scanner with a 10 minute interval between the scans. After the model was cleaned with a soft brush, the model was sprayed with Optispray (Sirona Dental Systems GmbH, Bensheim, Germany) according to the instructions of the manufacturer and 10 consecutive scans were performed with a 10 minute interval. All the scans of the different scanners were uploaded to the respective companies and returned after post-processing.

The physical model was cleaned with a soft brush and sent to Createch Medical (Mendaro, Spain) where it was scanned under strictly controlled conditions (temperature, humidity and vibrations) with a ultra-precision contact scanner with a precision of 0.1 μm (Leitz PMM 12106). The latter digital model formed the reference data set.

3D measurements

The distance and the angle between the centres of the high precision cylinders were used to assess the accuracy of the different scanners (Figure 5). For this each of the scans was imported in industrial reverse engineering software Rapidform (Rapidform, INUS Technology Inc, Seoul, Korea), where each of the cylinders was isolated as a separate object. Three 3D CAD models of the cylinders were subsequently imported and registered with each of the scanned equivalents. This was done to enable the proper construction of the centre-line of each cylinder.

To validate the precision of the registration algorithm a CAD cylinder, like the one used in the study, was imported in the Rapidform software. There it was duplicated and the second cylinder was subsequently moved to another location in the 3D space. The two cylinders were then registered and the difference between surfaces of the two cylinders was calculated by the software. As the cylinders are perfectly identical, the surfaces of the cylinders should ideally match perfectly. The experiment was repeated ten times and the mean of the registration error was calculated. The mean error of the registration procedure was 1.4 nm (+/−0.9 nm).

The distance between the centre-lines was measured in the software using a linear measurement tool. The angular deflection of the cylinders was measured with an angular measurement tool, using the cylinder at the location of the lower right molar as the baseline. The measurements were not broken down in x-, y- and z-components as the objects coordinate system could not properly be matched with a world coordinate system. As there is no true common coordinate system, the different models could only be registered in a virtual common coordinate system. As the registration is based on the surface of the models and as these will show minor errors, the positions of the models will differ slightly. This will introduce an error in their relative positions and makes it unreliable to compare measurements broken down in x-, y- and z-components. The measurements were noted in a table and compared to the same measurements made on the reference data set. A one-way ANOVA was performed to compare the differences between the 3 systems ($P<0.05$).

Results

The results are summarized in Table 1 and Table 2. The absolute distance errors ranged from 2,2 μm (Lava COS) to 287,5 μm (CEREC) (Figures 6 and 7). The mean of the distance errors of both the measured distances of the Lava COS, respectively 14,6 μm (95% confidence interval: 6,7 μm–22,4 μm) for the distance 1–2 and 23,5 μm (95% confidence interval: 14,7 μm–32,3 μm) for the distance 1–3. These values were the smallest compared to the CEREC and the iTero scanner. The confidence interval for the Lava COS was the smallest demon-

Table 2. Absolute errors in the angle between the cylinders in degrees.

	CEREC		iTero		Lava COS	
	ABS Error 1-2	ABS Error 1-3	ABS Error 1-2	ABS Error 1-3	ABS Error 1-2	ABS Error 1-3
MEAN	0,6303	0,4378	0,3451	0,4192	0,2049	0,4722
SD	0,5499	0,3211	0,3382	0,1667	0,0440	0,1436
CI (95%)	0,2894–0,9711	0,2388–0,6367	0,1355–0,5547	0,3159–0,5226	0,1776–0,2322	0,3831–0,5612

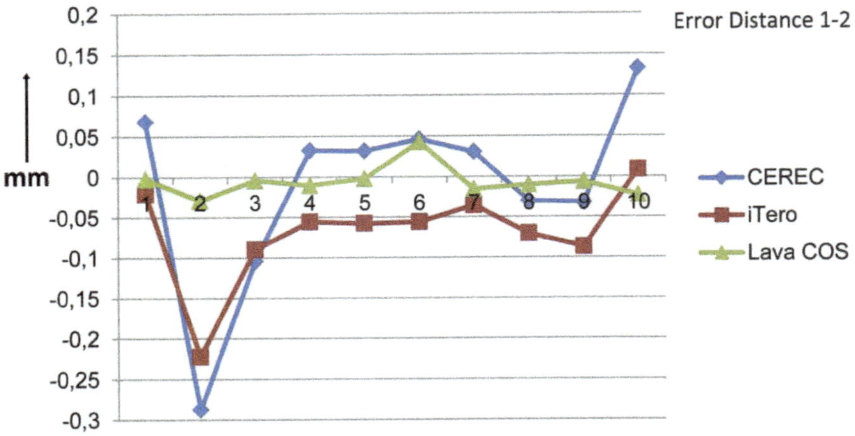

Figure 6. The distance errors between the cylinders 1 and 2 in millimeters for the three intra-oral scanners. The smallest distance error between cylinders 1 and 2 was −22,0 μm (Lava COS), while the largest error was −287,5 μm (CEREC). The Lava COS scanner showed the smallest mean distance error and also showed the smallest variations.

strating that the variations were the smallest. The distance errors of the CEREC were the largest, respectively 79,6 μm (95% confidence interval: 31,8 μm–127,4 μm) for the 1–2 distance and 81,6 μm (95% confidence interval: 49,1 μm–114,2 μm) for the 1–3 distance. All of the scanners had errors both in the positive and the negative range.

The angulation errors are shown in the figures 8 and 9. The mean of the absolute angulation errors ranged from 0,0061° (CEREC) to 1,8585° (CEREC). The mean absolute angulation errors for the cylinders 1–2 was the smallest for the Lava COS: 0,2049° (95% confidence interval: 0,1776°–0,2322°) and the largest for the CEREC: 0,6303° (95% confidence interval: 0,2894°–0,9711°). For the cylinders 1–3 the smallest mean absolute angulation error was provided by the iTero : 0,4192° (95% confidence interval: 0,3159°–0,5226°) and the largest by the Lava COS: 0,4722° (95% confidence interval: 0,3831°–0,5612°). The confidence interval for both the angulation errors 1–2 and 1–3 was the smallest for the Lava COS, indicating that the Lava COS had the smallest variations in its angulation errors. The CEREC had angulation errors in both the positive and negative range between the cylinders 1–2 and 1–3. The iTero showed a similar distribution for the angulation errors 1–2, but showed only negative values for the 1–3 measurements. The Lava COS was the only scanner that showed errors in the positive range for all measurements.

No statistical difference was found between the three groups.

Discussion

To our knowledge, this is the first study that compares three different intra-oral scanning technologies. The present study analysed the accuracy of three intra-oral scanners by determining the distance and angulation errors in vitro. The results show that the Lava COS has the smallest mean distance errors and the least variations in the measurements. In the angulation errors, the Lava COS showed the smallest mean error between cylinder 1–2 and the CEREC the largest mean error. The difference between the smallest and largest error was very small (0,4254°). Between

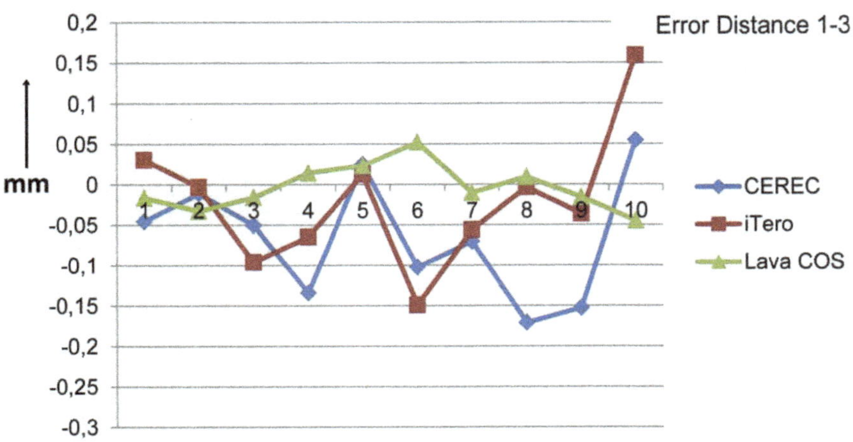

Figure 7. The distance errors between the cylinders 1 and 3 in millimeters for the three intra-oral scanners. The smallest distance error between cylinders 1 and 3 was −32,0 μm (iTero), while the largest error was −171,1 μm (CEREC). The Lava COS scanner showed the smallest mean distance error and also showed the smallest variations.

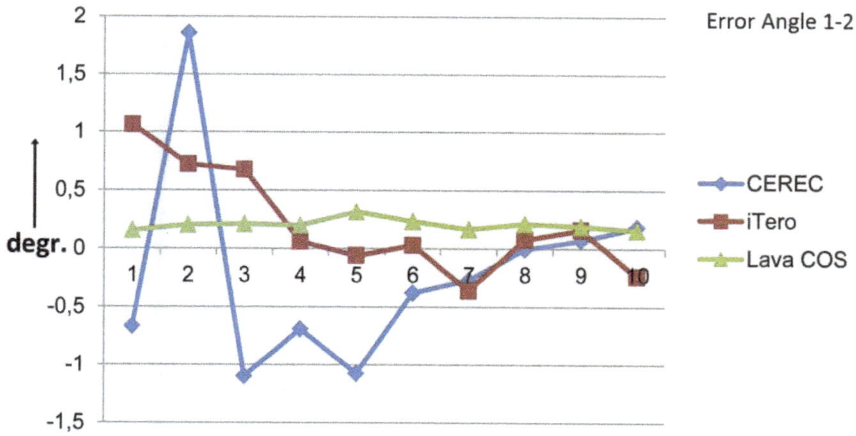

Figure 8. The angulation errors between the cylinders 1 and 2 in degrees for the three intra-oral scanners. The angulation errors were small and ranged from −0,0061° (CEREC) to 1,8585° (CEREC). The Lava COS showed the smallest mean angulation error and also the smallest variations. The Lava COS also showed only positive errors.

cylinders 1–3 the iTero showed the smallest mean error and the Lava COS the largest mean error. The difference between the smallest and the largest error was even smaller: 0,053°. The Lava COS had the smallest confidence interval in angular and linear measurements, indicating that this scanner has the lowest variation in its measurements. The Lava COS was also consistent in the angular errors as their range was small and all the values were positive. Only one other study has compared different intra-oral scanners. Ender and Mehl [19] have compared the Lava COS and the Cerec to determine which scanner is more accurate compared to the cast of an Impregum impression. In their study, the accuracy was defined by the terms "trueness": the deviation of the model with respect to the true size of the object, and "precision": the fluctuation of the different measurements. The "trueness" of the Lava COS was better than that of the CEREC and both were better than an Impregum impression. The "precision" of the CEREC was better than the Lava COS which was comparable to the Impregum impression. The high accuracy scanning protocol was not used in that study. Special software was used to superimpose datasets and the difference between the two models based on measuring points was calculated. This resulted in one value for the accuracy of the scanner.

The various scanners used in our study use different technologies to determine the spatial coordinates of the scanned object. Differences found between the three scanners may be related to measurement errors inherent to the technology employed. To improve the resolution of the 3D scan, CEREC has switched from white to blue light which has a shorter wavelength leading to a higher accuracy [18]. Apart from the differences in the technology of data acquisition, the CEREC and iTero scanners are point-and-click systems, while the Lava COS is a video system. This may explain both the similarities between the CEREC and iTero measurements and the differences with the results of the Lava COS. In the point-and-click systems, the 3D surfaces should be scanned with at least a one-third overlap of the adjoining surface. The registration of the neighbouring surfaces will occur on the basis of this overlap. In the video system with a frame rate of 20 images per second, the overlap of the images will most likely be larger than the aforementioned one-third which could lead to a better surface registration. Differences in the results may also occur

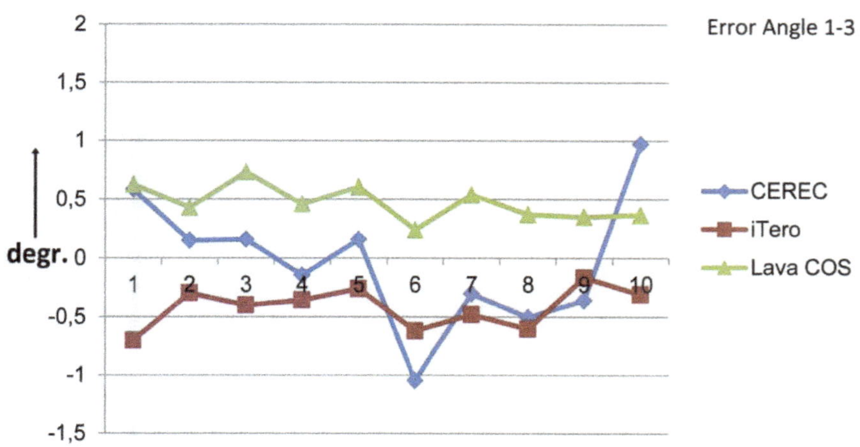

Figure 9. The angulation errors between the cylinders 1 and 3 in degrees for the three intra-oral scanners. The angulation errors were small and ranged from −0,1447° (CEREC) to 1,0456° (CEREC). The iTero showed the smallest mean angulation error. The Lava COS showed the smallest variations. The Lava COS showed only positive errors, while the iTero showed only negative errors. Only the Lava COS showed consistent positive errors in all cases, this could be regarded as an offset which may be compensated.

due to the registration of the 3D images and in the rest of the post-processing procedure. The Lava COS uses powder particles as markers as an extra toolfor the computer to join the different pieces of the 3D model. How the registration takes place and what algorithms are used in the different scanners is not shared knowledge. But algorithms that involve registration based on surface overlap are most likely. As registration errors, however minute, will always occur in registration procedures [26], one expects an additive effect of these errors over the length of the arch. When comparing intra-oral scanners in full arch impression procedures, it would be interesting to involve the influence of the length of the span to assess the expected additive effect of the registration errors that may occur. The aforementioned effect could be observed in our experiments for the CEREC and the Lava COS when considering the distance accuracy and for the iTero and the Lava COS when considering the angular accuracy. The differences however were very small and statistically not significant. Mehl et al found a decreasing accuracy when comparing single tooth images to quadrant images for the CEREC Bluecam intra-oral scanner [18] which could be explained by an accumulation of registration errors. In the study of Ender and Mehl [19] an increase in the deviations between the models in certain areas were noted, but these can be explained by the registration procedure. The algorithm most likely tried to register the surfaces in such a way that the overall mean deviation between the surfaces is the smallest and this may conceal an increase in deviations between the surfaces and makes interpretation of deviations difficult. A best fit algorithm on basis only of the area where the scanning was started may have shown a possible increase in deviations in their study.

In the study of Ender and Mehl [19] a mean "trueness" of 49±14.2 μm was found for the CEREC and 40.3±14.1 μm for the Lava COS. The difference from our data is most likely resulting from a different research model in their study and a high accuracy scanning protocol for the Lava COS in our study. In their study a 3D comparison was made between the models, where the computer calculates the difference between the surface points of the models. These measurements are usually expressed in a mean value for the error between the surfaces. In our study the linear and angular measurements were made as the accuracy of the distance and the angulation between implants can show the error that will be introduced at the inlet of a digital workflow. Other methods, like the aforementioned 3D comparison of digital models, will also generate a number that will generally reflect the accuracy of a model. However this number will not express the exact error between implant positions nor will it show errors in angulation that may occur or a possible increase in the distance and angular errors over distance.

In future studies other video-scanners should be involved as we have compared two point-and-click systems (CEREC and iTero) with one video system (Lava COS) in the present study. Differences in outcome could be explained with differences between the technologies as explained above. The amount of cylinders on the model should be increase to gain a better insight in possible increase in deviations over the length of the span. The number scans may be increased to increase the reliability of the study. Also a comparison with a traditional impression material, like Impregum, should be added to enable a comparison with the traditional workflow. A comparison between the normal scanning protocol and the high accuracy scanning protocol should also be included.

Conclusions

1. The Lava COS in combination with a high accuracy scanning protocol resulted in the smallest and most consistent errors of all three scanners tested when considering mean distance errors in full arch impressions for both measured distances.
2. For the mean angulation errors of the three scanners tested, the Lava COS had smallest errors between cylinder 1–2 and the largest errors between cylinder 1–3, although the absolute difference with the best mean value (iTero) was very small (0,0529°).
3. In the Lava COS the angulation errors were very consistent with a small confidence interval value.
4. An expected increase in distance and/or angular errors over the length of the arch due to an accumulation of registration errors of the patched 3D surfaces could be observed in this study design, but the effects were statistically not significant.

Clinical relevance

For making impressions of implant cases for digital workflows, the most accurate scanner with the scanning protocol that will ensure the most accurate digital impression should be used. In our study model that was the Lava COS with the high accuracy scanning protocol.

Acknowledgments

The authors thank Createch Medical for producing the scanning abutments and making the ultra-precision scanner and software available for us to collect the data used in this study.

Author Contributions

Conceived and designed the experiments: WJM YR DW. Performed the experiments: WJM FA. Analyzed the data: WJM YR. Contributed reagents/materials/analysis tools: WJM YR DW. Wrote the paper: WJM YR DW FA.

References

1. Johnson GH, Craig RG (1985) Accuracy of four types of rubber impression materials compared with time of pour and a repeat pour of models. J Prosthet Dent 53: 484–490.
2. Millstein PL (1992) Determining the accuracy of gypsum casts made from type IV dental stone. J Oral Rehabil 19: 239–243.
3. Sahin S, Çehreli MC (2001) The significance of passive framework fit in implant prosthodontics: current status. Implant Dent 10: 85–92.
4. Kim Y, Oh TJ, Misch CE, Wang HL (2005) Occlusal considerations in implant therapy: clinical guidelines with biomechanical rationale. Clin Oral Implants Res 16: 26–35.
5. Sahin S, Cehreli M, Yalcin E (2002) The influence of functional forces on the biomechanics of implant-supported prostheses— A review J Dent 30: 271–282.
6. Wang T, Leu L, Wang J, Lin L (2002) Effects of prosthesis materials and prosthesis splinting on peri-implant bone stress around implants in poor-quality bone: A numeric analysis. Int J Oral Maxillofac Implants 17: 231–237.
7. Sones AD (1989) Complications with osseointegrated implants. J Prosthet Dent 62: 581–585.
8. Kunavisarut C, Lang L, Stoner B, Felton D (2002) Finite element analysis on dental-implant supported prostheses without passive fit. J Prosthodont 11: 30–40.
9. Brånemark P (1983) Osseointegration and its experimental background. J Prosthet Dent 50: 399–410.
10. Ongül D, Gökçen-Röhlig B, Sermet B, Keskin H (2012). A comparative analysis of the accuracy of different direct impression techniques for multiple implants. Aust Dent J 57: 184–189.
11. Abduo J, Bennani V, Waddell N, Lyons K, Swain M(2010) Assessing the fit of implant fixed prostheses: a critical review. Int J Oral Maxillofac Implants 25: 506–515.

12. Karl M, Rosch S, Graef F, Taylor T, Heckman S (2005) Strain situation after fixation of 3-unit ceramic veneered implant superstructures. Implant Dent 14:157–165.
13. Del'Acqua M, Arioli-Filho J, Compagnoni M, Mollo F (2008) Accuracy of impression and pouring techniques for an implantsupported prosthesis. Int J Oral Maxillofac Implants 23: 226–236.
14. Caputi S, Varvara G (2008) Dimensional accuracy of resultant casts made by a monophase, one-step and two-step, and a novel two-step putty/light-body impression technique: an in vitro study. J Prosthet Dent 99: 274–281.
15. Franco EB, da Cunha LF, Herrera FS, Benetti AR (2011) Accuracy of Single-Step versus 2-Step Double-Mix Impression Technique. ISRN Dent 2011 : 341546. Epub 2011 Jul 25.
16. Kang AH, Johnson GH, Lepe X, Wataha JC (2009) Accuracy of a reformulated fast-set vinyl polysiloxane impression material using dual-arch trays. J Prosthet Dent 101: 332–341.
17. Luthardt RG, Loos R, Quaas S (2005) Accuracy of intraoral data acquisition in comparison to the conventional impression. Int J Comput Dent 8: 283–294.
18. Mehl A, Ender A, Mormann W, Attin T (2009) Accuracy testing of a new intraoral 3D camera. Int J Comput Dent 12: 11–28.
19. Ender A, Mehl A (2011) Full arch scans: conventional versus digital impressions-an in vitro study. Int J Comput Dent 14: 11–21.
20. Besl PJ, McKay ND (1992) A method for registration of 3-D shapes. IEEE Transactions on Pattern Analysis and Machine Intelligence, 14:239–256.
21. Chen Y, Medioni G (1992). Object modeling by registration of multiple range images. Image and Vision Computing, 14(2):145–155.
22. Park J, DeSouza GN (2005) 3-D Modeling of Real-World Objects Using Range and Intensity Images. In: Apolloni B, Ghosh A, Alpaslan F, Jain LC, Patnaik S, editors. Machine Learning and Robot Perception. Heidelberg: Springer Berlin. pp. 203–264.
23. Schenk O (2009) The new acquisition unit Cerec AC. Int J Comput Dent 12: 41–46.
24. Kachalia PR, Geissberger MJ (2010) Dentistry a la carte: in-office CAD/CAM technology. J Calif Dent Assoc 38: 323–330.
25. Syrek A, Reich G, Ranftl D, Klein C, Cerny B, et al (2010) Clinical evaluation of all-ceramic crowns fabricated from intraoral digital impressions based on the principle of active wavefront sampling. J Dent 38: 553–559.
26. Maintz JB, Viergever MA (1998) A survey of medical image registration. Med Image Anal 2:1–36.

14

Serum Antibodies to *Porphyromonas gingivalis* Chaperone HtpG Predict Health in Periodontitis Susceptible Patients

Charles E. Shelburne[1]*, P. Sandra Shelburne[1], Vishnu M. Dhople[1¤], Domenica G. Sweier[2], William V. Giannobile[3], Janet S. Kinney[3], Wilson A. Coulter[4], Brian H. Mullally[4], Dennis E. Lopatin[1]

1 Department of Biologic and Materials Sciences, The University of Michigan School of Dentistry, Ann Arbor, Michigan, United States of America, **2** Department of Cariology, Restorative Sciences and Endodontics, The University of Michigan School of Dentistry, Ann Arbor, Michigan, United States of America, **3** Department of Periodontics and Oral Medicine and The Michigan Center for Oral Health Research, The University of Michigan School of Dentistry, Ann Arbor, Michigan, United States of America, **4** Centre for Oral Research, Queen's University, Belfast, Northern Ireland

Abstract

Background: Chaperones are ubiquitous conserved proteins critical in stabilization of new proteins, repair/removal of defective proteins and immunodominant antigens in innate and adaptive immunity. Periodontal disease is a chronic inflammatory infection associated with infection by *Porphyromonas gingivalis* that culminates in the destruction of the supporting structures of the teeth. We previously reported studies of serum antibodies reactive with the human chaperone Hsp90 in gingivitis, a reversible form of gingival disease confined to the oral soft tissues. In those studies, antibodies were at their highest levels in subjects with the best oral health. We hypothesized that antibodies to the HSP90 homologue of *P. gingivalis* (HtpG) might be associated with protection/resistance against destructive periodontitis.

Methodology/Principal Findings: ELISA assays using cloned HtpG and peptide antigens confirmed gingivitis subjects colonized with *P. gingivalis* had higher serum levels of anti-HtpG and, concomitantly, lower levels of attachment loss. Additionally, serum antibody levels to *P. gingivalis* HtpG protein were higher in healthy subjects compared to patients with either chronic or aggressive periodontitis. We found a negative association between tooth attachment loss and anti-*P. gingivalis* HtpG ($p = 0.043$) but not anti-*Fusobacterium nucleatum* (an oral opportunistic commensal) HtpG levels. Furthermore, response to periodontal therapy was more successful in subjects having higher levels of anti-*P. gingivalis* HtpG before treatment ($p = 0.018$). There was no similar relationship to anti-*F. nucleatum* HtpG levels. Similar results were obtained when these experiments were repeated with a synthetic peptide of a region of *P. gingivalis* HtpG.

Conclusions/Significance: Our results suggest: 1) anti-*P. gingivalis* HtpG antibodies are protective and therefore predict health periodontitis-susceptable patients; 2) may augment the host defence to periodontitis and 3) a unique peptide of *P. gingivalis* HtpG offers significant potential as an effective diagnostic target and vaccine candidate. These results are compatible with a novel immune control mechanism unrelated to direct binding of bacteria.

Editor: Debbie Fox, The Research Institute for Children at Children's Hospital New Orleans, United States of America

Funding: Supported by NIH/NIDCR DE11117 (DEL) and patient sample collections were supported by NIH grants NIH/NIDCR U01-DE-14961 and NIH/NCRR M01-RR000042 (WVG). The sponsors of this work had no role in the design and conduct of the study, in the collection, analysis, and interpretation of the data and in the preparation, review, or approval of the manuscript.

Competing Interests: The authors have declared that no competing interests exist.

* E-mail: ceshelbu@umich.edu

¤ Current address: The Centre for Cellular and Molecular Biology, Hyderabad, India

Introduction

Porphyromonas gingivalis is a gram negative obligate anaerobe that has a major etiological role in human periodontitis. The bacterium is found with high frequency in persons with periodontitis where it participates in the initiation and establishment of chronic, infectious biofilms [1,2]. These biofilms facilitate the long term survival of *P. gingivalis* and induces an inflammatory reaction that is responsible for the destruction of the hard and soft tissue supporting structures of the teeth. In addition *P. gingivalis* can invade and persist in the cells of the gingival tissue[3]. It also can escape the oral cavity and has been found in atherosclerotic plaque where it may have a role in the pathophysiology of cardiovascular disease [4].

P. gingivalis produces a number of chaperones as essential tools in normal cellular processes and in response to environmental stresses [5]. In addition, the role of chaperones, like the *P. gingivalis* HSP90 homologue HtpG, in immune response dynamics has become an area of intense investigation because immunomodulation by chaperones has been demonstrated [6,7]. HtpG, like most chaperones tested [8], induces a strong humoral response that may have consequences in the pathogenesis of periodontitis [9]. These functions are important in the establishment and perpetuation of chronic inflammatory diseases.

Recent studies have shown that antibodies to periodontal disease associated pathogens may have protective effects although the exact mechanism is still unclear. Rams et al [10] demonstrated that serum levels of IgG antibodies against *A. actinomycetemcomitans* or *P. gingivalis* in periodontitis-stable patients were higher than those in patients with active periodontitis suggesting that these antibodies have a protective effect against periodontal infections. Yamasaki et al have shown that antibodies to *P. gingivalis* Hsp60 homologue increases with successful treatment [11]. We have recently described experiments that indicate that antibodies to HtpG may mitigate some of the induction of inflammatory chemokines through TLR4 and CD91 [12], a receptor expressed in human atherosclerotic lesions [13]. Taken together, these findings suggest a role for antibodies to *P. gingivalis* chaperones in both periodontal and cardiovascular disease.

The possible protective role of antibodies to chaperones in periodontitis is controversial. It has been suggested that these antibodies simply reflected the high level of homology between human and bacterial proteins, a hallmark of these evolutionarily conserved molecules [14]. Other results suggest that the conserved nature of the chaperones might lead to autoimmune phenomenon due to "immune mimicry". Earlier results from this laboratory suggested that high levels of anti-Hsp90 antibodies could have protective qualities [9]. However, that study utilized a group of individuals with minimal periodontal disease. Here we describe findings from a study of periodontitis subjects with more extensive disease that are similar to those reported earlier and support the notion of a protective role for anti-HtpG antibodies in untreated subjects. In addition, these studies suggest that the levels of these antibodies also may predict the response to treatment. These results may also reflect an immune control mechanism in chronic infections unrelated to direct binding of bacteria.

Results

Colonization of plaque by *P. gingivalis* and *F. nucleatum*

Initially we reported [9] that in gingivitis subjects probing depth and the levels of *P. gingivalis* were both associated with serum anti-Hsp90 antibody levels. Subjects from the gingivitis group were tested for the presence of *P. gingivalis* by slot immunoblot; 82 % of the subjects were positive for *P. gingivalis* [15,16]. Genomic DNA of pooled plaque samples from all teeth for each subject in the CP and AP groups were tested; 71% of the healthy subjects and 86% of individuals with periodontitis were positive for *P. gingivalis* 16S rRNA genes by PCR. The low end sensitivity of the assay was between 10 and 100 bacterial cells per sample. The mean percentage of *P. gingivalis* was 0.11 and 0.98 ($p<0.001$, *t*-test) in the controls and periodontitis subjects respectively. Both CP groups were 96% positive for *F. nucleatum*; the mean percentage of *F. nucleatum* was 2.77 and 3.78 ($p=0.07$; *t*-test) in the controls and periodontitis subjects respectively (Table 1). Plaque samples from the normal controls for the AP group were not available for *F. nucleatum* testing and as reported previously 17% of the AP subjects were positive for *P. gingivalis* 16S rRNA [17].

Antibodies to *P. gingivalis* and *F. nucleatum* total cell lysates

The level of antibodies to total cell lysates of *P. gingivalis* and *F. nucleatum* was determined as a measure of the long term colonization experience that each subject had with these bacteria. These two bacteria have different roles in periodontitis, *P. gingivalis* as a pathogen while *F. nucleatum* is an opportunistic commensal in the subgingival biofilm. Anti-*P. gingivalis* antibodies were detected in 38 of 45 samples obtained from gingivitis subjects. All CP and AP subjects had levels of anti-*P. gingivalis* and anti-*F. nucleatum* more than 3 standard deviations above the background of the assay. In the CP group there was a statistically significant elevated levels of antibodies to *P. gingivalis* ($p=0.01$, *t*-test) and *F. nucleatum* ($p=0.02$, *t*-test) in the diseased subjects compared to the control group; there was no difference between levels of antibody to total *P. gingivalis* in the AP group (Table 2). Similar results were found in CP subjects that were colonized by *P. gingivalis* (Table 3) and CP subjects not colonized by *P. gingivalis* (Table 4) at the time the serum samples were obtained. These results suggest that most subjects in the study were likely to have been colonized with *P. gingivalis* prior to their participation in this study.

Total IgG Antibodies to *P. gingivalis* HtpG and *F. nucleatum* HtpG

Levels of IgG-class antibodies that specifically reacted with recombinant HtpG proteins of *P. gingivalis* and *F. nucleatum were* measured. Anti-HtpG antibody levels were measured in gingivitis subjects; subjects with more CAL (more tissue loss) had lower levels of anti-*P. gingivalis* HtpG.

In the CP subjects we hypothesized that the pattern of anti-HtpG would be different for the two bacteria. However, there was a trend, both in CP individuals colonized (Table 3) or uncolonized (Table 4) by *P. gingivalis*, to higher antibody levels to HtpG from both species in healthy subjects than in subjects with disease even though this trend did not reach statistical significance.

There were substantial and significant differences between the healthy and diseased AP subjects in all the variables tested. The three clinical measurements were all significantly higher in the

Table 1. Research Subject Demographics

Group (n)	*Gingvitis (50)*	*CP-Healthy (49)*	*CP-Diseased (50)*	*AP-Healthy (21)*	*AP-Diseased (24)*
% Female	58	54	58	62	68
Age Range in years (mean)	18-66 (31.6)	20-78(43.0)	30-77(51.3)	18-35 (34.4)	22-40(32.0)
Attachment Loss (mm, mean±SD)	1.56±0.70	0.68±0.52	2.24±1.07	0.72±0.52	3.25±0.63
Probing Depth (mm, mean±SD)	2.64±0.54	1.60±0.21	2.60±0.71	1.50±0.22	2.83±1.32
Bleeding on Probing (%, mean±SD)	ND	0.24±0.12	0.57±0.17	0.13±0.06	0.33±0.16
Gingival Index (%, mean±SD)	0.2±0.17	0.18±0.19	0.52±0.23	ND	ND

ND–not determined

Table 2. Antibody responses to *P. gingivalis* and *F. nucleatum* in subjects.

Group (n)	*Gingivitis (50)*	*CP-Healthy (49)*	*CP-Diseased (50)*	*AP-Healthy (21)*	*AP-Diseased (24)*
% positive for *P. gingivalis*	82	71	86	ND	17
% positive for *F. nucleatum*	ND	96	96	ND	ND
Antibody to total *P. gingivalis* (Log mean ELISA Units±S.D.)	4.39±0.17	3.68±0.23	3.92±0.26	4.47±0 .07	4.39±0.15
Antibody to total *F. nucleatum* (Log mean ELISA Units±S.D.)	ND	3.95±0.62	4.86±0.81	ND	ND

ND–not determined

Table 3. Serum antibody (IgGγ) levels to bacterial antigens in CP subjects colonized by *P. gingivalis.*

	ELISA Units			
	Health (mean)	**Disease (mean)**	**p-value (*t*-test)**	**Valid N (Health/ Disease)**
Anti-*P.gingivalis* HtpG	10,200	9,882	NS	35/41
Anti-*F.nucleatum* HtpG	19,959	19,817	NS	35/38
Anti-*P.gingivalis* HtpG p18	7,138	6,254	0.047	35/40
Anti-*P.gingivalis* W83	5,654	10,076	0.002	35/40
Anti-*F.nucleatum* 22586	27,735	13,701	0.009	35/41

NS-not significant

Table 4. Serum antibody (IgGγ) levels to bacterial antigens in CP subjects not colonized by *P. gingivalis.*

	ELISA Units		**p-value (*t*-test)**	**Valid N (Health/ Disease)**
	Health (mean)	**Disease (mean)**		
Anti-*P.gingivalis* HtpG	9,224	8,594	NS	13/6
Anti-*F.nucleatum* HtpG	19,818	15876	NS	13/7
Anti-*P.gingivalis* HtpG p18	6,812	6,477	NS	13/7
Anti-*P.gingivalis* W83	5,347	11,008	0.002	13/7
Anti-*F.nucleatum* 22586	17,917	8,473	0.009	13/7

NS-not significant

diseased groups (Table 5) while the anti-HtpG levels were significantly lower in the diseased subjects ($p<0.002$, ANOVA).

Antibodies to *P. gingivalis* HtpG peptide p18

Previous studies [18] suggested that a peptide antigen, p18, of the HtpG molecule was responsible for eliciting the apparent protective effect found in the serum of healthy subjects. Therefore the serum response to a synthetic peptide antigen of this region was investigated in the CP and AP subjects. We expected that the levels of antibody to the peptide would be higher in control subjects compared to periodontitis subjects of both groups and that elimination of the majority of the epitopes in the HtpG molecules, most of which are highly conserved between bacterial species, would clarify the trend observed using the whole HtpG proteins as ELISA target antigens. As expected, subjects in both the CP (Table 3 & 4) and AP (Table 5) groups diagnosed with periodontitis had lower levels of anti-p18 than their respective control groups. Although the same trend was observed in both colonized and un-colonized individuals using the HtpG molecule only the differences in p18 antibody levels in CP subjects colonized by *P. gingivalis* reached statistical significance (Table 3 & 4).

Cluster Analysis by Disease Subgroups

There were trends supporting our hypothesis when the results of the assays were compared between groups as they were recruited into the studies, basically health or disease status. However, examination of those groupings showed that there was overlap between the groups based on clinical measures, especially in the CP subjects, the most complete study. Therefore the subjects were regrouped in line with their clinical measures by K-means clustering, irrespective of recruitment groups. The clusters were used as a basis for ANOVA analysis of differences in the clinical measures and antibody levels.

Gingivitis subjects were regrouped into three clusters and differences in four clinical measures (PD, CAL, GI, PL) and two antibody levels (anti-*P. gingivalis* HtpG, anti-P. gingivalis whole cell lysate) sought. Cluster 1 had the greatest PD and CAL; there were significant differences between the clusters for PD and CAL. Antibody levels against *P. gingivalis* HtpG were lowest in the subjects with the highest disease measures, similar to earlier findings [9] for human Hsp90, but did not reach statistical significance (Table 6).

CP Subjects were regrouped into 4 clusters and differences sought in four clinical measures (PD, CAL, BOP, GI) and three antibody levels (anti-*P. gingivalis* HtpG, anti-Fn HtpG and anti-Pg p18). There were significant differences between the groups in all clinical measures (Table 7). Cluster 2 had the highest levels of all clinical measures and the lowest levels of anti-*P. gingivalis* HtpG and anti-*P. gingivalis* HtpG p18, the latter being significant ($p = 0.00056$, ANOVA).

AP subjects were regrouped into 3 clusters and differences sought in three clinical measures (PD, CAL, BOP) and three antibody levels (anti-Pg whole bacteria, anti-*P. gingivalis* HtpG and anti-Pg P18). There were significant differences in all the clinical measures between groups and in anti-*P. gingivalis* HtpG and anti-*P. gingivalis* HtpG p18, but not anti-Pg whole bacteria (Table 8). Cluster 2 had the highest levels of clinical measures and lowest levels of anti-*P. gingivalis* HtpG p18. Both clusters 1 and 2 had substantially lower levels of anti-*P. gingivalis* HtpG compared to cluster 3.

Table 5. Serum antibody (IgGγ) levels to bacterial antigens in AP subjects.

	Health (mean±S.D)	*Disease (mean±S.D.)*	*p-value (ANOVA)*	*Valid N*
PD (mm)	1.51±0.22	3.31±0.67	<0.002	45
AL (mm)	0.719±0.52	2.85±1.45	<0.002	45
BOP (%)	0.125±0.07	0.29±0.17	<0.002	45
Log anti-p18	4.11±0.27	3.97±0.16	0.041	45
Log anti-HtpG	4.25±0.04	3.96±0.13	<0.002	45
Log anti-W83 cells	4.47±0.07	4.39±0.15	0.032	45

Table 6. Analysis of clustered subjects in the Gingivitis group.

	Cluster 1	*Cluster 2*	*Cluster 3*	*p*-value (ANOVA)
	Mild perio. n = 22	**Gingivitis n = 10**	**Healthy n = 18**	
PD	3.1±0.2	2.8±0.4	2.05±0.2	<0.001
AL	2.2±0.6	1.0±0.0	1.11±0.3	<0.001
GI	27.3±5.5	30.0±4.8	5.5±2.7	NS
PI	45.5±5.9	8.0±6.3	27.8±4.6	NS
Anti-*P. gingivalis* HtpG	9825±4720	14973±10178	12676±6928	NS
Anti-P. gingivalis W83	3100±6898	1301±177	7488±11008	NS

NS–not significant
Subjects were clustered by K-means clustering and differences sought in means (±S.D.) of variables by ANOVA. PD and AL measured in mm; GI is the % sites with gingival redness; PI values are % sites with accumulated plaque. Antibody values are expressed in ELISA units.

Table 7. Cluster analysis of CP subjects.

	Cluster 1	*Cluster 2*	*Cluster 3*	*Cluster 4*	*p*-value (ANOVA)
	Moderate CP n = 31	**Severe CP n = 10**	**Gingivitis n = 29**	**Healthy n = 27**	
PD	2.4±0.4	3.6±0.8	1.7±0.2	1.6±0.2	<0.001
AL	1.9±0.1	4.0±0.9	1.2±0.3	0.3±0.2	<0.001
BOP	56.8±16.2	68.4±16.6	27.7±.12.7	24.6±14.6	<0.001
GI	54.3±21.1	60.6±24.6	20.2±17.9	21.4±21.0	<0.001
Anti-*P. gingivalis* HtpG	10531±4791	7877±3906	9311±3833	10358±4443	NS
Anti-F. *nucleatum* HtpG	20053±806	18530±9346	18231±5752	20748±6540	NS
Anti-*P. gingivalis* HtpG p18	6485±1920	4793±2120	7171±1782	6957±1068	0.006

NS–not significant
Subjects were clustered by K-means clustering and differences sought in means (±S.D.) of variables by ANOVA. PD and AL measured in mm; GI is the % sites with gingival redness. Antibody values are expressed in ELISA units.

Correlation of Anti-*P. gingivalis* HtpG antibodies to clinical measures in Chronic and Aggressive Periodontitis

The supposition that antibodies to *P. gingivalis* HtpG may be protective is based on the hypothesis that high levels of antibodies should be found in subjects exhibiting healthier clinical signs and lower levels in subjects exhibiting more periodontitis related damage. Clinical measurements from each site in all the subjects were obtained and the average value determined for each subject. Relationships between those measurements and the levels of *P. gingivalis* and *F. nucleatum* anti-HtpG were sought using Pearson's R to compare baseline antibody levels in both AP and CP groups with the clinical signs obtained at the baseline were compared. When anti-*P. gingivalis* HtpG levels from CP subjects were analyzed with four clinical measurements in each of the same patients there was a trend for pocket depth and attachment loss measurements to inversely correlate with antibody levels, but the correlations were small and not statistically significant. Similar results were found with anti-*F. nucleatum* HtpG values. However, in the AP subjects there were substantial negative associations three

Table 8. Cluster analysis of AP subjects.

	Cluster 1	*Cluster 2*	*Cluster 3*	*p-value (ANOVA)*
	Localized AP n = 11	**Generalized AP n = 12**	**Healthy n = 21**	
PD	3.0±0.6	3.6±0.7	1.5±0.2	<0.001
AL	2.2±1.2	3.4±1.5	0.7±0.5	<0.001
BOP	21.4±11.2	37.9±18.1	12.5±5.7	<0.001
Anti-P. gingivalis HtpG p18	10182±2437	8371±2114	12390±5318	0.0283
Anti-*P. gingivalis* HtpG	8853±2493	10165±3479	17742±1349	<0.001
Anti-P. gingivalis W83	26899±9509	26040±12191	30041±4977	NS

NS–not significant
Subjects were clustered by K-means clustering and differences sought in means (±S.D.) of variables by ANOVA. PD and AL measured in mm; BOP is the % sites bleeding on probing. Antibody values are expressed in ELISA units. NS–not significant.

clinical measurements and anti-HtpG levels, all of which were statistically significant (Table 9). Similar experiments using HtpG cloned from *F. nucleatum* gave no significant correlations to the clinical signs (data not shown).

Correlation of Anti-*P. gingivalis* HtpG p18 antibodies to clinical measures in Chronic and Aggressive Periodontitis

We then sought relationships between the same measurements and the levels of *P. gingivalis* anti-HtpG p18 by comparing antibody levels in both AP and CP groups with the clinical measurement using Pearson's R analysis. Sera from the CP group and controls showed that levels of anti-p18 were significantly ($p = 0.047$) inversely correlated to CAL but not correlated to the other indices. In the AP group antibodies to p18 were significantly inversely correlated to PD ($p = 0.008$), CAL ($p = 0.018$) and BOP ($p = 0.046$), Table 10. Lastly, associations were sought between changes in clinical measurements 6 months after SRP treatment and the anti-p18 levels 6 months before treatment to determine if they might predict treatment success or failure. There was a significant positive correlation ($p = 0.05$) between the pre-treatment levels of anti-HtpG p18 and reduction in CAL.

Discussion

Chaperones are simultaneously highly conserved and immunodominant antigens which may have important roles in the pathogenesis of numerous human diseases. Although a subject of intense investigation, the role of the immune response to chaperones in human disease is currently not well understood. Periodontal diseases present a unique opportunity to examine the

Table 9. Correlation of Anti-*P. gingivalis* HtpG antibody levels with clinical measurements.

		A. Pretreatment				*B. Post-treatment*			
		Anti-*P. gingivalis* HtpG		**Anti-*F. nucleatum* HtpG**		**Anti-*P. gingivalis* HtpG**		**Anti-*F. nucleatum* HtpG**	
		Pearson's R	***p*-value**	**Pearson's R**	***p*-value**	**Pearson's R**	***p*-value**	**Pearson's R**	***p*-value**
Gingivitis									
	PD	−0.111	0.440						
	AL	−0.341	0.012						
	GI	−0.101	0.483						
	PI	−0.130	0.367						
CP									
	PD	−0.050	NS	−0.019	NS	0.361	0.002	0.076	NS
	AL	−0.108	NS	−0.113	NS	0.273	0.020	0.144	NS
	BOP	0.144	NS	0.057	NS	0.381	0.001	0.113	NS
	GI	0.093	NS	0.001	NS	0.263	0.026	0.140	NS
AP									
	PD	−0.787	<0.001	ND					
	AL	−0.628	<0.001	ND					
	BOP	−0.388	<0.01	ND					

NS–not significant
ND–not determined

Table 10. Correlation of Anti-*P. gingivalis* HtpG p18 antibody levels with clinical measurements.

		Pre-treatment		Post-treatment	
		Anti-*P. gingivalis* HtpG *p18*		Anti-*P. gingivalis* HtpG *p18*	
		Pearson's R	*p*-value	Pearson's R	*p*-value
Gingivitis					
	PD	−0.135	NS		
	AL	0.066	NS		
	GI	−0.081	NS		
	PI	0.136	NS		
CP					
	PD	−0.063	NS	0.072	NS
	AL	−0.204	0.047	0.153	NS
	BOP	−0.100	NS	−0.119	NS
	GI	−0.111	NS	−0.084	NS
AP					
	PD	−0.393	0.008		
	AL	−0.361	0.015		
	BOP	−0.298	0.046		

NS–not significant

immune response to chaperones in a distinctive and readily accessible human environment. A few reports of antibody levels to *P. gingivalis* chaperones (particularly GroEL) have been published but this is the first comprehensive analysis of anti-*P. gingivalis* HtpG in multiple periodontal disease states. Results reported here and earlier [9,12] suggest that anti-*P. gingivalis* HtpG antibodies predict health in patients susceptible to periodontal disease and are protective in the untreated periodontal disease patient. These results may also reflect a previously uncharacterized immune control mechanism unrelated to direct binding of bacteria. Further, these antibodies may augment periodontitis treatment and *P. gingivalis* HtpG might be an attractive vaccine candidate. These results appear to be unique to *P. gingivalis* as they are directed at a segment of HtpG unique to *P. gingivalis*; parallel experiments with the HtpG homologue of *F. nucleatum* did not manifest these same qualities. In addition, there is reason to believe that these results may be extended to other chronic infectious diseases.

Earlier studies of a population of subjects with minimal periodontal disease suggested that antibodies to human Hsp90 related chaperones might have a protective effect. This report expands on that notion by examining the response of periodontitis subjects to the Hsp90 homologue in *P. gingivalis*, HtpG. In gingivitis subjects as a whole it was found that there was a distinctive, but not statistically significant, trend in support of the hypothesis. Interestingly, when anti-*P. gingivalis* HtpG levels and clinical measures are compared on an individual basis there is a discernable correlation with CAL. At the opposite end of the periodontitis disease spectrum, the AP subjects, there is considerable support for the hypothesis. At the group level, there are substantial and significant differences between both anti-*P. gingivalis* HtpG and anti-*P. gingivalis* HtpG p18 between clusters based on clinical measures, but no differences in the response to the whole bacterium. On an individual basis, both anti-*P. gingivalis* HtpG and anti-*P. gingivalis* HtpG p18 are inversely and significantly correlated to the clinical measures.

Support of the hypothesis was somewhat tenuous in the initial examination of the CP subjects. Those recruited as either healthy or with CP and colonized by *P. gingivalis* possessed a humoral response to *Pg* HtpG p18 higher in subject groups with less periodontal destruction and inversely related to the level of attachment loss ($p<0.05$). A similar relationship was not found in un-colonized individuals. This was the opposite of antibody levels to the whole bacterium which were significantly higher is subjects with disease than controls ($p\leq0.01$), a finding reported by many other laboratories. Similar trends were found when we examined the humoral response to HtpG from *F. nucleatum* but there was no relationship to disease status. In addition, correlations between the same antibodies and clinical measures when considered in the context of individual subjects were not found, except for a correlation between ant-*P. gingivalis* HtpG p18 and CAL ($R=-0.205$, $p<0.05$). This dilemma was resolved when the subjects were clustered by clinical measures. In a cluster of 10 subjects with the most severe disease there was a substantial and significantly lower level of anti-*P. gingivalis* HtpG and anti-*P. gingivalis* HtpG p18 compared to the other clusters in the CP subjects. As might be expected, the clinical measures of these subjects resemble those of the AP subjects. In summary, there is a trend for both anti-*P. gingivalis* HtpG and anti-*P. gingivalis* HtpG p18 to be lower in subjects with the more serious disease in each of the 3 periodontal disease groups. Neither trend reaches statistical significance in the gingivitis group. In the CP group anti-*P. gingivalis* HtpG p18 is significantly lower in the most diseased cluster; anti-*P. gingivalis* HtpG trends in the same direction but does not reach statistical significance. In the AP group both anti-*P. gingivalis* HtpG and anti-*P. gingivalis* HtpG p18 are significantly lower in the diseased clusters of subjects. Our initial observations (16) were probably due to the response of the most diseased individuals in that group of subjects. However, we believe that the current results are not fortuitous because 1) the relationship between the antibody levels and disease is evident not only in the original group but in groups with more serious disease in an almost dose dependent manner; 2) there is a relationship between these antibody levels and response to periodontal treatment; 3) there is a link through these antibodies to cellular receptors involved in antigen recognition and inflammation; 4) similar results have been noted in other chronic bacterial infections. In addition, there is no evidence that the lower levels of anti-*P. gingivalis* HtpG are due to adsorption by high circulating levels of either human Hsp90. There was no significant correlation between individual serum levels of human Hsp90 protein and anti-*P. gingivalis* HtpG, anti-*F. nucleatum* HtpG or anti-*P. gingivalis* HtpG p18 (Table S1). In fact, there was a trend to higher levels of anti-*P. gingivalis* HtpG in subjects with higher levels of human Hsp90, the opposite of what be expected if such absorption was taking place. There was also no significant difference between levels of human Hsp90 in healthy subjects with high levels of anti-*P. gingivalis* HtpG antibodies and severe periodontitis subjects with low levels of anti-*P. gingivalis* HtpG (Table S2). Lastly, while it is possible that a subset of anti-*P. gingivalis* HtpG antibodies might bind other HSP90 homologues, including human Hsp90, the *P. gingivalis* HtpG p18 epitope is unique and antibodies to that peptide could not be adsorbed by other HSP90 family proteins (see discussion below).

Subjects with CP who were given periodontal treatment responded more effectively to that treatment the higher their original pretreatment levels of anti-*P. gingivalis* HtpG. There was no similar effect with antibodies to *F. nucleatum* HtpG. Notably, the serum samples, which are time-averaged values, correlate best

Table 11. Alignment of oral bacterial species HtpG amino acid sequences.

A. actinomycetemcom. HtpG	TPAVVSTDNDQMTTQMAKLFAAAG--QPVPEVKYTFELNPEHHLVKKVAEIAD-588
F.nucleatum HtpG	SASSLLAKGG-LSLEMEKTLSEMTNNNDMPKAEKVLAINPEHVLFNRLKSSVN 569
P.gingivalis HtpG	AILITQAEFMRRMRDMAQLQPGMSFYGELPDS-YNLVLNTDHPLIDRVLSGEK 582
A. actinomycetemcom. HtpG	IAD-------EAQFADWVELLLEQAMLAERGSLENP----------------- 614
F.nucleatum HtpG	SVN-------TEDFNKLVDVLYNQALLLEGFNIENP----------------- 595
P.gingivalis HtpG	GEKESVEPSLTELRAKIAELKAEEAKLLDEEKGKKPEEIPVATKEAKENNAVE **632**
A. actinomycetemcom. HtpG	--AAFIKRINKLLG 626
F.nucleatum HtpG	--AEFIKNLNSLI 606
P.gingivalis HtpG	*QAKTEGSINDQLTK*YAQDNELIGQLIDLALLGSGLLTGEALAEFIRRSQRLL 684

Alignment of oral bacterial species HtpG amino acid sequences in the region of the 65 amino acid "Bacteroidacae insert" (Bold, underlined characters). The insert has not been described outside the Cytophaga, Flavobacteria and Bacteroides (CFB) group. Italic, bold–p18.

with clinical indices related to tissue destruction and less with indices related to inflammation. This suggests that these antibodies are found in subjects predisposed to a better treatment outcome or they may somehow facilitate healing after treatment. Interestingly, drugs that inhibit Hsp90 have been shown to prolong survival, attenuate inflammation, and reduce lung tissue injury in murine sepsis [19].

These findings are also worthy of note because despite high homology among chaperones in diverse organisms, the *P. gingivalis* HtpG is dissimilar from *A. actinomycetemcomitans* and *F. nucleatum* HtpG proteins: the C-terminus contains an extra inserted sequence (Table 11. bold in alignment). This insert appears to be exclusive to the Cytophaga-Flavobacterium-Bacteroides group HtpG proteins sequenced to date, and contains both a portion unique to each species (p18, underlined in alignment) and a conserved portion (p19). In contrast, the DnaK and GroEL of *P. gingivalis, A. actinomycetemcomitans,* and *F. nucleatum* align closely and display high homology. Examination of an alignment of Bacertoidacae HtpG molecules (Table 12) shows the insert can be roughly divided into 2 sections of about 30 amino acids each. The first-which contains p18-has relatively little sequence homology to the other species, only 6 of 36 (17%) amino acids are exact matches to the other Bacteroidacae HtpGs. The adjacent segment, p19, has 13 of 25 (52%) amino acids that are identical, similar to that between whole HtpG molecules from all 5 species (60-63%). BLAST analysis of p18 against the entire non-redundant protein database at GeneBank results in no hits except *P. gingivalis* HtpG. Similar searches using p19 produce significant hits with species in each of the Bacteroidacae genera (*B. fragilis* group; Non-*B. fragilis* group, Prevotella, Porphyromonas, Tanerella and "other"). Taken together we have concluded it is reasonable to assume that p18 is or contains an epitope that is unique to *P. gingivalis* HtpG and are currently investigating that hypothesis.

The mechanism that may connect anti-HtpG antibodies and progression of periodontitis is not known, but we speculate that it may well be that these antibodies block an interaction between HtpG and cellular receptors on macrophage [12]. Interactions between HtpG and the TLR4 and CD91 receptors induce the chemokine CXCL8, a chemoattractant for phagocytic cells in periodontitis [20,21] and thus perpetuating the uncontrolled inflammation characteristic of periodontitis. Additionally, interactions between TLR4 and CD91 and HtpG induce inflammatory cytokines, including TNFα, as part of the innate immune response. Serum antibodies in 8 subjects with titers to *P. gingivalis* HtpG were found to reduce CXCL8 production in human monocytes in a dose dependent manner while serum antibodies from subjects without anti-HtpG activity did not [12].

Table 12. Alignment of Bacteroidiacae HtpG C-terminal inserts

B. thetaiotaomicron	LKDSQKDKKEEDIPTAEKDELNELDKKWDELKNKKEGIFAG 643
B. fragilis	LKKKQEGKKDEDIPTAEKDELNDLDKKWDELKQQKDSIFAG 643
P. intermedia	LRQEQGKKKAEEITQEEKDDLKNTEESLSKQRTEKNDVIAN 646
T. forsythia	LREAQNKKKEDEITASEKEDLTNTNRKLTELRGQQNAILAE 647
P. gingivalis	LLDEEKGKKPEEIPVATKEAKENNAVEQAKTEGSINDQLTK 646
Consensus	* . : ** ::*. *: : . : . . : ::
B. thetaiotaomicron	YASNNKVIRQLIDLALLQNNMLKGEALNNFVKRSIELI- 681
B. fragilis	YAGKNKVVRQLIDLALLQNNMLKGEALNNFVKRSIELI- 681
P. intermedia	YAKGNNAIHQLIDLALLQNGMLKGAALDKFIKRSVDLIK 685
T. forsythia	YAAGNPIIGQLIDLALLGNGLLKGEALSRFIRRSVDLIR 686
P. gingivalis	YAQDNELIGQLIDLALLGSGLLTGEALAEFIRRSQRLL- 684
Consensus	** * : ******** ..:*.* ** .*::** *:

Alignment of 65 amino insert found in most CFB group bacteria, but not other bacterial groups. Bacteroidiacae HtpG C-terminal inserts shows p18 is much less conserved than p19. Underline/bold–p18 sequence. Dashed underline–p19 sequence. Amino acid identities across all species-*.

The results reported here are similar to those of other chronic infections including *Heliobacter pylori*. World wide as much as 75% of the population has evidence of *H. pylori* infection but only subsets of these individuals manifest the peptic ulcers and stomach cancers associated with those chronic infections. The *H. pylori* chaperone hsp60 induces CXCL8 production in monocytic cells [22] and humoral immune response to a peptide epitope (pH9) of hsp60 is unique and seems to be associated with protection against *H. pylori* infection [23]. Intriguingly, when subjects with mucosa-associated lymphoid tissue lymphoma were examined for antibodies to the *H. pylori* hsp60 chaperone it was found that pre-treatment titers in patients whose tumors regressed after treatment were significantly higher than in patients whose tumors did not regress [24]. Low levels of antibodies to chaperones in disease subjects compared to controls has also been reported in inflammatory bowel disease [25], fungal infections [26] and other chronic bacterial infections [27].

The unique restriction of the *P. gingivalis* HtpG p18 peptide to the most important pathogen in periodontitis may have applications in vaccine and diagnostic arenas. The use of chaperones as vaccine candidates has been suggested by a number of investigators. Antibody to the Hsp90 homologue of *C. albicans* (Mycograb®, Novartis) has been shown to be effective in the treatment of disseminated fungal infections [28] in combination with amphotericin B. Other chaperones have been suggested as vaccine targets for diverse diseases in humans, cattle [29] and fish [30]. *P. gingivalis* GroEL has been used as a vaccine in a rat model of periodontitis that resulted in prevention of attachment loss [31], similar to that described here in humans. However, the authors cautioned that extensive homology between human and microbial chaperones may require use of peptides that do not induce cross-reactive antibodies with human hsp60 molecules. We believe this is the case with p18, which appears unique to *P. gingivalis* even to the exclusion of other Bacteroides species. The data presented here also suggests that serum antibodies to p18 may be useful in diagnosing periodontitis patients with extensive treatment requirements, identification of which would have substantial economic and epidemiological impact on the practice of periodontology.

Materials and Methods

Subjects

All work with human subjects was approved by the University of Michigan Institutional Review Board or the Queen's University, Belfast Ethics Committee, respectively. Each subject gave written individual informed consent and was advised that withdrawal from the study was available at their discretion at any time. The clinical condition of each subject was determined by examination of five clinical measurements: Probing pocket depth (PD) was determined to the nearest mm at six sites around each tooth and then averaged for all sites in each subject [32]. Bleeding on probing (BOP), was reported as a dichotomous measure and recorded as a percentage of the sites [33]. Clinical attachment loss (CAL) was determined at the same sites by measuring the distance between the cemento-enamel junction and the bottom of each pocket to the nearest mm and averaged [34]. The gingival index (GI) value represents the percentage of sites in each patient exhibiting redness associated with inflammation[35]. The plaque index value (PI) represents the percentage of sites found to have plaque biofilm accumulated at the gingival margin.

Gingivitis Subjects

This group was examined from archived samples described in a previous report and was included here to address the potential differences between response to *P. gingivalis* HtpG and human Hsp90. This retrospective study focused on a population of individuals living in southwestern Michigan [15,16] with gingivitis, a form of periodontal disease with no or minimal tissue destruction that is reversible with active oral hygiene. Subjects were recruited into the original study based on their membership in the rural community, not their oral health status, and all essentially presented with gingivitis or mild periodontitis. The clinical data and archived serum samples collected from 50 subjects were used. The average age was 31.6 years (range: 18–66) and 58% were female. Other characteristics of these subjects are found in Table 1.

Chronic Periodontitis Subjects

Subjects were recruited at the Michigan Center for Oral Health Research. Subject inclusion was based on: possession of at least 20 teeth, no periodontal treatment or antibiotic-related therapy for medical or dental reasons for 3 months before study inclusion, no history of long-term treatment with medications known to affect periodontal status, and no history of metabolic bone diseases. Healthy control subjects ($n = 49$) were recruited who had less than 3 mm of CAL, no pocket depth (PD)s greater than 4 mm, no radiographic bone loss, and less than 20 sites with bleeding on probing. Chronic periodontitis (CP) subjects ($n = 50$) exhibited at least 4 sites with evidence of radiographic bone loss, mean CAL >3mm, PD >4 mm and bleeding on probing (Table 1).

Aggressive Periodontitis Subjects

Studies were done with serum samples from an ongoing study of Aggressive Periodontitis (AP) subjects ($n = 24$) and age matched control subjects ($n = 21$) living in Northern Ireland. AP subjects included in this investigation were 30.3 ± 4.0 years of age at the time of clinical and radiographic examination, diagnosed with severe periodontitis, and had a minimum of 4 sites with a probing depth of at least 5 mm and CAL loss of at least 2 mm. Age matched controls without periodontitis were recruited from regular attendees at the Queen's University School of Dentistry. Colonization of AP subjects by *P. gingivalis* was determined by PCR using primers specific for the *P. gingivalis* 16S rRNA gene [17].

Bacterial strains and culture conditions

Porphyromonas gingivalis (ATCC 33277) and *Fusobacterium nucleatum* (ATCC 25586) were obtained from the American Type Culture Collection. *Porphyromonas gingivalis* strain W83 was a gift from Dr. Donald Clewell, University of Michigan School of Dentistry. The bacteria were maintained by weekly transfer in an anaerobe chamber (Coy Manufacturing, Grass Lake, MI) at 37°C on PRAS Brucella agar plates (Anaerobe Systems, Morgan Hill, CA) in a 5% hydrogen, 10% carbon dioxide, 85% nitrogen atmosphere. Broth cultures were grown in a mixture of 50% Brain Heart Infusion Broth, 50% Trypticase Soy Broth and 5 gram/L Yeast Extract supplemented with 0.01 gm/L Sodium Bisulfite, 5 mg/L hemin and 5ug/L Vitamin K.

Antigen preparation

Cloning and purification of *P. gingivalis* and *F. nucleatum* rHtpG. The full length sequence of *P. gingivalis* HtpG (GenBank ascension number AF176245) and *F. nucleatum* HtpG (GenBank ascension number EDK88176) were obtained from the National Center for Biotechnology Information (www,ncbi.nlm.nih.gov). PCR primers were designed to produce full-length products that were subsequently inserted into pCR®T7 TOPO® cloning vector following the manufacturer's instructions (Invitrogen, Carlsbad, CA.). Clones of One Shot® Chemically Competent *E. coli*

(Invitrogen) transformed with the vector were ampicillin selected and then screened by PCR. Inserts that produced amplicons of the correct size were sequenced to verify the full-length insert (Biomedical Research Core Facilities, University of Michigan, Ann Arbor, MI). Plasmids with in-frame inserts were used to transform TOP10F BL21(DE3)pLysS *E.coli* (Invitrogen) cells that were subsequently induced with 100 μM isopropyl β-D-1-thiogalactopyranoside for 4 hours to produce a fusion protein with 6 consecutive histidine (6xhis) residues preceding the N-terminal of the cloned proteins. The protein was purified to >95%, as determined by SDS-PAGE electrophoresis, by Ni-agarose chromatography (Ni-NTA™ Agarose, Qiagen, Valencia, CA).

Preparation of HtpG peptide (p18). A 36 amino aid peptide (KKPEEIPVATKEAKENNAVEQAKTEGSINDQLT-KYA) was synthesized on an Applied Biosystem 433A peptide synthesizer at the University of Michigan department of Chemistry using Fmoc amino acids from AnaSpec (San Jose, CA). The crude peptide was purified by HPLC and the purity (~98%) confirmed by MALDI-TOF analysis.

ELISA assays

All assays were carried out in 384-well microtiter plates (NUNC™ black MaxiSorp, Rochester, NY) using 4-methyumbliferone phosphate as a substrate for alkaline phosphatase-labeled tracers. Antigens were coated onto the plates in 25 μl/well volumes in sodium carbonate/bicarbonate buffer (0.05M, pH 9.5) and incubated overnight at 4°C. Plates were washed 3 times with 0.02 M phosphate buffered saline (PBS, pH 7.4) and PBS with 1% bovine serum albumin (PBS-BSA) added to block unoccupied protein binding sites (100 μL/well). After an additional hour of incubation at room temperature plates were washed with PBS with 0.125% NP40 three times and human serum (or control rabbit serum) diluted 1:100 in PBS-BSA (25 uL/well) added to the plates in triplicate and incubated overnight at 4°C. Plates were then washed 3 times with PBS with 0.125% NP40 and detection reagents added as described below. Blocked wells not coated with antigen were used as negative controls for each individual serum sample. Data is expressed as net relative florescent units (RFU) calculated by subtracting the average of 3 control wells from the average of 3 antigen coated wells and were repeated at least 3 times each.

Antibodies to *P. gingivalis* Whole Cell Lysate

P. gingivalis cells (strain W83) were grown to mid-log phase, washed by centrifugation at 10,000×g 3 times with sterile PBS and resuspended at an OD_{600} of 1.0 in water. The cells were sonicated for 2 minutes on ice three times and centrifuged at 10,000×g for 20 minutes. Total protein was determined and the clarified lysate diluted to 10 μg/mL for coating. Serum IgG binding was determined as described above using alkaline phophatase-labeled anti-human IgG(γ) antibodies and 4-methylubelliferyl phosphate (1 μg/mL in 0.2 M TRIS, pH 9.5) (Sigma, St. Louis).

Antibodies to *P. gingivalis* HtpG and *F. nucleatum* HtpG

Recombinant HtpG proteins were dissolved in carbonate buffer to 1 μg/mL for plate coating. Total IgG(γ) binding was determined using the same second antibodies as described for the whole cell lysate assay above.

Antibodies to *P. gingivalis* HtpG peptide 18

The peptide was dissolved in carbonate buffer to 10 μg/mL for plate coating. Total serum IgG(γ) binding was determined using the same second antibodies as above.

Detection of *P. gingivalis* and *F. nucleatum* colonization in plaque samples

The detection of *P. gingivalis* in pooled plaque samples from the gingivitis subjects was done using a slot immunoblotting method as described previously [36]. Colonization of plaque samples collected simultaneously with the serum in the CP groups were evaluated by real-time PCR as described [37] using primers specific for *P. gingivalis* (forward:5′-CATAGATATCACG-AGGAACTCCGATT-3′; reverse 5′-AAACTGTTAGCAACTACCGATGTGG-3′) and *F. nucleatum* (forward: 5′-AAATATGTTGAATTCTGGAAAGAGT-TTG-3′; reverse: 5′-TGAACTCCAGCTTTTATACTTCTAC-CAA-3′). Percentage of the total flora for each species was calculated by dividing the number of target organisms by the total number of bacteria as determined by realtime PCR using 16S rRNA primers that reacted with all bacterial species (forward: 5′-CCATGAA-GTCGGAATCGCTAG-3′; reverse: 5′-GCTTGACGGGCGG-TGT-3′). The presence of *P. gingivalis* in plaque from the AP subjects was determined by PCR as described earlier [17] using the same primers.

Statistical Analysis of anti-HtpG levels

Statistical computations were done using STATISTICA™ v. 6.0 (StatSoft, Omaha, NE). Comparison of two means was performed using *t*-tests. The relationships between specific indices of periodontal disease, antibody levels, and colonization were assessed by ANOVA. Fisher's method for multiple comparisons was used for group comparisons. Log transformation of data was performed where appropriate. Results with p-values of ≤ 0.05 were considered significant.

Supporting Information

Table S2 Antibody to *P. gingivalis* HtpG and human Hsp90 serum levels in CP subjects.

Table S1 Correlation of human Hsp90 levels to Anti-HtpG levels in 95 CP patients and healthy controls.

Acknowledgments

The authors wish to acknowledge the technical assistance of Florence Y-P An in cloning the *F. nucleatum* HtpG. The authors thank Dr. Vincent L. Pecoraro (University of Michigan Department of Chemistry) for use of the ABI 433A Peptide Synthesizer.

Author Contributions

Conceived and designed the experiments: DL CS. Performed the experiments: PS CS. Analyzed the data: WG CS. Contributed reagents/materials/analysis tools: WG VD DS JK WC BM DL CS. Wrote the paper: CS.

References

1. Socransky SS, Haffajee AD (1997) The nature of periodontal diseases. AnnPeriodontol 2: 3–10.
2. Socransky SS, Haffajee AD, Cugini MA, Smith C, Kent RL Jr (1998) Microbial complexes in subgingival plaque. JClinPeriodontol 25: 134–144.

3. Progulske-Fox A, Kozarov E, Dorn B, Dunn W Jr, Burks J, et al. (1999) Porphyromonas gingivalis virulence factors and invasion of cells of the cardiovascular system. J Periodontal Res 34: 393–399.
4. Kozarov E, Sweier D, Shelburne C, Progulske-Fox A, Lopatin D (2006) Detection of bacterial DNA in atheromatous plaques by quantitative PCR. Microbes Infect 8: 687–693.
5. Goulhen F, Grenier D, Mayrand D (2003) Oral microbial heat-shock proteins and their potential contributions to infections. Crit Rev Oral Biol Med 14: 399–412.
6. Prohaszka Z, Fust G (2004) Immunological aspects of heat-shock proteins-the optimum stress of life. Mol Immunol 41: 29–44.
7. Shamaei-Tousi A, D'Aiuto F, Nibali L, Steptoe A, Coates AR, et al. (2007) Differential regulation of circulating levels of molecular chaperones in patients undergoing treatment for periodontal disease. PLoS ONE 2: e1198.
8. Young D, Lathigra R, Hendrix R, Sweetser D, Young RA (1988) Stress proteins are immune targets in leprosy and tuberculosis. ProcNatlAcadSciUSA 85: 4267–4270.
9. Lopatin DE, Shelburne CE, Van Poperin N, Kowalski CJ, Bagramian RA (1999) Humoral immunity to stress proteins and periodontal disease. J Periodontol 70: 1185–1193.
10. Rams TE, Listgarten MA, Slots J (2006) Actinobacillus actinomycetemcomitans and Porphyromonas gingivalis subgingival presence, species-specific serum immunoglobulin G antibody levels, and periodontitis disease recurrence. J Periodontal Res 41: 228–234.
11. Yamazaki K, Ueki-Maruayama K, Honda T, Nakajima T, Seymour GJ (2004) Effect of periodontal treatment on the serum antibody levels to heat shock proteins. Clin Exp Immunol 135: 478–482.
12. Shelburne CE, Coopamah MD, Sweier DG, An FY, Lopatin DE (2007) HtpG, the Porphyromonas gingivalis HSP-90 homologue, induces the chemokine CXCL8 in human monocytic and microvascular vein endothelial cells. Cell Microbiol 9: 1611–1619.
13. Luoma J, Hiltunen T, Sarkioja T, Moestrup SK, Gliemann J, et al. (1994) Expression of alpha 2-macroglobulin receptor/low density lipoprotein receptor-related protein and scavenger receptor in human atherosclerotic lesions. J Clin Invest 93: 2014–2021.
14. Kinane DF, Mooney J, Ebersole JL (1999) Humoral immune response to Actinobacillus actinomycetemcomitans and Porphyromonas gingivalis in periodontal disease. Periodontol 2000 20: 289–340.
15. Bagramian RA, Farghaly MM, Lopatin D, Sowers M, Syed SA, et al. (1993) Periodontal disease in an Amish population. JClinPeriodontol 20: 269–272.
16. Bagramian RA, Farghaly MM, Lopatin D, Sowers M, Syed SA, et al. (1994) A comparison of periodontal disease among rural Amish and non-Amish adults. JClinPeriodontol 21: 386–390.
17. Mullally BH, Dace B, Shelburne CE, Wolff LF, Coulter WA (2000) Prevalence of periodontal pathogens in localized and generalized forms of early-onset periodontitis. JPeriodontal Res 35: 232–241.
18. Sweier DG, Shelburne CE, Cameron J, Lopatin DE (2004) Localizing antibody-defined immunoreactivity in Porphyromonas gingivalis HtpG recognized by human serum utilizing selective protein expression. J Immunol Methods 285: 165–170.
19. Chatterjee A, Dimitropoulou C, Drakopanayiotakis F, Antonova G, Snead C, et al. (2007) Heat shock protein 90 inhibitors prolong survival, attenuate inflammation, and reduce lung injury in murine sepsis. Am J Respir Crit Care Med 176: 667–675.
20. Hosokawa Y, Hosokawa I, Ozaki K, Nakae H, Matsuo T (2006) Proinflammatory effects of tumour necrosis factor-like weak inducer of apoptosis (TWEAK) on human gingival fibroblasts. Clin Exp Immunol 146: 540–549.
21. Okada H, Murakami S (1998) Cytokine expression in periodontal health and disease. Crit Rev Oral Biol Med 9: 248–266.
22. Lin SN, Ayada K, Zhao Y, Yokota K, Takenaka R, et al. (2005) Helicobacter pylori heat-shock protein 60 induces production of the pro-inflammatory cytokine IL8 in monocytic cells. J Med Microbiol 54: 225–233.
23. Yamaguchi H, Osaki T, Kai M, Taguchi H, Kamiya S (2000) Immune response against a cross-reactive epitope on the heat shock protein 60 homologue of Helicobacter pylori. InfectImmun 68: 3448–3454.
24. Takenaka R, Yokota K, Mizuno M, Okada H, Toyokawa T, et al. (2004) Serum antibodies to Helicobacter pylori and its heat-shock protein 60 correlate with the response of gastric mucosa-associated lymphoid tissue lymphoma to eradication of H. pylori. Helicobacter 9: 194–200.
25. Huszti Z, Bene L, Kovacs A, Fekete B, Fust G, et al. (2004) Low levels of antibodies against E. coli and mycobacterial 65kDa heat shock proteins in patients with inflammatory bowel disease. Inflamm Res 53: 551–555.
26. Matthews RC, Burnie JP, Howat D, Rowland T, Walton F (1991) Autoantibody to heat-shock protein 90 can mediate protection against systemic candidosis. Immunology 74: 20–24.
27. Zugel U, Kaufmann SH (1999) Role of heat shock proteins in protection from and pathogenesis of infectious diseases. ClinMicrobiolRev 12: 19–39.
28. Burnie JP, Carter TL, Hodgetts SJ, Matthews RC (2006) Fungal heat-shock proteins in human disease. FEMS Microbiol Rev 30: 53–88.
29. Koets A, Hoek A, Langelaar M, Overdijk M, Santema W, et al. (2006) Mycobacterial 70 kD heat-shock protein is an effective subunit vaccine against bovine paratuberculosis. Vaccine 24: 2550–2559.
30. Sudheesh PS, LaFrentz BR, Call DR, Siems WF, LaPatra SE, et al. (2007) Identification of potential vaccine target antigens by immunoproteomic analysis of a virulent and a non-virulent strain of the fish pathogen Flavobacterium psychrophilum. Dis Aquat Organ 74: 37–47.
31. Lee JY, Yi NN, Kim US, Choi JS, Kim SJ, et al. (2006) Porphyromonas gingivalis heat shock protein vaccine reduces the alveolar bone loss induced by multiple periodontopathogenic bacteria. J Periodontal Res 41: 10–14.
32. Loe H, Theilade E, Jensen SB (1965) Experimental gingivitis man. JPeriodontol 36: 177–187.
33. Offenbacher S (2005) Commentary: clinical implications of periodontal disease assessments using probing depth and bleeding on probing to measure the status of the periodontal-biofilm interface. J Int Acad Periodontol 7: 157–161.
34. Wolff LF, Liljemark WF, Pihlstrom BL, Schaffer EM, Aeppli DM, et al. (1988) Dark-pigmented Bacteroides species in subgingival plaque of adult patients on a rigorous recall program. J Periodontal Res 23: 170–174.
35. Silness J, Loe H (1966) Periodontal disease in pregnancy. 3. Response to local treatment. Acta OdontolScand 24: 747–759.
36. Van Poperin N, Lopatin DE (1991) Slot immunoblot assay for detection and quantitation of periodontal disease-associated microorganisms in dental plaque. JClinMicrobiol 29: 2554–2558.
37. Shelburne CE, Prabhu A, Gleason RM, Mullally BH, Coulter WA (2000) Quantitation of Bacteroides forsythus in subgingival plaque comparison of immunoassay and quantitative polymerase chain reaction. J Microbiol Methods 39: 97–107.

15

Artificial Neural Networks for the Diagnosis of Aggressive Periodontitis Trained by Immunologic Parameters

Georgios Papantonopoulos[1]*, Keiso Takahashi[2], Tasos Bountis[3], Bruno G. Loos[4]

1 Center for Research and Applications of Nonlinear Systems, Department of Mathematics, University of Patras, Patras, Greece, **2** Department of Conservative Dentistry, School of Dentistry, Ohu University, Fukushima, Japan, **3** Laboratory of Nonlinear Systems and Applied Analysis, Department of Mathematics, University of Patras, Patras, Greece, **4** Department of Periodontology, Academic Center for Dentistry Amsterdam (ACTA), University of Amsterdam and VU University, Amsterdam, The Netherlands

Abstract

There is neither a single clinical, microbiological, histopathological or genetic test, nor combinations of them, to discriminate aggressive periodontitis (AgP) from chronic periodontitis (CP) patients. We aimed to estimate probability density functions of clinical and immunologic datasets derived from periodontitis patients and construct artificial neural networks (ANNs) to correctly classify patients into AgP or CP class. The fit of probability distributions on the datasets was tested by the Akaike information criterion (*AIC*). ANNs were trained by cross entropy (*CE*) values estimated between probabilities of showing certain levels of immunologic parameters and a reference mode probability proposed by kernel density estimation (KDE). The weight decay regularization parameter of the ANNs was determined by 10-fold cross-validation. Possible evidence for 2 clusters of patients on cross-sectional and longitudinal bone loss measurements were revealed by KDE. Two to 7 clusters were shown on datasets of CD4/CD8 ratio, CD3, monocyte, eosinophil, neutrophil and lymphocyte counts, IL-1, IL-2, IL-4, INF-γ and TNF-α level from monocytes, antibody levels against A. *actinomycetemcomitans* (*A.a.*) and *P.gingivalis* (*P.g.*). ANNs gave 90%–98% accuracy in classifying patients into either AgP or CP. The best overall prediction was given by an ANN with *CE* of monocyte, eosinophil, neutrophil counts and CD4/CD8 ratio as inputs. ANNs can be powerful in classifying periodontitis patients into AgP or CP, when fed by *CE* values based on KDE. Therefore ANNs can be employed for accurate diagnosis of AgP or CP by using relatively simple and conveniently obtained parameters, like leukocyte counts in peripheral blood. This will allow clinicians to better adapt specific treatment protocols for their AgP and CP patients.

Editor: Ali Al-Ahmad, University Hospital of the Albert-Ludwigs-University Freiburg, Germany

Funding: The Academic Center for Dentistry Amsterdam (ACTA) (author B.G.L.) is supported in part by a grant from the University of Amsterdam for research into the focal point "Oral infections and Inflammation". This research has been co-financed by the European Union (European Social Fund, ESF) and Greek national funds through the Operational Program "Education and Lifelong Learning" of the National Strategic Reference Framework (NSRF) – Research Funding Program: THALES: Investing in knowledge society through the European Social Fund. The funders had no role in study design, data collection and analysis, decision to publish, or preparation of the manuscript.

Competing Interests: The authors have declared that no competing interests exist.

* E-mail: ppntnpls@otenet.gr

Introduction

Periodontitis is a bacterial-driven chronic inflammatory destructive disease of the tissues surrounding and supporting the dental root [1]. Severe periodontitis affects around 8.5% of the general population, while a moderate form of the disease is present in 30% and a mild form in 9% of adults aged 30 and older [2].

Periodontitis is a complex disease, where multiple causal factors simultaneously and interactively play a role. There are four main causal risk factors, i.e. the subgingival microbiota (the bacterial biofilm), individual genetic variations, life style and systemic factors [3]. It is a well-known fact that the behavior of a complex system cannot be explained by isolating its components [4]. Currently two clinical types of periodontitis are recognized; the aggressive (AgP) and the chronic (CP) form [5]. Due to the complexity of the pathogenesis of the disease, there is no single clinical, microbiological, histopathological, genetic test or combinations of them to discriminate AgP from CP patients [6].

Clinical identification of AgP cases is based on rapid attachment loss and bone destruction, the absence of systemic factors to explain this progression rate and familial aggregation [7]. Any age upper limit in discriminating AgP from CP is arbitrary. Nevertheless, given the same amount of periodontal destruction individuals with AgP are found considerably younger than CP patients. The age of 35 has been used as a cut-off point to discriminate between AgP and CP [8]. It is realized that is difficult to distinguish between the two phenotypes at the initial stages of periodontitis, thus preventing proper early clinical management of AgP, which is generally found more demanding.

Complexity is understood through modeling and simulation [4]. In a recent study [9] using cellular automata experiments, periodontitis was described as a system out of equilibrium with the level of the host immune response determining its entropy rate. In a subsequent study [10] a chaotic map was analyzed, expressed by a particular equation, which accurately models periodontitis progression in connection to the variation of the host immune response level. By renormalization arguments, two zones of disease activity were identified, a fast and a slow progressing zone, corresponding to AgP and CP respectively. Based on the above, we may now pose the hypothesis that different entropy rates might indeed reflect the presence of distinct patient clusters in immunologic and clinical datasets.

Histograms are the oldest probability density estimators [11], but suffer from certain important drawbacks; they are discontinuous and hardly appropriate for representing bivariate or trivariate data. Nonparametric kernel density estimation (KDE) methods on the other hand, reveal structure in datasets, such as skewness and multimodality that might be missed by classical parametric methods [12]. KDE is an unsupervised learning procedure that can be used for nonparametric classification tasks [13]. In general, when a desired outcome is known, a learning process is called supervised, otherwise it is unsupervised learning.

Artificial neural networks (ANNs) are considered powerful nonlinear statistical tools to model complex relationships between inputs and outputs. Therefore, they appear appropriate in searching for parameters that could achieve an accurate diagnosis of AgP or CP. ANNs consist of a set of simple units called neurons by analogy with the biological neurons [14]. Neurons are linked to each other by a weighted connection which is called synapsis, and are organized in layers: Information is fed to neurons of the input layer, and then processed in the hidden layer and finally exits to the neurons of the output layer. ANNs can be adaptive to external or internal changes and "learn" from the data entered into them. For instance, one type of ANN is the multilayer perceptron (MLP); this is a feedforward ANN trained by the backwards propagation of the error found in the outcome layer. It can be used for supervised learning classification procedures.

The first aim of this study was to estimate the probability density functions of a set of observed clinical and immunologic data in periodontitis patients. Secondly we investigated the fit of the data to various probability distribution models. Based on these findings we developed ANNs able to classify periodontitis patients belonging to either one of the two different clinical forms, aggressive or chronic form.

Materials and Methods

Study population

Data were retrieved from previous studies that provided 4 distinct patient samples. From one study [15], we obtained 29 periodontitis patients with severely advanced disease as evidenced by clinical and radiographic examination, which were clinically followed and maintained for 5 to 8 years (we designate this as sample-1). At baseline examination, they had ≥14 teeth present and at least 50% of their teeth showed bone loss of ≥50% of their root length. We used data on baseline radiographic mean bone loss and on longitudinal mean radiographic bone loss level change. From Loos et al. [16,17] studies from 76 periodontitis patients (the same group for both studies to which we will refer as sample-2) we derived datasets of total number of monocytes, lymphocytes, basophils, neutrophils and eosinophils in peripheral blood, as well as the total number of CD3, CD4, CD19 cells and the CD4/CD8 ratio. For sample-2 radiographic bone loss measurements were also available (% of teeth with bone loss of ≥50% of the tooth root length). From Graswinckel et al. [18] we used the datasets for IgA, IgM and IgG from 80 periodontitis patients (sample-3). From Takahashi et al. [19] (sample-4) we derived data of serum antibody levels in 162 periodontitis patients against *Aggregatibacter actinomycetemcomitans* (*A.a.*) (Y4 antigen), *A.a.* (ATCC 29523), *A.a.* (SUNY67), *Porphyromonas gingivalis* (*P.g.*) (FDC381), *P.g.* (SU63), *Eikenella corrodens* (*E.c.*) (ATCC 23834), *Prevotella intermedia* (*P.i.*) (ATCC 25611), *Prevotella nigrescens* (*P.i.*) (ATCC 33563), *Capnocytophaga ochracea* (*C.o.*) (S3), *Wolinella succinogens* (ATCC 29543), *Treponema Denticola* (*T.d.*) (ATCC 35405) and *Fusobacterium nucleatum* (*F.n.*) (ATCC 25586). In addition we derived data of IL-1, IL-2, IL-4, IL-6, TNF-α and INF-γ levels produced by mononuclear cells from peripheral blood.

The undefined periodontitis patients, those with adult periodontitis (AP) or those with localized (L) or generalized (G) early onset periodontitis (EOP) from the studies from which data were retrieved [16–19] were reclassified as previously described [9]. Those with an age at the time of diagnosis >35 years or originally having AP, were reclassified as CP; patients ≤35 years were classified as AgP; those with L- or G-EOP were all classified as AgP. EOP (a term used in the 1989 world workshop in clinical periodontics, preserved in the 1996 modification and changed to AgP in 1999) is considered to have its onset from puberty until 35 years [20].

Therefore from sample-2 we derived 23 AgP and 53 CP cases; from sample-3 18 AgP and 62 CP cases. For these two samples we had an exclusion of 20% of the initially recruited patients for various reasons that could affect their immunologic profile (like chronic medical disorder, pregnancy, trauma, recent tooth extraction, etc). From sample-4 we obtained 68 AgP and 43 CP cases. A group of 51 patients "suspected for EOP", was declared suspected for AgP with no definitive criteria for a final diagnosis; they had severe periodontitis and a disease history that suggested EOP, but were >35 years at the first examination and with no family members diagnosed with EOP. Patients in sample-4 were recruited as they presented at the Okayama University Dental Hospital over a period of 10 years.

Kernel density estimation

For the estimation of univariate or bivariate probability densities of the data distribution of the various parameters, an appropriate kernel function is needed [21]. The process of choosing a kernel function is described in Text S1 in File S1.

Fit of the data distributions to probability models

The fit of the available data distributions was tested in five well known probability models for continuous variables: the Normal, the Exponential, the Weibull, the Pareto and the Gamma models. They all have been extensively used and applied on biological systems [22]. A first visual appreciation of the fit was judged by quantile to quantile (Q-Q) plots. Subsequently, comparisons between models were based on the Akaike information criterion (*AIC*) [23,24], which safe-guards against overfitted models [25].

Construction of artificial neural networks

We built MLP ANNs to classify periodontitis patients. A diagram of the MLP ANN applied in this study is presented in Figure 1. It depicts the three types of layers, the input, the hidden and the output layer along with the interweaving of their neurons. We trained ANNs using cross entropy values (*CE*) [26] of immunological parameters of periodontitis patients in reference to a target probability value revealed by KDE.

The first step in the construction process was to calculate the probability $p(x)$ of demonstrating a certain level of an immunological parameter (x) in an individual patient. We used for that the cumulative probability function (cpf) of the corresponding probability model. At a second step, we computed cross entropy (*CE*) values [26] for each patient between the previously described probability $p(x)$ for selected immunologic parameters and a reference probability value, the target probability $t_{i(CP)}$. We used the formula

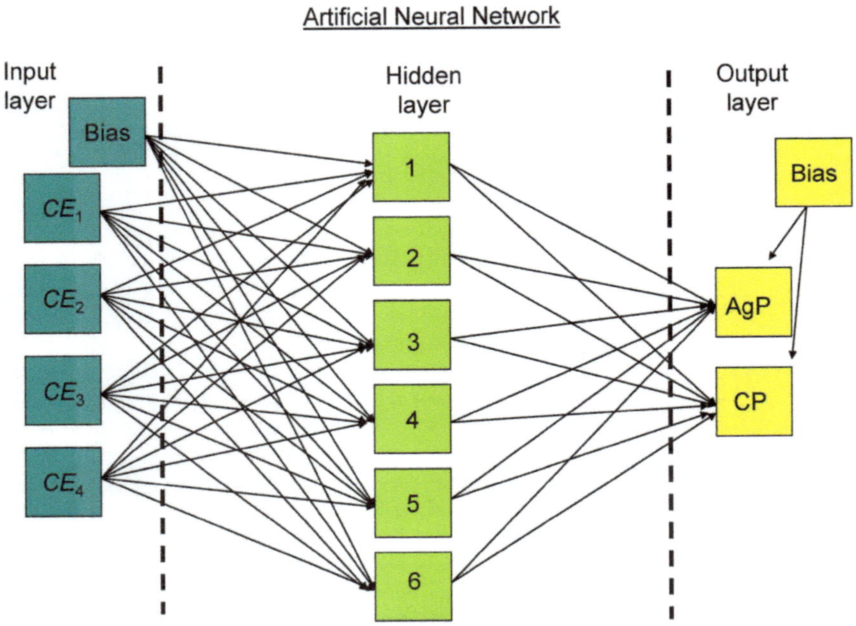

Figure 1. Multilayer perceptron feedforward neural network with error backpropagation. The information (cross entropy values of immunological parameters for each patient) is inserted in the input neurons. At the hidden layer, here with 6 neurons, we sum the information and transfer it (through the sigmoid function) to the outcome layer, where the sigmoid function exits an AgP or CP verdict. Bias neurons have a constant value and help the network to learn patterns. They are independent from other neurons and can shift the curve of the sigmoid function to the left or to the right. The classification error found at the outcome layer backpropagates in the network and synaptic weights are adapted accordingly as the network learns from its error and tries to minimize it.

$$CE_i = -\left(t_{i(CP)} \ln p(x_i)\right)$$

where i = 1, 2, ...N and N is the number of the immunological parameters (x) inserted into the ANN. *CE* is a nonsymmetric measure of the difference between two probability distributions. The target probability distribution $t_{i(CP)}$ was estimated by direct application of the appropriate cpf; we used the mode value of x with the highest density probability of the immunologic data distribution (indicated by KDE) as the reference point. We assumed that the highest density modes represent clusters inhabited mostly by the CP patients.

Our pruning strategy in feature selection at the input layer was based on automatic relevance determination (ARD) [27]. According to the method, features whose posterior weight distributions show low variance are discarded. The weight decay regularization parameter was determined by a 10-fold cross-validation process [28] (see text S1). If 10-fold cross validation is used for the determination of the weight decay regularization parameter, usually there is no need to use cross validation to determine the number of the hidden units [28]. We determined the number of hidden units and the maximum number of epochs by experimentation (we stopped increasing iterations when the sum of squares error stopped improving) [27,28]. Finally, since the results of the networks are sensitive to the initial weight values, we tried 10 random initial weight configurations and we computed the mean prediction rates [28]. We report the technical features of the ANNs, such as maximum number of epochs (iterations) and learning methods applied, as well as sensitivity, specificity and overall accuracy of the ANNs against the original clinical diagnosis.

Results

From 4 distinct samples we derived clinical and immunologic data and performed KDE. From sample-1 on baseline and longitudinal bone loss data KDE revealed possible evidence of two clusters of patients (Figure 2A, B). On sample-2 for the dataset of % of teeth with bone loss ≥50% of their root length, possible evidence of two main clusters was also found (Figure 2C). KDE on sample-2 revealed three to seven clusters for monocytes, basophils, neutrophils, eosinophils and lymphocytes counts (Figure 2Q, R, S, T & X) and two clusters for CD3 (Figure 2L). From sample-3, IgA and IgM data showed one mode (Figure 2V & W) while IgG data (Figure 2U) showed two clusters. From sample-4, KDE gave possible evidence of two main clusters for IL-2, IL-4, IL-6, TNF-α, INF-γ, (Figure 2D, E, F, H, J & K), and of 2 to 3 modes for antibody IgG titers against the 12 examined bacteria (graphs are shown for three of them) (Figure 2M, N & O).

Some bivariate KDE were generated. Using longitudinal bone loss data in relation to age (sample-1), we identified two clusters of patients (Figure 3A). The majority of patients clustered around the mode of 0.2 mm of longitudinal bone loss over the follow up period, while a small cluster of patients showed a mode with an almost 5 times higher value for this parameter. In the bivariate KDE of the CD4/CD8 ratio in relation to age (sample-2) (Figure 3B) or in relation to % of teeth with bone loss ≥50% of their root length (Figure 3C), two clusters at modes x = 1.5 and x = 1.9 are found.

We found the baseline and longitudinal bone loss measurements to fit to the Normal model (Table S1 in File S1). Most of the immunologic data fitted to the Gamma model (Figure S1, Table S1 in File S1). We built three ANNs with three kinds of immunologic parameters as inputs: leukocytes (ANN_1) (from sample-2), interleukins (ANN_2) and IgG antibody titers (ANN_3)

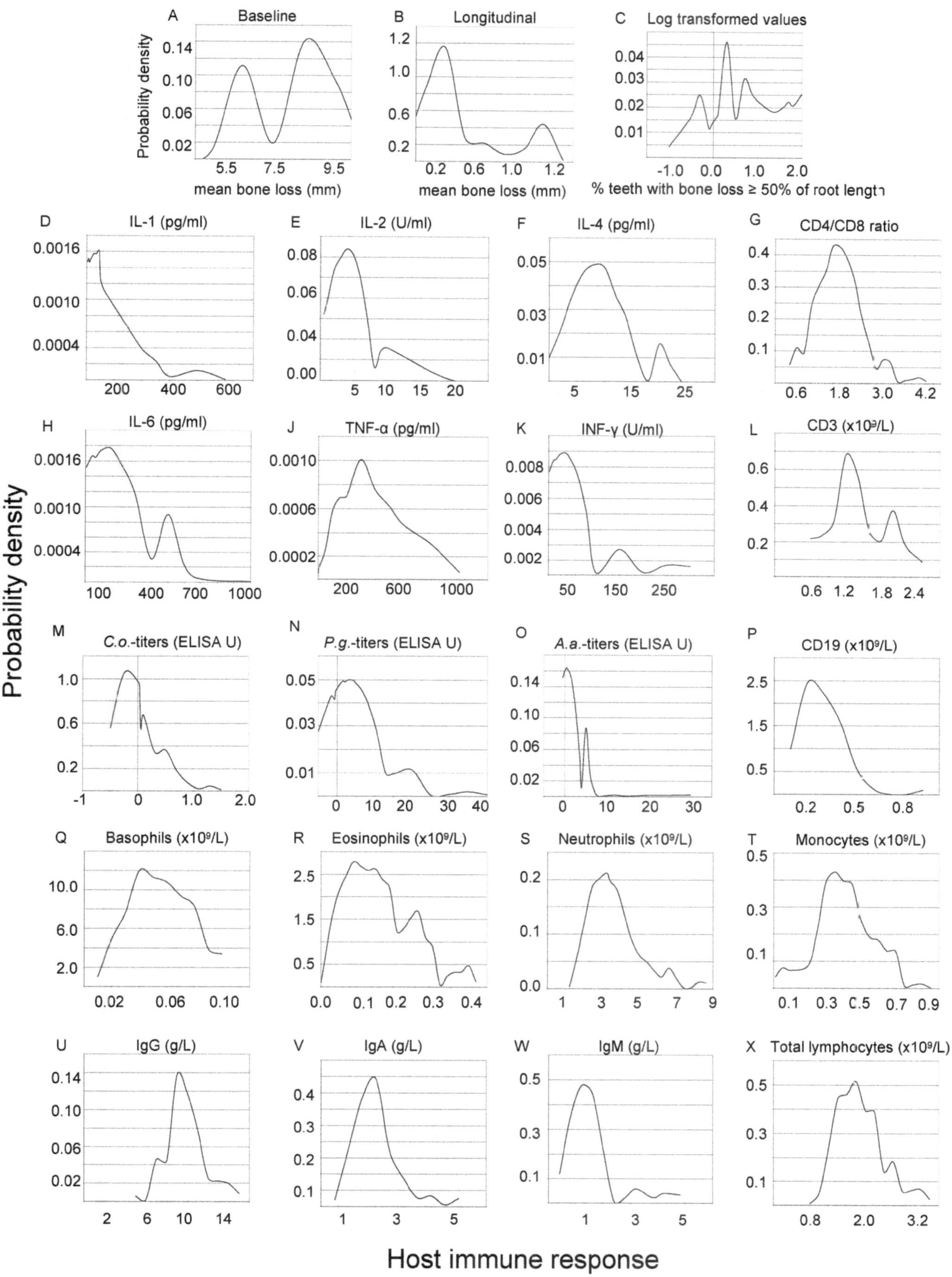

A Baseline
B Longitudinal
C Log transformed values
Probability density
mean bone loss (mm)
mean bone loss (mm)
% teeth with bone loss ≥ 50% of root length
D IL-1 (pg/ml)
E IL-2 (U/ml)
F IL-4 (pg/ml)
G CD4/CD8 ratio
H IL-6 (pg/ml)
J TNF-α (pg/ml)
K INF-γ (U/ml)
L CD3 (x10⁹/L)
M C.o.-titers (ELISA U)
N P.g.-titers (ELISA U)
O A.a.-titers (ELISA U)
P CD19 (x10⁹/L)
Q Basophils (x10⁹/L)
R Eosinophils (x10⁹/L)
S Neutrophils (x10⁹/L)
T Monocytes (x10⁹/L)
U IgG (g/L)
V IgA (g/L)
W IgM (g/L)
X Total lymphocytes (x10⁹/L)
Probability density
Host immune response

Figure 2. Univariate kernel density estimation (KDE) graphs. Graphs A to C. Univariate KDE for radiographic bone loss measurements: modes (single, bimodal or multimodal) are defined as the values that appear more frequent. Graphs A & B from sample-1. In graph C (sample-2) we log transformed the confined data to find support in the interval $(-\infty, +\infty)$ (see text S1). Graphs D to X. Univariate KDE for immunologic data: possible evidence of multimodality for the CD4/CD8 ratio, CD3, lymphocytes, monocytes, eosinophils, basophils and neutrophils counts (sample-2), IgG levels (sample-3), IL-2, IL-4, IL-6, INF-γ, TNF-α, IgG *A.a.* titers and IgG *C.o.* titers (sample-4). Mini clusters close to each other are detected for IL-1 and IgG *P.g* titers (sample-4).

(from sample-4). We didn't mix parameters from the two samples. The results of ARD on feature selection are presented in Table S2 in File S1. ANN_1 showed high accuracy (98.1%) followed close by ANN_2 (95.6%), while ANN_3 was left behind in overall accuracy (90%) (Table 1). For comparison to the ANNs performance, we conducted canonical discriminant analysis and binary logistic regression using the above selected inputs. They both displayed inferior results compared to the ANNs (Table S3 in File S1).

Discussion

We found by KDE techniques possible evidence of two modes in radiographic bone loss and selected immunologic data. We also fitted probability models to our datasets. In training ANNs we used *CE* values instead of original data. This might seem an unnecessary complication, but the ANNs were trained far better providing higher prediction accuracy. We can only speculate on the reason for that. It might have been that the smoothing parameter in KDE fine-tuned the complexity of ANNs via a shrinking effect on weights; increasing complexity directly relates to an increasing variance of ANNs test error and poorer prediction outcome [28,29]. The nonsymmetric nature of *CE* might also have facilitated the learning process.

ANNs have been used in monitoring medical conditions, where a complex combination of changes in multiple variables is associated with the onset of a disease [30]. ANNs simulate the *tabula rasa* or clean-slate learning we find associated with biological processes [14]. ANNs using the softmax transfer function and the *CE* error function are equivalent to linear logistic regression in the hidden units [28]. However, a growing number of studies in various scientific fields indicate that ANNs provide higher prediction accuracy than multiple regression models in solving classification problems [31]. This was also shown by our results (Table S3 in File S1). We must note however, that the performance of an ANN is variable, depending on the learning method used. In fact, ANNs in supervised machine learning methodology are found to approximate any function with arbitrary accuracy. However, they are susceptible to the overfitting problem [29]. Our results indicate that ANNs can be helpful in the diagnosis of AgP in a periodontal practice, while they appear unsuitable for monitoring the general population where a test with almost 100% specificity is required.

Clustering periodontal patients to gain insight into the pathogenesis of periodontitis is not a new idea. Among the vast literature, we can distinguish a study that analysed differences among 5 groups of patients [32]; grouping was based on pocket depth (PD) and bleeding on probing scores (BOP). Using logistic regression *C. rectus* antibody titers was the best single predictor among all IgG titers of one of the 5 phenotypes and *P. gingivalis* titers found the best single predictor of other three phenotypes. The study supported the microbial specificity of periodontitis pathogenesis. However, the discontinuity of the grouping method used in the study, like in the use of histograms, translates into inefficient use of the data and causes huge difficulties when derivatives of the estimates are required. The situation can be perplexed by the combination of two parameters (PD and BOP). In contrast, KDE when used as intermediate component of another method, like in the current study, is particularly justified as an alternative to histograms.

The main body of the periodontal literature relevant to cluster analysis is based on similarities of subgingival microbiota, followed by investigation of clinical and immunologic differences among clusters. For example, hierarchical cluster analysis identified 5 groups of AgP patients of similar subgingival microbiota [33]; IL-1β/IL-10 ratio in gingival crevicular fluid (GCF) was significantly different among groups. A recent review underscored the fact that although bacteria initiate periodontitis, disease progression is multidimensional and poorly understood [34]. Our unsupervised grouping method on immunologic parameters from peripheral blood determined clusters by local maxima of the overall density function. However, one can question the validity of the *in vitro* interleukin evaluation tests. Using parameters from GCF or saliva [35] is an alternative that may enhance the prediction or generalization ability of ANNs. Our hypothesis that the host immune response level is the determinant of periodontitis disease rate [8], agrees with the recently proposed paradigm for periodontitis pathogenesis [36]; it is suggested that even the immune response level mounted at the early stage of gingivitis is the determinant factor of periodontitis progression and not the presence of specific bacteria known for their virulent properties. On this basis it becomes meaningful to use immunologic parameters by nonlinear methods to discriminate AgP from CP.

It is currently understood that for the behavior of a complex disease many components intricately and dynamically interact; the emergence of the behavior of a complex system cannot be explained by considering its contributing parts separately (the whole does not equal the sum of the parts) [4]. The biological relevance of our results can be evaluated through the above realization. A complex system is not static: it undergoes continuous scale transformations. At one scale some factors compete to each other and at another scale below or above they act in synergy. That makes it difficult to find significant differences between AgP and CP when simple comparisons are made, for example by mean values of immunologic parameters. On the other hand, ANNs start nearly linear (with weights near zero) and become nonlinear as the weights increase [28]. As they grow they learn the nonlinear patterns of the data through the backpropagation of their misclassification error. However, the problem with ANNs remains their generalization ability and overfitting is always a concern [28,29].

The limitations of the methodology used in this study should be addressed. First of all, there are no rules for determining how large a sample should be for justifying the application of ANNs. However, having larger samples would allow us to leave a portion of the patients entirely out of the training process to finally evaluate upon this portion the general performance of the models. This seems to be an objective way to test the generalization ability of the models. Secondly, regarding the ANNs design, it is better to have too many hidden units than too few. The number of hidden units varies in relation to the number of inputs and the size of the training sample, usually being in the range of 5 to 100 [28]. With too few hidden units, the model might not have enough flexibility to capture the nonlinearities in the data; with too many hidden

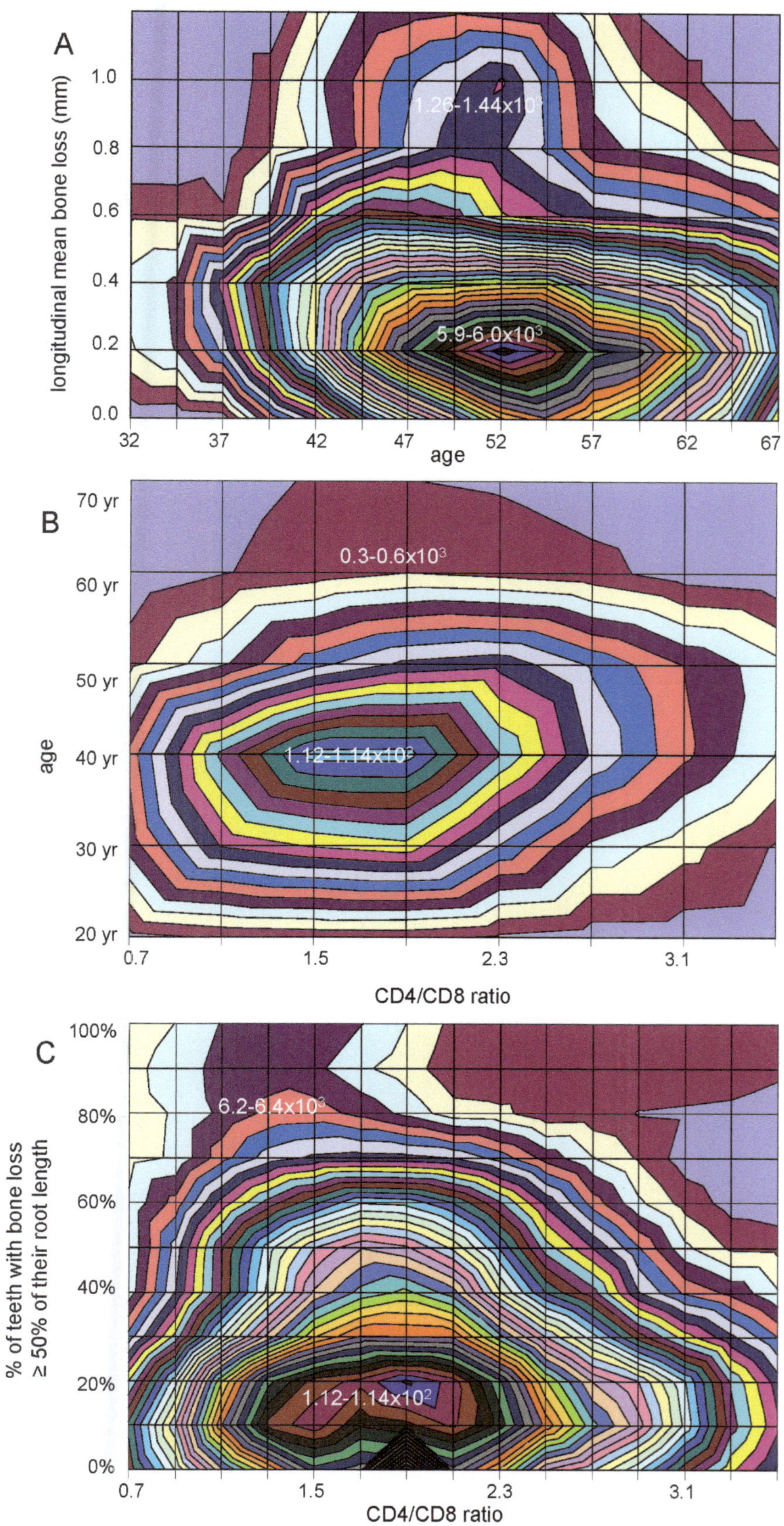

Figure 3. Bivariate kernel density estimation (KDE) for some selected parameters. (A) Contour plot for bivariate KDE of longitudinal radiographic bone loss level (sample-1) in relation to age: this topographical-like plot shows a main cluster with 0.2 mm longitudinal bone loss and a small cluster with almost five times greater bone loss. (B) Contour plot for bivariate KDE: By estimating probability density for CD4/CD8 ratio by age (sample-2), we see two clusters although not separated distinctly, at modes of 1.5 and 1.9. (C) Contour plot for bivariate KDE: By estimating

probability density for CD4/CD8 ratio (sample-2) by disease severity (% of teeth with bone loss ≥ of 50% of their root length), we reveal two distinct clusters of patients, with modes at *x* values of 1.5 and 1.9.

units the model will suffer from overfitting. Overfitting is avoided by early stopping or regularization. A common technique of regularization is to add a penalty in the error function, as we actually did (see text S1). By early stopping or by regularization we want to stop training well before we approach the global minimum, where neural networks with too many weights generally overfit the data. Third, not removing irrelevant input features would affect the classification accuracy of the network. Feature pruning typically increases the generalization ability of classifiers [29]. It is realized, however, that a variable, even though useless by itself, can be useful in combination with others [37]. Therefore, a limited set of candidate features may miss a potent combination of features. On the other hand, the variance-bias trade-off problem calls for our attention when we increase the complexity of the model. Too many features will decrease the training error by overfitting and at the same time will increase the test (generalization) error [28].

The diagnostic criteria for AgP and CP were different among the 4 patient groups used for this study. One sample [15] was selected on the basis of the presence of severe periodontitis with no discrimination of AgP or CP. The sole criterion of disease severity was obviously inadequate to predict the future behaviour of all patients. A small subgroup of patients showed a 5 times higher rate of longitudinal bone loss than the main cluster of patients (Figure 3A). This is definitely a group of patients with aggressive disease behavior. Takahashi's group [19] used the current classification scheme [5]; however, discrimination of AgP and CP was as much as possible precise, resulting in a group of "suspected" for AgP patients, which contributed to KDE but was not used in ANNs. The other two samples used in this study suffered of a crude method in designating patients into the AgP or CP group. Obviously one can argue why we should concern ourselves for a complicated method while by taking the age of 35 as a cutoff point, one has a classification [38]. However we demonstrated that even in "noisy" samples (some AgP cases are declared CP and vice versa) a host immune classifier can work with arbitrary accuracy. We assume this kind of noise is present even with the established criteria for AgP diagnosis [5]. Recently a

Table 1. Characteristics of three artificial neural networks (ANN) built on immunological parameters.

Input neurons	Network's description	Results[f]
ANN_1		
CE[a] values of	#[o] of hidden layers = 1,	Sensitivity = 98,6%,
1. CD4/CD8[b]	# of neurons in hidden layer = 9,	Specificity = 97.9%
2. Neutrophils	max. # of epochs[c] = 900,	Accuracy = 98.1%
3. Monocytes	weight decay regularization parameter[d] = 0.0001,	
4. Eosinophils	learning method = batch[e], gradient descent.	
ANN_2		
CE values of	# of hidden layers = 1,	Sensitivity = 92.3%,
1. IL-1[g]	# of neurons in hidden layer = 10,	Specificity = 96.9%
2. IL-4	max. # of epochs = 800,	Accuracy = 95.6%
3. IFN-γ[h]	weight decay regularization parameter = 0.0005,	
4. TNF-α[i]	learning method = batch, gradient descent.	
ANN_3		
CE values of	# of hidden layers = 1,	Sensitivity = 91.1%,
1. *A.a.*[k] titers	# of neurons in hidden layer = 10,	Specificity = 89.4%
2. *P.g.*[l] titers	max. # of epochs = 1000,	Accuracy = 90.0%
3. *C.o.*[m] titers	weight decay regularization parameter = 0.005,	
4. *F.n.*[n] titers	learning method = batch, gradient descent.	

[a]CE = Cross entropy. Feature selection by automatic relevance determination.
[b]CD = cluster of differentiation.
[c]epoch = iteration.
[d]Determined by 10-fold cross validation.
[e]Batch training passes all input data before updating the synaptic weights.
[f]The mean values of 10 random configurations of initial weights are reported (mean values of sensitivity, specificity and overall accuracy of the ANNs against the original clinical diagnosis).
[g]IL = interleukin.
[h]INF = interferon.
[i]TNF = tumor necrosis factor.
[k]*A.a.* = *Aggregatibacter actinomycetemcomitans*(Y4 antigen).
[l]*P.g.* = *Porphyromonas gingivalis*(FDC381 antigen).
[m]*C.o.* = *Capnocytophaga ochracea.*
[n]*F.n.* = *Fusobacterium nucleatum.*
[o]# = Number.

study using a transcriptome classifier with four supervised learning methods reported good prediction results by one of the four; AgP or CP diagnosis was strictly made by the established criteria [39]. The authors suggested possible heterogeneity within the AgP and CP classes based on the variability of the results of the four methods. The combined use of unsupervised with supervised learning methods can be an attempt to reduce true misclassification error [28]. We realize that the AgP diagnostic criteria for the patients of sample-2 limit the generalization ability of the ANN results based on it.

In conclusion, we demonstrated by KDE methods possible evidence of two clusters on clinical and most immunological data from periodontitis patients. By the use of ANNs we can effectively classify periodontitis patients by their immune response profile into the AgP or CP class. We anticipate that future work on bigger samples extending the results of the present study and employing a wider array of parameters can turn personalized treatment of periodontitis from concept to reality.

Supporting Information

File S1 This file includes the following: Text S1. Selection of a kernel function; Fitting clinical datasets to probability models; Constructing multilayer perceptron neural networks. **Table S1.** The fit of probability distribution models to clinical and immunological data. **Table S2.** Input feature selection by automatic relevance determination. **Table S3.** Comparison of two multivariate analyses to artificial neural networks.

Figure S1 An example of quantile to quantile plots.

Author Contributions

Conceived and designed the experiments: GP BGL. Performed the experiments: GP BGL KT. Analyzed the data: GP TB. Contributed reagents/materials/analysis tools: BGL KT. Wrote the paper: GP BGL TB.

References

1. Kinane DF, Berglund T, Lindhe J (2008) Pathogenesis of periodontitis. In: Lindhe J, Karring T, Lang NP, editors. Clinical Periodontology and Implant Dentistry. Blackwell Munksgaard: Oxford. pp. 285–306.
2. Eke PI, Dye BA, Wei L, Thornton-Evans GO, Genco RJ (2012) Prevalence of periodontitis in adults in the United States: 2009 and 2010. J Dent Res 91:914–920.
3. Laine ML, Crielaard W, Loos BG (2012) Genetic susceptibility to periodontitis. Periodontol 2000 58:37–68.
4. Nicolis G, Nicolis C (2012) Foundations of complex systems: emergence, information and prediction. World Scientific: Singapore. 12 p.
5. Armitage GC (1999) Developement of a classification system for periodontal diseases and conditions. Ann Periodontol 4:1–6.
6. Armitage GC (2013) Learned and unlearned concepts in periodontal diagnostics: a 50-year perspective. Periodontol 2000 62:20–36.
7. Tonetti MS, Mombelli A (2008) Aggressive periodontitis. In: Lindhe J, Karring T, Lang NP, editors. Clinical Periodontology and Implant Dentistry. Blackwell Munksgaard: Oxford. pp. 428–458.
8. Armitage GC, Cullinan MP (2010) Comparison of the clinical features of chronic and aggressive periodontitis. Periodontol 2000 53:12–27.
9. Papantonopoulos G, Takahashi K, Bountis T, Loos BG (2013a) Using cellular automata experiments to model periodontitis: A first step towards understanding the nonlinear dynamics of the disease. Int J Bifurcation Chaos 23:1350056.
10. Papantonopoulos G, Takahashi K, Bountis T, Loos BG (2013b) Mathematical modeling suggests periodontitis behaves as a nonlinear chaotic dynamical process. J Periodontol 84(10):e29–e39.
11. Silverman BW (1986) Density estimation for statistics and data analysis. Chapman and Hall: London. 6 p.
12. Simonoff JS (1996) Smoothing methods in statistics. New York: Springer-Verlag: New York. 13 p.
13. Sheather SJ (2004) Density estimation. Stat Science 19:588–597.
14. Abdi H (2003) Neural networks. In: Lewis-Beck M, Bryman A, Futing T, editors. Encyclopaedia of Social Sciences Research Methods. Sage: Thousand Oaks (CA). pp. 725–729.
15. Papantonopoulos G (2004) Effect of periodontal therapy in smokers and nonsmokers with advanced periodontal disease: Results after maintenance therapy for a minimum of 5 years. J Periodontol 75:839–843.
16. Loos BG, Craandijk J, Hoek FJ, Wertheim-van Dillen PME, van der Velden U (2000) Elevation of systemic markers related to cardiovascular diseases in the peripheral blood of periodontitis patients. J Periodontol 71:1528–1534.
17. Loos BG, Roos MT, Schellekens PT, van der Velden U, Miedema F (2004) Lymphocyte number and function in relation to periodontitis and smoking. J Periodontol 75:557–564.
18. Graswinckel JEM, van der Velden U,van Winkelhoff AJ, Hoek FJ, Loos BG (2004) Plasma antibody levels in periodontitis patients and controls. J Clin Periodontol 31:562–568.
19. Takahashi K, Ohyama H, Kitanaka M, Sawa T, Mineshiba J, et al. (2001) Heterogeneity of host immunological risk factors in patients with aggressive periodontitis. J Periodontol 72:425–437.
20. Kinane DF (2001) Periodontal disease in children and adolescents: introduction and classification. Periodontol 2000 26:7–15.
21. Hall P, Kang KH (2005) Bandwidth choice for nonparametric classification. Ann Statist 33:284–306.
22. Vose D (2008) Risk analysis: A quantitative guide. West Sussex: John Wiley & Sons. 115 p.
23. Sakamoto Y, Ishikuro M, Kitaqawa G (1986) Akaike information criterion statistics. Springer-Verlag: New York. 56 p.
24. Myung J (2003) Tutorial on maximum likelihood estimation. J Math Psychol 47:90–100.
25. Burnham KP, Anderson DR (2004) Multimodel inference: understanding AIC and BIC in model selection. Sociol Methods Res 33:261–304.
26. de Boer PT, Kroese DP, Mannor S, Rubinstein RY (2005) A tutorial on the cross-entropy method. Ann Oper Res 134:18–67.
27. Neal R, Zhang J (2006) High dimensional classification with bayesian neural networks and dirichlet diffusion trees. In: Guyon I, Gunn S, Nikravesh M, Zadeh L, editors. Feature Extraction, Foundations and Applications. Springer: New York. pp. 265–296.
28. Hastie T, Tibshirani R, Friedman J (2009) The elements of statistical learning: Data mining, inference, and prediction. Springer: New York. 389 p.
29. Zhang GP (2000) Neural networks for classification: A survey. IEEE Trans Syst Man Cybern 30:451–462.
30. Mazurowski MA, Habas PA, Zurada JM, Lo JY, Baker JA, et al. (2008) Training neural network classifiers for medical decision making; The effects of imbalanced datasets on classification performance. Neural Netw 21:427–436.
31. Shi H-Y, Lee K-T, Lee H-H, Ho W-H, Sun D-P, et al. (2012) Comparison of artificial neural network and logistic regression models for predicting in-hospital mortality after primary liver cancer surgery. PLOS ONE 7(4):e35781.
32. Offenbacher S, Barros SP, Singer RE, Moss K, Williams RC, et al. (2007) Periodontal disease at the biofilm-gingival interface. J Periodontol 78:1911–1925.
33. Teles RP, Gursky LC, Faveri M, Rosa EA, Teles FRF, et al. (2010) Relationships between subgingival microbiota and GCF biomarkers in generalized aggressive periodontitis. J Clin Periodontol 37: 313–323.
34. Razzouk S, Termechi O (2013) Host genome, epigenome, and oral microbiome interactions: towards personalized periodontal therapy. J Periodontol 84:1266–1271.
35. Loos BG, Tjoa S (2005) Host-derived diagnostic markers for periodontitis: do they exist in gingival crevicular fluid? Periodontol 2000 39:53–72.
36. Bartold PM, Van Dyke E (2013) Periodontitis: a host-mediated disruption of microbial homeostasis. Unlearning learned concepts. Periodontol 2000 62:203–217.
37. Guyon I, Elisseeff A (2003) An introduction to variable and feature selection. J Mach Learn Res 3:1157–1182.
38. Van der Velden U (2005) Purpose and problems of periodontal disease classification. Periodontol 2000 39:13–21.
39. Kebschull M, Guarnieri P, Demmer RT, Boulesteix AL, Pavlidis P, et al. (2013) Molecular Differences between Chronic and Aggressive Periodontitis. J Dent Res 92:1081–1088.

16

Inequalities in Oral Health for Children with Disabilities: A French National Survey in Special Schools

Martine Hennequin[1,2]*, Véronique Moysan[3], Didier Jourdan[4], Martine Dorin[3], Emmanuel Nicolas[1,2]

1 University of Auvergne (Clermont 1) EA 3847, Clermont-Ferrand, France, **2** CHU de Clermont-Ferrand, Clermont-Ferrand, France, **3** Caisse Nationale de l'Assurance Maladie des Travailleurs Salariés (CNAMTS), Paris, France, **4** Institut Universitaire de Formation des Maîtres, JE 2432, Clermont-Ferrand, France

Abstract

Background: Despite wide recognition that children with disability often have poor oral health, few high quality, controlled results are available.

Method: Twenty-four objective and subjective criteria covering feeding, autonomy, access to dental care, oral hygiene, oral disease, general health and behavior were evaluated in a observational cross-sectional study of 2,487 children with disability (DC group), 4,772 adolescents with disability (DA group) and 1,641 children without disability (NDC group). Five algorithms ranked the subjects according to clinical criteria in three original oral health indices: the Clinical Oral Health Index (COHI), indicating the level of oral health problems, the Clinical Oral Care Needs Index (COCNI) giving dental care need levels, and the Clinical Oral Prevention Index (COPI) determining possible needs in terms of dental education initiatives.

Results: DC-group children presented poorer oral health and had greater needs in both treatment and preventive oral health actions than NDC-group children (OR = 3.97, 95% CI = 3.25–4.86 for COHI; OR = 2.01, 95% CI = 1.77–2.28 for COCNI; OR = 5.25, 95% CI = 4.55–6.02 for COPI). These conditions were worse again in the DA group comparing to the DC group (OR = 3.52, 95% CI = 2.7–4.6 for COHI; OR = 1.52, 95% CI = 1.38–1.69 for COCNI; OR = 1.53, 95% CI = 1.39–1.69 for COPI).

Conclusion: Clinical indices generated by algorithmic association of various clinical indicators allow sensitive clinical measurement, and in this study demonstrated inequalities in oral health for children with disabilities schooling in institutions. Questions need now to be addressed as to the measures that could be taken to compensate for this situation.

Editor: An-Wen Chan, University of Toronto, Canada

Funding: The survey that provided the data for the DC and DA groups was given financial support by three French national health insurance schemes (the Caisse Nationale d'Assurance Maladie des Travailleurs Salariés (CNAMTS), the Mutualité Sociale Agricole (MSA) and the Assurance Maladie des Professions Indépendantes (RSI)) that had pooled their resources under a national research program (Programme National Inter Régimes 2004). The survey that provided the data for the NDC group was given financial support through two research teams: JE 2432 from the Auvergne region teacher training institute and EA 3847 from the University of Auvergne. The current analysis received financial support from the EA 3847 research team, which participated in building the methodology for both projects, designed the study, built the database, analyzed the data, wrote the paper, and managed the submission process for publication.

Competing Interests: The authors have declared that no competing interests exist.

* E-mail: martine.hennequin@u-clermont1.fr

Introduction

Oral health is often considered as a probable source of health inequalities in persons with neuromotor and mental deficiencies. The quality of the evidence base supporting this assumption is not high despite numerous studies reporting poor oral health in patient groups with disabilities. Many studies have no control group, use inappropriate indicators or report a partial evaluation of oral health. The 2001 National Survey of Children with Special Health Care Needs conducted in the USA showed that dental care was the most commonly-reported unmet service need [1]. However, none of the clinical data collected through a large sample was able to confirm the parents' declarations. Some studies have aimed to measure only the prevalence of infectious disease, such as carious process or periodontal disease [2–4], while others have focused on the occurrence of anatomical deficiencies [5–7], traumatic disease [8] or functional incapacity [9–12]. Oral health is, however, a far more complex concept that encompasses all aspects of health related to the mouth, the jaw, the teeth, the throat and related tissues [13,14]. Self-rated questionnaires on oral health-related quality of life aim to offer a global measure of the concept of health but their use is not feasible by the majority of people with intellectual disability [15–17]. Proxy questionnaires have been developed for use with persons presenting special medical conditions [18,19], but they remain too specific to be used universally across all disability groups. The lack of appropriate indicators has consequently made it impossible to compare oral health between groups with and without disabilities. This study was thus designed to provide epidemiological data on oral health gathered using original indicators from a representative sample of children and adolescents with disabilities in France.

Method

Database setting

This observational cross-sectional study compared data gathered in the same conditions through two surveys. The design for data base setting is shown in Figure 1. One dataset was taken from

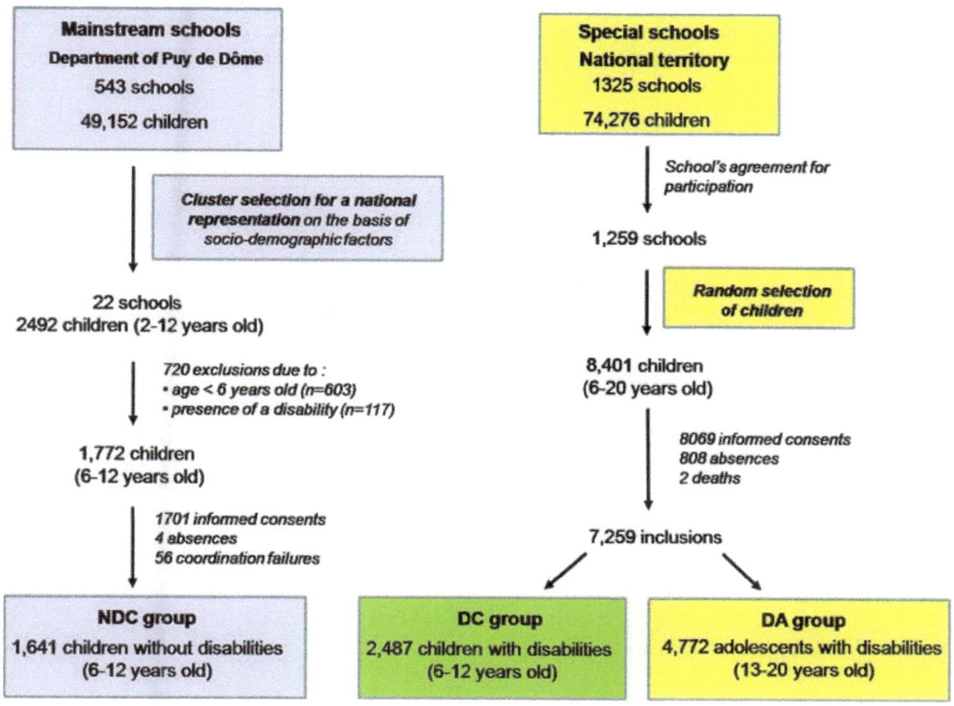

Figure 1. Design for data base setting.

a national survey that evaluated oral health in a sample of 6 to 20-year-old children and adolescents in special schooling. The second dataset was taken from a regional survey of a nationally representative sample of 6 to 12-year-old children without disabilities in mainstream schooling. The database thus included three groups differentiated by both age and presence of a disability: one group comprising of 6 to 12-year-old children without disability (NDC group), a second group made up of 6 to 12-year-old children with disability (DC group), and a third group comprising of 13 to 20-year-old adolescents and young adults with disability (DA group). Consent for participation was obtained from the school directors, class teachers, parents, and adult subjects. All legal conditions for epidemiological surveys were respected, and the French national commission governing the application of data privacy laws (the '*Commission Nationale Informatique et Libertés*') issued approval for both projects.

Children, adolescents and young adults with disability. The sample populations of children and adolescents with disability were derived from the databases of three national health insurance systems. The population comprised of all 74,276 children, adolescents and young adults born between the 1st October 1984 and the 31st January 1999 attending one of the 1,325 special schools registered in France. The sample size was calculated to determine the results with a 99% Confidence Interval and a precision of ±1.5% around the calculated value. Theoretical national sample size thus reached 7,373 statistical units. Since the risk of non-response was evaluated at between 25% and 35%, the sample size was raised to 10,000 statistical units. For random selection, all children born on a 4th, 7th, 21st or 27th day of the month were included. The survey was conducted between October 2004 and January 2005.

Children without disabilities. The sample of children without disabilities comprised the entire population of 2 to 12-year-old healthy children attending schools situated in the department of Puy de Dôme. This group was devised to be nationally representative, by performing a cluster evaluation design with the school as the intervention unit. The schools were selected on the basis of the following criteria: rural or urban location, socioeconomic status (4 standard groups from underprivileged to highly privileged) and size (more or less than 4 classes) in two school districts (corresponding to a population of 106,088 inhabitants). Twenty two schools were sampled based on these criteria. Comparison between the sample and national data [20] is showed in Table 1. Children under 6 years old and children

Table 1. Characteristics (expressed as %) of the sample compared to national data [20].

	Location of the schools		Socio-economic status				Number of classes in the school	
	rural	urban	1	2	3	4	<4 classes	>4 classes
Sample	54.6%	45.4%	13.0%	17.7%	26.8%	42.2%	40.9%	59.1%
France (#)	47.0%	53%	17.9%	14.1%	26.6%	41.4%	41.4%	58.6%

The location is based on the INSEE (National Institute for Statistics and Economic Studies) definition (more or less than 2000 inhabitants in the city), the socioeconomic status analysis is based on the standards of the education department (from 1: privileged to 4: underprivileged). There is no national data for the location, so the regional data were used.

Table 2. Conditions observed by algorithms ranking children among Clinical Oral Health Index values.

COHI Values		CRITERIA
0		**Having no criteria that had a medical impact:**
No oral health problems		No mucosal lesion on lips, tongue or jaw
		and Absence of dental plaque (Greene and Vermillon index = 0 for both arches) [35]
		and Absence of calculus (Greene and Vermillon index = 0 for both arches) [35]
		and No gingivitis (Loe and Silness index = 0 for both arches) [36]
		and No fractured anterior tooth
		and No missing anterior tooth
		and No missing posterior tooth
		and No dental caries
		and No infectious disease
		and No severe orofacial dysmorphology
		AND having no criteria that had a social impact:
		No halitosis
		and No drooling
		and No anterior tooth with a fractured, unrestored crown
1	OR	**Having no criteria that had a medical impact:**
Existence of one or more problems with a low to a moderate impact on health		No mucosal lesion on lips, tongue or jaw
		or Absence of dental plaque (Green and Vermillon index = 0 for both arches) [35]
		or Absence of calculus (Green and Vermillon index = 0 for both arches) [35]
		or No gingivitis (Loe and Silness index = 0 for both arches) [36]
		or No fractured anterior tooth
		or No missing anterior tooth
		or No missing posterior tooth
		or No dental caries
		or No infectious disease
		or No orofacial dysmorphology
		AND having at least one criteria that had a social impact:
		Presence of halitosis
		or Presence of drooling
		or At least one anterior tooth with a fractured unrestored crown
		Having at least one criterion that had a medical impact
		At least one mucosal lesion on lips, tongue or jaw
		or Dental plaque (Greene and Vermillon index >0, on a group of teeth or all the teeth of at least one arch) [35]
		or Calculus (Greene and Vermillon index >0, on a group of teeth or all the teeth of at least one arch) [35]
		or Localized gingivitis (Loe and Silness index >0 on a group of teeth or at least one arch) [36]
		or At least one anterior tooth with a fractured, unrestored crown
		or One limited anterior edentulous segment (1 or 2 anterior teeth)
		or At least one minor posterior edentulous segment (missing all molars and premolars on 1 or 2 half-arches with at least one residual inter-arch dental contact)
		or At least one incipient carious lesion, but no developed carious lesion (stage 1 or 2 according to the Eckstrand classification for carious lesions) [37]
		or Presence of a simple orofacial dysmorphology
		... regardless of the criteria that had a social impact
2		**Having at least one criteria that had an important medical impact**
Existence of one or more problems with important to severe impact on health		Generalized gingivitis (Loe and Silness index >0 for both arches) [35]
		or Missing at least 3 anterior teeth
		or At least one major posterior edentulous segment (missing all molar and premolars on at least 2 half-arches, without any residual inter-arch dental contact)

Table 2. Cont.

COHI Values		CRITERIA
	or	At least one developed carious lesion (stage 3 or 4 according to the Eckstrand classification for carious lesions) either on a deciduous or a permanent tooth [37]
	or	At least one infected lesion (presence of an abscess, or a tooth with pulpal exposure, or a fistula)
	or	Presence of complex orofacial dysmorphology
		... regardless of the criteria that had a social impact
Undetermined		At least one undetermined criteria that had a medical impact and regardless of the criteria that had a social impact.
Others conditions by elimination	or	Having no criteria that had a medical impact but having at least one undetermined criteria that had a social impact.

who received special schooling time for medical reasons were not included in the database. The survey was conducted between January and May 2005.

Data collection

Investigators. Examination of the children, adolescents and young adults with disability was conducted by 338 salaried dentists belonging to one of the three French national health insurance schemes. The investigator first conducted a structured interview with the child and his or her carer, and then examined the child. Any modification in the child's behavior or any declaration that suggested discomfort or distress led to the evaluation being interrupted. For the group of children without disability, the evaluation was conducted by 7 dentists who collected the data under these same conditions. All investigators underwent a one-day training course in their region prior to starting the study. The course consisted of three hours on the conditions for data collection and three hours on the psychosocial conditions of the population of children with disabilities.

Development of the list of indicators. A initial list of 36 indicators for examination was generated from literature review, interviews with professional experts in special care dentistry, in special education and with practitioners of the health insurance system. They were descriptions of global health, feeding, autonomy, access to dental care, oral hygiene, oral disease, and behavior. The feasibility of data collection and the clinical and social significance of the indicators were initially tested with a sample of 236 children and adolescents from 27 institutions distributed in 7 regions. Items resulting in a response rate of less than 70% were then deleted from the list that finally included 24 items. External consistency of the 24 item list was evaluated by comparing the prevalence of oral disease in the test group to the values founded in previous studies for different groups of children with disabilities. External consistency was good for food texture [21,18], difficulties in pain communication [22,23], halitosis [18] drooling [24,25], presence of dental plaque, calculus and gingivitis [18,26,27], missing teeth [28,29], fractured anterior tooth [30], caries decay [4,27,30,31], dental infectious process [29], severe dysmorphology [32], and lack of compliance during oral examination [4,33]. Cronbach's alpha was used to assess internal consistency of the list of 24 indicators for oral health evaluation. It was shown that the list was consistent ($\alpha = 0.93$).

The inclusion criteria for children with disabilities were based on the diagnoses that justified children being orientated towards special schooling. These diagnoses were defined according to standard ICD-10 criteria [34].

Subject examination. Among the 24 item list, 20 items were objective indicators that were evaluated by the investigator during the oral examination. Children and adolescents in DC and DA groups were examined in the school dispensary in presence of their carer. Children in the NDC group were examined in their classroom in the presence of their teacher. For the evaluation of objective criteria, the investigators used disposable gloves, a mouth mirror and a portable light. Drying teeth and the use of a dental probe, both of which are indicated for caries and periodontal disease screening in the general population [35–37], were prohibited so as to avoid discomfort or injury. Four subjective indicators of oral health were obtained during a structured interview with the carer for each subject with disability, and with the child him or herself for each child without disability.

Stability of the indicators. Considering the vulnerability of the target population, it would have been unethical to build a true sample of children with disability for the calibration of the investigators. A virtual sample was therefore simulated with a set of 144 photos of the mouths of 6 to 20-year-old children and young adults with and without oral disease. The investigators had to evaluate the pictures twice, with a one-week interval.

Internal reliability was verified by paired comparisons of consistency between the two evaluations for all 144 pictures (intra-class correlation coefficients (ICC, r), and kappa coefficients (k)). Among the investigators who evaluated the children and adolescents with disabilities, 269 (79.6%) participated in the reliability test. Test-retest revealed that internal reliability was acceptable for the 144 pictures (mean ICC 95%, $r = 0.65$; $k = 0.49$, ($p<0.001$)). The distribution of the investigators within the range of the ICC values was: $r>0.4$ for 6 investigators (2.2%); $0.4<r<0.6$ for 48 investigators (17.8%); $0.6<r<0.8$ for 211 investigators (78.4%); and $0.8<r$ for 4 investigators (1.5%). External reliability was verified by testing the agreement between the criteria values given for each picture by the group of 269 investigators (ICC 95%, $r = 0.63$). All 7 investigators examining the group of children without disabilities participated in the reliability test. Test-retest showed that internal reliability was acceptable for the set of 144 pictures (mean 95% ICC, $r = 0.74$; $k = 0.46$) and that external reliability was good (95% ICC, $r = 0.86$).

Data analysis. Indicators of oral health were then associated to produce 3 original indices for global oral health. Initially a series of 3 algorithms were performed using logical association (If... then... else...) to rank the subjects according to the 4 levels of the Clinical Oral Health Index (COHI) (Table 2). A fourth algorithm was then used to rank the subjects according to the 4 levels of the Clinical Oral Care Needs Index (COCNI) (Table 3). Finally,

Table 3. Conditions observed by algorithms ranking children among Clinical Oral Care Needs Index values.

COCNI Values	Suspected health conditions	CRITERIA
3 Urgent need for care or examination	Marker of local infectious disease	During the last three months the child expressed discomfort or pain in his/her mouth and consecutively he/she had no dental visit. or At least one mucosal lesion on lips, tongue or jaw or At least one infected lesion (presence of an abscess, or a tooth with pulp exposure cavity, or a fistula) AND absence of any systemic disease* requiring specific oral health monitoring.
	Marker of focal infectious disease	During the last three months the child expressed discomfort or pain in his/her mouth and consecutively he/she had no dental visit. or Presence of at least one mucosal lesion on lips, tongue or jaw or At least one infected lesion (presence of an abscess, or a tooth with a pulp exposure, or a fistula) or Presence of generalized gingivitis (Loe and Silness index >0 for both arches) AND Existence of a systemic disease requiring specific oral health monitoring*
	Marker of traumatic lesions	During the last three months the child expressed discomfort or pain in his/her mouth and consecutively he/she had no dental visit. or Presence of at least one mucosal lesion on lips, tongue or jaw
	Marker of oral disease with functional or social consequences	During the last three months the child expressed discomfort or pain with his/her mouth and consecutively he/she had no dental visit.
2 Need for care or examination	Marker of local infectious disease	Presence of calculus or Presence of gingivitis or Presence of at least one anterior tooth with a fractured, unrestored crown or Presence of at least one developed carious lesion. AND Absence of a systemic disease* requiring specific oral health monitoring
	Marker of focal infectious disease	Presence of calculus. or Presence of a localized gingivitis or Presence of at least one anterior tooth with a fractured, unrestored crown or Presence of at least one developed carious lesion. AND Existence of a systemic disease* requiring specific oral health monitoring
	Marker of traumatic lesions	Presence of at least one anterior tooth with a fractured, unrestored crown
1 Need for examination	Marker of local infectious disease	No dental visit over the last 12 months or Presence of dental plaque or Presence of at least one incipient carious lesion. AND Absence of a systemic disease* requiring specific oral health monitoring
	Marker of focal infectious disease	No dental visit over the last 12 months or Presence of dental plaque or Presence of at least one incipient carious lesion. AND Existence of a systemic disease* requiring specific oral health monitoring
	Marker of traumatic lesions	No dental visit over the last 12 months
	Marker of oral disease with functional or social consequences	No dental visit over the last 12 months or Presence of an anterior edentulous segment from 1 to 6 teeth on at least one arch. or Presence of a posterior edentulous segment for children up to 13 years old) or Presence of untreated severe orofacial dysmorphology
0 No need for care nor examination		Other conditions by elimination

*Epilepsy, congenital cardiac disease, bronchopneumopathy (including asthma), internal prosthesis, immunodeficiency and hematological disease, or diabetes.

preventive health or oral health education needs were determined by applying a fifth algorithm that ranked the subjects according to the two levels of the Clinical Oral Prevention Index (COPI) (Table 4).

The distributions of the NDC and DC groups across the various levels of the COHI, COCNI and COPI indices were compared to determine whether having a disability is a risk factor for poor oral health. The impact of age on oral health status was determined by comparing the distributions of the DC and DA groups across the different levels of the COHI, COCNI and COPI oral health indices. Odds ratios (OR) were calculated at 95% confidence intervals for inter-group comparisons.

The impact of 69 (untrained) out of 338 (trained) examiners for the DC and NDC group not participating in the test retest exercise, was evaluated by comparing the distributions of the subjects evaluated by untrained and trained examiners across the different levels of the COHI, COCNI and COPI oral health indices.

Results

Descriptive results

A total of 8,401 children, adolescents and young adults with disability were randomly selected among the 1,259 institutions that

Table 4. Conditions observed by algorithms ranking children among Clinical Oral Prevention Index values.

COPI Values	CRITERIA
1	Existence of systemic disease requiring specific oral health monitoring*
Existence of at least one preventive or dental health education action need	or Presence of dental plaque
	or Lack of autonomy for feeding
	or Being fed by tube or parenteral nutrition
	or Restriction to puréed foods
	or Eating hyper-calorific food complements or drinking sweetened drinks
	or Coughing regularly during meals
	or Presence of halitosis
	or Having difficulties communicating pain
	or Drooling
	or Being uncooperative during oral examination [38]
0	
No need for either preventive health action or dental education	Other conditions, by elimination

*as defined in the descriptive results section.

agreed to participate. Refusals to participate were declared in 332 cases, absence from the institution at the time of evaluation was recorded in 808 cases, and two children died before the investigator visit. Hence, 2,487 children aged 6 to 12 years old were included in the DC group (935 males, 552 females; mean age±SD: 9.75±1.88 years (95% CI = 9.68–9.82)), and 4,772 adolescents and young adults aged 13 to 20 years old were included in the DA group (2,920 males, 1,852 females; mean age±SD: 15.85±1.92 years (95% CI = 15.79–15.90)). Medical grounds for special schooling were categorized into 8 groups as follows: 1) any intellectual disability, regardless of severity (45.4%); 2) autism (4.6%), other psychological developmental problems (11.5%), schizophrenia and delusional disorders (2%), other mental and behavioral diseases (6.8%); 3) Down syndrome (9.5%) and other chromosome anomalies (2.4%); 4) developmental disorder (3.1%) and neonatal or maternal disease (3%); 5) epilepsy (1.9%) and other anomalies of the central nervous system (3%); 6) other diseases (3.9%); 7) unfavorable family and social background (1.6%); 8) missing data (0.5%). Systemic diseases requiring oral health monitoring were recorded in both the DC and DA groups (maximum 3 per subject). Epilepsy, congenital cardiac disease, bronchopneumopathy (including asthma), internal prosthesis, immunodeficiency and hematological disease, and diabetes, were recorded for 1027, 410, 287, 32, 32 and 31 subjects, respectively. Others miscellaneous systemic diseases were recorded in 408 cases. There were no distribution-based differences either in medical conditions or in gender between the DC and DA groups.

The NDC population consisted of 1,772 healthy children aged 6 to 12 years old from 22 mainstream schools. Among this group, refusals to participate were received from either parents or teachers of 71 children, evaluation failed for lack of coordination between school staff and investigators for another 56 children, and 4 children were absent from school at the time of evaluation. Hence, 1,641 children without disability aged between 6 and 12 year old were included (862 males, 779 females; mean age±SD: 7.98±1.61 years (95%CI = 7.91–8.06)). Gender and age distribution differed significantly between DC and NDC groups with both prevalence of boys (Chi Square test, $p<0.001$) and mean age being greater in the DC group than in NDC group (Chi Square test, $p<0.01$).

Oral health status

Subject distributions in terms of oral health criteria and the indices are presented in tables 5 and 6, respectively. Distribution comparisons between the NDC and DC groups showed that more children with disability were rated COHI level 1 or 2 than level 0 (OR = 3.97; 95% CI = 3.25–4.86). Moreover, the number of children for whom some oral health indicators could not be estimated was greater in the DC group than in the NDC group (OR = 2.41; 95% CI = 1.74–3.32). Comparisons of COCNI distributions showed that more children with disability were in need of urgent care or examination (level 3) or non-urgent care (level 2) than those without disability (OR = 2.01; 95%CI = 1.77–2.28). COPI index distribution comparisons showed that more children with disability were in need of preventive oral health care or oral health education than children without disability (OR = 5.25, 95% CI = 4.55–6.02).

COHI index distribution comparisons between the DC and DA groups showed that a higher number of adolescents and young adults were rated COHI level 1 or 2 than level 0 (OR = 3.52; 95% CI = 2.7–4.6). Moreover, the number of subjects who could not be rated due to unspecified criteria was significantly higher in the DA group than in the DC group (OR = 1.3; 95% CI = 1.08–1.56). COCNI index distribution comparisons showed that more adolescents and young adults were in need of urgent care or examination (level 3) or non-urgent care (level), whereas slightly more younger children were either in need of examination (level 1) or were not in need of care or examination (level 0) than children with disabilities (OR = 1.52; 95% CI = 1.38–1.69). COPI index distribution comparisons showed that adolescents and young adults with disabilities had greater needs for preventive oral health care or oral health education actions than children (OR = 1.53, 95% CI = 1.39–1.69).

A stratified comparison between the DC and NDC groups was performed testing for the impact of gender and age on child distribution between COHI, COCNI and COPI. It was shown that the distribution of children between the DC and NDC groups remained different regardless of gender (Chi Square test, $p<0.001$, for distribution in COHI, COCNI and COPI) and age for all age classes (Chi Square test, $p<0.05$ COHI, COCNI and COPI),

Table 5. Subject distribution among the oral health criteria for the three groups of children or adolescents.

Criteria for oral health	Children without disability (NDC group) 6–12 yrs old			Children with disability (DC group) 6–12 yrs old			Adolescents with disability (DA group) 13–20 yrs old		
	n	Yes	*95%CI*	n	Yes	*95%CI*	n	Yes	*95%CI*
Lack of autonomy for feeding	1,625	2.2%	*1.5–2.9*	2,487	18.6%	*17.1–20.1*	4,772	9.6%	*8.8–10.4*
Eating puréed foods	1,621	1.2%	*0.7–1.7*	2,466	8.4%	*7.3–9.5*	4,743	4.5%	*3.9–5.1*
Being fed by tube or parenteral nutrition	1,641	0.0%	*0*	2,487	0.8%	*0.5–1.2*	4,772	0.6%	*0.4–0.8*
Drinking sweetened drinks regularly	1,625	25.9%	*23.8–28.0*	2,483	11.9%	*10.7–13.2*	4,768	10.6%	*9.7–11.5*
Coughing often during meals	1,621	7.4%	*6.1–8.7*	2,188	31.9%	*30–33.9*	4,263	21.5%	*20.3–22.7*
Having recent discomfort or pain in the mouth	1,374	29.0%	*26.6–31.4*	2,330	7.5%	*6.4–8.9*	4,599	6.6%	*5.9–7.3*
Lack of a dental consultation consecutive - recent pain or discomfort*	401	42.0%	*37.2–46.8*	177	33.8%	*26.8–40.8*	188	57.8%	*50.7–64.9*
Difficulty expressing pain	1,366	15.8%	*13.9–17.7*	2,390	30.5%	*28.7–32.4*	4,664	20.6%	*19.4–21.8*
No dental visit over the last 12 months	1,277	52.5%	*49.8–55.2*	1,670	55.7%	*53.3–58.1*	3,560	55.7%	*54.1–57.3*
Presence of hali-sis	1,641	6.6%	*5.4–7.8*	2,465	6.0%	*5.1–6.9*	4,767	8.6%	*7.8–9.4*
Presence of drooling	1,641	0.0%	*0*	2,320	12.7%	*11.4–14.1*	4,599	8.4%	*7.6–9.2*
Presence of dental plaque	1,641	2.6%	*1.8–3.4*	2,376	11.5%	*10.2–12.8*	4,655	17.9%	*16.8–19*
Presence of calculus	1,631	1.5%	*0.9–2.1*	2,359	3.3%	*2.6–4*	4,644	6.0%	*5.3–6.7*
Presence of gingivitis	1,641	10.4%	*8.9–11.9*	2,358	36.5%	*34.6–38.4*	4,644	50.0%	*48.6–51.4*
Presenting at least one missing anterior -oth	1,641	0.0%	*0*	2,484	0.9%	*0.6–1.3*	4,766	1.0%	*0.7–1.3*
Presenting at least one missing posterior segment†	1,641	0.0%	*0*	2,484	0.3%	*0.1–0.5*	4,766	0.2%	*0.1–0.3*
Presence of at least one fractured anterior -oth left unres-red	1,620	0.9%	*0.4–1.4*	2,382	6.7%	*5.7–7.7*	4,671	8.1%	*7.3–8.9*
Presence of at least one incipient carious lesion ‡	1,641	12.7%	*11.1–14.3*	2,223	18.1%	*16.5–19.7*	4,525	24.3%	*23.1–25.6*
Presence of at least one developed carious lesion §	1,641	1.9%	*1.2–2.6*	2,223	9.4%	*8.2–10.6*	4,525	16.5%	*15.4–17.6*
Presence of at least one mucosal lesion on lips, -ngue or jaw	1,641	1.8%	*1.2–2.4*	2,366	8.9%	*5.3–12.5*	4,636	10%	*9.1–10.9*
At least one dental infectious process ‖	1,641	2.7%	*1.9–3.5*	2,297	9.3%	*8.1–10.5*	4,555	7.3%	*6.5–8.1*
Presence of severe orofacial dysmorphology **	1,611	37.6%	*35.2–40*	2,290	63.5%	*61.5–65.5*	4,631	58.1%	*56.7–59.5*
Lack of treatment for dysmorphology *	605	83.0%	*80–86*	1,454	94.1%	*92.9–95.3*	2,598	89.7%	*88.5–90.9*
Being uncooperative during oral examination††	1,641	10.5%	*9–12*	2,487	26.4%	*24.7–28.1*	4,772	15.8%	*14.8–16.8*

*for those having pain.
†absence of molars or premolars in at least one quarter of the mouth.
‡stage 1 or 2 according to the Eckstrand classification for carious lesions without stage 3 or 4 caries, either on a deciduous or permanent tooth [37].
§stage 3 or 4 according to the Eckstrand classification for carious lesions either on a deciduous or permanent tooth [37].
‖presence of an abscess, or a tooth with pulp exposure, or a fistula related to dental disease.
**Four groups of malocclusion were defined:
G1: Complete overjet of one or more than one tooth.
G2: 1) Overjet of 6 mm or more than 6 mm; or 2) Labial or buccal openbite concerning three pairs of teeth or more than three; or 3) Significant or considerable crowding or overcrowding in labial or buccal arch sectors.
G3: 1) Reverse overbite of at least one upper incisor or reverse overbite of at least one lower incisor; or 2) reverse overbite of post-canine teeth on one side or overbite of a complete or half arch buccal sector, provoking deflection or deviation of the mandible on contact through the intercuspal position or 3) overcoupled teeth.
G4: 1) Deep overbite of front teeth associated with an overjet; or 2) Bilateral reverse overbite associated with an early deviating contact during the mandibular closing phase.
Malocclusions of types G1 and G3 are considered as simple when not associated with malocclusions pertaining to G2 or G4.
Malocclusions of types G2 and G4 and those associated with other malocclusions are considered as complex.
††according to the modified Venham scale [38] score ≥1.
The modalities of subject distribution among the criteria were dichotomized for simplification. n: number of subjects for whom the criteria was evaluated; Yes: percentage of subjects experiencing the disorder.

except for the distribution of 7 to 8 year old children in COPI (Chi Square test, non significant).

The distributions of the children who did not participate in the evaluation for refusal for participation, absence from school or death did not differ between the group of 269 trained investigators and those 69 untrained investigators (Chi Square test, non significant). A total of 1343 subjects with disabilities were evaluated by the 69 untrained examiners (Table 7) The distributions across the different levels of COHI, COCNI and COPI of the 395 DC group children who were evaluated by the 69 untrained examiners did not differ from those of the other 2092 DC group children who were evaluated by the 269 trained examiners. The distributions across the oral health indices of the 948 adolescents in the DA group who were evaluated by the

Table 6. Distribution of the children with and without disabilities according to the values of the Clinical Oral Health Index (COHI), the Clinical Oral Care Needs Index (COCNI) and the Clinical Oral Prevention Index (COPI).

	Children without disability 6–12 yrs old (NDC group)			Children with disability 6–12 yrs old (DC group)			Adolescents with disability 13–20 yrs old (DA group)		
Clinical Oral Health Index	number	%	*95% CI*	number	%	*95% CI*	number	%	*95% CI*
0: no problem	357	21.8	*19.8–23.7*	157	6.3	*1.3–5.3*	88	1.8	*1.4–2.2*
1: at least one low to moderate problem	790	48.1	*45.7–50.5*	941	37.8	*35.9–39.7*	1 984	41.6	*40.2–42.9*
2: at least one important to severe problem	445	27.1	*24.9–29.3*	1 218	49.0	*45.3–50.9*	2 282	47.8	*46.3–49.2*
Unspecified level	49	3.0	*2.1–3.8*	171	6.9	*5.9–7.9*	418	8.8	*7.9–9.6*
Total	*1641*	*100%*		*2487*	*100%*		*4772*	*100%*	
Clinical Oral Care Needs Index	number	%	*95% CI*	number	%	*95% CI*	number	%	*95% CI*
0: No need for care nor examination	296	18.0	*16.4–19.8*	244	9.8	*8.6–10.9*	390	8.2	*7.4–8.9*
1: Need for examination	668	40.7	*37.6–42.3*	787	31.6	*29.7–33.4*	1123	23.5	*22.3–24.7*
2: Need for care	391	23.8	*21.7–25.8*	1013	40.7	*38.7–42.6*	2413	50.6	*48.6–52.0*
3: Urgent need for care or examination	286	17.4	*15.5–19.2*	443	17.8	*16.3–19.3*	846	17.7	*14.3–18.8*
Total	*1641*	*100%*		*2487*	*100%*		*4772*	*100%*	
Clinical Oral Prevention Index	number	%	*95% CI*	number	%	*95% CI*	number	%	*95% CI*
0: No need for prevention or dental education	1292	78.7.	*76.7–80.7*	1459	58.7	*56.8–60.7*	2297	48.1	*46.7–49.5*
1: Need for prevention or dental education	349	21.3	*19.3–23.3*	1028	41.3	*39.3–43.3*	2475	51.9	*50.4–53.3*
Total	*1641*	*100%*		*2487*	*100%*		*4772*	*100%*	

untrained examiners differ significantly from those of the 3824 other DA group children who were evaluated by the trained examiners for COHI (Chi square test, $p<0.005$) and COCNI (Chi square test, $p<0.001$). There were fewer subjects in both level 2 for COHI and level 3 for COCNI among the DA group subjects who were evaluated by the untrained examiners. The distribution across COPI did not differ significantly depending on whether the examiners were trained or not.

Discussion

This is the largest cross-sectional study to report oral health status for children and adolescents with disability. It demonstrates that the prevalence of poor oral health is increased in children with disability than in children without, and that this situation worsens with age. This study is also the first attempt to produce an original biopsychosocial indicator for oral health. The construct validity of the list of indicators could discriminate between subjects by age and presence of a disability. The concept of a clinical index generated by an algorithmic association of various clinical indicators is completely new in oral health, and offers a sensitive clinical measurement that could be used transversally in different populations.

Improving oral health is a specific concern for individuals with disability as oral health has both local and systemic consequences. Poor oral health is a factor for co-morbidity when associated with systemic disease. It increases the risk of infectious complications for patients presenting systemic diseases such as congenital cardiac disease, immunodeficiency or diabetes, or those with internal prostheses, and plays a direct role in the aggravation of chronic respiratory disease that is the main cause of mortality in people with disability [39–41]. For patients with epilepsy or mental deficiencies, both neurological and behavioral problems may be related to undiagnosed and untreated oral pain. This survey raises questions as to the measures that could be taken to decrease inequalities in oral health for children and adolescents with disability. There are three main strands to improving oral health in this population: improving oral hygiene, defining specific training for dental professionals, and allocating funds to cover dental care access and service utilization [42]. Oral hygiene decreases bacterial load by eliminating the lung pathogens present on the tongue, gum tissue and other oral mucosa or contained in dental plaque. Persons with disability, however, do not always have the neuromotor abilities required to independently and effectively perform oral hygiene [43]. Consequently, care staff and families who help with daily dental hygiene tasks should be targeted for educative programs [44,45]. In some countries, including France, the healthcare system does not currently identify the professionals needed to teach care staff. Training of hygienists and tutoring special care issues during dental education could help to improve oral hygiene and care standards for people with disability [46].

There are both political and economic choices to be made before specific funds can be allocated for this population. It has been shown in the USA that children with the most limited functional ability were 50% less likely to meet the health insurance core outcome than those without limitations [47]. In France, the national health insurance system does not cover specific oral care procedures for people with disability, despite the fact that the State has declared its obligation to provide administrative facilitators to compensate for disability issues in the 2002 Disability Rights Bill. Other countries, including the USA, are examining the adoption of new standards and studying the continuing obstacles of limited government support for dental services [48].

There were many potential methodological biases that could undermine this study. The first question is related to the representativity of our sample against national populations of children with and without disabilities. The sample of children and adolescents with disabilities was randomly selected from a child

Table 7. Distribution of children and adolescents with disabilities (respectively DC and DA groups) across the values of the Clinical Oral Health Index (COHI), the Clinical Oral Care Needs Index (COCNI) and the Clinical Oral Prevention Index (COPI) dependant on the training of the examiners.

	DC GROUP					DA GROUP				
Clinical Oral Health Index	Trained Examiners (n = 269)		Untrained examiners (n = 69)		Chi Square	Trained Examiners (n = 269)		Untrained examiners (n = 69)		Chi Square
0: no problem	131	*6.26%*	26	*6.58%*	p = 0.35	64	*1.67%*	24	*2.53%*	p<0.05
1: at least one low to moderate problem	777	*37.14%*	164	*41.52%*		1594	*41.68%*	390	*41.14%*	
2: at least one important to severe problem	1043	*49.86%*	175	*44.30%*		1852	*48.43%*	430	*45.36%*	
Unspecified level	141	*6.74%*	30	*7.59%*		314	*8.21%*	104	*10.97%*	
Total	2092	*100%*	395	100%		3824	*100%*	948	*100%*	
Clinical Oral Care Needs Index	Trained Examiners (n = 269)		Untrained examiners (n = 69)		Chi Square	Trained Examiners (n = 269)		Untrained examiners (n = 69)		Chi Square
0: No need for care nor examination	199	*9.51.%*	45	*11.39%*	p = 0.10	292	*7.64%*	98	*10.34%*	p<0.01
1: Need for examination	670	*32.039%*	117	*29.62%*		882	*23.06%*	241	*25.42%*	
2: Need for care	836	*39.96%*	177	*44.81%*		1945	*50.86%*	468	*49.37%*	
3: Urgent need for care or examination	387	*18.50%*	56	*14.18%*		705	*18.44%*	141	*14.87%*	
Total	2092	*100%*	395	*100%*		3824	*100%*	948	*100%*	
Clinical Oral Prevention Index	Trained Examiners (n = 269)		Untrained examiners (n = 69)		Chi Square	Trained Examiners (n = 269)		Untrained examiners (n = 69)		Chi Square
0: No need for prevention or dental education	1231	*58.84%*	228	57.72%	p = 0.85	1853	*48.46%*	444	*46.84%*	p = 0.45
1: Need for prevention or dental education	861	*41.16%*	167	42.28%		1971	*51.54%*	504	*53.16%*	
Total	2092	*100%*	395	100%		3824	*100%*	948	*100%*	

Chi square test compared the subjects' distribution between subgroups.

population in 1279 out of 1325 special schools. In France, the vast majority of children with learning disabilities are schooled in institutions, following a decision by a special commission which evaluates their medical condition. Special schools therefore offer an ideal context in order to gain access to a large national sample of these children. It was however impossible to compare the sample of children and adolescents with disability to the national population of children with disabilities, as we had no information on the population from the 46 institutions that did not consent to participate in the study. In addition we have no demographic information on the population of children with severe disabilities who are schooled either at home, or in ordinary schools. This discrepancy in the constitution of samples cannot be controlled and could induce bias. It was however the only practical way to undertake the study, as it was impossible to constitute a wider sample of children with disabilities in the usual conditions that are respected for epidemiological studies. An even greater degree of difficulty was found in constituting a sample of adolescents and young adults with disabilities. Ethical, political, financial and technical difficulties were barriers that led to abandon the project of comparing the oral health conditions in DA group to those of a control sample.

Secondly, the methodology for the reliability tests was based on photograph-based evaluations rather than on clinical examinations. Compared to a subject based examination, the photos gave a partial view of the subject, reducing him/her to a part of his/her mouth or face. In these conditions, the quality of the computer screens that served for photo evaluation was a factor that might affect the external reliability, in addition to the psychometric characteristics of each individual investigator. Despite these conditions, internal and external reliability remained acceptable.

Thirdly, the examination/interview of children and adolescents with disability was conducted by 338 dentists working for a French national health insurance scheme while those without disability were examined/interviewed by 7 other dentists. In addition, the investigators were not isolated, and independent assessments for both groups cannot be expected. As these conditions could not be modified, we tried to control them by giving the same training to each group of investigators. In particular and in order to limit the psychological impact of contact with children suffering from severe disability on the investigators' evaluation, specific training was provided regarding patients with special needs prior to the survey.

Fourth, a total of 69 out 338 examiners did not participate in the test retest exercise. It was however demonstrated that this point did not alter the distribution across the COHI, COCNI and COPI indices in the DC group children but that it could affect the subjects distribution across COHI and COCNI for the DA group (Table 7). The untrained examiners who did not participate in the test-retest exercise underestimated the severity of the oral health disease and the needs for treatment in the group of adolescents with disabilities. Consequently it could be assumed that the differences between the DA and DC groups would be increased if all the examiners had completed the test-retest exercise.

Fifth, among the 24 indicators for examination/interviews, four (coughing often during meals, having recent discomfort or pain, difficulties expressing pain, and being uncooperative during oral examination) were subjectively evaluated using either care staff report for the DC and DA groups, or self report for the NDC groups. The information thus compiled might not be exactly the same in these different conditions. For this reason, these subjective indicators were not included in the items determining the COHI and COCNI indices but featured exclusively in the COPI index.

Despite these limitations, the COHI, COCNI and COPI indices offer sensitive clinical measurements of oral health status in epidemiological surveys. Further developments are needed to increase the field of application of these biopsychosocial indices for oral health.

Author Contributions

Conceived and designed the experiments: MH VM MD. Performed the experiments: MH VM EN. Analyzed the data: MH VM MD EN. Contributed reagents/materials/analysis tools: MH VM MD EN. Wrote the paper: MH. Other: Coordinated the survey that produced the data from children without disabilities: DJ. Coordinated the survey that produced the data from children and adolescents with disabilities: MD.

References

1. Waldman HB, Perlman SP (2006) Children with special health care needs: results of a national survey. J Dent Child 73: 57–62.
2. Shaw MJ, Shaw L, Foster TD (1990) The oral health in different groups of adults with mental handicaps attending Birmingham (UK) adult training centres. Community Dent Health 7: 135–141.
3. Rodriquez Vazquez C, Garcillan R, Rioboo R, Bratos E (2002) Prevalence of dental caries in an adult population with mental retardation in Spain. Spec Care Dentist 22: 65–69.
4. Nunn JH, Gordon PH, Carmichael CL (1993) Dental Disease and current treatment needs in a group of physically handicapped children. Community Dent Health 10: 389–396.
5. Oreland A, Heijbel J, Jagell S (1987) Malocclusions in physically and/or mentally handicapped children. Swed Dent J 11: 103–119.
6. Fischer-Brandies H (1988) Cephalometric comparison between children with and without Down's syndrome. Eur J Orthod 10: 255–263.
7. Hobson RS, Nunn JH, Cozma I (2005) Orthodontic management of orofacial problems in young people with impairments: review of the literature and case reports. Int J Paediatr Dent 15: 355–363.
8. Shyama M, al-Mutawa SA, Honkala S (2001) Malocclusions and traumatic injuries in disabled schoolchildren and adolescents in Kuwait. Spec Care Dentist 21: 104–108.
9. Frazier JB, Friedman B (1996) Swallow function in children with Down syndrome: a retrospective study. Dev Med Child Neuro 38: 695–703.
10. Spender Q, Stein A, Dennis J, Reilly S, Percy E, et al. (1996) An exploration of feeding difficulties in children with Down syndrome. Dev Med Child Neurol 38: 681–94.
11. Dos Santos MT, Nogueira ML (2005) Infantile reflexes and their effects on dental caries and oral hygiene in cerebral palsy individuals. J Oral Rehabil 32: 880–885.
12. Hennequin M, Allison PJ, Faulks D, Orliaguet T, Feine JS (2005) A comparison of chewing indicators between adults with Down syndrome and controls. J Dent Res 84: 1057–1061.
13. Locker D (1988) Measuring oral health: a conceptual framework. Community Dent Health 5: 3–18.
14. McEntee MI (2006) An existential model of oral health from evolving views on health, function and disability. Community Dent Health 23: 5–14.
15. Slade GD, Spencer AJ (1994) Development and evaluation of the Oral Health Impact Profile. Community Dent Health 11: 3–11.
16. Allison P, Locker D, Jokovic A, Slade G (1999) A cross-cultural study of oral health values. J Dent Res 78: 643–649.
17. Foster Page LA, Thomson WM, Jokovic A, Locker D (2005) Validation of the Child Perceptions Questionnaire (CPQ 11–14). J Dent Res 84: 649–652.
18. Hennequin M, Allison PJ, Veyrune JL (2000) Prevalence of oral health problems in a group of individuals with Down syndrome in France. Dev Med Child Neurol 42: 691–698.
19. Trulsson U, Klingberg G (2003) Living with a child with a severe orofacial handicap: experiences from the perspectives of parents. Eur J Oral Sci 111: 19–25.
20. Ministère de l'Education Nationale (2007) Repères et références statistiques sur les enseignements, la formation et la recherche. Available: http://www.education.gouv.fr/cid5490/le-systeme-educatif.html.
21. Sullivan PB, Lambert B, Rose M, Ford-Adams M, Johnson A, et al. (2000) Prevalence and severity of feeding and nutritional problems in children with neurological impairment: Oxford Feeding Study. Dev Med Child Neurol 42: 674–680.
22. Hennequin M, Faulks D, Allison PJ (2003) Pain perception by parents of children with Down syndrome. J Orofac Pain 17: 347–353.
23. Hennequin M, Morin C, Feine J (2000) Pain expression and stimulus localization for individuals with Down syndrome. The Lancet 356: 1882–1887.
24. Tahmassebi JF, Curzon ME (2003) Prevalence of drooling in children with cerebral palsy attending special schools. Dev Med Child Neurol 45: 613–617.
25. Donnell DO, Sheiham A, Wai YK (2002) Dental findings in 4-, 14-, and 25-to 35-year-old Hong Kong residents with mental and physical disabilities. Spec Care Dentist 22: 231–234.
26. Lancashire P, Jansen J, Zach GA, Addy M (1997) The oral hygiene and gingival health of paraplegic inpatients- a cross-sectional survey. J Clin Periodontol 24: 198–200.
27. Stabholz A, Mann J, Sela M, Schurr D, Steinberg D, et al. (1991) Caries experience, periodontal treatment needs, salivary pH and Streptococcus mutans counts in a preadolescent Down syndrome population. Spec Care Dentist 11: 203–208.
28. Maestre C (1996) The use of general anaesthesia for tooth extraction in young handicapped adults in France. Br Dent J 180: 297–302.
29. Hennequin M, Faulks D, Roux D (2000) Accuracy of estimation of dental treatment needs in special care patients. J Dent 28: 131–136.
30. Shyama M, al-Mutawa SA, Honkala S (2001) Malocclusions and traumatic injuries in disabled schoolchildren and adolescents in Kuwait. Spec Care Dentist 21: 104–108.
31. Muller M, Jasmin JR (1988) The oro-dental status of a population of school children in the southeast of France. J Biol Buccale 16: 239–244.
32. Franklin DL, Luther F, Curzon ME (1996) The prevalence of malocclusion in children with cerebral palsy. Eur J Orthod 18: 637–643.
33. Gordon SM, Dionne RA, Snyder J (1998) Dental fear anxiety as a barrier to accessing oral health care among patients with special health care needs. Spec Care Dent 18: 88–92.
34. World Health Organisation (1993) ICD 10, International Classification for Disabilities, 10th version, Genève, Switzerland. 1243 p.
35. Greene JC, Vermillion JR (1960) The oral hygiene index: a method of classifying oral hygiene status. J Am Dent Assoc 61: 172–179.
36. Löe H, Silness J (1963) Periodontal disease in pregnancy. I. Prevalence and severity. Acta Odontol Scand 21: 533–551.
37. Ekstrand KR, Kuzmina I, Bjorndal L, Thylstrup A (1995) Relationship between external and histologic features of progressive stages of caries in the occlusal fossa. Caries Res 29: 243–250.
38. Venham L, Bengston D, Cipes M (1977) Children's response to sequential dental visits. J Dent Res 56: 455–459.
39. Mojon P (2002) Oral health and respiratory infection. J Can Dent Assoc 68: 340–345.
40. Yoneyama T, Yoshida M, Ohrui T, Mukaiyama H, Okamoto H, et al. (2002) Oral Care Working Group Oral care reduces pneumonia in older patients in nursing homes. J Am Geriatr Soc 50: 430–433.
41. Adachi M, Ishihara K, Abe S, Okuda K (2007) Professional oral health care by dental hygienists reduced respiratory infections in elderly persons requiring nursing care. Int J Dent Hyg 5: 69–74.
42. Young NL, Steele C, Fehlings D, Jutai J, Olmsted N, et al. (2005) Use of health care among adults with chronic and complex physical disabilities of childhood. Disabil Rehabil 27: 1455–1460.
43. Faulks D, Collado V, de Fréminville B, Newton TJ, Hennequin M (2006) A controlled national survey of difficulty encountered by persons with Down syndrome during hygiene and health care. Nursing Outlook 54: 345–352.
44. Frenkel HF, Harvey I, Needs KM (2002) Oral health care education and its effects on caregivers' knowledge and attitudes: a randomised controlled trial. Community Dent Oral Epidemi 30: 91–100.
45. Glassman P, Miller CE (2003) Preventing dental disease for people with special needs: the need for practical preventive protocols for use in community settings. Spec Care Dentist 23: 165–167.
46. Allison PJ, Hennequin M, Faulks D (2000) Dental care access among individuals with Down syndrome in France. Spec Care Dentist 20: 28–34.

47. Honberg L, McPherson M, Strickland B, Gage JC, Newacheck PW (2005) Assuring adequate health insurance: results of the National Survey of Children with Special Health Care Needs. Pediatrics 115: 1233–1239.

48. Waldman HB, Perlman SP (2006) Mandating education of dental graduates to provide care to individuals with intellectual and developmental disabilities. Ment Retard 44: 184–188.

Global Metabolomic Analysis of Human Saliva and Plasma from Healthy and Diabetic Subjects, with and without Periodontal Disease

Virginia M. Barnes[1], Adam D. Kennedy[3], Fotinos Panagakos[1], William Devizio[1], Harsh M. Trivedi[1], Thomas Jönsson[3], Lining Guo[3], Shannon Cervi[2], Frank A. Scannapieco[2]*

1 Colgate Palmolive Technology Center, Piscataway, NJ, United States of America, **2** Metabolon, Durham, NC, United States of America, **3** Department of Oral Biology, School of Dental Medicine, University at Buffalo, State University of New York, Buffalo, NY, United States of America

Abstract

Recent studies suggest that periodontal disease and type 2 diabetes mellitus are bi-directionally associated. Identification of a molecular signature for periodontitis using unbiased metabolic profiling could allow identification of biomarkers to assist in the diagnosis and monitoring of both diabetes and periodontal disease. This cross-sectional study identified plasma and salivary metabolic products associated with periodontitis and/or diabetes in order to discover biomarkers that may differentiate or demonstrate an interaction of these diseases. Saliva and plasma samples were analyzed from 161 diabetic and non-diabetic human subjects with a healthy periodontium, gingivitis and periodontitis. Metabolite profiling was performed using Metabolon's platform technology. A total of 772 metabolites were found in plasma and 475 in saliva. Diabetics had significantly higher levels of glucose and α-hydroxybutyrate, the established markers of diabetes, for all periodontal groups of subjects. Comparison of healthy, gingivitis and periodontitis saliva samples within the non-diabetic group confirmed findings from previous studies that included increased levels of markers of cellular energetic stress, increased purine degradation and glutathione metabolism through increased levels of oxidized glutathione and cysteine-glutathione disulfide, markers of oxidative stress, including increased purine degradation metabolites (e.g. guanosine and inosine), increased amino acid levels suggesting protein degradation, and increased ω-3 (docosapentaenoate) and ω-6 fatty acid (linoleate and arachidonate) signatures. Differences in saliva between diabetic and non-diabetic cohorts showed altered signatures of carbohydrate, lipid and oxidative stress exist in the diabetic samples. Global untargeted metabolic profiling of human saliva in diabetics replicated the metabolite signature of periodontal disease progression in non-diabetic patients and revealed unique metabolic signatures associated with periodontal disease in diabetics. The metabolites identified in this study that discriminated the periodontal groups may be useful for developing diagnostics and therapeutics tailored to the diabetic population.

Editor: Özlem Yilmaz, University of Florida, United States of America

Funding: This study was funded by a grant from Colgate Palmolive Co. The funder and Metabolon provided support in the form of salaries for authors VMB, FP, WD, HMT, and TJ, LG, ADK respectively, but did not have any additional role in the study design, data collection and analysis, decision to publish, or preparation of the manuscript. The specific roles of these authors are articulated in the "author contributions" section.

Competing Interests: This research was supported by Colgate Palmolive Co. VMB, FP, WD, and HMT are employed by Colgate. Other authors (TJ, LG, and ADK) are employed by Metabolon, a commercial company specializing in metabolomic analysis. Both Metabolon and the University at Buffalo (FAS and SC) received funding from Colgate Palmolive to complete these studies. There are no patents, products in development, or marketed products to declare.

* Email: fas1@buffalo.edu

Introduction

Periodontal disease is a chronic bacterial infection causing persistent gingival inflammation, and in some cases connective tissue destruction and bone resorption around the teeth. It is also characterized by pocket formation and recession. Although advances in dental care has resulted in improved periodontal status in certain populations, disparities persist as severe periodontitis is often found to be exaggerated in certain segments of the population, for example those from a low socio-economic background [1]. It is well known that bacteria colonize the teeth to form a biofilm, called dental plaque, which initiates gingivitis, and sometimes progresses to periodontitis. Release of bacterial products from the biofilm induces local inflammation. Without treatment, periodontal tissue destruction, bone resorption and tooth loss may ensue [1]. Periodontal disease also has been associated with several systemic diseases, including cardiovascular disease, diabetes mellitus, respiratory disease, rheumatoid arthritis, chronic kidney disease, and adverse pregnancy outcomes [2–6].

The gingival epithelium forms a crevice around each tooth that provides a protected space for bacterial colonization and proliferation [7–10]. Analysis of gingival crevicular fluid (GCF) [11] and saliva [12–14] from periodontal patients has identified a variety of inflammatory mediators and tissue-destructive molecules, including metalloproteinases [15–23] and metabolic signatures associated with host-bacterial interactions to be elevated when compared to periodontally health patients.

Diabetic patients have a high prevalence of gingivitis, periodontitis, oral candidiasis, and xerostomia, and the severity of these diseases are correlated with the duration of diabetes and degree of glycemic control [24,25]. Poor glycemic control has been shown to be associated with poor periodontal health, of which the molecular signatures may be monitored using modern "omics" -based methods [26–30].

Saliva is a complex secretory fluid that contains trace metals, metabolites, biochemicals, proteins, glycoproteins, lipds, etc., that serve a spectrum of physiological needs. Saliva is a critical source of tissue lubricants, tooth mineralizing factors, acid buffers, toxin neutralizers, and antimicrobial components [31–35]. The ability to use saliva to evaluate physiological conditions, follow disease progression, and monitor post-treatment therapeutic results through noninvasive methods is an important objective for healthcare in general and periodontology in particular. We have previously performed a series of untargeted global metabolomic profiling tests of GCF and saliva samples from subjects with healthy gingiva, gingivitis, and periodontitis that have suggested a rigorous set of potential biomarkers for monitoring periodontal disease status and examining the effectiveness of oral care treatment that resolves the metabolic signature of inflammation [11,12,36,37]. Many metabolites associated with inflammation, oxidative stress, tissue degradation, and bacterial metabolism were found to be significantly elevated in periodontal disease and reduced by treatment [37]. Validation of such biomarkers will provide an objective phenotype to allow practitioners to diagnose disease, monitor patient disease activity and determine the effectiveness of treatment.

Metabolomic profiling is a rapidly evolving technology that has been increasingly used to discover early markers of disease [11,12,37–40]. Whole saliva can be easily collected through noninvasive means and has considerable potential to monitor general health and disease status. With the advancement of technological means such as metabolomics, saliva can be leveraged as a clinical and diagnostic tool because of its potential to mirror oral and systemic health conditions [41–45]. To this end, metabolomic signatures were determined in saliva and compared to those in plasma from orally healthy subjects and periodontal subjects, with and without type 2 diabetes, in an effort to identify unique metabolomic profiles and biomarkers of periodontal disease in both systemic health and diabetes. Based on our previous results from biomarker identification of periodontal disease progression [11,12,37], we performed a discovery study to identify biomarkers of decreased periodontal health as monitored by biochemical profiling of saliva and plasma collected from orally healthy subjects and those with gingivitis and periodontitis using an unbiased metabolomic profiling approach based on liquid and gas chromatography/mass spectrometry (LC/MS and GC/MS).

Materials, Participants, and Methods

Experimental Design and Participants

This cross-sectional clinical study enrolled adult male and female subjects from the Buffalo, New York area and was conducted in accordance with the Helsinki Declaration. The Institutional Review Board at the University at Buffalo approved the protocol (ORB0650111E), including the clinical examination, collection of saliva and plasma samples. All subjects read and signed a written informed consent before their enrollment into the study. The inclusion criteria were: age between 18 and 65 years, in good general health (n = 81), or subjects diagnosed with diabetes (n = 80); and a minimum of 20 natural teeth (excluding third molars) present. Exclusion criteria included: inability or unwillingness to sign the informed consent form, diagnosis of a medical condition which required pre-medication prior to dental visits/procedures, 5 or more decayed untreated teeth at screening (cavities), diagnosis of other diseases of the hard or soft oral tissues, impaired salivary function, use of antibiotics or antimicrobial drugs within 30 days prior to the first study visit, a history of uncharacterized systemic disease, pregnant or nursing women, participation in any other clinical study within 1 week prior to enrollment into this study, present use of tobacco products, subjects who required dental treatment during the duration of the study, immune compromised individuals (e.g. those diagnosed with HIV, AIDS, or taking immunosuppressive drug therapy), or subjects who received periodontal treatment within the previous 30 days.

Subjects were evaluated by a single dental examiner (SC) for inclusion/exclusion criteria. At the first visit, participants received a tube of standard, non-anti-microbial fluoridated toothpaste with instructions for use, in order to minimize variations in results that might be driven by the use of different toothpastes. A fasting blood sample was then collected from subjects self-identifying as diabetic to confirm diabetic status. During the second visit, subjects gave an update on their medical and medication history, contributed saliva and blood samples, had an assessment of their oral tissues to assess periodontal status, to monitor adverse events since the first visit and answer questions regarding their compliance as to the use of the standard toothpaste. A minimum of 0.5 ml of unstimulated saliva and 10 ml of blood was collected. Subjects were asked to refrain from eating or drinking (excluding water) from 11:00 PM the previous night; to brush their teeth and entire mouth the evening before the saliva donation, but not the morning of collection. Blood samples were obtained after collection of the saliva. Saliva was collected into sterile polypropylene tubes and immediately frozen in a dry ice bath and stored at −80 degrees C until shipped to Metabolon. No preservatives were added to the saliva samples

Definition of oral status groups

Within the diabetic or non-diabetic cohorts, three sub-groups were established: periodontal health, gingivitis and periodontitis. Subjects were stratified according to the gingivitis index: Healthy: These subjects had an average full mouth Modified Gingival Index (MGI) [46] score below 1.0, with fewer than 3 bleeding on probing (BOP) sites and minimal dental plaque present as scored by the method of Sillness and Lõe [47]. Gingivitis: These subjects had an average full mouth MGI score between 1 and 2 with multiple BOP sites and periodontal pockets <4 mm. Periodontitis: These subjects had an average full mouth MGI of 2.0 or greater with multiple BOP sites, and 2 or more periodontal pockets with probing depths of 5 mm or more in at least two quadrants. Plaque at any level was present. Measurement of oral indices was performed as per Lobene et al. [46] as follows: 0 = normal, 1 = mild inflammation of the gingival unit (slight change in color, little change in texture of any portion of the gingival unit), 2 = mild inflammation of the entire gingival unit, 3 = moderate inflammation (moderate change in texture, redness, edema and hypertrophy of the gingival unit, 4 = severe inflammation (marked redness and edema/hypertrophy, spontaneous bleeding or ulceration) of the gingival unit. Plaque indices were assessed for 6 surfaces on each tooth and the plaque index score was the average of the scores obtained from all teeth. The amount of plaque observed on each tooth was scored 0 to 3 as follows: 0 = no plaque notes; 1 = plaque seen only on the tip of an explorer passed over the tooth surface;

Table 1. Sample Size of Study Groups.

	Healthy	Gingivitis	Periodontal	Totals
Diabetic	28	27	26	**81**
Non-Diabetic	25	26	29	**80**
Totals	**53**	**53**	**55**	**161**

2 = plaque obvious with the naked eye; 3 = gross deposits of plaque present over the entire tooth.

Systemic Health Selection Criteria/Assessment for Diabetes Status

For this study, diabetes status was established by self-reported history. Subjects who reported a history of diabetes were asked to confirm diabetic status by providing blood samples to measure HbA1c values. An individual was defined with Type 2 diabetes if hemoglobin A1C≥6.5%. Due to financial limitations, HbA1c levels were not assessed for those not reporting a history of diabetes. As a recent study suggested, the prevalence of diabetes (as measured by HbA1c>6.4) is likely low (extrapolated to be 5.0% with diabetes and 9.5% with pre-diabetes) in dental patients unaware of their diabetes status [48], we assumed that the prevalence of diabetes in the non-diabetes subject in this study would be similar and therefore not compromise the analysis.

Saliva and Plasma Sample Collection

Saliva was collected in 50 mL polypropylene tubes and plasma was collected in Vacutainer tubes and anti-coagulated with EDTA. Samples were immediately frozen in a dry ice bath and stored at −80°C.

Metabolomic Profiling Technology

Metabolomic profiling was performed as described previously [12,49]. In summary, after the extraction of metabolites from each sample, the extracts were analyzed by GC/MS and LC/MS. We carried out chromatographic separation, followed by full-scan mass spectroscopy, to record and quantify all detectable ions presented in the samples [50]. We identified metabolites with

Table 2. Demographics of Study Subjects.

Healthy n = 53		
	Non DM	**DM**
Total	**28**	**25**
Male	9	14
Female	19	11
Mean Age	37.5 (15.2)	50.2 (11.0)
Mean BMI	26.1 (4.2)	33.6 (9.9)
Mean HbA1C*	no data	7.1 (1.1)
Gingivitis n = 53		
	Non DM	**DM**
Total	**27**	**26**
Male	11	10
Female	16	16
Mean Age	35.9 (12.0)	53.8 (7.5)
Mean BMI	26.9 (5.7)	33.1 (7.6)
Mean HbA1C	no data	7.2 (1.5)
Periodontal n = 55		
	Non DM	**DM**
Total	**26**	**29**
Male	11	19
Female	15	10
Mean Age	49.7 (10.8)	54.5 (6.8)
Mean BMI	30.3 (6.0)	32.8 (7.9)
Mean HbA1C	no data	7.7 (1.9)

*HbA1c testing was done on purported diabetic subjects only.

Table 3. Overall statistical analysis of saliva and plasma samples from the healthy periodontal cohorts.

Summary of Altered Metabolites	*t*-Test Saliva (Diabetic vs. Non-diabetic)	*t*-Test Plasma (Diabetic vs. Non-diabetic)
Total number of comparisons $p \leq 0.05$	69	174
Biochemical direction of change	66 ↑/3 ↓*	115 ↑/59 ↓**

*66 metabolites were increased in saliva from subjects with diabetes, 3 metabolites were increased in saliva from non-diabetic subjects.
**115 metabolites were increased in plasma from subjects with diabetes, 59 metabolites were increased in plasma from non-diabetic subjects.

known chemical structure by matching the ions' chromatographic retention index and mass spectral fragmentation signatures with reference library entries created from authentic standard metabolites under the identical analytical procedure as the experimental samples [51]. For ions that were not covered by the standards, additional library entries were added based on their unique ion signatures (chromatographic and mass spectral). After this, these ions could be routinely detected and quantified.

Statistical Analysis

After normalization and imputation, the data were log-transformed. We then performed ANOVA and *t* tests to compare data obtained from the healthy, gingivitis, and periodontitis samples. Multiple comparisons were accounted for with the false discovery (FDR) rate method, and each FDR was estimated by *q*-values.

Results

A total of 174 subjects were enrolled in this study (Table 1). The mean age of the non-diabetic subjects tended to be younger than the diabetic subjects (Table 2). Diabetic subjects had a higher BMI for all groups (Table 2). HbA1C testing confirmed diabetic status of the subjects self-reporting as diabetic.

An untargeted metabolomic profiling approach was used to assess the chemical milieu of saliva and plasma. In total, 161 individual saliva samples were collected, 80 from subjects with diabetes and 81 from subjects without diabetes. We detected 475 and 772 metabolites in saliva and plasma, respectively, of which 370 and 430 could be mapped to known chemical structures (Tables S1 and S2).

Characterization of Diabetic and Non-Diabetic Samples

Welch's two sample *t* tests and ANOVA identified statistically significant differences in these saliva samples between non-diabetic subjects and those with diabetes. Approximately 14% of the detected metabolites (69 of 475) in saliva showed altered levels ($p \leq 0.05$) among the healthy samples when compared to the diabetic cohort, suggesting that these may be markers of diabetic status in humans (Table 3). Alternatively, comparison of the plasma from the same subjects resulted in 174 statistically significant changes. ANOVA analysis with either matrix did not produce a list of metabolites largely different from the *t* tests (data not shown).

Glycemic control can be monitored by changes in 1,5-anhydroglucitol (1,5-AG). 1,5-AG is reabsorbed in the renal tubules, a process competitively inhibited by glucosuria, which leads to a reduction in its level in plasma. Thus, the greater the degree of glucosuria, the lower the amount of 1,5-AG present in the plasma [52–54]. The correlation between this reduction and the amount of glucose present in urine is so close that 1,5-AG represents a sensitive, real-time marker of glycemic control [55]. Thus, elevations of 1,5-AG in plasma are highly indicative of reduced glucosuria as a consequence of improved glycemic control. Not surprisingly, subjects with diabetes had significantly lower 1,5-AG and significantly higher levels of glucose in their plasma (Table 4). Additionally, diabetic subjects had significantly lower 1,5-AG in their saliva for all periodontal disease groups and higher levels of glucose in their saliva (Table 4). These observations lend confidence to the appropriateness of the control group, which was based on self-report of diabetes. None of the non-diabetic subjects had metformin in their plasma or saliva (data not shown).

α-hydroxybutyrate (AHB) is an early marker for insulin resistance in humans [52] as it arises from states of lactic and ketoacidosis or disrupted energy metabolism [56–61]. AHB levels were increased significantly in the diabetic cohort in plasma (Table 4) and were increased significantly in saliva in the healthy and gingivitis cohorts (data not shown). This may be a reflection of the increased energetic stress induced by the infection during the development of periodontitis or a translation of insulin resistance markers to saliva.

High-Level Characterization of Diabetic and Non-Diabetic Periodontal Cohorts

The analysis of each periodontal cohort (diabetic and non-diabetic) separately resulted in the identification of several

Table 4. Relative levels of biochemicals linked to diabetic status in saliva and plasma*.

Matrix	Biochemical Name	Fold Change (Diabetc/Non-diabetic)	P value	Q value
Saliva	1-5 anhydroglucitol (1,5-AG)	0.93	0.0417	0.3041
	Glucose	2.66	0.0074	0.2228
	α-hydroxybutyrate (AHB)	2.14	0.0009	0.0958
Plasma	1-5 anhydroglucitol (1,5-AG)	0.61	0.0007	0.0168
	Glucose	1.35	9.46×10^{-6}	0.0009
	α-hydroxybutyrate (AHB)	1.59	0.0012	0.0255

*Metformin was not detected in any of the non-diabetic samples.

Table 5. Overall statistical analysis of saliva samples comparing periodontal cohorts from diabetics and non-diabetics.

Summary of Altered Biochemicals	*t*-Test Saliva (Diabetic Gingivitis vs. Diabetic Healthy)	*t*-Test Saliva (Diabetic Periodontitis vs. Diabetic Healthy)	*t*-Test Saliva (Non-diabetic gingivitis vs. Non-diabetic Healthy)	*t*-Test Saliva (Non-diabetic periodontitis vs. Non-diabetic Healthy)
Total number of comparisons $p \leq 0.05$	35	54	20	64
Biochemical direction of change	25 ↑/10 ↓*	12 ↑/42 ↓**	17 ↑/3 ↓***	62 ↑/2 ↓****

*25 metabolites were increased in saliva from subjects with gingivitis, 10 metabolites were increased in saliva from diabetic, non-gingivitis subjects.
**12 metabolites were increased in saliva from diabetic subjects with periodontitis, 42 metabolites were increased in saliva from diabetic, periodontally healthy subjects.
***17 metabolites were increased in saliva from non-diabetic gingivitis subjects without diabetes, 3 metabolites were increased in saliva from non-diabetic, periodontally healthy subjects.
****62 metabolites were increased in saliva from non-diabetic periodontitis subjects, 2 metabolites were increased in saliva from non-diabetic, periodontally healthy subjects.

metabolites that were associated with the progression of gingival status (Table 5). The most striking find in the study was the direction of change in the periodontitis samples in the diabetic cohort. In the non-diabetic cohort, metabolites increased in abundance through disease progression, whereas many biochemicals increased in abundance when comparing the healthy to gingivitis groups, but then decreased in abundance in the diabetic subjects with periodontal disease suggesting an interaction between the diabetes signature and the periodontal signature.

Both periodontal status and diabetes status of the subjects were major driving factors in the biochemical changes observed. For the majority of metabolites with altered concentrations in the non-diabetic cohort, the levels at gingivitis samples were found to be intermediate between those levels found in healthy and periodontitis samples (Table S1). This suggests that the metabolic changes induced by gingivitis are a continuum of those of periodontitis.

Analysis of the Non-Diabetic Saliva Samples

Barnes et al. found differences in the biochemical signatures in saliva between non-diabetic subjects with healthy gingiva or periodontitis [12]. This report showed increased levels of metabolites in the saliva of the periodontal population reflecting enhanced degradation of macromolecules, including proteins, lipids, nucleotides and polysaccharides. Comparison of the non-diabetic cohort from the current study with these previous studies showed similar results (Table 6). This metabolic signature, which includes elevated levels of ω-6 fatty acids, is indicative of a hyper-inflammatory environment resulting from chronic bacterial infection and further support for increased macromolecular degradation of the periodontal tissues resulting from inflammation. Several metabolic signatures supported the notion that a more diverse and active microbial flora accompanied the inflammatory response resulting in gingivitis and periodontitis. Aromatic amino acid metabolites likely derived from bacteria were increased in periodontitis samples (Table 6). Moreover, carnitine, which is often the sole source of carbon and nitrogen for bacteria, was also elevated. Periodontal saliva samples also contained elevated levels of 3-dehydrocarnitine, a bacterial degradation product of carnitine, further supporting the utilization of carnitine in oral bacterial metabolism.

Table 6. Comparison of biochemical changes to previously published results.

Biochemical Pathway/Name	Barnes et al., J. Dent. Res. [12] Saliva Periodontitis vs. Healthy	Current Study Saliva (Non-diabetic subjects only) Periodontitis vs. Healthy
Purine Degradation (Link to Oxidative Stress)	Increased*	Increased
Dipeptides (Macromolecular degradation of proteins)	Increased	Increased
Amino Acid Metabolites (p-cresol sulfate, Bacterial)	Increased	Increased
Carbohydrates (monosaccharides indicative of amylase activity)	Increased	Increased
Energy Metabolites (TCA cycle, indicative of energetic stress)	Unchanged	Increased
Uridine (DNA/RNA Degradation)	Increased	Increasing trend**
Allantoin	Increased	Increasing trend
ω-6 fatty acids (link to inflammation)	Increased	Increased
Fatty Acids	Increased	Increased
Acetylcarnitine	Increased	Increased
Carnitine	Increased	Unchanged
3-dehydrocarnitine	Increased	Increased

*Increased with statistically significant differences ($p \leq 0.05$) in biochemicals from those pathways. I
**Increasing trend reflects differences ($0.05 < p \leq 0.10$) in biochemicals from those pathways.

Table 7. Relative levels of biochemicals linked to purine degradation and anti-oxidant status in saliva samples from diabetics.

Biochemical Name	Fold Change (Diabetic -Gingivitis/Diabetic - Healthy)	P value	Q value
Adenosine	1.37	0.0943	0.6881
Inosine	1.70	0.0294	0.629
Guanine	2.40	0.0673	0.6546
Guanosine	2.06	0.0343	0.629
Xanthine	1.49	0.0434	0.629
Glutathione, oxidized (GSSG)	1.40	0.07	0.6546
Cysteine-glutathione disulfide	1.57	0.061	0.6444

Comparison of Biochemical Signatures in Saliva Samples from Diabetics vs Non-Diabetic subjects

Oxidative Stress and Anti-Oxidant Capacity. Purine degradation is regulated, in part, by oxidative stress [62], and increased purine degradation serves as an indication of an increased inflammatory response. Specifically, the conversion of hypoxanthine to xanthine and the subsequent conversion of xanthine to uric acid require O_2 to activate xanthine oxidase [63,64] and these reactions are coupled with a reduction of oxygen to generate superoxides in the form of O_2^- and H_2O_2. Urate is known to function in redox balance as a radical scavenger or antioxidant under conditions of oxidative stress and in the process converted to other products (e.g. allantoin). In the context of gingival disease, increased oxidative stress would result in higher levels of purine degradation metabolites, reflected in increased levels of hypoxanthine and xanthine. The results of this study are consistent with the results from previous studies [11,37]. Metabolites in the purine degradation pathway were statistically elevated in the diabetic cohort compared to the non-diabetic cohort (Table 7).

The levels of cysteine-glutathione disulfide and oxidized glutathione increased with gingival disease in non-diabetics and diabetics (Table 7). Glutathione plays a central role in the cellular defense against free radicals and xenobiotics. The increased levels of these oxidized glutathione species in saliva indicated increased oxidative stress.

Lipid and Sphingolipid Metabolism. Several lipid inflammatory mediators increased significantly in saliva from both the non-diabetic and diabetic groups during periodontal disease progression (Table 8). In this state of oxidative stress, lipoxygenase enzymes oxidize fatty acids to generate lipid signaling molecules such as 12-HETE. In saliva, arachidonate and 12-HETE increased in the non-diabetic cohort with periodontal disease and also increased in the diabetic gingivitis cohort compared to the healthy group, but was reduced in periodontitis (Table 8). Sphingomyelin, ceramides and glycosphingolipids are molecules that reside in the plasma membrane and participate in intracellular signaling cascades. Palmitoyl sphingomyelin was elevated in saliva of diabetic and non-diabetic subjects periodontitis (Table 8).

Discussion

We used metabolomic profiling technology to analyze saliva from subjects with and without diabetes who had a healthy gingiva, gingivitis, or periodontitis. In addition to verifying previously published observations in saliva [12] and GCF [11,37], we also identified in the present study salivary biochemical changes associated with diabetes, as well as changes associated with periodontal disease. The results from this analysis show that human diabetic subjects with periodontal disease have an increased purine degradation signature, a decreased redox balance capacity (Table 7) and altered ω-3/ω-6 fatty acid profiles (Table 8) in saliva.

Redox balance is vital for maintaining cellular homeostasis. Oxidative stress, caused by over production of reactive oxygen species and insufficient cellular anti-oxidant capabilities, can lead to cell damage. Glutathione and other anti-oxidant molecules serve to protect cellular proteins and structures from oxidative stress caused by reactive oxygen species. Glutathione is a thiol-containing tripeptide that plays a central role in cellular defense against free radicals and xenobiotics [65–68] and is the major intracellular redox mediator and it is pivotal for controlling the electrical or redox gradient across the mitochondrial inner-membrane [69,70]. Glutathione in the mitochondrial intermembrane space plays a intricate role in the mechanism of redox balance in living cells through its linkage to the redox milieu in the cytosol [71]. Oral interventions that enhance redox balance have been shown to be effective at relieving oral symptoms. For

Table 8. Fatty acids and sphingomyelins inreased in saliva from subjects with diabetes and periodontal disease.

Biochemical Name	Fold Change (Diabetic - Gingivitis/Diabetic - Healthy)	P value	Q value
12-HETE	2.41	0.0127	0.629
Linoleate (18:2n6)	3.22	0.0269	0.629
Linolenate [α or γ; (18:3n3 or 6)]	4.52	0.0476	0.629
Docosapentaenoate (n3 DPA; 22:5n3)	1.63	0.0483	0.629
Arachidonate (20:4n6)	2.00	0.0631	0.6517
Palmitoyl sphingomyelin	1.65	0.0422	0.629

example, Hansen and Grunnet showed that taurine plays a significant role in mitochondria in pH buffering that not only affects the status of glutathione, but also the NADH/NAD+ redox pair [72]. These molecules were all found to be elevated in saliva from the diabetic subjects.

Several lipid compounds are important for the initiation and propagation of inflammatory signaling in cells and tissues. Linoleic acid and arachidonic acid give rise to many of these metabolites. These lipid signaling inflammatory mediators are liberated from the plasma membrane phospholipids by phospholipase A_2 enzymes ultimately resulting in the production of linoleic and arachidonic acid-derived eicosanoids which help to mediate the inflammatory response [73]. Arachidonic acid release can also be initiated by collagen, thrombin, bradykinin, serotonin, and adrenaline, which increase in tissues during tissue damage and the early stages in inflammation and oxidative stress. Immune cells such as macrophages and neutrophils produce reactive oxygen species and reactive nitrogen species during cell activation that have the potential to damage lipids, proteins, and other molecules. Interestingly, these compounds were found to be elevated in the saliva of diabetic subjects with gingivitis.

Mobilization of lipid signaling pathways results in the synthesis of ceramides or the liberation of ceramides from intracellular stores. The activity of ceramidases results in the formation of sphingosine and sphingomyelin molecules that function in an array of intracellular signaling or maintenance of cell membrane architecture including apoptosis [74,75]. Depending on the specific cellular type and mechanism of activation, sphingomyelins and ceramides can serve activation or inhibitory purposes [76]. The formation of ceramides and sphingomyelins has been linked to cell death through nutrient starvation [74–76] as well as an important signaling molecule for cell differentiation and polarity [77]. *Porphyromonas gingivalis* is known to induce and alter sphingomyelin and ceramide signaling during infection [78].

Prediction of risk and accurate diagnosis of current disease activity may facilitate effective prevention and treatment of gingival diseases. GCF and saliva have been extensively examined in attempts to assess the oral disease status. The markers identified in this study may be leveraged to monitor the effectiveness of interventions as well as identify the mechanisms of action for these interventions. Several different approaches have confirmed that identifying a single marker characteristic of a disease is unlikely; rather, a combination of biomarkers would likely constitute an effective clinical test. For example, insulin resistance is a feature if the pre-diabetes stage in humans prior to the development of diabetes. Untargeted biochemical profiling to identify biomarkers of insulin resistance following the development of targeted assays and validation of the targeted assays in a clinical cohort resulted in the development of a diagnostic that monitors insulin sensitivity status in humans [52,79]. By monitoring selected metabolites representing the diverse biochemical pathways, it is therefore possible to identify unique biomarkers and to monitor during the course of periodontal treatment in diabetics. In conclusion, this study demonstrated that biochemical profiling technology is a powerful tool for dental research and the results provide new mechanistic insights and treatment strategies that could be specific for oral health of diabetics. Additionally, the biochemicals identified in this study that segregated the individuals by periodontal status could be leveraged or developed into a rapid diagnostic to monitor periodontal disease activity.

Supporting Information

Table S1 Saliva Metabolic Profiling and Pathway Analysis. Statistical analyses for each biochemical detected in saliva between each of the gingival and diabetic cohorts.

Table S2 Plasma Metabolic Profiling and Pathway Analysis. Statistical analyses for each biochemical detected in plasma between each of the gingival and diabetic cohorts.

Author Contributions

Conceived and designed the experiments: VMB FP WD HMT TJ LG FAS. Performed the experiments: TJ LG ADK SC FAS. Analyzed the data: VMB LG ADK FAS. Contributed reagents/materials/analysis tools: LG ADK. Contributed to the writing of the manuscript: ADK FAS VMB FP LG.

References

1. Leyden JJ, Thiboutot D, Shalita A (2004) Photographic review of results from a clinical study comparing benzoyl peroxide 5%/clindamycin 1% topical gel with vehicle in the treatment of rosacea. Cutis 73: 11–17.
2. Gutman DA, Cooper LA, Hwang SN, Holder CA, Gao J, et al. (2013) MR imaging predictors of molecular profile and survival: multi-institutional study of the TCGA glioblastoma data set. Radiology 267: 560–569.
3. Demmer RT, Desvarieux M (2006) Periodontal infections and cardiovascular disease: the heart of the matter. J Am Dent Assoc 137 Suppl: 14S–20S; quiz 38S.
4. Tonetti MS, D'Aiuto F, Nibali L, Donald A, Storry C, et al. (2007) Treatment of periodontitis and endothelial function. N Engl J Med 356: 911–920.
5. Pussinen PJ, Tuomisto K, Jousilahti P, Havulinna AS, Sundvall J, et al. (2007) Endotoxemia, immune response to periodontal pathogens, and systemic inflammation associate with incident cardiovascular disease events. Arterioscler Thromb Vasc Biol 27: 1433–1439.
6. Pussinen PJ, Paju S, Mantyla P, Sorsa T (2007) Serum microbial- and host-derived markers of periodontal diseases: a review. Curr Med Chem 14: 2402–2412.
7. Nieman DC, Shanely RA, Gillitt ND, Pappan KL, Lila MA (2013) Serum metabolic signatures induced by a three-day intensified exercise period persist after 14 h of recovery in runners. J Proteome Res 12: 4577–4584.
8. Scannapieco FA (1994) Saliva-bacterium interactions in oral microbial ecology. Crit Rev Oral Biol Med 5: 203–248.
9. Scannapieco FA, Bergey EJ, Reddy MS, Levine MJ (1989) Characterization of salivary alpha-amylase binding to Streptococcus sanguis. Infect Immun 57: 2853–2863.
10. Scannapieco FA, Solomon L, Wadenya RO (1994) Emergence in human dental plaque and host distribution of amylase-binding streptococci. J Dent Res 73: 1627–1635.
11. Barnes VM, Teles R, Trivedi HM, Devizio W, Xu T, et al. (2009) Acceleration of purine degradation by periodontal diseases. J Dent Res 88: 851–855.
12. Barnes VM, Ciancio SG, Shibly O, Xu T, Devizio W, et al. (2011) Metabolomics reveals elevated macromolecular degradation in periodontal disease. J Dent Res 90: 1293–1297.
13. Christodoulides N, Floriano PN, Miller CS, Ebersole JL, Mohanty S, et al. (2007) Lab-on-a-chip methods for point-of-care measurements of salivary biomarkers of periodontitis. Ann N Y Acad Sci 1098: 411–428.
14. Miller CS, King CP Jr, Langub MC, Kryscio RJ, Thomas MV (2006) Salivary biomarkers of existing periodontal disease: a cross-sectional study. J Am Dent Assoc 137: 322–329.
15. Akalin FA, Baltacioglu E, Alver A, Karabulut E (2007) Lipid peroxidation levels and total oxidant status in serum, saliva and gingival crevicular fluid in patients with chronic periodontitis. J Clin Periodontol 34: 558–565.
16. Akalin FA, Isiksal E, Baltacioglu E, Renda N, Karabulut E (2008) Superoxide dismutase activity in gingiva in type-2 diabetes mellitus patients with chronic periodontitis. Arch Oral Biol 53: 44–52.
17. Pradeep AR, Kumar MS, Ramachandraprasad MV, Shikha C (2007) Gingival crevicular fluid levels of neopterin in healthy subjects and in patients with different periodontal diseases. J Periodontol 78: 1962–1967.
18. Pradeep AR, Manjunath SG, Swati PP, Shikha C, Sujatha PB (2007) Gingival crevicular fluid levels of leukotriene B4 in periodontal health and disease. J Periodontol 78: 2325–2330.
19. Waddington RJ, Embery G, Samuels RH (1994) Characterization of proteoglycan metabolites in human gingival crevicular fluid during orthodontic tooth movement. Arch Oral Biol 39: 361–368.
20. Embery G, Waddington R (1994) Gingival crevicular fluid: biomarkers of periodontal tissue activity. Adv Dent Res 8: 329–336.

21. Alpagot T, Bell C, Lundergan W, Chambers DW, Rudin R (2001) Longitudinal evaluation of GCF MMP-3 and TIMP-1 levels as prognostic factors for progression of periodontitis. J Clin Periodontol 28: 353–359.
22. Alpagot T, Silverman S, Lundergan W, Bell C, Chambers DW (2001) Crevicular fluid elastase levels in relation to periodontitis and metabolic control of diabetes. J Periodontal Res 36: 169–174.
23. Kardesler L, Buduneli N, Cetinkalp S, Lappin D, Kinane DF (2011) Gingival crevicular fluid IL-6, tPA, PAI-2, albumin levels following initial periodontal treatment in chronic periodontitis patients with or without type 2 diabetes. Inflamm Res 60: 143–151.
24. Acker-Hewitt TL, Shafer BM, Saunders MJ, Goh Q, Luden ND (2012) Independent and combined effects of carbohydrate and caffeine ingestion on aerobic cycling performance in the fed state. Appl Physiol Nutr Metab 37: 276–283.
25. Garcia-German D, Viloria F, Menendez P, Canillas F (2012) [Letter in reference to the article "surgery on the wrong side: implication for the patient and the professional. Experience in a major ambulatory surgery of the foot unit"]. Rev Esp Cir Ortop Traumatol 56: 421; author reply 422.
26. Keles GC, Cetinkaya BO, Eroglu C, Simsek SB, Kahraman H (2010) Vascular endothelial growth factor expression levels of gingiva in gingivitis and periodontitis patients with/without diabetes mellitus. Inflamm Res 59: 543–549.
27. Salvi GE, Franco LM, Braun TM, Lee A, Rutger Persson G, et al. (2010) Pro-inflammatory biomarkers during experimental gingivitis in patients with type 1 diabetes mellitus: a proof-of-concept study. J Clin Periodontol 37: 9–16.
28. Sima C, Rhourida K, Van Dyke TE, Gyurko R (2010) Type 1 diabetes predisposes to enhanced gingival leukocyte margination and macromolecule extravasation in vivo. J Periodontal Res 45: 748–756.
29. Xiang X, Duarte PM, Lima JA, Santos VR, Goncalves TD, et al. (2013) Diabetes-Associated Periodontitis Molecular Features in Infrared Spectra of Gingival Crevicular Fluid. J Periodontol.
30. Yoon AJ, Cheng B, Philipone E, Turner R, Lamster IB (2012) Inflammatory biomarkers in saliva: assessing the strength of association of diabetes mellitus and periodontal status with the oral inflammatory burden. J Clin Periodontol 39: 434–440.
31. Mandel ID (1989) The role of saliva in maintaining oral homeostasis. J Am Dent Assoc 119: 298-304.
32. Stuchell RN, Blitzer A, Mandel ID (1984) Medical management of non-neoplastic salivary gland disease. Otolaryngol Clin North Am 17: 697–703.
33. Tabak LA, Levine MJ, Mandel ID, Ellison SA (1982) Role of salivary mucins in the protection of the oral cavity. J Oral Pathol 11: 1–17.
34. Dunn W, Griffith JW, Morrison MT, Tanquary J, Sabata D, et al. (2013) Somatosensation assessment using the NIH Toolbox. Neurology 80: S41–44.
35. Hargreaves CE, Grasso M, Hampe CS, Stenkova A, Atkinson S, et al. (2013) Yersinia enterocolitica provides the link between thyroid-stimulating antibodies and their germline counterparts in Graves' disease. J Immunol 190: 5373–5381.
36. Barnes VM, Arvanitidou E, Szewczyk G, Richter R, DeVizio W, et al. (2011) Evaluation of the antiplaque efficacy of two cetylpyridinium chloride-containing mouthwashes. J Clin Dent 22: 200–203.
37. Barnes VM, Teles R, Trivedi HM, Devizio W, Xu T, et al. (2010) Assessment of the effects of dentifrice on periodontal disease biomarkers in gingival crevicular fluid. J Periodontal 81: 1273–1279.
38. Ganti S, Weiss RH (2011) Urine metabolomics for kidney cancer detection and biomarker discovery. Urol Oncol 29: 551–557.
39. Lobene RR, Kashket S, Soparkar PM, Shloss J, Sabine ZM (1979) The effect of cetylpridinium chloride on human plaque bacteria and gingivitis. Pharmacol Ther Dent 4: 33–47.
40. Fredericks MA, Lobene RR, Mundy P (1971) A model for teaching social concepts to dental auxiliaries. J Dent Educ 35: 232–235.
41. Bessonneau V, Bojko B, Pawliszyn J (2013) Analysis of human saliva metabolome by direct immersion solid-phase microextraction LC and benchtop orbitrap MS. Bioanalysis 5: 783–792.
42. Zhang A, Sun H, Wang X (2012) Saliva metabolomics opens door to biomarker discovery, disease diagnosis, and treatment. Appl Biochem Biotechnol 168: 1718–1727.
43. Al-Tarawneh SK, Border MB, Dibble CF, Bencharit S (2011) Defining salivary biomarkers using mass spectrometry-based proteomics: a systematic review. OMICS 15: 353–361.
44. Rathnayake N, Akerman S, Klinge B, Lundegren N, Jansson H, et al. (2013) Salivary biomarkers for detection of systemic diseases. PLoS ONE 8: e61356.
45. Rathnayake N, Akerman S, Klinge B, Lundegren N, Jansson H, et al. (2013) Salivary biomarkers of oral health: a cross-sectional study. J Clin Periodontol 40: 140–147.
46. Lobene RR, Weatherford T, Ross NM, Lamm RA, Menaker L (1986) A modified gingival index for use in clinical trials. Clin Prev Dent 8: 3–6.
47. Silness J, Loe H (1964) Periodontal Disease in Pregnancy. Ii. Correlation between Oral Hygiene and Periodontal Condtion. Acta Odontol Scand 22: 121–135.
48. Genco RJ, Schifferle RE, Dunford RG, Falkner KL, Hsu WC, et al. (2014) Screening for diabetes mellitus in dental practices: A field trial. J Am Dent Assoc 145: 57–64.
49. Judice PB, Matias CN, Santos DA, Magalhaes JP, Hamilton MT, et al. (2013) Caffeine intake, short bouts of physical activity, and energy expenditure: a double-blind randomized crossover trial. PLoS ONE 8: e68936.
50. Evans A, DeHaven CD, Barrett T, Mitchell M, Milgram E (2009) Integrated, nontargeted ultrahigh performance liquid chromatography/electrospray ionization tandem mass spectrometry platform for the identification and relative quantificationof the small-molecule complement of biological systems. Anal Chem 81: 6656–6667.
51. DeHaven CD, Evans AM, Dai H, Lawton KA (2010) Organization of GC/MS and LC/MS metabolomics data into chemical libraries. J Cheminformatics 2: 9–21.
52. Gall WE, Beebe K, Lawton KA, Adam KP, Mitchell MW, et al. (2010) Alpha-hydroxybutyrate is an early biomarker of insulin resistance and glucose tolerance in a nondiabetic population. PLoS ONE 5: 1–10.
53. Nerby CL, FStickle DF (2009) 1,5-anhydroglucitol monitoring in diabetes: A mass balance perspective. Clin Biochem 42: 158–167.
54. Toth BI, Geczy T, Griger Z, Dozsa A, Seltmann H, et al. (2009) Transient receptor potential vanilloid-1 signaling as a regulator of human sebocyte biology. J Invest Dermatol 129: 329–339.
55. Buse JB, Freeman JL, Edelman SV, Jovanovic L, McGill JB (2003) Serum 1,5-anhydroglucitol (GlycoMark): a short-term glycemic marker. Diabetes Technol Ther 5: 355–363.
56. Brass EP (1986) Effect of alpha-ketobutyrate on palmitic acid and pyruvate metabolism in isolated rat hepatocytes. Biochim Biophys Acta 888: 18–24.
57. Landaas S (1975) The formation of 2-hydroxybutyric acid in experimental animals. Clin Chim Acta 58: 23–32.
58. Landaas S, Pettersen JE (1975) Clinical conditions associated with urinary excretion of 2-hydroxybutyric acid. Scand J Clin Lab Invest 35: 259–266.
59. Pettersen JE, Landaas S, Eldjarn L (1973) The occurrence of 2-hydroxybutyric acid in urine from patients with lactic acidosis. Clin Chim Acta 48: 213–219.
60. Silva AR, Ruschel C, Helegda C, Wyse AT, Wannmacher CM, et al. (2001) Inhibition of in vitro CO2 production and lipid synthesis by 2-hydroxybutyric acid in rat brain. Braz J Med Biol Res 34: 627–631.
61. Yang W, Roth KS (1985) Defect in alpha-ketobutyrate metabolism: a new inborn error. Clin Chim Acta 145: 173–182.
62. Quinlan GJ, Lamb NJ, Tilley R, Evans TW, Gutteridge JM (1997) Plasma hypoxanthine levels in ARDS: implications for oxidative stress, morbidity, and mortality. Am J Respir Crit Care Med 155: 479–484.
63. Quick KL, Hardt JI, Dugan LL (2000) Rapid microplate assay for superoxide scavenging efficiency. J Neurosci Methods 97: 139–144.
64. Becker BF (1993) Towards the physiological function of uric acid. Free Radic Biol Med 14: 615–631.
65. Forman HJ, Dickinson DA (2003) Oxidative signaling and glutathione synthesis. Biofactors 17: 1–12.
66. Pastore A, Federici G, Bertini E, Piemonte F (2003) Analysis of glutathione: implication in redox and detoxification. Clin Chim Acta 333: 19–39.
67. Wu G, Fang YZ, Yang S, Lupton JR, Turner ND (2004) Glutathione metabolism and its implications for health. J Nutr 134: 489–492.
68. Townsend DM, Tew KD, Tapiero H (2003) The importance of glutathione in human disease. Biomed Pharmacother 57: 145–155.
69. Garcia-Ruiz C, Colell A, Morales A, Kaplowitz N, Fernandez-Checa JC (1995) Role of oxidative stress generated from the mitochondrial electron transport chain and mitochondrial glutathione status in loss of mitochondrial function and activation of transcription factor nuclear factor-kappa B: studies with isolated mitochondria and rat hepatocytes. Mol Pharmacol 48: 825–834.
70. Garcia-Ruiz C, Morales A, Colell A, Ballesta A, Rodes J, et al. (1995) Feeding S-adenosyl-L-methionine attenuates both ethanol-induced depletion of mitochondrial glutathione and mitochondrial dysfunction in periportal and perivenous rat hepatocytes. Hepatology 21: 207–214.
71. Kojer K, Bien M, Gangel H, Morgan B, Dick TP, et al. (2012) Glutathione redox potential in the mitochondrial intermembrane space is linked to the cytosol and impacts the Mia40 redox state. Embo J 31: 3169–3182.
72. Hansen SH, Grunnet N (2013) Taurine, glutathione and bioenergetics. Adv Exp Med Biol 776: 3–12.
73. Calder PC (2006) n-3 polyunsaturated fatty acids, inflammation, and inflammatory diseases. Am J Clin Nutr 83: 1505S–1519S.
74. Guenther G, Peralta E, Rosales K, Wong S, Siskind L, et al. (2008) Ceramide starves cells to death by downregulating nutrient transporter proteins. Proc Natl Acad Sci U S A 105: 17402–17407.
75. Peralta E, Edinger A (2009) Ceramide-induced starvation triggers homeostatic autophagy. Autophagy 5: 407–409.
76. Mao C, Obeid LM (2008) Ceramidases: regulators of cellular responses mediated by ceramide, sphingosine, and sphingosine-1-phosphate. Biochim Biophys Acta 1781: 424–434.
77. Bieberich E (2011) Ceramide in stem cell differentiation and embryo development: novel functions of a topological cell-signaling lipid and the concept of ceramide compartments. J Lipids In Press.
78. Nichols FC, Rojanasomsith K (2006) Porphyromonas gingivalis lipids and diseased dental tissues. Oral Microbiol Immunol 21: 84–92.
79. Cobb J, Gall W, Adam KP, Nakhle P, Button E, et al. (2013) A novel fasting blood test for insulin resistance and prediabetes. J Diabetes Sci Technol 7: 100–110.

18

Risk Factors of Developmental Defects of Enamel-A Prospective Cohort Study

Hai Ming Wong[1]*, Si-Min Peng[1,4], Yi Feng Wen[1], Nigel M. King[2], Colman P. J. McGrath[3]

1 Paediatric Dentistry & Orthodontics, Faculty of Dentistry, The University of Hong Kong, Hong Kong, **2** Paediatric Dentistry, School of Dentistry, University of Western Australia, Perth, Australia, **3** Dental Public Health, Faculty of Dentistry, The University of Hong Kong, Hong Kong, **4** Department of Paediatric Dentistry, Guanghua School of Stomatology, Hospital of Stomatology, Sun Yat-sen University, Guangzhou, China

Abstract

Background and objective: Current studies on the aetiology of developmental defects of enamel (DDE) are subject to recall bias because of the retrospective collection of information. Our objective was to investigate potential risk factors associated with the occurrence of DDE through a prospective cohort study.

Methods: Using a random community sample of Hong Kong children born in 1997, we performed a cohort study in which the subjects' background information, medical and dental records were prospectively collected. A clinical examination to identify DDE was conducted in 2010 when the subjects were 12 years old. The central incisor, lateral incisor and first molar in each quadrant were chosen as the index teeth and were examined 'wet' by two trained and calibrated examiners using the modified FDI (DDE) Index.

Results: With a response rate of 74.9%, the 514 examined subjects had matched data for background information. Diffuse opacites were the most common type of DDE. Of the various possible aetiological factors considered, only experience of severe diseases during the period 0–3 years was associated with the occurrence of 'any defect' ($p = 0.017$) and diffuse opacities ($p = 0.044$). The children with experience of severe diseases before 3 years of age were 7.89 times more likely to be affected by 'any defect' compared with those who did not have the experience (OR 7.89; 95% CI 1.07, 58.14; $p = 0.043$). However, after adjusting for confounding factors, the association no longer existed.

Conclusion: No variables could be identified as risk factors of DDE in this Hong Kong birth cohort.

Editor: Sompop Bencharit, University of North Carolina at Chapel Hill, United States of America

Funding: The work described in this paper was supported by a grant from the Research Grants Council of the Hong Kong Special Administrative Region, China (Project No. 782811; http://www.ugc.edu.hk/eng/rgc/). HMW received the funding. The funders had no role in study design, data collection and analysis, decision to publish, or preparation of the manuscript.

Competing Interests: The authors have declared that no competing interests exist.

* Email: wonghmg@hku.hk

Introduction

Developmental defects of enamel (DDE) are regions of enamel with altered quality and quantity as a consequence of insults to the enamel organ at the time of enamel formation [1]. DDE occur frequently on the incisors [2,3], and may thereby lead to major aesthetic concerns [4]. Common complications of DDE include tooth sensitivity and occlusal dysfunction [4,5]. Furthermore, DDE have been reported to predispose the teeth to early childhood caries [6] and increased attrition [7]. Despite the distinct treatment need of teeth affected by DDE, it is unfortunate that the treatment has frequently been unsuccessful because the altered enamel structure in DDE creates difficulties with anaesthetizing the tooth and bonding of the restoration to the enamel [5].

Faced with such a dilemma, we may consider directing our focus to the prevention of DDE, which in itself requires a substantial understanding of relevant aetiological factors. Although the aetiology of DDE has been studied for many years and that over 90 different factors have been identified [3,9], the best available data have been gained from animal studies and individual case reports of children with systemic disorders. Thus, reliable evidence for the involvement of specific risk factors remains equivocal.

According to published studies seeking possible risk factors for DDE, low socio-economic status, respiratory infections, exposure to cigarette smoking, asthma, otitis media, urinary tract infection, chickenpox and early life health problems have been said to be associated with enamel defects [10–14]. However, these results have always been challenged. For example, while amoxicillin has been reported to significantly increase the probability of DDE [15,16], such an effect was not found among a random sample of Western Australian children [17]. Similar conflicting results have also been reported for the impacts of otitis media [10,12], chicken pox [12,17], and maternal factors [16,17]. Furthermore, some New Zealand researchers failed correlate any early life health problems and the occurrence of DDE in the permanent dentition [18].

Conclusions from these studies should therefore be interpreted with caution. Primarily because information about past childhood diseases was mainly collected retrospectively after a relatively long interval and was hence dependent on the reliability of parental recall which can be notoriously poor. In addition, small sample sizes and the low prevalence of DDE limit the ability to differentiate the effects of the exposures on the creation of specific type of defects. Hence, the lack of robust data makes the results of these studies inconclusive.

The paucity of reliable information on possible causal factors of DDE supports the need for further investigations into the causes of these defects. Thus, the present study aimed to investigate the prevalence of DDE among a random group of Hong Kong adolescents aged 12 years old and to explore potential risk factors associated with the occurrence of DDE in these children who had prospectively maintained health records.

Methods

Ethics Statement

The study protocol was approved by the Institutional Review Board of the University of Hong Kong/Hospital Authority Hong Kong West Cluster (IRB reference number: UW 09-437, UW 11-070).

Patient Selection

This was a prospective, population-representative study. The eligible subjects were Hong Kong children born during April and May of 1997 when the fluoride in public water supply system was 0.5 ppm. The study was carried out in 2010 when the subjects were 12 years old. The sampling frame was all local secondary schools in Hong Kong (by law all children are required to attend secondary school). A random sample of 45 schools (approximately 10% of all local secondary schools) from 18 districts in Hong Kong, SAR, was selected. The secondary schools were the primary sampling unit. Within each school all Form 1 and Form 2 (equivalent to US Grade 6 and 7) students born between April 1st and May 31st, 1997 were invited to participate in the study. Parents/primary caregivers provided their written consent and students were asked to provide their assent. A sample size of 497 was calculated based on the prevalence of DDE at 89% in Hong Kong adolescents [19], and an odds ratio of 3.31 for having DDE among subjects with and without infection during the neonatal period [17]. The statistical power was 0.8 and the significance level was set at 0.05. Anticipating a response rate of 75%, 668 subjects were invited to participate in the study.

Information Collection

Background information solicited from the parents/guardians covered several aspects including socio-economic status, family history, infant and early childhood exposures, and oral hygiene habits. In addition, medical and dental records of the children, in particular their birth characteristics and history of oral diseases were also sought. Health care background information and data were obtained for these children immediately after birth and then on yearly basis through active follow-up surveys in the form of self-reported questionnaires; medical and dental records of the subjects were retrieved by passive follow-up via record linkage [20].

DDE Clinical Examination

Examinations were performed on the central incisors, lateral incisors and first permanent molars of the subjects. Two trained and calibrated examiners, who were blind to the subjects' information and the objectives of this study, completed all of the clinical examinations. Approximately 5% of the children were re-examined to test the intra- and inter-examiner reliabilities.

The children were instructed to lie in a supine position on a portable dental chair in classrooms in the schools. Before the examination, all of the incisors and first molars were cleaned with gauze in order to remove any gross plaque or food deposits that may have been present. These teeth were then examined under 'wet' conditions using a plane intra-oral disposable mouth mirror with a built in LED light source and a blunt probe. The probe was used to detect, or confirm the presence of any discontinuity of the enamel surface of the teeth.

Diagnostic Criteria of DDE

The diagnostic criteria were based on the modified version of the FDI (DDE) Index for use in general purpose epidemiological studies [21]. Three main types of enamel defects, based on their macroscopic appearance, were recognized, namely demarcated opacities, diffuse opacities and hypoplasia [21]. The demarcated opacities included the white/cream and the yellow/brown subtypes. Under the main type of diffuse opacities, there were subtypes of diffuse lines, diffuse patchy, diffuse confluent, and confluent/patchy plus staining and/or loss of enamel. Hypoplasia included subtypes of pits and missing enamel.

Statistical Analysis

Sample size was calculated using SAS software for windows, v9.2 (SAS Institute, Inc., CARY, NC, USA). Data collected were coded and entered into IBM SPSS Statistics v20.0 (IBM Corp., Armonk, NY, USA) for analysis. Information on the DDE status at the tooth surface level was used to generate information at the tooth level and the subject level. In the analysis, the eight different subtypes of DDE recorded were grouped into the three main types. 'Any defect' denoted the presence of DDE regardless of the main types. Frequency distributions of DDE by type at tooth and subject level were calculated. Bivariate associations between the occurrence of DDE and potential causal factors were tested using chi-square test for categorical independent variables and ANOVA for continuous independent variables. The statistical significance level was set at 0.05.

To assess the relative strength of the association between the presence of different types of DDE and various potential risk factors, unadjusted and adjusted logistic regression analyses were performed. In the unadjusted model, separate logistic regression was undertaken for each individual aetiological factor; while for the adjusted model, all explanatory variables were simultaneously entered into the model and a backward stepwise logistic regression was performed. The model building strategy for the adjusted logistic regression analysis was as follows: (i) variables with a p value no greater than 0.25 in bivariate analysis were included in the regression model; and (ii) at the significance level of 0.05, variables that did not contribute to the model as calculated by the likelihood ratio test were backward eliminated, until all retained variables were of significant impact on the model. For both models, the unadjusted and adjusted odds ratio (OR) and 95% confidence intervals (CI) were estimated. Poisson regression models were also been conducted to assess the association between the rarer main types of DDE and potential causal factors.

Results

There were a total of 668 children who had been randomly selected into this study and all of them completed the clinical examinations. Among these children, 514 had the matched background information, which represented a response rate of

76.9%. Twenty seven subjects (756 tooth surfaces) were re-examined to measure the level of examiner reliability throughout the study. At the tooth surface level, the intra-examiner reliabilities for the diagnoses of the various subtypes of DDE were 0.87 and 0.85, while the inter-examiner reliability was 0.82 (unweighted κ values).

Table 1 shows the frequency distribution of various types of DDE by types of tooth and at the subject level. Diffuse opacities were found to be the most prevalent of the three main types of DDE both at the tooth and at subject level. First permanent molars were more frequently affected by DDE than the incisors.

Bivariate associations of the occurrence of DDE and each independent variable are presented in Table 2. A higher proportion of demarcated opacities was observed among male subjects ($p<0.05$), while no gender difference was found for 'any defect', diffuse opacities or hypoplasia ($p>0.05$). The experience of severe diseases during the 0–3 year period was associated with a higher prevalence of 'any defect' ($p=0.017$) and diffuse opacities ($p=0.044$). The reported severe diseases prior to 3 years of age included spinal bifida, congenital heart disease, neonatal lupus erythematosus, Kawasaki disease, thalassemia, hepatitis B, meningitis, pneumonia, nephritis, pancreatitis, and severe asthma. While no statistical significant associations were found for other variables, higher proportion of 'any defect' and diffuse opacities were observed among subjects with lower levels of household monthly income ($p>0.05$). In addition, children who used an adult type toothpaste before 5 years of age were more susceptible to 'any defect' and diffuse opacities than those who used a toothpaste formulated for children ($p>0.05$).

In the unadjusted logistic regression model (Table 3), only the independent variable of 'child severe disease 0–3 years old' was associated with the occurrence of 'any defect'. Subjects with experience of severe diseases during the 0–3 years period were 7.89 times more likely to be affected by 'any defect' compared to those children who did not have the experience (OR 7.89; 95% CI 1.07, 58.14; $p=0.043$). No associations were found between any of the three main types of DDE and various independent variables in the unadjusted model. After controlling for potential confounding factors in the adjusted model, 'child severe disease 0–3 years old' was no longer associated with the presence of 'any defect'. As a result, no variable remained significant in the final adjusted model. Poisson regression models confirmed the above results for the main types of demarcated opacities and hypoplasia.

Discussion

The present prospective cohort study collected the subjects' background information and health care related records from a random community sample of Hong Kong children born in 1997, and the prevalence of DDE was assessed when the subjects were aged 12-year-old. Bivariate analyses were performed to screen for possible aetiological factors responsible for the presence of DDE and subsequent multinomial logistic regression was undertaken to control for potential confounding factors.

To date, most studies that investigated risk factors of DDE were case-control studies [10,11,16] or cross-sectional surveys [14,17], and the subjects' information was collected retrospectively. Recall bias was thereby introduced into these studies. In a carefully designed study by Arrow [17], information was collected prior to eruption of the teeth of interest. While reporting bias was avoided, recall bias still existed due to the retrospective nature of the study. To the best of the authors' knowledge, there is only one antecedent prospective study that investigated the potential causal factors for DDE. A group of 696 New Zealand children participated in the

Table 1. Frequency distribution [n (%)] of DDE by type at tooth and subject level.

	Tooth level									
	Central incisor			Lateral incisor			1st permanent molar			
Type of DDE	Upper (N = 1000)	Lower (N = 988)	Total (N = 1988)	Upper (N = 1000)	Lower (N = 981)	Total (N = 1981)	Upper (N = 1002)	Lower (N = 1004)	Total (N = 2006)	Subject level (N = 514)
No defects	200 (19.2)	430 (46.5)	630 (31.7)	219 (21.9)	380 (38.7)	599 (30.2)	157 (15.7)	241 (24.0)	398 (19.8)	52 (10.1)
Any defects	800 (80.8)	558 (56.5)	1358 (68.3)	781 (78.1)	601 (61.3)	1382 (69.8)	845 (84.3)	763 (76.0)	1608 (80.2)	462 (89.9)
Demarcated opacities	20 (2.0)	17 (1.7)	37 (1.9)	2 (0.2)	3 (0.3)	5 (0.3)	11 (1.1)	16 (1.6)	27 (1.3)	44 (8.6)
Diffuse opacities	795 (79.5)	555 (56.2)	1350 (67.9)	780 (78.0)	600 (61.2)	1380 (69.7)	844 (84.2)	757 (75.4)	1601 (79.8)	460 (89.5)
Hypoplasia	0 (0)	4 (0.4)	4 (0.2)	0 (0)	1 (0.1)	1 (0.1)	5 (0.5)	2 (0.2)	7 (0.3)	9 (1.8)

Table 2. Distribution of variables among children with different types of DDE.

Variable	No defects		Any defects		Demarcated opacities		Diffuse opacities		Hypoplasia	
Gender (N = 514)										
Male	28	(10.8)	231	(89.2)	30	(11.6)*	229	(88.4)	4	(1.5)
Female	24	(9.4)	231	(90.6)	14	(5.5)*	231	(90.6)	5	(2.0)
Gestation; weeks (N = 514)[a]	39.1	(1.6)	38.9	(1.7)	38.8	(1.1)	38.9	(1.7)	39.0	(1.2)
Birth weight; kg (N = 514)[a]	3.2	(0.5)	3.2	(0.5)	3.2	(0.5)	3.2	(0.5)	3.3	(0.4)
Maternal age (N = 501)										
<30 years	20	(9.4)	193	(90.6)	16	(7.5)	191	(89.7)	4	(1.9)
≥30 years	31	(10.8)	257	(89.2)	25	(8.7)	257	(89.2)	5	(1.7)
Paternal age (N = 495)										
<30 years	4	(4.7)	81	(95.3)	7	(8.2)	80	(94.1)	1	(1.2)
≥30 years	47	(11.5)	363	(88.5)	34	(8.3)	362	(88.3)	8	(2.0)
Small-for-gestational age infants (N = 512)										
No	46	(10.2)	404	(89.8)	38	(8.4)	402	(89.3)	9	(2.0)
Yes	6	(9.7)	56	(90.3)	5	(8.1)	56	(90.3)	0	(0)
Mode of delivery (N = 497)										
Natural labour	21	(7.9)	245	(92.1)	26	(9.8)	244	(91.7)	7	(2.6)
Assisted natural labour	15	(14.4)	89	(85.6)	6	(5.8)	88	(84.6)	2	(1.9)
Caesarean birth	14	(11.0)	113	(89.0)	9	(7.1)	113	(89.0)	0	(0)
Breast feeding (N = 507)										
No	28	(10.0)	252	(90.0)	19	(6.8)	250	(89.3)	5	(1.8)
Yes	24	(10.6)	203	(89.4)	24	(10.6)	203	(89.4)	4	(1.8)
Maternal education (N = 505)										
Grade 9 or below	22	(10.6)	185	(89.4)	16	(7.7)	183	(88.4)	3	(1.4)
Grade 10–11	24	(10.6)	202	(89.4)	21	(9.3)	202	(89.4)	4	(1.8)
Grade 12 or above	5	(6.9)	67	(93.1)	6	(8.3)	67	(93.1)	2	(2.8)
Paternal education (N = 505)										
Grade 9 or below	19	(8.5)	204	(91.5)	17	(7.6)	203	(91.0)	5	(2.2)
Grade 10–11	24	(13.0)	161	(87.0)	15	(8.1)	160	(86.5)	2	(1.1)
Grade 12 or above	8	(8.2)	89	(91.8)	11	(11.3)	89	(91.8)	2	(2.1)
Mother's place of birth (N = 475)										
Hong Kong	30	(9.7)	279	(90.3)	28	(9.1)	278	(90.0)	5	(1.6)
Others	14	(8.4)	152	(91.6)	14	(8.4)	152	(91.6)	3	(1.8)
Father's place of birth (N = 483)										
Hong Kong	37	(10.4)	320	(89.6)	31	(8.7)	319	(89.4)	6	(1.7)
Others	8	(6.3)	118	(93.7)	11	(8.7)	118	(93.7)	2	(1.6)
Type of birth hospital (N = 497)										
Public	38	(10.1)	340	(89.9)	31	(8.2)	338	(89.4)	7	(1.9)

Table 2. Cont.

Variable	No defects		Any defects		Demarcated opacities		Diffuse opacities		Hypoplasia	
Private	14	(11.8)	105	(88.2)	11	(9.2)	105	(88.2)	1	(0.8)
Household monthly income (N = 493)										
Less than HK$10,000	9	(7.7)	108	(92.3)	10	(8.5)	107	(91.5)	1	(0.9)
HK$10,000–HK$40,000	31	(10.5)	264	(89.5)	26	(8.8)	263	(89.2)	6	(2.0)
Over HK$40,000	11	(13.6)	70	(86.4)	7	(8.6)	70	(86.4)	2	(2.5)
Parents smoking pattern during the child aged 0–3years (N = 375)										
father	11	(10.3)	96	(89.7)	11	(10.3)	96	(89.7)	2	(1.9)
mother	1	(16.7)	5	(83.3)	1	(16.7)	5	(83.3)	0	(0)
both	1	(7.7)	12	(92.3)	1	(7.7)	11	(84.6)	1	(7.7)
none	22	(8.8)	227	(91.2)	17	(6.8)	226	(90.8)	5	(2.0)
Mother's severe disease during pregnancy (N = 372)										
No	34	(9.4)	327	(90.6)	29	(8.0)	326	(90.3)	8	(2.2)
Yes	1	(9.1)	10	(90.9)	0	(0)	10	(90.9)	4	(0)
Mother's medication during pregnancy (N = 195)										
No	21	(12.8)	143	(87.2)	13	(7.9)	143	(87.2)	4	(2.4)
Amoxicillin and/or other antibiotics	0	(0)	4	(100.0)	1	(25.0)	4	(100.0)	0	(0)
Others	2	(7.4)	25	(92.6)	1	(3.7)	25	(92.6)	1	(3.7)
Infant special medical maintenance (N = 373)										
No	26	(8.1)	294	(91.9)	25	(7.8)	293	(91.6)	7	(2.2)
Yes	8	(15.1)	45	(84.9)	5	(9.4)	45	(84.9)	1	(1.9)
Child severe disease 0–3 years old (N = 508)										
No	50	(11.2)	395	(88.8)*	42	(9.4)	394	(88.5)*	7	(1.6)
Yes	1	(1.6)	62	(98.4)*	2	(3.2)	61	(96.8)*	2	(3.2)
Medication 0–3 years old (N = 133)										
No	10	(15.2)	56	(84.8)	3	(4.5)	56	(84.8)	1	(1.5)
Amoxicillin and/or other antibiotics	3	(7.5)	37	(92.5)	5	(12.5)	37	(92.5)	1	(2.5)
Others	3	(11.1)	24	(88.9)	1	(3.7)	24	(88.9)	1	(3.7)
Dental trauma 0–3 years old (N = 373)										
No	33	(8.9)	337	(91.1)	30	(8.1)	336	(90.8)	8	(2.2)
Yes	1	(33.3)	2	(66.7)	0	(0)	2	(66.7)	0	(0)
Tooth extraction due to caries 1–3 years old (N = 373)										
No	33	(8.9)	328	(91.1)	29	(8.1)	327	(90.8)	8	(2.2)
Yes	1	(33.1)	11	(84.6)	1	(7.7)	11	(84.6)	0	(0)
Age begin to use toothpaste (N = 507)										
Before 4 years old	41	(10.2)	359	(89.8)	35	(8.8)	357	(89.2)	7	(1.8)
4 years old or older	10	(9.3)	97	(90.7)	8	(7.5)	97	(90.7)	2	(1.9)

Table 2. Cont.

Variable	No defects		Any defects		Demarcated opacities		Diffuse opacities		Hypoplasia	
Toothpaste type before 5 years old (N = 506)										
Adult toothpaste	3	(7.7)	36	(92.3)	2	(5.1)	36	(92.3)	0	(0)
Children toothpaste	48	(10.3)	419	(89.7)	41	(8.8)	417	(89.3)	9	(1.9)
Toothpaste contained fluoride before 5 years old (N = 506)										
No	6	(12.0)	44	(88.0)	3	(6.0)	44	(88.0)	0	(0)
Yes	16	(10.6)	135	(89.4)	10	(6.6)	135	(89.4)	5	(3.3)
Don't know	29	(9.5)	276	(90.5)	30	(9.8)	274	(89.8)	4	(1.3)
Amount of tooth paste applied before 5 years old (N = 500)										
Smear	13	(8.7)	136	(91.3)	16	(10.7)	136	(91.3)	1	(0.7)
Pea size	32	(10.6)	271	(89.4)	23	(7.6)	269	(88.8)	5	(1.7)
Larger than pea size	6	(12.5)	42	(87.5)	3	(6.2)	42	(87.5)	3	(6.2)
Toothbrushing habits before 5 years old (N = 499)										
Less than once daily	3	(7.9)	35	(92.1)	2	(5.3)	35	(92.1)	1	(2.6)
At least once daily	48	(10.4)	413	(89.6)	39	(8.5)	411	(89.2)	8	(1.7)

*$p<0.05$.
mean (SD)[a] or frequency distribution, n (%).

Table 3. Multinomial logistic regression of DDE.

	Unadjusted[1]			Adjusted[2]		
Variable	OR	95% C.I.	p-value	OR	95% C.I.	p-value
Any defects						
Child severe disease 0–3 years old						
no	1			-	-	-
yes	7.89	1.07, 58.14	0.043*	-	-	-

[1]Unadjusted: separate logistic regression analysis.
[2]Adjusted: adjusted for gender; gestation age; birth weight; maternal age (<30 years, ≥30 years); paternal age (<30 years, ≥30 years); small-for-gestational age infants (no, yes); mode of delivery (natural labour, assisted natural labour, caesarean birth); breast feeding (no, yes); maternal education (grade 9 or below, grade 10–11, grade 12 or above); paternal education (grade 9 or below, grade 10–11, grade 12 or above); mother's place of birth (Hong Kong, outside Hong Kong); father's place of birth (Hong Kong, outside Hong Kong); type of birth hospital (public, private); household monthly income (less than HK$10,000, HK$10,000–HK$40,000, over HK$40,000); parent smoking pattern during the child aged 0–3 years (father, mother, both, and none); mother's severe disease during pregnancy (no, yes); mother's medication during pregnancy (no, amoxicillin and/or other antibiotics, and others); infant special medical maintenance (no, yes); child severe disease 0–3 years old (no, yes); medication 0–3 years old (no, amoxicillin and/or other antibiotics, and others); dental trauma 0–3 years old (no, yes); tooth extraction due to caries 1–3 years old (no, yes); age begin to use toothpaste (before 4 years old, 4 years old or older); toothpaste type before 5 years old (adult toothpaste, children toothpaste); toothpaste contained fluoride before 5 years old (no, yes); amount of toothpaste applied before 5 years old (smear, pea size, larger than pea size); tooth brushing habits before 5 years old (less than once daily, at least once daily).
*p<0.05.

Dunedin Multidisciplinary Child Developmental Study in which the medical and dental histories were correlated with the presence of DDE; only chicken pox before the age of 3 years and trauma to the primary incisors were identified as risk factors [12]. However, only bivariate analyses were undertaken without control of other potential confounding factors. Moreover, there might have been dramatic changes over the past two decades in the pattern of children's health profiles due to immunization, the use of medication and readily available medical facilities. Therefore, it is difficult to compare the present results with those of other older studies.

Male subjects were found at an increased risk of demarcated opacities (Table 2). We speculate that this might have arisen because of the small number of subjects with demarcated opacities in our sample. Results on gender differences of DDE have been inconsistent and warrant further exploration. While some researchers found male subjects more likely to be affected [22], others [14,17] reported no gender differences.

The associations of DDE with birth characteristics, including gestational weeks, birth weight, mode of delivery and parental age, were not significant (Table 2). Our results confirmed findings from previous studies [16,23], but were in contrast with a pilot study by van Amerongen and Kreulen [24], where subjects born prematurely were common among the subjects affected by enamel defects. Since no premature babies were recruited in the current study, further research is required to clarify the association of DDE with gestational weeks.

Investigations into the effect of breastfeeding on DDE are interesting. Developing enamel has been reported to be especially sensitive to even a minute amount of dioxin [25], which is expressed in breast milk [26]. Duration of breastfeeding has been associated with the presence of DDE in permanent teeth [26] and DDE have even been suggested as a biomarker of dioxin exposure [27]. However, our results (Table 2), which are in agreement with several other epidemiologic studies [14,16,17], suggested that the duration of breastfeeding did not affect the occurrence of DDE.

Since our subjects were drawn from a random community sample, we expect the socio-economic status, including the levels of parental education and household monthly incomes, of our subjects to be proportionately distributed and so be a reflection of the society's socio-economic status as a whole. Even though there were reports stating that subjects of lower socio-economic status had a higher chance of developing DDE [10,28], we were unable to find significant associations in this study. Thus our results were in line with those reported by Arrow [17] and other researchers [29,30].

Contrary to the findings reported by Ford and colleagues [10], which indicated that parental cigarette smoking was correlated with DDE, we failed to identify any statistically significant associations between DDE and any of the prenatal exposure factors, such as parental smoking, maternal severe disease and medication during pregnancy. Early life health problems have consistently been reported to be associated with DDE. Arrow [17] found subjects who had had an illness during the neonatal period were at increased risk of DDE. Health problems in the first three years of life were also found to increase the likelihood of DDE [11,14]. Data on severe diseases experienced by children during the first three years of life were collected in this study because this is the period when the index teeth were undergoing formation [31,32] overlaps with the time period when children are most susceptible to various diseases. As a result, we revealed the significant effects of 'child severe disease 0–3 years old' on 'any defect' and diffuse opacities. However, this association disappeared in the adjusted logistic model when confounding factors were controlled for.

Fluoride consumption has been related to the occurrence of DDE in terms of diffuse opacities [2,33] and a significant association between the use of adult toothpaste and DDE was reported from a case-control study that was conducted in Australia [10]. Therefore, oral hygiene habits such as the age when toothpaste usage commenced, the type of toothpaste, amount of toothpaste applied, and the frequency of tooth brushing were studied in this investigation. We found no significant associations between the various oral hygiene habits and the occurrence of DDE. Although the children in this study who used an adult type toothpaste before 5 years of age were more susceptible to 'any defect' and diffuse opacities than those who used a child formula toothpaste, the result was not statistically significant ($p>0.05$).

Inevitably the present study had several limitations. Due to the low prevalence of demarcated opacities and hypoplasia in the Hong Kong population, the number of subjects affected by these two types of DDE was very limited. This decreased the statistical power of the analyses; therefore, the findings on demarcated opacities and hypoplasia should be interpreted with caution. Future research into the aetiological factors of demarcated opacities and hypoplasia in situations where the prevalence is rather low could adopt a case-control study as the study design. The neonatal period is a very important stage of a child's development. Under the item 'child severe disease 0–3 years old', we did not differentiate between the neonatal period and the remainder of this age range. In addition, while different types of diseases experienced by the children were recorded, statistical analysis was not performed with respect to each specific disease type. This may explain why the impact of childhood severe disease on DDE disappeared after controlling for potential confounding factors. Future studies could be designed to gather specific detailed information and other potential risk factors for DDE. Furthermore, investigations into the effect of antibiotics on DDE are not straightforward because the illness for which the antibiotic was prescribed may have caused the DDE and thereby serve as a confounding factor.

Conclusions

Our uniquely large prospective cohort study among randomly selected Hong Kong children expands the current knowledge on the aetiology of DDE. Experiences of severe diseases experienced during 0–3 years of age were associated with 'any defect' and diffuse opacities. Children with severe diseases in early life were found to be almost 8 times more likely than healthy children to be affected by DDE. However, after adjusting for confounding factors, no variable was associated with the occurrence of DDE.

Acknowledgments

The authors would like to give our great appreciation to the children who participated in this study. We would also like to thank the Academic Editor and the anonymous reviewers for their constructive suggestions and valuable comments. The work described in this paper was fully supported by a grant from the Research Grants Council of the Hong Kong Special Administrative Region, China (Project No. 782811).

Author Contributions

Conceived and designed the experiments: HMW NMK CPJM. Performed the experiments: HMW SMP. Analyzed the data: HMW SMP YFW. Contributed reagents/materials/analysis tools: HMW CPJM. Contributed to the writing of the manuscript: HMW SMP YFW NMK CPJM.

References

1. Suckling G (1989) Developmental defects of enamel–historical and present-day perspectives of their pathogenesis. Adv Dent Res 3: 87–94.
2. Wong HM, McGrath C, Lo EC, King NM (2006) Association between developmental defects of enamel and different concentrations of fluoride in the public water supply. Caries Res 40: 481–486.
3. Seow WK, Ford D, Kazoullis S, Newman B, Holcombe T (2011) Comparison of enamel defects in the primary and permanent dentitions of children from a low-fluoride District in Australia. Pediatr Dent 33: 207–212.
4. Wong HM, McGrath C, King NM (2007) Dental practitioners' views on the need to treat developmental defects of enamel. Community Dent Oral Epidemiol 35: 130–139.
5. Jälevik B, Klingberg G (2002) Dental treatment, dental fear and behaviour management problems in children with severe enamel hypomineralization of their permanent first molars. Int J Paediatr Dent 12: 24–32.
6. Seow WK, Clifford H, Battistutta D, Morawska A, Holcombe T (2009) Case-control study of early childhood caries in Australia. Caries Res 43: 25–35.
7. Kazoullis S, Seow WK, Holcombe T, Newman B, Ford D (2007) Common dental conditions associated with dental erosion in schoolchildren in Australia. Pediatr Dent 29: 33–39.
8. Small B, Murray J (1978) Enamel opacities: prevalence, classifications and aetiological considerations. J Dent 6: 33–42.
9. Pindborg J (1982) Aetiology of developmental enamel defects not related to fluorosis. Int Dent J 32: 123–134.
10. Ford D, Seow WK, Kazoullis S, Holcombe T, Newman B (2009) A controlled study of risk factors for enamel hypoplasia in the permanent dentition. Pediatr Dent 31: 382–388.
11. Tapias-Ledesma MA, Jiménez R, Lamas F, González A, Carrasco P, et al. (2003) Factors associated with first molar dental enamel defects: a multivariate epidemiological approach. ASDC J Dent Child 70: 215–220.
12. Suckling GW, Herbison GP, Brown RH (1987) Etiological factors influencing the prevalence of developmental defects of dental enamel in nine-year-old New Zealand children participating in a health and development study. J Dent Res 66: 1466–1469.
13. Arnadóttir IB, Sigurjóns H, Holbrook WP (2005) Enamel opacities in 8-year-old Icelandic children in relation to their medical history as infants. Community Dent Health 22: 279–281.
14. Jälevik B[1], Norén JG, Klingberg G, Barregård L (2001) Etiologic factors influencing the prevalence of demarcated opacities in permanent first molars in a group of Swedish children. Eur J Oral Sci 109: 230–234.
15. Hong L, Levy SM, Warren JJ, Dawson DV, Bergus GR (2005) Association of amoxicillin use during early childhood with developmental tooth enamel defects. Arch Pediatr Adolesc Med 159: 943–948.
16. Whatling R, Fearne J (2008) Molar incisor hypomineralization: a study of aetiological factors in a group of UK children. Int J Paediatr Dent 18: 155–162.
17. Arrow P (2009) Risk factors in the occurrence of enamel defects of the first permanent molars among schoolchildren in Western Australia. Community Dent Oral Epidemiol 37: 405–415.
18. Suckling G, Pearce E (1984) Developmental defects of enamel in a group of New Zealand children: their prevalence and some associated etiological factors. Community Dent Oral Epidemiol 12: 177–184.
19. King N (1989) Developmental defects of enamel in Chinese girls and boys in Hong Kong. Adv Dent Res 3: 120–125.
20. Schooling CM, Hui LL, Ho LM, Lam TH, Leung GM (2012) Cohort profile: 'children of 1997': a Hong Kong Chinese birth cohort. Int J Epidemiol 41: 611–620.
21. FDI Commission on Oral Health (1992) A review of the developmental defects of enamel index (DDE Index). Int Dent J 42: 411–426.
22. Robles MJ, Ruiz M, Bravo-Perez M, González E, Peñalver MA (2013) Prevalence of enamel defects in primary and permanent teeth in a group of schoolchildren from Granada (Spain). Med Oral Patol Oral Cir Bucal 18: e187–e193.
23. Beentjes VE, Weerheijm KL, Groen HJ (2002) Factors involved in the aetiology of molar-incisor hypomineralisation (MIH). Eur J Paediatr Dent 3: 9–13.
24. van Amerongen W, Kreulen CM (1995) Cheese molars: a pilot study of the etiology of hypocalcifications in first permanent molars. ASDC J Dent Child 62: 266–269.
25. Billings RJ, Berkowitz RJ, Watson G (2004) Teeth. Pediatrics 113: 1120–1127.
26. Alaluusua S, Lukinmaa PL, Koskimies M, Pirinen S, Hölttä P, et al. (1996) Developmental dental defects associated with long breast feeding. Eur J Oral Sci 104: 493–497.
27. Alaluusua S, Lukinmaa PL, Torppa J, Tuomisto J, Vartiainen T (1999) Developing teeth as biomarker of dioxin exposure. Lancet 353: 206.
28. Oliveira AF, Chaves AM, Rosenblatt A (2006) The influence of enamel defects on the development of early childhood caries in a population with low socioeconomic status: a longitudinal study. Caries Res 40: 296–302.
29. Ellwood R, O'Mullane D (1994) The demographic and social variation in the prevalence of dental enamel opacities in north Wales. Community Dent Health 11: 192–196.
30. Elley K, Charlton J (1993) Prevalence of dental enamel defects in 6, 7 and 8-year-old children resident in West Bromwich, Sandwell, UK. Community Dent Health 10: 11–21.
31. Haavikko K (1970) The formation and the alveolar and clinical eruption of the permanent teeth. An orthopantomographic study. Suom Hammaslaak Toim 66: 103–170.
32. Logan W, Kronfeld R (1933) Development of the human jaws and surrounding structures from birth to the age of fifteen years. J Am Dent Assoc 20: 379–427.
33. Wong HM, McGrath C, King NM (2014) Diffuse opacities in 12-year-old Hong Kong children - four cross-sectional surveys. Community Dent Oral Epidemiol 42: 61–69.

19

Whole Genome Sequencing Reveals Novel Non-Synonymous Mutation in Ectodysplasin A (*EDA*) Associated with Non-Syndromic X-Linked Dominant Congenital Tooth Agenesis

Tanmoy Sarkar[1], Rajesh Bansal[2], Parimal Das[1]*

1 Centre for Genetic Disorders, Faculty of Science, Banaras Hindu University, Varanasi, Uttar Pradesh, India, 2 Faculty of Dental Sciences, Institute of Medical Sciences, Banaras Hindu University, Varanasi, Uttar Pradesh, India

Abstract

Congenital tooth agenesis in human is characterized by failure of tooth development during tooth organogenesis. 300 genes in mouse and 30 genes in human so far have been known to regulate tooth development. However, candidature of only 5 genes viz. *PAX9, MSX1, AXIN2, WNT10A* and *EDA* have been experimentally established for congenitally missing teeth like hypodontia and oligodontia. In this study an Indian family with multiple congenital tooth agenesis was identified. Pattern of inheritance was apparently autosomal dominant type with a rare possibility to be X-linked. Whole genome sequencing of two affected individuals was carried out which revealed 119 novel non-synonymous single nucleotide variations (SNVs) distributed among 117 genes. Out of these only one variation (**c.956G>T**) located at exon 9 of X-linked *EDA* gene was considered as pathogenic and validated among all the affected and unaffected family members and unrelated controls. This variation leads to p.Ser319Ile change in the TNF homology domain of EDA (transcript variant 1) protein. *In silico* analysis predicts that this Ser319 is well conserved across different vertebrate species and a part of putative receptor binding site. Structure based homology modeling predicts that this amino acid residue along with four other amino acid residues nearby, those when mutated known to cause selective tooth agenesis, form a cluster that may have functional significance. Taken together these results suggest that c.956G>T (p.Ser319Ile) mutation plausibly reduces the receptor binding activity of EDA leading to distinct tooth agenesis in this family.

Editor: Vladimir N. Uversky, University of South Florida College of Medicine, United States of America

Funding: The authors acknowledge the financial support from Department of Biotechnology, Govt. Of India (Grant Number: BT/PR12638/MED/12/467/2009 dated 18/03/2010; http://dbtindia.nic.in/index.asp) for the present work. TS acknowledges the receipt of Senior Research Fellowship from University Grants Commission, Govt. Of India (http://www.ugc.ac.in/). The funders had no role in study design, data collection and analysis, decision to publish, or preparation of the manuscript.

Competing Interests: The authors have declared that no competing interests exist.

* Email: parimal@bhu.ac.in

Introduction

Congenital tooth agenesis (CTA) is one of the most common cranio-facial disorders in human. Considering third molar (Wisdom teeth) agenesis, it affects up to 20% of the population. Among other teeth mandibular second premolar shows highest frequency of agenesis (2.9% to 3.2%) followed by maxillary lateral incisor (1.5% to 1.8%) and maxillary second premolar (1.4% to 1.6%).[1] Depending upon the severity, congenital tooth agenesis in human can be classified into three different forms: Hypodontia (Congenital absence of six or few teeth), oligodontia (Congenital absence more than six teeth), Anodontia (Congenital absence of all primary and/or permanent teeth).

Occurrence of hypodontia differs among population. A meta-analysis suggests that Saudi Arabian white people are less susceptible [2.5% (1.9% to 3.1%)] to tooth agenesis compared to North Americans [3.9% (3.1%–4.6%)], Europeans [5.5% (5.3%–5.6%)], Australians [6.3% (5.4%–7.2%)] and Chinese (Mongoloid) [6.9% (5.3%–.4%)]. It also shows clear gender bias; females are more susceptible for congenital tooth agenesis than males in all population except Saudi Arabia.[1] It has also been shown that most frequently missing tooth excluding 3rd molars is mandibular second premolars (2.91%–3.22%) followed by maxillary lateral incisors (1.55%–1.78%) and maxillary second premolars (1.39%–1.66%) [1].

Congenital tooth agenesis in human may be syndromic as well as non-syndromic. In syndromic cases it is found to be associated with various forms of ectodermal displasia,[2,3] oral-facial clefting like Pierre Robin syndome, [4] Van Der Woude syndrome [5] Hypodontia is also one of the cranio-facial features in several other syndromes such as Stickler's syndrome, [6] Down's syndrome [7,8] and number of other syndromes [9].

Beside the syndromic cases congenital tooth agenesis is a well established birth defect that occurs as an isolated disorder. Non-syndromic tooth agenesis may be sporadic or familial. In familial cases it may show autosomal dominant, autosomal recessive or X-linked mode of inheritance. So far five major genes are found to be associated with CTA in human. These are Paired box 9 (*PAX9*) (MIM *167416),[10] Muscle segment homology homeobox 1 (*MSX1*) (MIM *142983),[11] Ectodisplasin A (*EDA*) (MIM *300451),[12] Axis inhibitor 2 (*AXIN2*) (MIM *604025),[13] Wingless type MMTV integration site family member 10A (*WNT10A*) (MIM *606268).[14,15].

In the present study we have reported a novel non-synonymous mutation in *EDA* gene detected by whole genome sequencing and assessment of its pathogenic potential for determining the plausible cause for severe non-syndromic oligodontia (Tooth agenesis, selective, X-linked 1 MIM #313500) in an Indian family.

Materials and Methods

Family with congenital tooth agenesis

All the individuals investigated in this study belong to an Indian family (Figure 1A) showing multiple missing teeth. Following clinical diagnosis of the individuals as oligodontia patients at the faculty of Dental Sciences, Banaras Hindu University, an informed written consent was signed from patients and their unaffected family members for their participation in the present study. For minors (bellow 18 years of age) written consent was signed by their parent for their participation in this study. The study protocol and subject consent were approved by Institutional Review Board of Banaras Hindu University (No. Dean/2008-09/484). The severity of tooth agenesis was determined using the orthopentamogram (OPG). All available patients were critically screened for any other congenital disorders related with hair, skin, nails, tooth and other birth defect by interview. Blood samples were collected in heparinised syringe from four affected and two unaffected family members of DEN12 family.

Whole Genome sequencing

Genomic DNA was extracted from whole blood using the protocol introduced by Grimberg *et al.*[16] with slight modifications and purified by standard phenol-chloroform-isoamyl alcohol method. Two affected members of DEN12 family were selected for performing whole genome sequencing. Genomic DNA sample was processed for library preparation using TruSeq DNA Sample Preparation Kit (Illumina) and sequencing was performed using Illumina HiSeq 2500 platform with an average of 10X depth; base calling was performed using CASAVA software v1.8.2 (Illumina) and variant calling was performed based on Human reference Sequence v19 (NCBI) database using Avadis NGS v.1.5.1 (Strand scientific intelligence, Inc).

DNA Sequencing

To screen *PAX9* and *MSX1*; exon 2 to 4 along with exon-intron boundaries and a previously reported putative promoter region [chr14:37129645-37130161, refNC_000014.8, *H. sapiens* chr 14, GRCh37.p10 Primary Assembly] of *PAX9* and exon 1 through 2 along with exon-intron boundaries of *MSX1* were initially amplified from four affected and two unaffected individuals of DEN12 family using polymerase chain reaction (PCR). PCR was carried out using 50 ng genomic DNA in ABI Veriti 96 well thermal cycler (Applied Biosystems, USA) programmed with initial denaturation at 95°C for 5 min., followed by 30 cycles of 94°C for 1 min., 60°C to 62°C for 1 min., 72°C for 1 min. and one final hold at 72°C for 10 min. All the PCR products were purified by exonuclease I and recombinant Shrimp alkaline phosphatase (rSAP) (USB Affimetrix, USA). All the primers for amplifying *PAX9* putative promoter, *PAX9* and *MSX1* exon were designed previously by Mendoza-Fandino *et al.* (2010),[17] Das *et al.* (2003)[18] and Wang *et al.* (2011)[19] respectively. PCR products were labeled with ABI Big Dye Terminator V3.1 cycle sequencing kit followed by automated sequencing in ABI 3130 Genetic Analyzer according to manufacturer's protocol. All the sequences were analyzed using Sequencing analysis software version 5.2 (Applied Biosystems, USA). To identify any sequence variation(s), all the sequences of putative promoter region, exon 2 to 4 of *PAX9* and exon 1 to 2 of *MSX1*, were compared with available National Center for Biotechnology Information (NCBI) GenBank database using NCBI- Basic Local Alignment Search (BLAST) tool.

For genotyping c.956G>T variation of *EDA* gene (NM_001399), primers h*EDA*ex8F1 (5′-GATTCTGTCAATT-CACCACAG-3′) and h*EDA*ex8R1 (5′-ATCTTGACGGC-GATCTT CTG-3′) were designed using Primer3web v4.0.0 software and used to amplify and sequence (Sanger dideoxy chain termination sequencing) an amplicon of 250 bp, harboring the variant 115 bp downstream from 5′ side of the amplicon, from all the affected and unaffected individuals of the family.[20,21] The PCR and sequencing protocol is same as mentioned above.

Genotyping of c.956G>T nucleotide variant

For cross validation of c.956G>T variant detected in *EDA*, PCR-Restriction Fragment Length Polymorphism (PCR-RFLP) and Single-Strand Conformational Polymorphism (SSCP) were designed using the same 250 bp amplicon. For SSCP amplicon from case and control samples were denatured at 95°C for 5 min in the presence of denaturing buffer (5% formamide; 0.01N NaOH; 20 mM di-Na-EDTA, pH8.0; 0.05% bromophenol blue and 0.05% xylene cyanol) followed by rapid chilling on ice. Electrophoresis was performed using 10% non-denaturing midi (14 cm×15 cm) polyacrylamide gel containing 10% glycerol and 1× TBE at 25°C for 13 hr under 250V. Gel was stained using standard silver staining protocol. For PCR-RFLP, 250 bp amplicons from patients and controls were digested using 3U of *Alu*I restriction endonuclease (New England BioLabs Inc.) at 37°C for 8 hr. Digested products were resolved using 4% agarose gel and stained with Ethidium Bromide.

In silico analysis of EDA1 c.956G>T (p.Ser319Ile) and its effect on protein structure

In order to determine the inheritance pattern of X-linked *EDA* c.956G>T variant, sequences from all the affected and unaffected individuals through Sanger sequencing were aligned using NCBI-BLAST tool. PolyPhen-2 (Polymorphism Phenotype v2.2.2) tool was used to predict pathogenic potential of p.Ser319Ile mutation in EDA1 protein (NP_001390.1).[22] Multiple sequence alignment of the wild type and mutated EDA1 protein (UniProtKB/Swiss-Prot: Q92838.2) with Protein Data Bank (PDB) was carried out using blastp algorithm of NCBI BLAST tool. Subsequent conserved domain was mapped using NCBI Conserve Domain Database (CDD) [23,24].

Further analysis for assessment of probable consequence/s of Ser319Ile mutation on EDA1 function, three dimensional model has been created using PDB atomic coordinate file (1RJ7) for EDA1 protein [25]. Four amino acids (Gln331, Met364, Val365 and Ser374) for which mutation has been known to cause non-syndromic tooth agenesis and Ser319 (present study) were used to create stick model; surface electrostatic potential for those residues

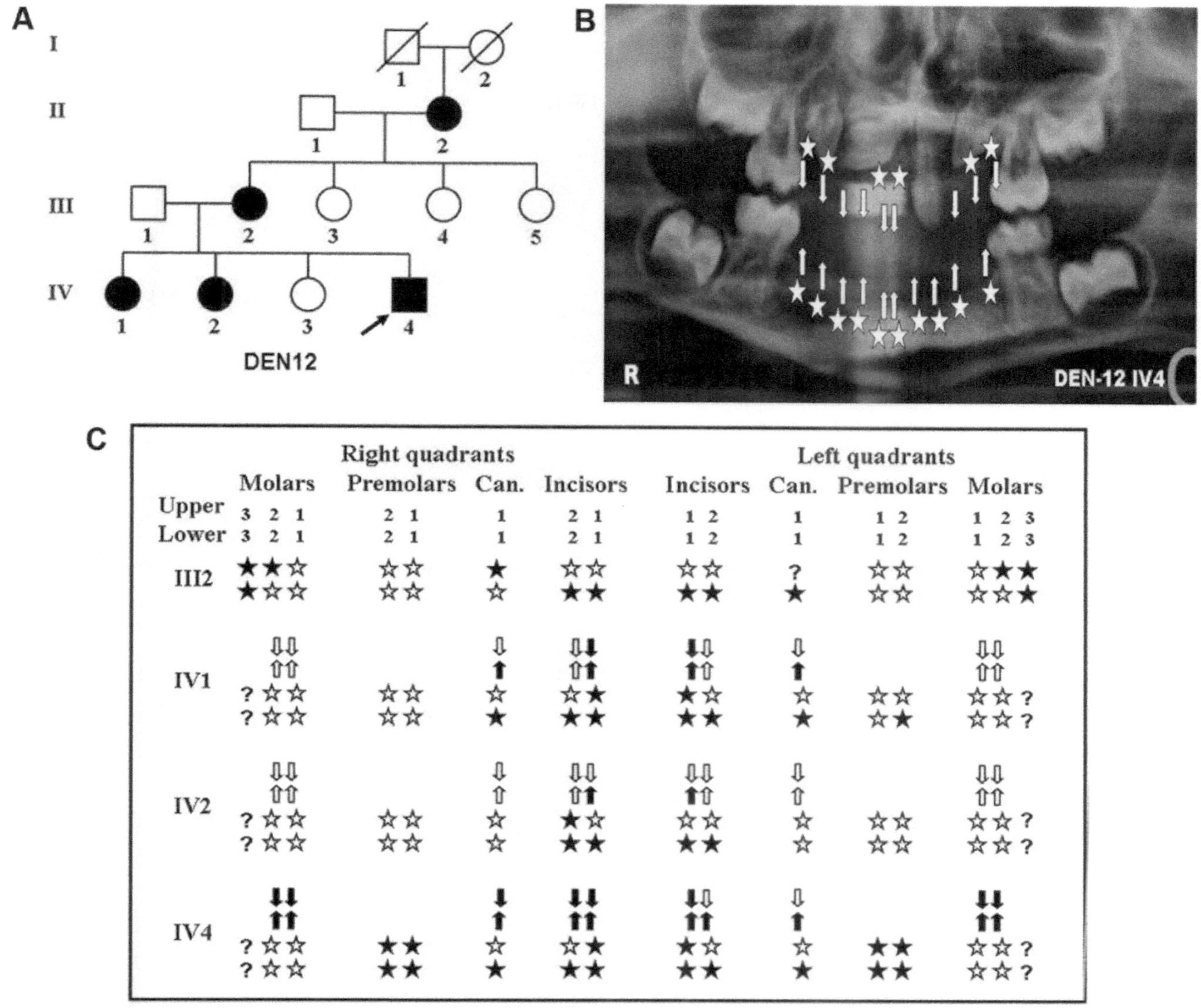

Figure 1. Pedigree structure and tooth agenesis pattern in affected individuals of DEN12 family. (A) Pedigree showing pattern of inheritance of congenital tooth agenesis in DEN12 family. (*squares* males, *circles* females, *blackened* affected, *clear* unaffected, *arrow* proband, *slash* deceased). Note that phenotype of deceased individuals is according to the memory of living relatives and phenotype of II2 of DEN12 is according to the information provided by the family members. (B) Representative orthopantomograph (OPG) of the proband showing the tooth agenesis pattern (*Star* missing permanent teeth, *arrow* missing deciduous teeth). (C) Deciduous and permanent dentition pattern of representative affected individuals. (*Arrow* position of deciduous teeth, *filled arrow* position of missing of deciduous teeth *star* position of permanent teeth, filled *star* missing permanent teeth). Note: status of the upper left canine (?) of DEN12 III2 is undetermined.

were also calculated. All of this modeling was performed using Swiss-PdbViewer 4.1.0 tool [26].

Results

Clinical findings and mode of inheritance

In this family (DEN12), six years old boy (IV4), his two elder sisters (IV1 and IV2), who were under age of 12 years, and his mother (III2) showed non-syndromic incisors-canine tooth agenesis while his father (III1) and another elder sister (IV3) were unaffected. The pattern of inheritance was seems to be autosomal dominant with a rare possibility of being X linked dominant type (Figure 1A). All the affected children showed deciduous as well as permanent teeth agenesis. The 6 years old boy, who was the proband, was most severely affected than others. All mandibular deciduous and permanent teeth except first and second permanent molars were missing. Among maxillary deciduous dentition, all but one incisor teeth were missing. Among maxillary permanent teeth two incisors and all four premolars were missing. One maxillary permanent incisor was larger in size as appeared in OPG (Figure 1B). However, two of his elder sisters were less severely affected. In one of his sisters (IV1) all the deciduous maxillary and mandibular central incisors along with mandibular canines were missing. Regarding permanent teeth all her mandibular incisors, canines, one second premolar and two maxillary central incisors were missing. In his other sister (IV2) two mandibular deciduous central incisors, all four mandibular permanent incisors and one maxillary permanent lateral incisor were missing However, the site for tooth agenesis in their affected mother (III2) confined to all mandibular incisors, one mandibular and one maxillary canine

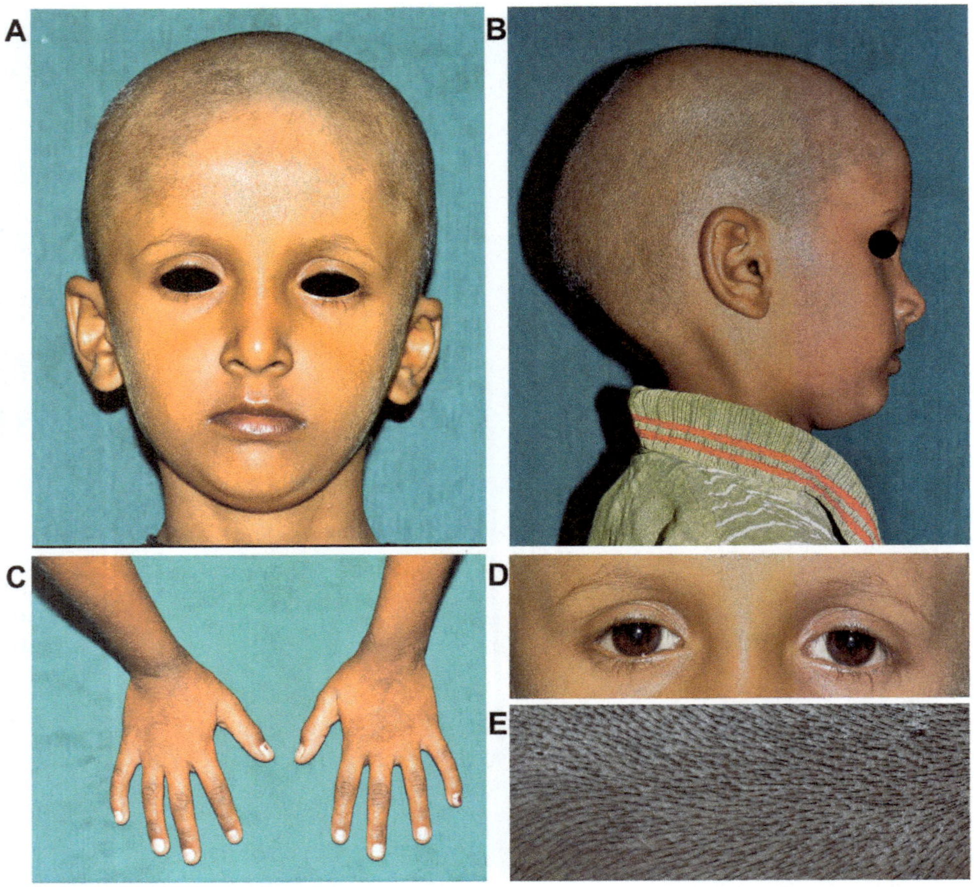

Figure 2. Facial and dermatological features of the proband (DEN12:IV4). (A–B) Frontal and lateral view of proban's face. (C) Hands (D) Eyes and (E) Scalp hair.

along with both the maxillary second molars and all third molars (Figure 1C).

Besides tooth agenesis scalp hair density, body hair, eyes, nail, skin and facial appearance of the proband and all the affected individuals were normal. There was no family history of thermal intolerance and problem in perspiration (Figure 2).

Whole genome sequencing

50 bp reads generated through whole genome sequencing was initially filtered through dbSNP (NCBI) database which remove all the annotated single nucleotide polymorphisms, intronic, intergenic and synonymous changes were also filtered out. In all 119 novel non-synomous variants, distributed in 117 different genes, were detected which were unique to this two affected individuals [Supplementary data file (Table S1)]. Further screening for all the known candidate genes for congenital non-syndromic tooth agenesis viz. *PAX9*, *MSX1*, *AXIN2*, *WNT10A* and *EDA*, only one novel non-synonymous variant resulting in G to T transversion was identified at c.956 position (NM_001399) of *EDA* gene exon 9 (Figure 3A) leading to p.Ser319Ile (UniProtKB/Swiss-Prot: Q92838.2) change.

Exclusion of *PAX9* and *MSX1* genes and analysis of c.956G>T mutation status in all the cases and controls

Through NCBI-BLAST and UCSC-BLAT search, no pathogenic mutation had been identified in all the coding exons and exon-intron boundaries of *PAX9* and *MSX1* genes except a few reported polymorphisms (data not shown).

The c.956G>T mutation (ClinVar ID SCV000148371 and dbSNP ID rs483352804) in *EDA*, detected through whole genome sequencing, was cross validated using Sanger sequencing in all the affected and unaffected individuals of the family. This change was present in heterozygous ($X^GX^{\underline{T}}$) condition in all three affected females (III2, IV1 and IV2) and in the affected male (IV4) as hemizygous ($X^{\underline{T}}Y$) condition (Figure 3B). None of the unaffected individuals (III1 and IV3) had the mutant T allele. Further RFLP and/or SSCP were also used to cross validate the findings. 104 normal unrelated controls with same ethnic background which include 18 females and 86 males with 25 to 30 years age group with all the affected and unaffected individuals were screened using allele specific PCR-RFLP. A 250 bp amplified product of *EDA* exon 9 encompassing this said DNA variation get digested into 115 bp and 135 bp products with *Alu I* in presence of wild type allele (G) while presence of mutant allele (T) destroys the *Alu I* restriction site resulting only 250 bp product. (Figure 4A). In SSCP distinct polymorphic bands were observed associated with disease phenotype (Figure 4B). These two assays showed that this nucleotide variation was segregated with disease phenotype only and was not present in any of the unaffected family members and 104 unrelated normal control individuals suggesting this nucleotide variation (c.956G>T) as a novel and potentially pathogenic mutation.

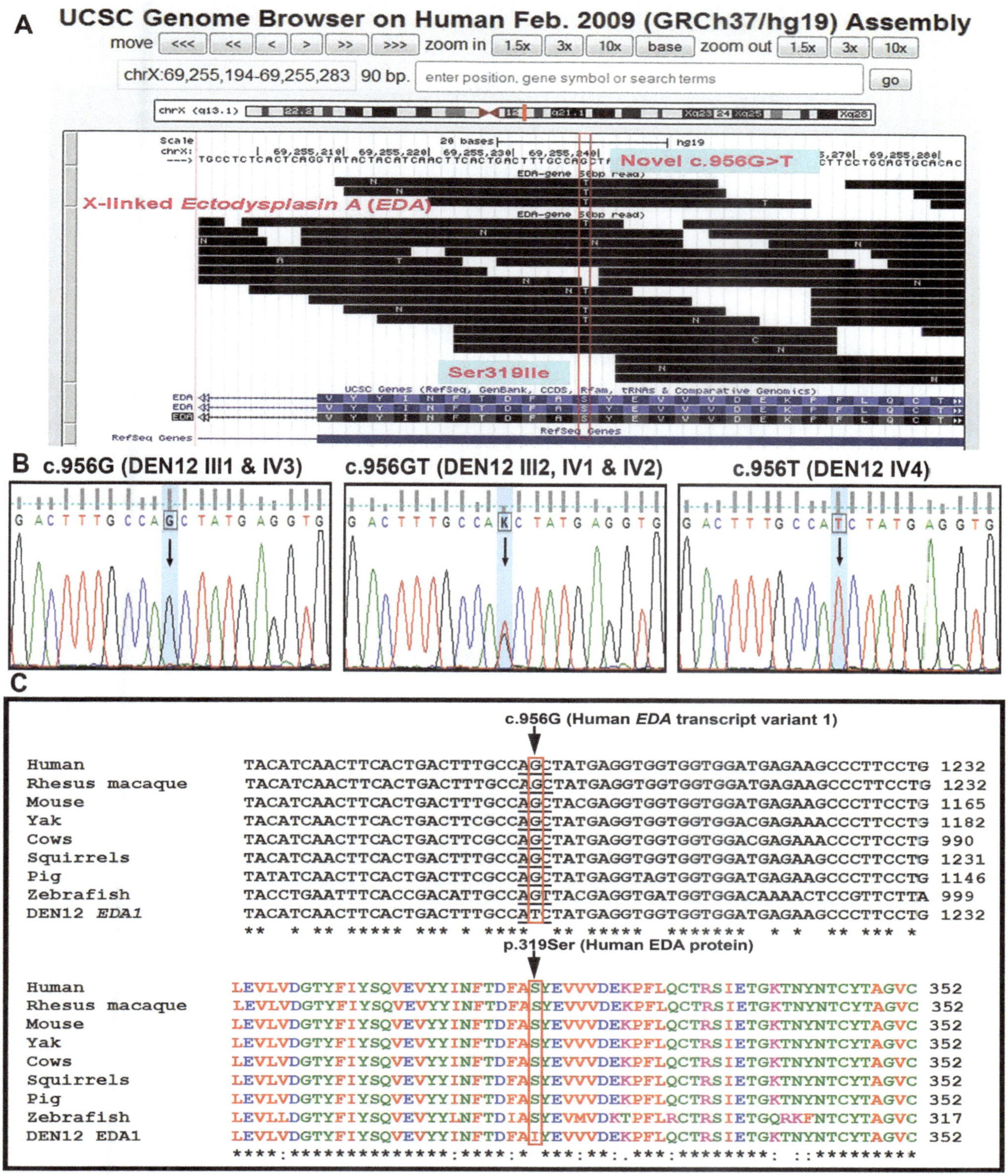

Figure 3. Novel mutation identification at evolutionarily conserved c.956/p.319 position of *EDA*. (A) Over view of 50 base pair reads, generated through whole genome sequencing, from patient samples flanking c.956 position located in *EDA* exon 9. Highlighted 'T' base indicating the mismatched base at c.956 position when aligned to human genome data base using UCSC Genome Browser. (B) Representative chromatogram of Sanger sequencing confirming nucleotide transversion form G to T at c.956 in exon 9 of *EDA1* gene identified through whole genome sequencing in affected members of DEN12 family. (C) Multiple sequence alignment of a portion of TNF-homology domain of human EDA1 orthologs and mutant EDA1 (DEN12- EDA1) reported in this study at mRNA lavel (upper panel) and protein lavel (lower panel) showing conserved c.956G and p.319Serine across different vertebrate species.

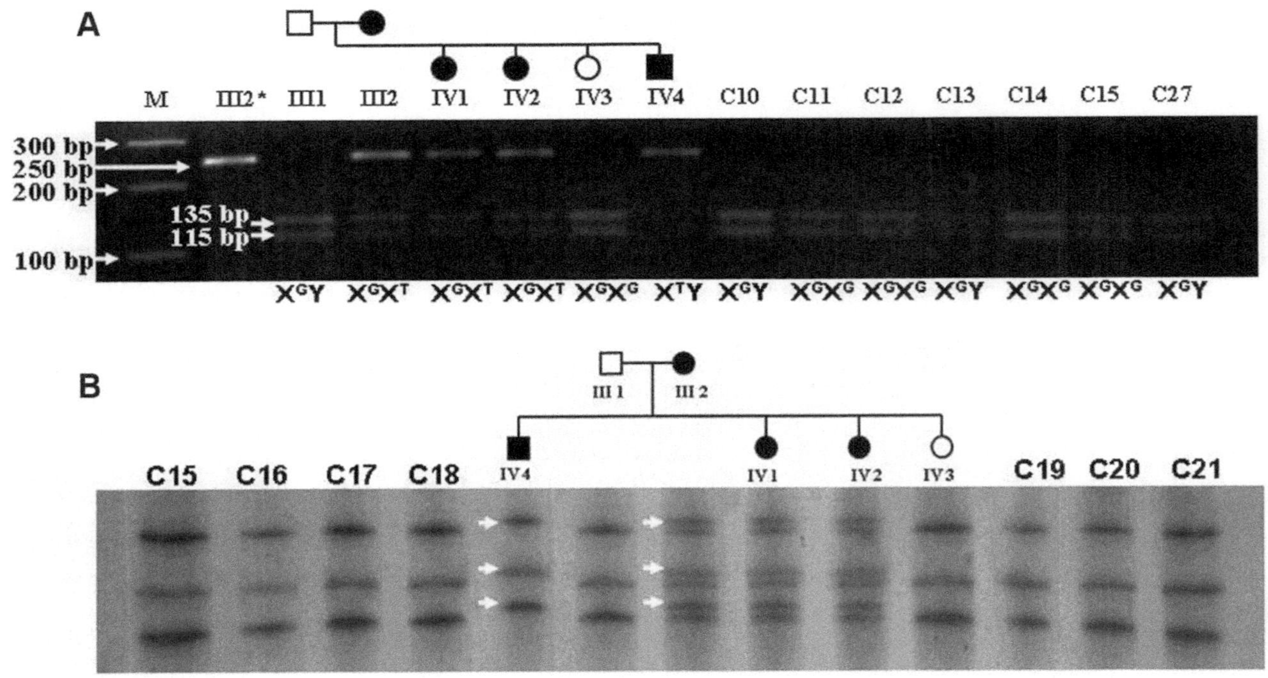

Figure 4. SSCP and PCR-RFLP analysis of c.965 G>T change in *EDA*. (A) Representative SSCP gel picture showing abnormal band (*white arrow*) co-segregated with disease phenotype which are absent in normal individuals. (B) PCR-RFLP pattern after resolving Alu I digested 250 bp PCR product which generate 135 bp and a 115 bp fragment. * indicate undigested PCR product.

In silico functional characterization of novel *EDA1* mutation

In silico analysis using UCSC genome browser and NCBI data base showed that *EDA* c.956G>T change caused a substitution from uncharged polar amino acid Serine to hydrophobic non-polar Isoleucine at 319 position of EDA transcript variant 1 (EDA1). Multiple sequence alignment of human *EDA1* mRNA and amino acid sequences with its orthologs using ClustalW2 software, showed that the c.956G and Ser319 residue is evolutionary conserved across different vertebrate species (Figure. 3C). PolyPhen-2 tool denotes EDA1 Ser319Ile mutation as potentially damaging. Multiple sequence alignment with Protein Data Bank proteins (PDB) database showed that Ser319 is one among the five residues maintaining the conserved feature of receptor binding site of TNF homology domain of EDA. NCBI-CDD analysis showed that due to the mutation of p.319 Ser to Ile number of residues maintaining the conserved feature domain for receptor binding was reduced down from five to four (Data not shown).

Localization of Ser319 on previously reported three dimensional structure of EDA TNF homology region (PDB ID: 1RJ7) showed that this amino acid is located towards the periphery of EDA monomer with in the monomer-monomer interface (Figure 5A). Stick model and surface electrostatic potential calculation through *in silico* analysis showed that four amino acid residues (Gln331, Met364, Val365 and Ser374) for which mutation have been known to cause non-syndromic congenital tooth agenesis along with Ser319 resides in close proximity to each other and form overlapping surface with slightly negative potential (Figure 5D, E). Out of those five residues Ser319 form hydrogen bonding with Gln331 and Val365. So due to the novel Ser319Ile mutation the mutant Ile319 unable to form hydrogen bond with Gln331 (Figure 5B, C).

Discussion

In our present study we have identified a novel c.956G>T mutation in *EDA1* gene in an Indian family with X-linked dominant type of non-syndromic tooth agenesis affecting both primary and permanent dentition. While tooth agenesis was mainly restricted to incisors and canines in all the affected females, affected male child also showed agenesis of deciduous molar and permanent premolar which indicates that the male child is more susceptible to the pathogenic affect of the mutation. Careful clinical study unable to identify any features of Ectodermal dysplasia or mental retardation, as mentioned in available literatures in any of the affected family members including proband [27]. Initially the pattern of inheritance was seems to be autosomal dominant type but sequence of all the coding exons and exon-intron boundaries of two major candidate genes *viz. PAX9* and *MSX1* failed to reveal any pathogenic mutation, leading to possible association of novel candidate gene/s with the disease phenotype. Whole genome sequence analysis by next generation or third generation sequencing techniques has become a powerful tool for identification of novel gene or mutation underlying disease condition.

Two of the affected family members (III2 and IV4) selected for whole genome sequencing showed 119 novel non-synonymous DNA sequence variants compared to the unaffected and those were distributed in 117 different genes across the genome. However, among those 119 sequence variants a c.956G>T mutation in X-linked *EDA1* was the unique one among six candidate genes (*viz.PAX9, MSX1, AXIN2, WNT10A, EDAR* and *EDA1*) associated with non-syndromic tooth agenesis known so far.

Functional EDA1 is a type-II trimeric transmembrane protein belonging to TNF ligand superfamily. It has four distinct functional parts; an N-terminal intracellular domain, a collagen

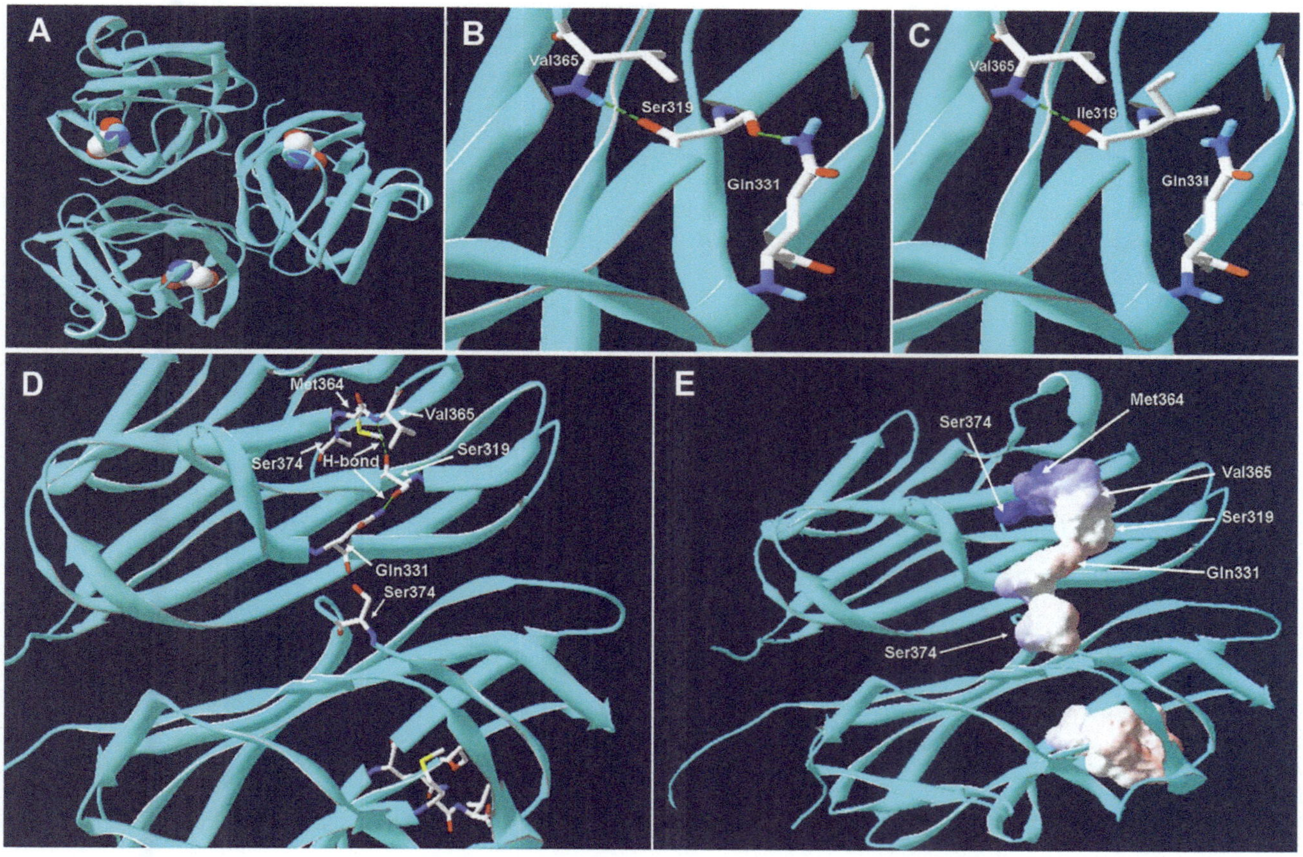

Figure 5. *In silico* analysis of p.Ser319Ile mutation on protein structure. (A) Model showing homo trimer of TNF homology domain of wild type EDA1 protein Ser319 residue is indicated by space filling structure. (B) Ser319 form hydrogen bond (*green line*) with Gln331 and Val365 (C) After getting substituted Ile319 unable form hydrogen bond (*green line*) with Gln331 (D) Location of five amino acid (Ser319, Gln331, Met364, Val365 and Ser374) with in the monomer-monomer interface of two EDA1 monomer, mutations in those amino acids are associated with non-syndromic tooth agenesis. (C) Surface electrostatic potentiality of those five residues shows an overlapping region that may involved in receptor binding activity. All the images are produced through Swiss-PdbViewer 4.1.0 software using PDB file 1RJ7.

like repeat domain, a furin cleavage site and a C-terminal TNF homology domain [28]. The C-terminal domain subsequently cleaved off at the furin cleavage site and binds with EDAR and subsequently regulates cellular physiology by NF-κB pathway [29]. The amino acid variation (p.S319I) observed in DEN12 family is located with in the TNF homology domain which shows 100% amino acid sequence similarity with mouse Eda. Several studies recognize TNF homology domain along with collagen sub-domain as a mutational hotspot for EDA protein. Sequence homology modeling of EDA protein using PDB entries showed that TNF homology domain has two distinct regions, one consists of seven trimer forming residues (H252, F302, Y304, Y347, C352, F379 and I383) and another consists of five receptor binding residues (S275, I277, S319, 326E and 328P). So far 74 mutations have been identified out of which 47 are located in conserved TNF homology domain. 13 mutations among those 47 are responsible for non-syndromic tooth agenesis.[30,31,32,33] Out of those, four residues (Gln331, Met364, Val365 and Ser374) and Ser319 (present study) can form a cluster with slightly negative surface potential. This being located with in the monomer-monomer interface plays critical role during receptor binding activity of EDA and several other TNF domain containing protein.[34,25,35] Several studies showed that mutations which affect the structural stability of EDA protein mainly contribute in X linked hypohidrotic ectodermal dysplasia (XLHED) on the other hand mutations which slightly alter the receptor binding activity have their role in milder form of XLHED and/or non-syndromic tooth agenesis. Ser319, which is a part of five receptor binding resides as observed from NCBI Conserve Domain Database (CDD), also form hydrogen bond with Gln331 and Val365 (mutation in this two residues are reported to be associated with non-syndromic tooth agenesis). Due to mutation in Ser to Ile, hydrogen bond between Ser319 and Gln331 get disrupted and the receptor binding residues thus reduced from five to four.

In this family a total of three females and one male showed congenital tooth agenesis and all of them have c.956G>T mutation in X linked *EDA* gene resulting p.Ser319Ile change in EDA1 protein. Unlike other X linked phenotype, in which most of the females remain protected from the effect of X-linked mutation due to X inactivation phenomenon, in our study all the females carrying this mutation (c.956G>T) in heterozygous condition (X^GX^T) showed mutant phenotype along with the male child who has only one copy of X linked *EDA* and so showed the mutant type (X^TY). Although this mutation shows complete penetrance but the expressivity differs not only between male and female, which is obvious due to presence of mutant genotype in hemizygous (X^TY) condition, but also among females. To explain this rear behavior of this X-linked mutation careful study of available literatures had been carried out. In one study, a Chinese family with p.Asp316Gly mutation in EDA1 protein was found to be associated with non-syndromic congenital tooth agenesis affecting all tooth type. All the children, three females and one male showed hypodontia phenotype with differential expressivity.[36] This affection status closely resembles to that of the family we had identified. Further, functional analysis of p.Asp316Gly along with five other mutations associated with non-syndromic tooth agenesis showed that this mutation, unlike other five, drastically reduces interaction between EDA receptor (EDAR) and mutant EDA1 protein.[31] These two studies clearly indicate that mutation(s) which severely affect the receptor binding activity of EDA protein may show almost complete penetrance for male and female in spite of the X inactivation. One possible explanation of this may lies during the course of tooth development. In female embryo there is equal chance of inactivation either of mutant or of wild type gene (eg. *EDA*) located in X chromosome leading to mosaicism. Thus at the site of tooth development amount of bioactive protein will become almost half if the activity of the mutant protein reduced down to near zero which subsequently leads to milder form of hypodontia phenotype in females compared to males with only the mutant copy of the gene.

Thus in our study the novel p.Ser319Ile mutation located in a putative receptor binding region may almost completely abolish the receptor binding activity of mutant EDA1 protein. In females (DEN12 III2, IV1 and IV2) due to mosaic pattern of X-inactivation the pathogenic activity of this mutation could be diluted leading to milder phenotype compared to the affected male (DEN12 IV4), with single X chromosome bearing the mutant *EDA*. In a resent study by Piccione *et al.* (2012), identify mutation in same amino acid position associated with X-linked hypohidrotic ectodermal dysplasia with keratoconus.[37] Further expression and functional analysis of p.Ser319Ile mutation could provide direct evidence regarding the pathogenic property of this mutation.

Accession Numbers

c.956G>T mutation in human gene EDA transcript variant 1: NCBI ClinVar database (SCV000148371) and NCBI dbSNP database (rs483352804).

Web Resources

The URLs for data presented herein are as follows:

NCBI BLAST tool, http://blast.ncbi.nlm.nih.gov/Blast.cgi.

UCSC-BLAT tool, http://genome.ucsc.edu/cgi-bin/hgBlat.

Polymorphism phenotype-2, http://genetics.bwh.harvard.edu/pph2/.

NCBI Conserved domain search tool, http://www.ncbi.nlm.nih.gov/Structure/cdd/wrpsb.cgi.

Online Mendelian Inheritance in Man (OMIM), http://www.ncbi.nlm.gov/Omim/.

ClustalW2 software, http://www.ebi.ac.uk/Tools/msa/clustalw2/.

Primer3web software, http://primer3.ut.ee/.

Supporting Information

Table S1 Novel non-synonymous nucleotide variations detected in two affected individuals (DEN12-III2, IV4) through Whole Genome Sequencing.

Acknowledgments

We are thankful to all the members of DEN12 family and all control individuals who provided their valuable time and material for this research work. Next Generation Sequencing Facility of Banaras Hindu University is also acknowledged for providing whole genome sequencing facility.

Author Contributions

Conceived and designed the experiments: PD TS. Performed the experiments: TS. Analyzed the data: PD RB TS. Contributed reagents/materials/analysis tools: PD RB. Contributed to the writing of the manuscript: PD RB TS.

References

1. Polder BJ, Van't Hof MA, Van der Linden FP, Kuijpers-Jagtman AM (2004) A meta-analysis of the prevalence of dental agenesis of permanent teeth. Community Dent Oral Epidemiol 32: 217–226.
2. Silengo MC, Davi GF, Bianco R, Costa M, DeMarco A, et al. (1982) Distinctive hair changes (pili torti) in Rapp-Hodgkin ectodermal dysplasia syndrome. Clin Genet 21: 297–300.
3. Bala M, Pathak A (2011) Ectodermal dysplasia with true anodontia. J Oral Maxillofac Pathol 15: 244–246.
4. Rintala A, Ranta R, Stegars T (1984) On the pathogenesis of cleft palate in the Pierre Robin syndrome. Scand. J Plast Reconstr Surg 18: 237–240.
5. Ranta R (1983) Hypodontia and delayed development of the second premolars in cleft palate children. Eur J Orthod 5: 145–148.
6. Temple IK (1989) Stickler's syndrome. J Med Genet 26: 119–126.
7. Cohen MM, Blitzer FJ, Arvystas MG, Bonneau RH (1970) Abnormalities of the permanent dentition in trisomy G. J Dent Res 49 Suppl: 1386–1393.
8. Suri S, Tompson BD, Atenafu E (2011) Prevalence and patterns of permanent tooth agenesis in Down syndrome and their association with craniofacial morphology. Angle Orthod 81: 260–269.
9. De Coster PJ, Marks LA, Martens LC, Huysseune A (2009) Dental agenesis: genetic and clinical perspectives. J Oral Pathol Med 38: 1–17.
10. Stockton DW, Das P, Goldenberg M, D'Souza RN, Patel PI (2000) Mutation of PAX9 is associated with oligodontia. Nat Genet 24: 18–19.
11. Vastardis H, Karimbux N, Guthua SW, Seidman JG, Seidman CE (1996) A human MSX1 homeodomain missense mutation causes selective tooth agenesis. Nat Genet 13: 417–421.
12. Tao R, Jin B, Guo SZ, Qing W, Feng GY, et al. (2006) A novel missense mutation of the EDA gene in a Mongolian family with congenital hypodontia. J Hum Genet 51: 498–502.
13. Lammi L, Arte S, Somer M, Jarvinen H, Lahermo P, et al. (2004) Mutations in AXIN2 cause familial tooth agenesis and predispose to colorectal cancer. Am J Hum Genet 74: 1043–1050.
14. Kantaputra P, Sripathomsawat W (2011) WNT10A and isolated hypodontia. Am J Med Genet A 155A: 1119–1122.
15. van den Boogaard MJ, Creton M, Bronkhorst Y, van der Hout A, Hennekam E, et al. (2012) Mutations in WNT10A are present in more than half of isolated hypodontia cases. J Med Genet 49: 327–331.
16. Grimberg J, Nawoschik S, Belluscio L, McKee R, Turck A, et al. (1989) A simple and efficient non-organic procedure for the isolation of genomic DNA from blood. Nucleic Acids Res 17: 8390.
17. Mendoza-Fandino GA, Gee JM, Ben-Dor S, Gonzalez-Quevedo C, Lee K, et al. (2011) A novel g.-1258G>A mutation in a conserved putative regulatory element of PAX9 is associated with autosomal dominant molar hypodontia. Clin Genet 80: 265–272.
18. Das P, Hai M, Elcock C, Leal SM, Brown DT, et al. (2003) Novel missense mutations and a 288-bp exonic insertion in PAX9 in families with autosomal dominant hypodontia. Am J Med Genet A 118A: 35–42.
19. Wang J, Jian F, Chen J, Wang H, Lin Y, et al. (2011) Sequence analysis of PAX9, MSX1 and AXIN2 genes in a Chinese oligodontia family. Arch Oral Biol 56: 1027–1034.
20. Untergrasser A, Cutcutache I, Koressaar T, Ye J, Faircloth BC, et al. (2012) Primer3 - new capabilities and interfaces. Nucleic Acids Res 40(15): e115.
21. Koressaar T, Remm M (2007) Enhancements and modifications of primer design program Primer3 Bioinformatics 23(10): 1289–1291.
22. Adzhubei IA, Schmidt S, Peshkin L, Ramensky VE, Gerasimova A, Bork P, Kondrashov AS, Sunyaev SR (2010) A method and server for predicting damaging missense mutations. Nat Methods 7: 248–249.
23. Marchler-Bauer A, Bryant SH (2004) CD-Search: protein domain annotations on the fly. Nucleic Acids Res 32: W327–331.
24. Marchler-Bauer A, Zheng C, Chitsaz F, Derbyshire MK, Geer LY, et al. (2013) CDD: conserved domains and protein three-dimensional structure. Nucleic Acids Res 41: D348–352.

25. Hymowitz SG, Compaan DM, Yan M, Wallweber HJ, Dixit VM, et al. (2003) The crystal structures of EDA-A1 and EDA-A2: splice variants with distinct receptor specificity. Structure 11: 1513–1520.
26. Guex N, Peitsch MC (1997) SWISS-MODEL and the Swiss-PdbViewer: an environment for comparative protein modeling. Electrophoresis 18: 2714–2723.
27. Clarke A (1987) Hypohydrotic ectodermal dysplasia. J Med Genet 24: 659–663.
28. Ezer S, Bayes M, Elomaa O, Schlessinger D, Kere J (1999) Ectodysplasin is a collagenous trimeric type II membrane protein with a tumor necrosis factor-like domain and co-localizes with cytoskeletal structures at lateral and apical surfaces of cells. Hum Mol Genet. 8: 2079–2086.
29. Mikkola ML, Thesleff I (2003) Ectodysplasin signaling in development. Cytokine Growth Factor Rev 14: 211–224.
30. Yang Y, Luo L, Xu J, Zhu P, Xue W, et al. (2013) Novel EDA p.Ile260Ser mutation linked to non-syndromic hypodontia. J Dent Res 92: 500–506.
31. Mues G, Tardivel A, Willen L, Kapadia H, Seaman R, et al. (2010) Functional analysis of Ectodysplasin-A mutations causing selective tooth agenesis. Eur J Hum Genet 18: 19–25.
32. Tarpey P, Pemberton TJ, Stockton DW, Das P, Ninis V, et al. (2007) A novel Gln358Glu mutation in Ectodysplasin A associated with X-linked dominant incisor hypodontia. Am J Med Genet A 143: 390–394.
33. Lee KE, Ko J, Shin TJ, Hyun HK, Lee SH, et al. (2014) Oligodontia and curly hair occur with Ectodysplasin A mutations. J Dent Res 93, 371–375.
34. Hymowitz SG, O'Connell MP, Ultsch MH, Hurst A, Totpal K, et al. (2000) A unique zinc-binding site revealed by a high-resolution X-ray structure of homotrimeric Apo2L/TRAIL. Biochemistry 39: 633–640.
35. Kowalczyk-Quintas C, Willen L, Dang AT, Sarrasin H, Tardivel A, et al. (2014) Generation and characterization of function-blocking anti-Ectodysplasin A (EDA) monoclonal antibodies that induce Ectodermal Dysplasia. J Biol Chem 289: 4273–4285.
36. Li S, Li J, Cheng J, Zhou B, Tong X, et al. (2008) Non-syndromic tooth agenesis in two Chinese families associated with novel missense mutations in the TNF domain of EDA (ectodysplasin A). PLoS One 3: e2396.
37. Piccione M, Serra G, Sanfilippo C, Andreucci E, Sani I, et al. (2012) A new mutation in EDA gene in X-linked hypohidrotic ectodermal dysplasia associated with keratoconus. Minerva Pediatr 64: 59–64.

20

The Effect of Periodontal Treatment on Hemoglobin A1c Levels of Diabetic Patients

Xingxing Wang[1], Xu Han[1], Xiaojing Guo[2], Xiaolong Luo[1], Dalin Wang[1]*

1 Department of Stomatology, Changhai Hospital, The Second Military Medical University, Shanghai, China, 2 Department of Health Statistics, The Second Military Medical University, Shanghai, China

Abstract

Background: There is growing evidence that periodontal treatment may affect glycemic control in diabetic patients. And several systematic reviews have been conducted to assess the effect of periodontal treatment on diabetes outcomes. Researches of this aspect are widely concerned, and several new controlled trials have been published. The aim of this study was to update the account for recent findings.

Methods: A literature search (until the end of January 2014) was carried out using various databases with language restriction to English. A randomized controlled trial (RCT) was selected if it investigated periodontal therapy for diabetic subjects compared with a control group received no periodontal treatment for at least 3 months of the follow-up period. The primary outcome was hemoglobin A1c (HbA1c), and secondary outcomes were periodontal parameters included probing pocket depth (PPD) and clinical attachment level (CAL).

Results: Ten trials of 1135 patients were included in the analysis. After the follow-up of 3 months, treatment substantially lowered HbA1c compared with no treatment after periodontal therapy (–0.36%, 95%CI, −0.52% to −0.19%, $P<0.0001$). Clinically substantial and statistically significant reduction of PPD and CAL were found between subjects with and without treatment after periodontal therapy (PPD −0.42 mm, 95%CI: −0.60 to −0.23, $P<0.00001$; CAL −0.34 mm, 95%CI: −0.52 to −0.16, $P=0.0002$). And there is no significant change of the level of HbA1c at the 6-month comparing with no treatment (–0.30%, 95%CI, −0.69% to 0.09%, $P=0.13$).

Conclusions: Periodontal treatment leads to the modest reduction in HbA1c along with the improvement of periodontal status in diabetic patients for 3 months, and this result is consistent with previous systematic reviews. And the effect of periodontal treatment on HbA1c cannot be observed at 6-month after treatment.

Editor: Yu-Kang Tu, National Taiwan University, Taiwan

Funding: These authors have no support or funding to report.

Competing Interests: The authors have declared that no competing interests exist.

* Email: Wang_Dento@163.com

Introduction

Periodontitis is a multi-factorial infectious disease of the soft tissues and bone that support the teeth [1], and it is a major cause of tooth loss in adults [2]. Periodontitis may lead to the development of a high systemic disease burden [3] and possibly affect general health [4]. It is reported that periodontitis is associate with rheumatoid arthritis [5]. cardiovascular disease [6] and even the patients in the periodontitis cohort exhibit a higher risk of developing oral cancer than those in the gingivitis cohort [7].

Diabetes mellitus is a chronic, non-communicable disease and also one of the major global public health issues [8]. The distinguishing features of diabetes mellitus type 1 and type 2 are autoimmunity and chronic low-grade inflammation, respectively [9]. A large number of studies support the point that there is an association between diabetes and periodontal disease [10]: Firstly, individuals with diabetes have a higher prevalence of periodontitis [11–13]. Nelson et al. [14] reported that the incidence of periodontitis was 2.6 times higher in subjects with diabetes than those without. Tsai et al. [11] reported that patients with poorly controlled diabetes have a 2.9 times higher risk to have sever periodontitis compared to no-diabetic subjects. Secondly, diabetes mellitus can increase the severity of periodontitis [15–17] and the severity of the periodontitis is always greater than individuals without diabetes [10,11]. And periodontitis is considered to be one of the diabetic complications [18,19].

Although strong evidence tends to support the adverse effects of diabetes on periodontitis, numerous reports indicate that periodontitis can adversely affect glycemic control in diabetics [20,21]. It is considered that this close association between periodontitis and diabetes is established on the reciprocal influence [22]. So a number of potential mechanisms for the two-way relationship between them have been proposed. It is known that periodontitis is a kind of inflammatory process which can generate localized and systemic infections, and emerging evidence implicates inflammation in the pathogenesis of type 2 diabetes [23,24]. But the exact relationship between periodontitis and diabetes remains unclear.

Some intervention studies concerning the effects of periodontal disease on glycemic control of diabetic patients report more direct evidence. Iwamoto et al. [25] showed that antimicrobial periodontal therapy can cause a significant reduction of HbA1c value in type 2 diabetic patients. Gaikwad et al. [26] also found that scaling and root planning can improve glycemic control in patients with type 2 diabetes mellitus with or without adjunctive systemic doxycycline therapy. Bharti et al. [27] gave diabetic patients with periodontitis a periodontal treatment with topical antibiotics and found that this kind of therapy protocol can improve glycemic control and elevate serum adiponectin with improvement of periodontal status in type 2 diabetic patients. However, a recent phase III randomized controlled clinical trial (RCT) with 514 patients by Engebretson et al. [28] revealed that nonsurgical periodontal therapy did not improve glycemic control in patients with type 2 diabetes.

HbA1c is related to the mean blood glucose concentration over the past 1–3 months [8], and it is also associated with an increased risk for diabetes complications [29]. So the periodic monitoring of HbA1c in diabetic patients was proposed [30]. It is considered to be a standardized measurement used to estimate the effect of diabetes treatment on control of glucose metabolism [31–33], and is widely used in trials to monitor diabetes status [34].

Several recent systematic reviews [35,36] have been conducted to assess the evidence that periodontal treatment influences the level of HbA1c. Due to several new research reports with bigger sample size, we therefore performed this meta-analysis of RCTs to evaluate the effect of periodontal treatment on glycemic control of diabetic patients.

Research Design and Methods

Search strategy

Three databases, PubMed, Embase and Cochrane Library were searched according to a method previously described by Teeuw et al. [35] and Engebretson et al. [36], using identical search criteria and terms: ((periodontal disease) OR (periodont*[Text Word]) OR (periodontitis)) AND ((diabetes[Text Word]) OR (diabet*[Text Word]) OR (diabetic*[Title]) OR (diabetic patient*[Text Word]) OR (diabetes patient[Text Word]) OR (non insulin dependent diabetes) OR (niddm[Text Word]) OR (insulin dependent diabetes[Text Word]) OR (iddm[Text Word]) OR (type 1 diabetes) OR (t1 dm) OR (type 2 diabetes) OR (t2 dm)) AND ((therapy) OR (treatment) OR (intervention)) AND ((controlled clinical trial) OR (randomized controlled trial) OR (RCT)) AND (english[Language]) until the end of the January of 2014. Additional searches were conducted in PubMed's medical subject headings with: (periodontal diseases) AND (diabetes mellitus) AND (therapeutics OR therapy OR intervention studies). Moreover, we searched the World Health Organization (http://www.who.int/triasearch) and Clinical Trials.gov (http://wwwClinicalTrials.gov.) Web sites for information on registered RCTs.

Study selection criteria

The studies to be included in the systematic review had to meet the following criteria: (1) randomized controlled trial; (2) participants over the age of 18 with both diabetes (both type 1 and type 2) and periodontitis; (3) intervention consisting of non-surgical treatment with or without adjunctive use of local drug delivery and systemic antibiotics; (4) comparator group with no periodontal treatment or delayed treatment; (5) study duration ≥3 months; (6) outcome consisting of mean change in HbA1c level, or pre- and post-treatment HbA1c levels.

Two independent reviewers (Xingxing Wang and Xiaolong Luo) evaluated all retrieved articles. Titles and abstracts were scanned to rule out studies that did not meet inclusion criteria. From the selected articles, the full texts were reviewed followed by a decision on their eligibility for inclusion.

Data extraction and quality assessment

Data extraction and quality assessment were independently conducted by two authors (Xingxing Wang and Xiaojing Guo) using a standardized approach, and disagreements were adjudicated by a third reviewer (Dalin Wang) after referring back to the original articles.

Data retrieved from the studies included publication details (year of publication, name of first author and country) and trial characteristics (Patients' types and treatment of diabetes, study design, sample size, interventions, follow-up duration, change of HbA1c and periodontal parameters). The quality of the included studies was assessed by Risk of Bias tool according to the Cochrane handbook for systematic reviews of interventions (Version 5.1.0) [37].

Statistical analyses

The absolute difference of HbA1c percentage in each treatment arm was recorded. When not reported, it was calculated for the intervention and the control groups by means of the formula [35]:

$$\Delta HbA1c = HbA1c_f - HbA1c_b,$$

where $HbA1c_f$ is the mean HbA1c value after treatment and $HbA1c_b$ is the mean HbA1c value before treatment. And if the standard deviation was not reported, it was obtained by the formula [35,38]:

$$SD_c = \sqrt{SD_b^2 + SD_f^2 - (2 \times Corr \times SD_b \times SD_f)}$$

Where SD_c is the standard deviation of mean change of HbA1c, SD_b is the standard deviation of mean baseline HbA1c values, SD_f is the standard deviation of mean end HbA1c values. Corr is the correlation between the baseline and end values, it was set at 0.5, consistent with the previous reviews [35,38].

For the three-arm studies, the two treatment groups or the two control groups, which were assumed to be "group 1" and "group 2", were firstly combined into a single group according to the "Cochrane handbook for systematic reviews of interventions (Version 5.1.0)" [37] and "Introduction to meta-analysis" [39].

Sample size: $N = N_1 + N_2$

Mean: $M = \dfrac{N_1 M_1 + N_2 M_2}{N_1 + N_2}$

SD: $SD =$

$$\sqrt{\frac{(N_1-1)SD_1^2 + (N_2-1)SD_2^2 + \frac{N_1 N_2}{N_1+N_2}\left(M_1^2 + M_2^2 - 2M_1 M_2\right)}{N_1+N_2-1}}$$

For periodontal clinical parameters, according to the Cochrane handbook for systematic reviews of interventions (Version 5.1.0) [37]: if the value of Corr less than 0.5 is obtained, then there is no value in using change from baseline and an analysis of final values

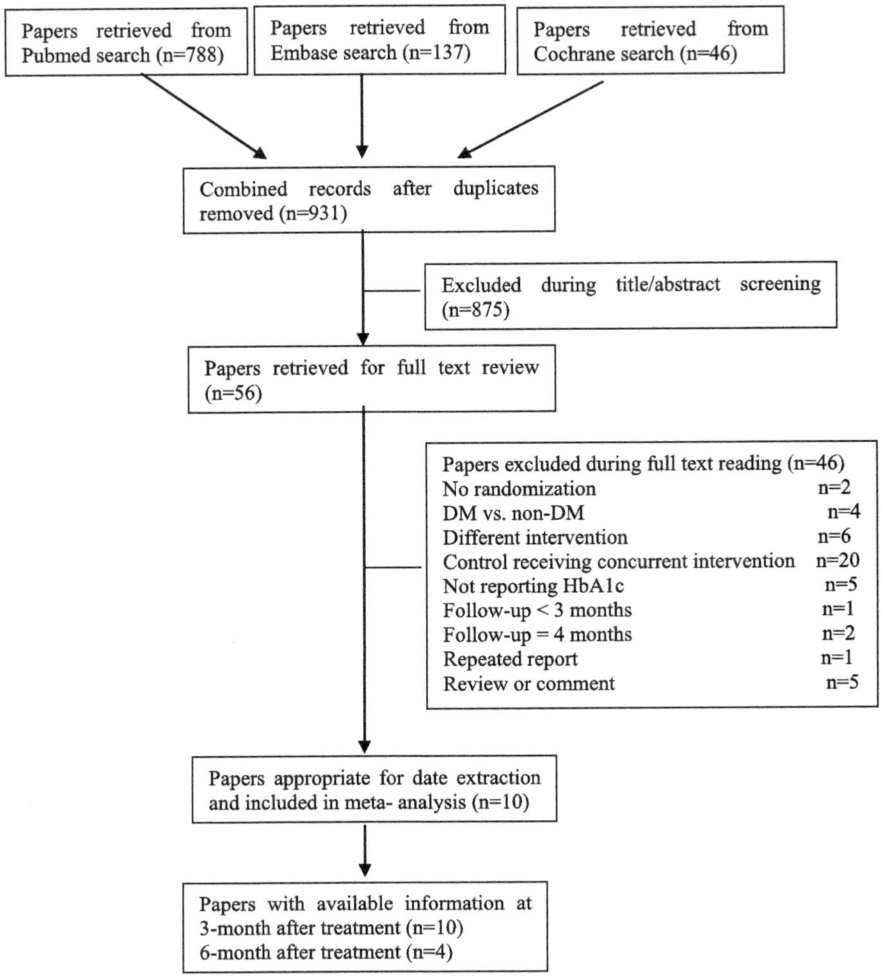

Figure 1. Flow diagram of the trials search and selection process.

will be more precise. We obtained the values of Corr by using the data extracted from Sun et al. 2011 [40] and Telgi et al. 2013 [8], and they were all less than 0.5, so we took the SD_f as the standard deviation of mean change of PPD and CAL.

The weighted mean difference (WMD) was calculated, Chi-square (χ^2) and I^2 tests were used to assess the heterogeneity of the studies included in this meta-analysis. The heterogeneity of the trials will be regarded as low-level when $P>0.10$ for the χ^2 test and $I^2<25\%$, and a fixed-effects model analysis was used to calculate a pooled effect; otherwise, a random-effects model was applied.

Forest plots showing the point estimate and confidence intervals for each study were created. Statistical significance was defined as a two-tailed $P<0.05$. All numerical data for meta-analysis were conducted using RevMan version 5.3 from the Cochrane collaboration.

Results

Study characteristics

The literature search resulted in 931 potentially relevant articles. The titles and abstracts of these articles were scanned for relevance. And the second level full text search was initiated on those remaining studies. Fifty-six potentially eligible trials were identified for full-text review, 46 of which were excluded for specific reasons listed in Figure 1. The remaining ten trials of 1135 patients (614 in the treated group and 521 in the control group) [8,28,39–46] that met the inclusion criteria were included in the meta-analysis, and the characteristics of each study were shown in Table 1. Of the ten trials, seven studies [39,41–46] were also included in the previous analysis [35,36]. Whereas two other studies [48,49] that were included in the previous systematic reviews [35,36] were excluded because their study duration were 4 months and the outcomes of the 3 months were not available.

All studies included were reported as RCTs, and the durations of the follow-up period were at least 3 months. Of the ten studies, five were of 6-month duration [28,41–43,45], but the data is not available in Katagiri et al. [43], we wrote to the author and we were not answered. And there was also one study was of 9-month duration [41]. All studies described a study population having type 2 diabetes and suffering from periodontitis, and also one study included type 1 diabetes [41]. Eight studies were single centre [8,40–42,44–47], two were multi-centered [28,43]. The largest in terms of sample size of the study is Engebretson et al. [28] with 514 participants. Four trials were three-arm studies, [8,41,42,47] and three of them [41,42,47] reported two intervention groups, while the other one [8] reported two control groups. And they were combined into a single group firstly.

Overall, all included studies had different levels of bias. Six studies [28,41–43,45,46] showed a clear randomization scheme, the other four studies [8,40,44,47] did not give out sufficient

Table 1. Characteristics of included trials.

Author(s)	Country Number of subjects (tx, ctr) Single versus multicenter	HbA1c inclusion criteria Treatment in test and control group	Inclusion criteria	Periodontitis evaluation	HbAlc(%) (mean±SD) at baseline and at 3 months (mean change)	HbAlc(%) (mean±SD) at 6 months (mean change)	PPD (mm)(mean±SD), CAL (mm)(mean±SD) at baseline and at 3 months(mean change)	Number of subjects with diabetic medication at baseline Change in diabetic medication
Kiran M et al. 2005	Turkey 44DM2 (tx:22 ctr:22) single center	HbA1c 6%–8% tx:SRP+OH ctr: no treatment	not reported	PPD, CAL, GR, PI, GI, BOP	tx:7.31±0.74~6.51±0.80(−0.86) ctr:7.00±0.72~7.31±2.08(0.31)	NA	tx:PPD 2.29±0.49~1.80±0.25(−0.49) CAL 3.19±1.13~2.80±1.03 (−0.39) ctr:PPD 2.24±0.70~2.26±0.63 (0.02) CAL 2.92±1.10~2.87±1.03(−0.05)	Diet control:3 Oral medication:30 Insulin:4 Insulin + oral:7 no change in the medication or diet
Singh S et al. 2008	India 45 DM2 (tx1:15 tx2:15 ctr:15) single center	HbAlc not reported tx1:SRP TX2:SRP+ doxycycline ctr:no treatment	30% or more of the teeth examined having ≥4 mm PD	PPD, CAL, PI, GI	tx1:7.9±0.7~7.3±0.6(−0.6) tx2:8.3±0.7~7.5±0.6(−0.7) ctr:8.08±0.7~8.1±0.74(0.06)	NA	tx1:PPD 2.67±0.35~2.33±0.35(−0.34) CAL 3.44±0.45~3.14±0.45 (−0.30) tx2: PPD 2.52±0.47~2.14±0.46 (−0.38) CAL 3.22±0.63~2.88±0.61 (−0.34) ctr:PPD 2.44±0.26~2.40±0.46 (−0.04) CAL 2.78±0.33~2.83±0.35 (0.04)	Baseline medication not reported no change in the medication or diet
Katagiri S et al. 2009	Japan 49 DM2 (tx:32 ctr:17) multicenter	HbAlc 6.5–10 tx1:SRP+ topical minocycline ctr:OH	≥11 teeth ≥2 sites with PD≥4 mm	PPD, BOP	tx:7.2±0.9~7.06* ctr:6.9±0.9~6.81	reported in a graph	tx:PPD 3.0±0.9~2.2±0.5 CAL NA ctr: PPD 2.8±0.9~2.6±0.7 CAL NA	Diet control:3 Oral medication:27 Insulin:19 anti-diabetic drugs were not changed
Koromantzos PA et al. 2011	Greece 60DM2 (tx:30 ctr:30) single center	HbA1c 7.0%–9.9% tx:SRP+OH ctr: supragingival+OH	≥16 teeth, PD≥6 mm in≥8 sites, CAL≥5 mm, in≥2 quadrants	PPD, CAL, BOP, GI	tx:7.87±0.74~7.14±0.54* ctr:7.59±0.66~7.41±0.48	tx:(−0.72±0.93)* ctr:(−0.13±0.46)	tx:PPD NA CAL NA ctr:PPD NA CAL NA	Oral medication 48 insulin 19 change in medication reported
Sun WL et al. 2011	China 157DM2 (tx:82 ctr:75) single center	HbA1c 7.5%–9.5% tx:SRP+OH+flap when indicated+ antibiotics ctr: OH	≥20 teeth, PD>5 mm, CAL≥4 mm in ≥30% teeth or PD>4 mm, CAL>3 mm in ≥60% teeth	PPD, CAL, BI, PI	tx:8.75±0.67~8.25±0.72(−0.50±0.18) ctr:8.70±0.65~8.56±0.69(−0.14±0.12)	NA	tx:PPD 4.53±0.83~2.97±0.78 (−1.15±0.66) CAL 4.85±1.38~4.12±0.95 (−0.73±0.51) ctr:PPD 4.49±0.85~4.28±0.81 (−0.21±0.19) CAL 4.88±1.39~4.73±1.29 (−0.15±0.13)	Diet or oral medication no medication changes

Table 1. Cont.

Author(s)	Country Number of subjects (tx, ctr) Single versus multicenter	HbA1c inclusion criteria Treatment in test and control group	Inclusion criteria	Periodontitis evaluation	HbAlc(%) (mean±SD) at baseline and at 3 months (mean change)	HbAlc(%) (mean±SD) at 6 months (mean change)	PPD (mm)(mean±SD), CAL (mm)(mean±SD) at baseline and at 3 months(mean change)	Number of subjects with diabetic medication at baseline Change in diabetic medication
Chen L et al. 2012	China 126DM2 (tx1:42 tx2:43 ctr:41) single center	HbA1c not reported tx1:SRP+subgingival debridement at 3-month tx2:SRP+ supragingival prophylaxis at 3-month ctr:no treatment+no OH	≥16 teeth, CAL≥1 mm	PPD, CAL, PI, BOP	tx1:7.31±1.23~7.30±1.50 tx2:7.29±1.55~7.43±1.53 ctr:7.25±1.49~7.59±1.54	tx1:7.09±1.34 tx2:6.87±1.12 ctr:7.38±1.57	tx1:PPD 2.66±0.68~2.27± 0.50 CAL 3.57±1.31~3.28± 1.25 tx2:PPD 2.57±0.66~2.20±0.39 CAL 2.95±1.21~2.55±1.15 ctr:PPD 2.47±0.57~2.38± 0.47 CAL 3.37±1.24~ 3.29±1.23	Diet control:4 Oral medication:109 Insulin:13 no medication changes
Moeintaghavi A et al. 2012	Iran 40DM2 (tx:22 ctr:18) single center	HbA1c >7% tx: SRP+OH ctr: OH	not reported	PPD, CAL, PI, GI	tx:8.15±1.18~7.41±1.18 ctr:8.72±2.22~8.97±1.82	NA	tx:PPD 2.31±0.65~ 2.21±0.6 CAL 3.14±1.08~2.8±1.09 ctr:PPD 2.06±0.24~ 2.33±0.3 CAL 3.1±1.05~3.47±1.44	Oral medication Medical treatment unchange
Botero JE et al. 2013[†]	Colombia 39DM1, 66DM2(tx1:33 tx2:37 ctr:35) single center	HbA1c not reported tx1:scaling+ azithromycin tx2:scaling+placebo ctr:supragingival prophylaxis+ azithromycin	CAL≥4 mm in ≥2 interproximal sites, or PD≥5 mm in ≥2 interproximal sites	PPD, CAL, PI, BOP	tx1:7.92±1.58~±1.36(–0.8)* tx2:7.98±2.16~±1.91(–0.6) ctr:7.87±1.81~±2.48(0.2)	tx1:(–0.4) tx2:(0) ctr:(0.2)	tx1:PPD 2.7±0.6~2.3± 0.6 CAL 2.8±0.8~2.5± 0.8 tx2:PPD 2.6±0.7~ 2.5±0.5 CAL 3.1± 1.16~3.0±1.1 ctr:PPD 2.4±0.6~2.2±0.4 CAL 2.9±1.1~2.8±0.9	Baseline medication not reported change not reported
Telgi RL et al. 2013	India 60DM2 (tx:20 ctr1:20 ctr2:20) single center	HbA1c not reported tx:scaling+CHX+brush ctr1:CHX+brush ctr2:brush	PD 4–5 mm, ≥28 teeth	PPD, PI, GI	tx:7.68±0.63~7.10±0.64 (–0.58±0.27) ctr1:7.56±0.59~ 7.31±0.59(–0.25±0.14) ctr2:7.74±0.59~7.75±0.58 (0.004±0.12)	NA	tx:PPD 5.05±0.70~ 4.59±0.72(–0.46±0.26) CAL NA ctr1:PPD 5.11±0.57~4.87±0.55 (–0.25±0.11) CAL NA ctr2:PPD 5.05±0.69~ 5.03±0.69(–0.02±0.05) CAL NA	Oral medication change in medication not reported
Engebretson SP et al. 2013	USA 275DM2 (tx:240 ctr:235) multicenter	HbA1c 7%–9% tx:SRP+CHX+OH ctr:OH	PD≥5 mm in ≥2 quadrants, ≥16 teeth	PPD, CAL, PI, BOP	tx:7.84±0.65~(0.13) ctr:7.77±0.60~(0.08)	tx:(0.15) ctr:(0.09)	tx:PPD 3.3±0.6~2.8 CAL 3.5±0.8~3.2 ctr:PPD 3.3±0.7~ 3.2 CAL 3.5±0.9~3.4	No diatetes medications:11 Oral medication:244 Insulin:80 Combination:179 Changes between treatment groups were similar

PI, plaque index; GI, gingival index; PPD, probing pocket depth; CAL, clinical attachment loss; GR, gingival recession; BOP, bleeding on probing; NA, not available; CHX, chlorhexidine gluconate; OH, oral hygiene; SRP, scaling and root planning.
*reported in a graph.
[†]data obtained by calculation.

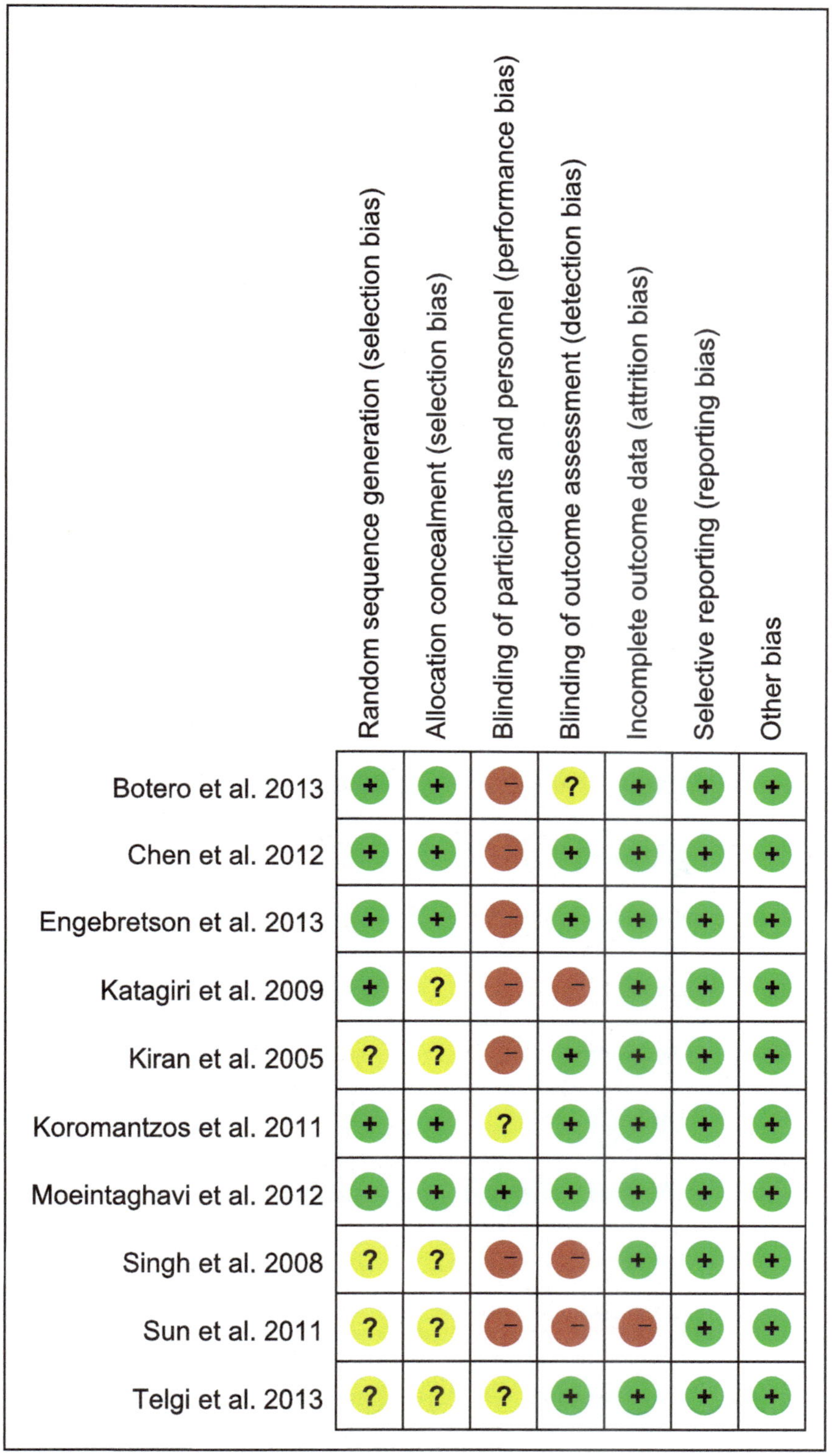

Figure 2. Judgements about each risk of bias item for each included study.

information about the generation of a randomized sequence. Concealment was inadequate in five of the included studies [8,40,43,44,47]. In one of the studies treatments were performed under the supervision of an expert [46]. Six studies were outcome assessment blinded [8,28,42,44–46]. One study [46] excluded the data of the patients who did not finish the study at the baseline. (Fig. 2, 3).

Since the heterogeneity of every outcomes was assessed and shown as P for χ^2 test and I^2, as they were shown in Fig. 4, 5–7 that all of the P<0.10 for χ^2 test and I^2>25%, so there were heterogeneity among the included trials, and a random-effects

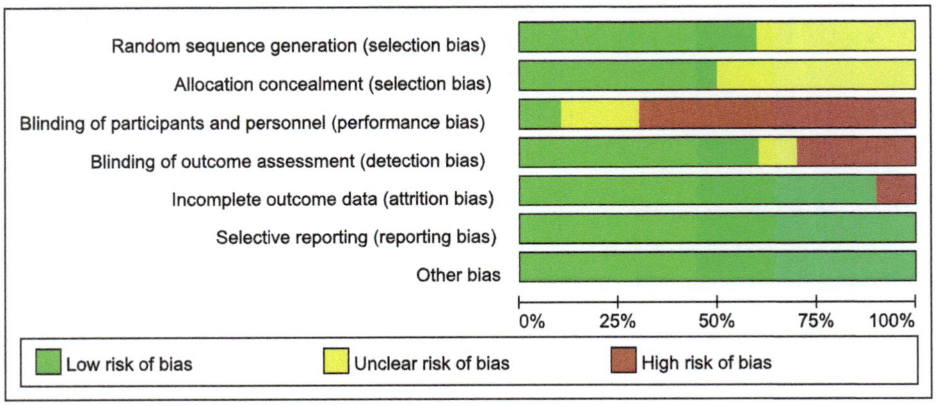

Figure 3. Each risk of bias item presented as percentages across all included studies.

model analysis was used. In addition, the results analyzed with the fixed-effects model, including the relevant forest plots (Fig. S1–S4), were provided as online supplements.

Change of HbA1c at 3-month

Data on change of HbA1c were available for analysis in 1135 patients enrolled in ten trials investigating the effect of non-surgical periodontal treatment on glycemic control of diabetic patients. The change of HbA1c for 3 months ranged from −0.86% to 0.13%, with a mean change of HbA1c from baseline of −0.36% (95%CI: −0.52%, −0.19%). As it was showed in Fig. 4, the forest plot described the effect on HbA1c in terms of mean reduction from baseline, and standard deviation, as a comparison between treatment and control groups. Nevertheless, there might be substantial heterogeneity in the change of HbA1c across studies ($P = 0.0003$, $I^2 = 71\%$). Furthermore, publication bias may exist as the funnel plot (Fig. 8) displayed an asymmetrical distribution.

Change of periodontal parameters at 3-month

Non-surgical periodontal treatment demonstrated a significant benefit on the periodontal status. Nine trials [8,28,40–44,46,47] reported the mean change of PPD in 1077 patients. The mean change of PPD from baseline to the 3-month after treatment was −0.42 mm (95%CI: −0.60, −0.23) (Fig. 5); seven trials [28,40–42,44,46,47] reported the mean change of CAL in 968 patients, and the mean change of CAL 3 months after treatment was −0.34 mm (95%CI: −0.52, −0.16) (Fig. 6).

Change of HbA1c at 6-month

Data on the change of HbA1c for 6 months in diabetic patients with periodontitis were available for 754 patients enrolled in four trials [28,41,42,45]. The change of HbA1c for 6 months ranged from −0.72% to 0.15%, and the result presented no statistical difference between the treatment and control groups (−0.30%, 95%CI: −0.69 to 0.09, $P = 0.13$), and there might be heterogeneity in the change of HbA1c for 6 months across studies ($P = 0.02$, $I^2 = 68\%$) (Fig. 7).

Treatment modalities

All treatment group interventions consisted of non-surgical periodontal therapy with or without adjunctive topical or systemic antibiotics, and/or topical antiseptics. Six trials [28,40,43–46] were two-arm studies, and four trials [8,41,42,47] were three-armed. Of the three-arm studies, Boter et al. [41] and Singh et al. [47] reported that both treatment arms received non-surgical therapy with or without adjunctive antibiotics; Chen et al. [42] reported that both treatment arms received scaling and root planning only; while in the Telgi et al. [8] study only one arm received scaling. Of the two arm studies, two studies' treatment included scaling and root planning only [44,46], Koromantzos et al. [45] treatment included scaling and root planning plus extraction of hopeless teeth, and Sun et al. [40] treatment also included flap surgery ("when indicated") and systemic Tinidazole plus ampicillin. The remaining studies included adjunctive treatment of chlorhexidine oral rinse [28] or topical use of

Study or Subgroup	Treatment Mean	Treatment SD	Treatment Total	Control Mean	Control SD	Control Total	Weight	Mean Difference IV, Random, 95% CI
Botero et al. 2013	-0.68	1.84	60	0.2	2.22	35	3.2%	-0.88 [-1.75, -0.01]
Chen et al. 2012	0.06	2.05	83	0.34	2.14	41	3.7%	-0.28 [-1.07, 0.51]
Engebretson et al. 2013	0.13	1.09	233	0.08	1	228	18.1%	0.05 [-0.14, 0.24]
Katagiri et al. 2009	-0.14	0.63	32	-0.09	0.57	17	11.7%	-0.05 [-0.40, 0.30]
Kiran et al. 2005	-0.86	0.77	22	0.31	1.83	22	3.4%	-1.17 [-2.00, -0.34]
Koromantzos et al. 2011	-0.73	0.91	30	-0.18	0.82	30	9.0%	-0.55 [-0.99, -0.11]
Moeintaghavi et al. 2012	-0.74	1.67	22	0.25	2.87	18	1.2%	-0.99 [-2.49, 0.51]
Singh et al. 2008	-0.65	0.91	30	0.06	1.02	15	5.7%	-0.71 [-1.32, -0.10]
Sun et al. 2011	-0.5	0.18	82	-0.14	0.12	75	23.3%	-0.36 [-0.41, -0.31]
Telgi et al. 2013	-0.58	0.27	20	-0.12	0.18	40	20.7%	-0.46 [-0.59, -0.33]
Total (95% CI)			**614**			**521**	**100.0%**	**-0.36 [-0.52, -0.19]**

Heterogeneity: Tau² = 0.03; Chi² = 30.64, df = 9 (P = 0.0003); I² = 71%
Test for overall effect: Z = 4.19 (P < 0.0001)

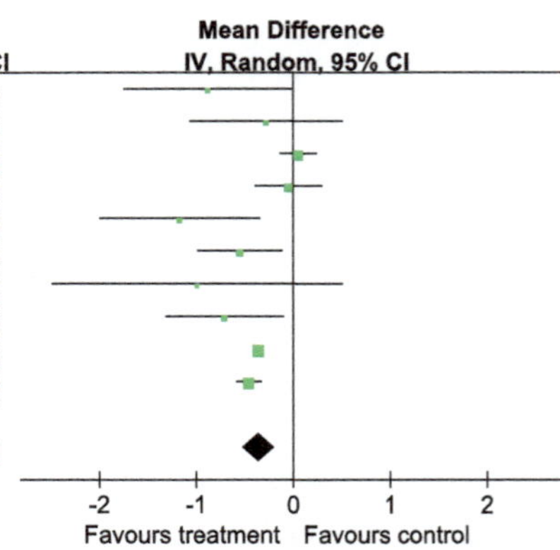

Figure 4. Forest plot presenting change in HbA1c (%) at 3-month.

Study or Subgroup	treatment Mean	treatment SD	treatment Total	Control Mean	Control SD	Control Total	Weight	Mean Difference IV, Random, 95% CI
Botero et al. 2013	-0.22	0.56	60	-0.2	0.4	35	11.6%	-0.02 [-0.21, 0.17]
Chen et al. 2012	-0.38	0.45	85	-0.09	0.47	41	11.9%	-0.29 [-0.46, -0.12]
Engebretson et al. 2013	-0.5	0.61	233	-0.1	0.6	228	12.7%	-0.40 [-0.51, -0.29]
Katagiri et al. 2009	-0.8	0.51	32	-0.2	0.7	17	8.5%	-0.60 [-0.98, -0.22]
Kiran et al. 2005	-0.49	0.25	22	0.02	0.63	22	10.1%	-0.51 [-0.79, -0.23]
Moeintaghavi et al. 2012	-0.1	0.6	22	0.27	0.3	18	10.0%	-0.37 [-0.66, -0.08]
Singh et al. 2008	-0.36	0.4	30	-0.04	0.46	15	10.3%	-0.32 [-0.59, -0.05]
Sun et al. 2011	-1.15	0.66	82	-0.21	0.19	75	12.3%	-0.94 [-1.09, -0.79]
Telgi et al. 2013	-0.46	0.26	20	-0.14	0.14	40	12.6%	-0.32 [-0.44, -0.20]
Total (95% CI)			**586**			**491**	**100.0%**	**-0.42 [-0.60, -0.23]**

Heterogeneity: Tau² = 0.07; Chi² = 69.78, df = 8 (P < 0.00001); I² = 89%
Test for overall effect: Z = 4.46 (P < 0.00001)

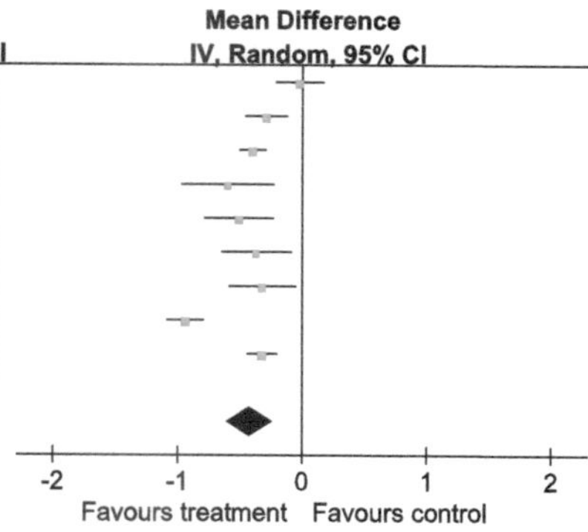

Figure 5. Forest plot presenting change in PPD (mm) at 3-month.

minocycline ointment [43]. And five trials [28,41–43,45] reported the additional supra- or subgingival debridement at the post-treatment appointment.

Discussion

There have been several excellent systematic reviews [35,36] reported about the effect of periodontal treatment on glycemic control of diabetic patients, the previous studies used for analysis in the reviews except those couldn't meet the inclusion criteria were included, and three new studies have been added. In all, ten randomized clinical trials were included in this review, with more than 3 months of follow-up period. The total number of subjects within the studies included in this review was 1135. And we could conclude from the current systematic review that non-surgical periodontal treatment for diabetic patients is beneficial in glycemic control and can reduce HbA1c levels by 0.36% 3 months after treatment, the effect at 6-month post-treatment is not obvious. It might present that non-surgical periodontal treatment may play a role on glycemic control for diabetic patient for just a period of time. But because of the difference of the treatment modalities the number of included studies is limited, the sample size is insufficient, and there is significant heterogeneity across studies, it is worthy of attention in future studies.

Although not all literature reported the related change of periodontal parameter, the available data extracted from the included studies was analyzed. The results showed that there was an overall 0.42 mm reduction in PPD and 0.34 mm reduction in CAL at 3-month post-treatment. It is generally considered that inflammation cytokines like C-reactive protein (CRP) may play an important role between diabetes and periodontitis [50], and a meta-analysis made by Teeuw et al. [51] find that periodontal treatment can significantly reduce the level of CRP. Katagiri et al. [43] revealed that there is a relationship between the change of CRP and HbA1c level. Therefore, we believe that periodontal therapy can certainly reduce systemic inflammation by improvement of the periodontal status, then impact the glycaemic control for a period of time. And when the inflammation is under control, the effect of periodontal therapy on glycaemic control may not obvious.

It is reported that although dental prophylaxis including removal of supragingival calculus and plaque can improve periodontal health, it cannot influence HbA1c levels [52]. So we considered the group in Boter et al. [41] received removal of supragingival calculus and plaque as the control group.

High risk of bias of the included studies especially the "blinding of participants and personnel", should be explained by the fact that the intervention of the studies was periodontal treatment, such as scaling and root planning etc., while the control group without treatment, so it was difficult to mask the therapists and subjects.

Compared with the previous reports, there are some certain improvements in this study. Firstly, a phase 3, multi-center, randomized trial with a number of 514 participants was included [28]. Although the results of that trial was that non-surgical periodontal therapy did not improve glycaemic control in patients with type 2 diabetes, and was not exactly the same with this review, the difference made us to look for the reasons. Three significant reasons should be considered. One reason was that the characteristics of the participants in Engebretson et al. [28] and the previous studies were different. Although the participants were all diabetics, they were different in many aspects, such as ethnic and geographic, severity of periodontitis, compliance of the

Study or Subgroup	treatment Mean	treatment SD	treatment Total	Control Mean	Control SD	Control Total	Weight	Mean Difference IV, Random, 95% CI
Botero et al. 2013	-0.18	0.99	60	-0.1	0.9	35	11.7%	-0.08 [-0.47, 0.31]
Chen et al. 2012	-0.35	1.19	85	-0.08	0.23	41	16.6%	-0.27 [-0.53, -0.01]
Engebretson et al. 2013	-0.3	0.92	233	-0.1	0.9	228	21.0%	-0.20 [-0.37, -0.03]
Kiran et al. 2005	-0.39	1.03	22	-0.05	1.03	22	6.6%	-0.34 [-0.95, 0.27]
Moeintaghavi et al. 2012	-0.34	1.09	22	0.37	1.44	18	4.2%	-0.71 [-1.52, 0.10]
Singh et al. 2008	-0.32	0.53	30	0.04	0.35	15	16.7%	-0.36 [-0.62, -0.10]
Sun et al. 2011	-0.73	0.51	82	-0.15	0.13	75	23.2%	-0.58 [-0.69, -0.47]
Total (95% CI)			**534**			**434**	**100.0%**	**-0.34 [-0.52, -0.16]**

Heterogeneity: Tau² = 0.03; Chi² = 19.21, df = 6 (P = 0.004); I² = 69%
Test for overall effect: Z = 3.72 (P = 0.0002)

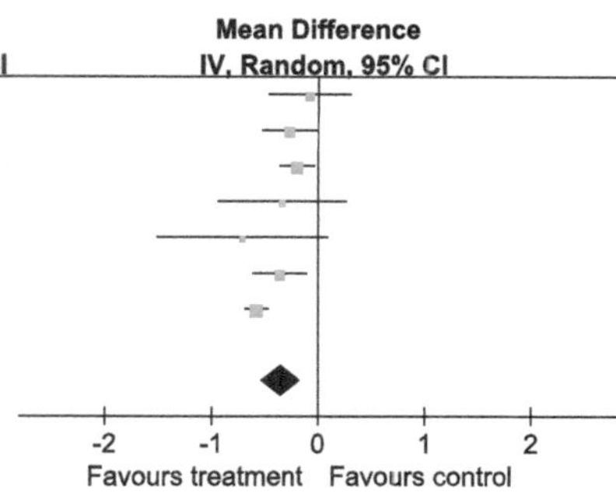

Figure 6. Forest plot presenting change in CAL (mm) at 3-month.

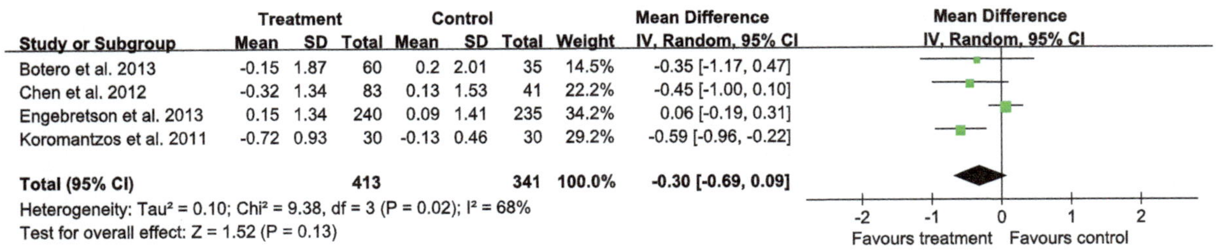

Figure 7. Forest plot presenting change in HbA1c (%) at 6-month.

participants, oral hygiene habits, etc. Especially, the concern about the treatment of diabetes was different. Only the participants enrolled in Engebretson et al. [28] were reported under the supervision of the physician for the diabetes, and the change of diabetic medicine was monitored. Six of the other studies instructed the participants not to modify the medication or diet [40,42–44,46,47], two did not reported the change of diabetic medication [8,41] and the other one [45] reported that only 13.3% for treatment group and 10% for control group participants increased their insulin dosages. It was considered that many factors, including whether the diabetic patients were under the supervision of physicians, and the different regions, the level of medical institutions (medical centers or primary clinics), and the different types that the supervisors belong to [53], can influent the level of HbA1c. So we think that the concern about the treatment of diabetes may have an impact on the outcome of the studies. Although the author disproved, Chapple et al. [54] pointed out that almost 60% patients having HbA1c level less than 8% at the baseline in Engebretson et al. Another reason was that the sample size of Engebretson et al. [28] was much more bigger than the other included studies, and the range of standard deviation of the change from baseline of HbA1c was wide. This point also increases the difficulty for us to explain the heterogeneity. When the heterogeneity cannot be readily explained, random-effects model is one of the strategies for addressing heterogeneity according to the Cochrane handbook for systematic reviews of interventions (Version 5.1.0) [37]. So a random-effects model was used for the analysis. The other reason was that the treatment of the periodontitis was not completely the same with the other studies, this study did not use the adjunctive topical or systemic antibiotics [55,56]. Since the effect of scaling and root planning with the adjunctive topical or systemic antibiotics on reduction of HbA1c level has been shown in several studies [41,43,47], we believe that it may be a potential factor affecting the results of the study.

Secondly, the follow-up period of the studies included in this review was more than 3 months, and all of the studies reported about the HbA1c values at the 3-month after treatment. Two studies [48,49] included in the previous review reported on a 4-month follow-up outcome, and they were excluded.

Thirdly, One of the strengths of the present meta-analysis is that it takes into account the change of periodontal parameters at 3-month after treatment. It allows us to be more intuitive understanding of the effect of periodontal treatment on glycaemic control while improving periodontal status. The change of HbA1c for 6 months was also analyzed. The result can help us to

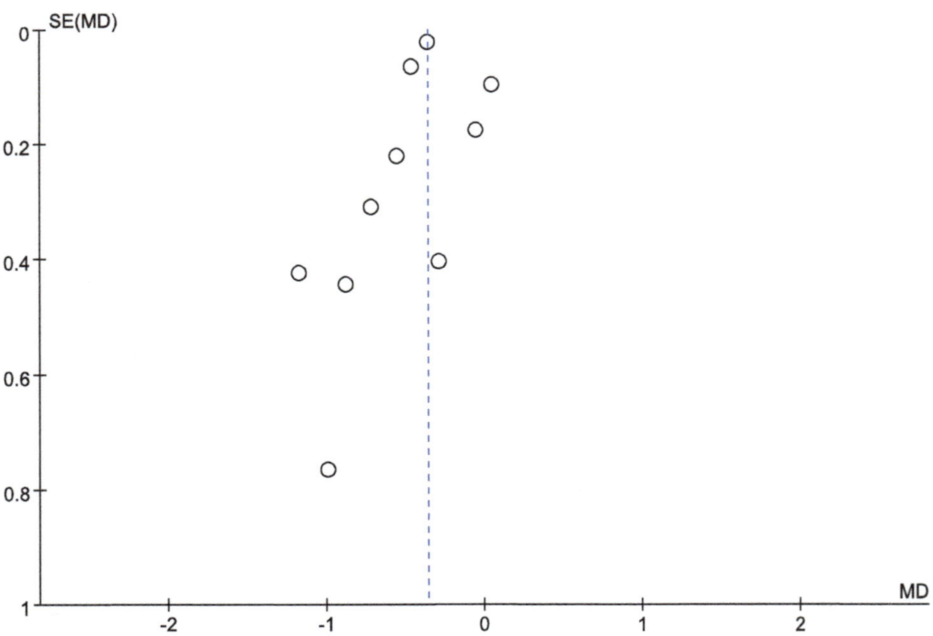

Figure 8. Funnel plot presenting change in HbA1c (%) at 3-month.

understand the long-term effect of periodontal treatment on HbA1c level in subjects with diabetes and periodontitis.

There are also several limitations to this review. The first is that the effect of periodontal treatment on glycaemic control of different type of diabetes with periodontitis cannot be analyzed in subgroups. One study [41] included participants with type 1 diabetes. But the sample size was small, and the outcomes were not reported separately, so it was analyzed as a part of treatment and control group. Another limitation is that adjunctive treatments such as: topical or systemic antibiotics and topical antiseptics were taken in many trials. And the systemic antibiotics could potentially mask the effect of scaling and root planning on HbA1c [28]. And it was not reported in this study. The other limitation of the present meta-analysis is that several studies did not reported the standard deviation of the change of HbA1c, and the data included in the analysis were obtained by calculation. The last but not the least is that only one recent trials was included in this update systemic review.

In conclusion, we demonstrate that periodontal treatment leads a reduction of HbA1c in diabetic patients with periodontitis while the improvement of periodontal status for 3 months after treatment. But the treatment may have no obvious effect on glycemic control for diabetic patient for 6 months after treatment. So physicians and dentists should carefully interpret these results when they apply them in clinical practice. And we look forward to more large randomized controlled trials with clear intervention design.

Supporting Information

Figure S1 Forest plot presenting change in HbA1c (%) at 3-month (fixed-effects model).

Figure S2 Forest plot presenting change in PPD (mm) at 3-month (fixed-effects model).

Figure S3 Forest plot presenting change in CAL (mm) at 3-month (fixed-effects model).

Figure S4 Forest plot presenting change in HbA1c (%) at 6-month (fixed-effects model).

Checklist S1 Prisma Checklist.

File S1

Flow Diagram S1

Author Contributions

Conceived and designed the experiments: W-DL W-XX. Performed the experiments: W-XX H-X L-XL W-DL. Analyzed the data: W-XX H-X G-XJ L-XL W-DL. Contributed reagents/materials/analysis tools: W-XX G-XJ. Contributed to the writing of the manuscript: W-XX H-X L-XL G-XJ W-DL.

References

1. Persson GR (2006) What has ageing to do with periodontal health and disease? Int Dent J 56: 240–249.
2. Thornton-Evans G, Eke P, Wei L, Palmer A, Moeti R, et al. (2013) Periodontitis among adults aged >/ = 30 years - United States, 2009–2010. 62 Suppl 3: 129–135.
3. Shangase SL, Mohangi GU, Hassam-Essa S, Wood NH (2013) The association between periodontitis and systemic health: an overview. Sadj 68: 8, 10–12.
4. Hung HC, Willett W, Ascherio A, Rosner BA, Rimm E, et al. (2003) Tooth loss and dietary intake. J Am Dent Assoc 134: 1185–1192.
5. Chen HH, Chen DY, Lai KL, Chen YM, Chou YJ, et al. (2013) Periodontitis and etanercept discontinuation risk in anti-tumor necrosis factor-naive rheumatoid arthritis patients: a nationwide population-based cohort study. J Clin Rheumatol 19: 432–438.
6. Holtfreter B, Empen K, Glaser S, Lorbeer R, Volzke H, et al. (2013) Periodontitis is associated with endothelial dysfunction in a general population: a cross-sectional study. PLoS One 8: e84603.
7. Wen BW, Tsai CS, Lin CL, Chang YJ, Lee CF, et al. (2013) Cancer risk among gingivitis and periodontitis patients: a nationwide cohort study. Qjm.
8. Telgi RL, Tandon V, Tangade PS, Tirth A, Kumar S, et al. (2013) Efficacy of nonsurgical periodontal therapy on glycaemic control in type II diabetic patients: a randomized controlled clinical trial. J Periodontal Implant Sci 43: 177–182.
9. Sanchez-Zamora YI, Rodriguez-Sosa M (2014) The Role of MIF in Type 1 and Type 2 Diabetes Mellitus. 2014: 804519.
10. Soskolne WA, Klinger A (2001) The relationship between periodontal diseases and diabetes: an overview. J Diabetes Res 6: 91–98.
11. Tsai C, Hayes C, Taylor GW (2002) Glycemic control of type 2 diabetes and severe periodontal disease in the US adult population. Community Dent Oral Epidemiol 30: 182–192.
12. Pucher J, Stewart J (2004) Periodontal disease and diabetes mellitus. Curr Diab Rep 4: 46–50.
13. Mealey BL, Oates TW (2006) Diabetes mellitus and periodontal diseases. J Periodontol 77: 1289–1303.
14. Nelson RG, Shlossman M, Budding LM, Pettitt DJ, Saad MF, et al. (1990) Periodontal disease and NIDDM in Pima Indians. Diabetes Care 13: 836–840.
15. Meenawat A, Punn K, Srivastava V, Meenawat AS, Dolas RS, et al. (2013) Periodontal disease and type I diabetes mellitus: Associations with glycemic control and complications. J Indian Soc Periodontol 17: 597–600.
16. Stanko P, Izakovicova Holla L (2014) Bi directional association between diabetes mellitus and inflammatory periodontal disease. A review. Biomed Pap Med Fac Univ Palacky Olomouc Czech Repub.
17. Al-Khabbaz AK (2014) Type 2 diabetes mellitus and periodontal disease severity. Oral Health Prev Dent 12: 77–82.
18. Loe H (1993) Periodontal disease. The sixth complication of diabetes mellitus. Diabetes Care 16: 329–334.
19. Mirnic J, Djuric M, Predin T, Gusic I, Petrovic D, et al. (2013) [Impact of the level of metabolic control on the non-surgical periodontal therapy outcomes in diabetes mellitus type 2 patients–clinical effects]. Srp Arh Celok Lek 141: 738–743.
20. Santacroce L, Carlaio RG, Bottalico L (2010) Does it make sense that diabetes is reciprocally associated with periodontal disease? Endocr Metab Immune Disord Drug Targets 10: 57–70.
21. Taylor GW, Borgnakke WS (2008) Periodontal disease: associations with diabetes, glycemic control and complications. Oral Dis 14: 191–203.
22. Moodley A, Wood NH, Shangase SL (2013) The relationship between periodontitis and diabetes: a brief review. Sadj 68: 260, 262–264.
23. Goldfine AB, Fonseca V, Jablonski KA, Pyle L, Staten MA, et al. (2010) The effects of salsalate on glycemic control in patients with type 2 diabetes: a randomized trial. Ann Intern Med 152: 346–357.
24. Goldfine AB, Fonseca V, Shoelson SE (2011) Therapeutic approaches to target inflammation in type 2 diabetes. Clin Chem 57: 152–167.
25. Iwamoto Y, Nishimura F, Nakagawa M, Sugimoto H, Shikata K, et al. (2001) The effect of antimicrobial periodontal treatment on circulating tumor necrosis factor-alpha and glycated hemoglobin level in patients with type 2 diabetes. J Periodontol 72: 774–778.
26. Gaikwad SP, Gurav AN, Shete AR, Desarda HM (2013) Effect of scaling and root planing combined with systemic doxycycline therapy on glycemic control in diabetes mellitus subjects with chronic generalized periodontitis: a clinical study. J Periodontal Implant Sci 43: 79–86.
27. Bharti P, Katagiri S, Nitta H, Nagasawa T, Kobayashi H, et al. (2013) Periodontal treatment with topical antibiotics improves glycemic control in association with elevated serum adiponectin in patients with type 2 diabetes mellitus. Obes Res Clin Pract 7: e129–e138.
28. Engebretson SP, Hyman LG, Michalowicz BS, Schoenfeld ER, Gelato MC, et al. (2013) The effect of nonsurgical periodontal therapy on hemoglobin A1c levels in persons with type 2 diabetes and chronic periodontitis: a randomized clinical trial. Jama 310: 2523–2532.
29. Zhang Y, Hu G, Yuan Z, Chen L (2012) Glycosylated hemoglobin in relationship to cardiovascular outcomes and death in patients with type 2 diabetes: a systematic review and meta-analysis. PLoS One 7: e42551.
30. Koenig RJ, Peterson CM, Jones RL, Saudek C, Lehrman M, et al. (1976) Correlation of glucose regulation and hemoglobin AIc in diabetes mellitus. N Engl J Med 295: 417–420.
31. Group UPDSU (1998) Intensive blood-glucose control with sulphonylureas or insulin compared with conventional treatment and risk of complications in

patients with type 2 diabetes (UKPDS 33). UK Prospective Diabetes Study (UKPDS) Group. Lancet 352: 837–853.
32. Nathan DM, Cleary PA, Backlund JY, Genuth SM, Lachin JM, et al. (2005) Intensive diabetes treatment and cardiovascular disease in patients with type 1 diabetes. N Engl J Med 353: 2643–2653.
33. Jones A, Gladstone BP, Lubeck M, Lindekilde N, Upton D, et al. (2014) Motivational interventions in the management of HbA1c levels: A systematic review and meta-analysis. Prim Care Diabetes.
34. Tricco AC, Ivers NM, Grimshaw JM, Moher D, Turner L, et al. (2012) Effectiveness of quality improvement strategies on the management of diabetes: a systematic review and meta-analysis. Lancet 379: 2252–2261.
35. Teeuw WJ, Gerdes VE, Loos BG (2010) Effect of periodontal treatment on glycemic control of diabetic patients: a systematic review and meta-analysis. Diabetes Care 33: 421–427.
36. Engebretson S, Kocher T (2013) Evidence that periodontal treatment improves diabetes outcomes: a systematic review and meta-analysis. J Periodontol 84: S153–169.
37. Higgins JPT, Green S (1996) Cochrane Handbook for Systematic Reviews of Interventions Version 5.1.0 [updated March 2011]. The Cochrane Collaboration, 2011. Available from www.cochrane-handbook.org. Control Clin Trials 17.
38. Liew AK, Punnanithinont N, Lee YC, Yang J (2013) Effect of non-surgical periodontal treatment on HbA1c: a meta-analysis of randomized controlled trials. Aust Dent J 58: 350–357.
39. Borenstein M, Hedges LV, Higgins JPT, Rothstein HR (2009) Independent Subgroups within a Study. Introduction to Meta-Analysis: John Wiley & Sons, Ltd. pp. 217–223.
40. Sun WL, Chen LL, Zhang SZ, Wu YM, Ren YZ, et al. (2011) Inflammatory cytokines, adiponectin, insulin resistance and metabolic control after periodontal intervention in patients with type 2 diabetes and chronic periodontitis. Intern Med 50: 1569–1574.
41. Botero JE, Yepes FL, Ochoa SP, Hincapie JP, Roldan N, et al. (2013) Effects of periodontal non-surgical therapy plus azithromycin on glycemic control in patients with diabetes: a randomized clinical trial. J Periodontal Res 48: 706–712.
42. Chen L, Luo G, Xuan D, Wei B, Liu F, et al. (2012) Effects of non-surgical periodontal treatment on clinical response, serum inflammatory parameters, and metabolic control in patients with type 2 diabetes: a randomized study. J Periodontol 83: 435–443.
43. Katagiri S, Nitta H, Nagasawa T, Uchimura I, Izumiyama H, et al. (2009) Multi-center intervention study on glycohemoglobin (HbA1c) and serum, high-sensitivity CRP (hs-CRP) after local anti-infectious periodontal treatment in type 2 diabetic patients with periodontal disease. Diabetes Res Clin Pract 83: 308–315.
44. Kiran M, Arpak N, Unsal E, Erdogan MF (2005) The effect of improved periodontal health on metabolic control in type 2 diabetes mellitus. J Clin Periodontol 32: 266–272.
45. Koromantzos PA, Makrilakis K, Dereka X, Katsilambros N, Vrotsos IA, et al. (2011) A randomized, controlled trial on the effect of non-surgical periodontal therapy in patients with type 2 diabetes. Part I: effect on periodontal status and glycaemic control. J Clin Periodontol 38: 142–147.
46. Moeintaghavi A, Arab HR, Bozorgnia Y, Kianoush K, Alizadeh M (2012) Non-surgical periodontal therapy affects metabolic control in diabetics: a randomized controlled clinical trial. Aust Dent J 57: 31–37.
47. Singh S, Kumar V, Kumar S, Subbappa A (2008) The effect of periodontal therapy on the improvement of glycemic control in patients with type 2 diabetes mellitus: A randomized controlled clinical trial. Int J Diabetes Dev Ctries 28: 38–44.
48. Jones JA, Miller DR, Wehler CJ, Rich SE, Krall-Kaye EA, et al. (2007) Does periodontal care improve glycemic control? The Department of Veterans Affairs Dental Diabetes Study. J Clin Periodontol 34: 46–52.
49. Yun F, Firkova EI, Jun-Qi L, Xun H (2007) Effect of non-surgical periodontal therapy on patients with type 2 diabetes mellitus. Folia Med (Plovdiv) 49: 32–36.
50. Choi YH, McKeown RE, Mayer-Davis EJ, Liese AD, Song KB, et al. (2014) Serum C-reactive Protein and Immunoglobulin G Antibodies to Periodontal Pathogens may be Effect Modifiers of Periodontitis and Hyperglycemia. J Periodontol.
51. Teeuw WJ, Slot DE, Susanto H, Gerdes VE, Abbas F, et al. (2014) Treatment of periodontitis improves the atherosclerotic profile: a systematic review and meta-analysis. J Clin Periodontol 41: 70–79.
52. Lopez NJ, Quintero A, Casanova PA, Martinez B (2013) Three-Monthly Routine Prophylaxes Improves Chronic Periodontitis Status in Type 2 Diabetes. J Periodontol.
53. Huang LY, Shau WY, Yeh HL, Chen TT, Hsieh JY, et al. (2014) A model measuring therapeutic inertia and the associated factors among diabetes patients: A nationwide population-based study in Taiwan. J Clin Pharmacol.
54. Chapple IL, Borgnakke WS, Genco RJ (2014) Hemoglobin A1c levels among patients with diabetes receiving nonsurgical periodontal treatment. Jama 311: 1919–1920.
55. Vergnes JN (2014) Hemoglobin A1c levels among patients with diabetes receiving nonsurgical periodontal treatment. Jama 311: 1920–1921.
56. Merchant AT (2014) Hemoglobin A1c levels among patients with diabetes receiving nonsurgical periodontal treatment. Jama 311: 1919.

21

Involvement of Trigeminal Transition Zone and Laminated Subnucleus Caudalis in Masseter Muscle Hypersensitivity Associated with Tooth Inflammation

Kohei Shimizu[1,3]*, Kunihito Matsumoto[2,3], Noboru Noma[4,5], Shingo Matsuura[1], Kinuyo Ohara[1], Hiroki Komiya[1], Tetsuro Watase[1], Bunnai Ogiso[1,3], Yoshiyuki Tsuboi[6,7], Masamichi Shinoda[6,7], Keisuke Hatori[1,3], Yuka Nakaya[4], Koichi Iwata[6,7,8]

1 Department of Endodontics, Nihon University School of Dentistry, Tokyo, Japan, **2** Department of Radiology, Nihon University School of Dentistry, Tokyo, Japan, **3** Divisions of Advanced Dental Treatment, Dental Research Center, Nihon University School of Dentistry, Tokyo, Japan, **4** Department of Oral Diagnosis, Nihon University School of Dentistry, Tokyo, Japan, **5** Divisions of Clinical Research, Dental Research Center, Nihon University School of Dentistry, Tokyo, Japan, **6** Department of Physiology, Nihon University School of Dentistry, Tokyo, Japan, **7** Division of Functional Morphology, Dental Research Center, Nihon University School of Dentistry, Tokyo, Japan, **8** Division of Applied System Neuroscience Advanced Medical Research Center, Nihon University Graduate School of Medical Science, Tokyo, Japan

Abstract

A rat model of pulpitis/periapical periodontitis was used to study mechanisms underlying extraterritorial enhancement of masseter response associated with tooth inflammation. Periapical bone loss gradually increased and peaked at 6 weeks after complete Freund's adjuvant (CFA) application to the upper molar tooth pulp (M1). On day 3, the number of Fos-immunoreactive (IR) cells was significantly larger in M1 CFA rats compared with M1 vehicle (veh) rats in the trigeminal subnucleus interpolaris/caudalis transition zone (Vi/Vc). The number of Fos-IR cells was significantly larger in M1 CFA and masseter (Mass) capsaicin applied (M1 CFA/Mass cap) rats compared with M1 veh/Mass veh rats in the contralateral Vc and Vi/Vc. The number of phosphorylated extracellular signal-regulated kinase (pERK)-IR cells was significantly larger in M1 CFA/Mass cap and M1 veh/Mass cap rats compared to Mass-vehicle applied rats with M1 vehicle or CFA in the Vi/Vc. Pulpal CFA application caused significant increase in the number of Fos-IR cells in the Vi/Vc but not Vc on week 6. The number of pERK-IR cells was significantly lager in the rats with capsaicin application to the Mass compared to Mass-vehicle treated rats after pulpal CFA- or vehicle-application. However, capsaicin application to the Mass did not further affect the number of Fos-IR cells in the Vi/Vc in pulpal CFA-applied rats. The digastric electromyographic (d-EMG) activity after Mass-capsaicin application was significantly increased on day 3 and lasted longer at 6 weeks after pulpal CFA application, and these increase and duration were significantly attenuated by i.t. PD98059, a MEK1 inhibitor. These findings suggest that Vi/Vc and Vc neuronal excitation is involved in the facilitation of extraterritorial hyperalgesia for Mass primed with periapical periodontitis or acute pulpal-inflammation. Furthermore, phosphorylation of ERK in the Vi/Vc and Vc play pivotal roles in masseter hyperalgesia after pulpitis or periapical periodontitis.

Editor: Theodore J. Price, University of Texas at Dallas, United States of America

Funding: This study was supported in part by Research grants from Sato and Uemura Funds from Nihon University School of Dentistry, and Grant from Dental Research Center, Nihon University School of Dentistry; Nihon University multidisciplinary research grant and Individual Research Grant; a Grant from the Ministry of Education, Culture, Sports, Science and Technology to promote multi-disciplinary research Projects (KAKENHI (Grant-in-Aid for Young Scientist (B)) # 21791868 and # 23792192 to KS, # 22792021 to MS, KAKENHI (Challenging Exploratory Research) #24659832 to KI); grants from the Ministry of Education, Culture, Sports, Science, Technology to promote multidisciplinary research projects "Brain Mechanisms for Cognition, Memory and Behavior" and "Translational Research Network on Orofacial Neurological Disorders" at Nihon University. The funders had no role in study design, data collection and analysis, decision to publish, or preparation of the manuscript.

Competing Interests: The authors have declared that no competing interests exist.

* Email: shimizu.kouhei01@nihon-u.ac.jp

Introduction

Orofacial persistent pain following trigeminal nerve injury or orofacial inflammation is known to cause various motor as well as sensory disorders in the orofacial regions such as mastication or swallowing dysfunction [1]. Orofacial dysesthesia is known as the secondary hyperalgesia often associated with pulpitis and/or periapical periodontitis [2], suggesting that oral and craniofacial organs are target regions for ectopic pain following intraoral inflammation. Furthermore, it has been reported that the chronic orofacial pain associated with pulpitis and/or periapical periodontitis is one of the most frequent referred pain in the orofacial region, and pulpitis or periapical periodontitis is also known to be involved in the referred pain in various intraoral structures [3,4]. Referred pain in non-inflamed orofacial areas associated with pulpitis or periapical periodontitis is often accounted for misdiagnosis or inappropriate clinical treatment. Thus, it is very important to understand the mechanisms underlying orofacial-referred pain associated with pulpitis or periapical periodontitis to develop appropriate diagnosis and treatment of these patients.

The spinal trigeminal subnucleus caudalis (Vc) has been known as a key nucleus to relay tooth pulp afferent inputs to the higher central nervous system, and a large number of nociceptive neurons in the Vc are activated by orofacial noxious stimulation as well as tooth pulp stimulation [5,6]. Electrical stimulation of the tooth pulp produces Fos protein expression in many neurons in the transition zone between the subnucleus interpolaris (Vi) and Vc (Vi/Vc) and the caudal Vc and upper cervical cord [5]. These two areas are thought to play differential roles in processing noxious information from the tooth pulp as well as orofacial skin or muscles [7,8]. It has been reported that Vi/Vc and Vc have a role to process masseter muscle pain [9]. Furthermore, many neurons in these two areas are also known to receive noxious as well as non-noxious inputs from the orofacial regions [7,10]. Therefore, it is highly possible that nociceptive neurons in the Vi/Vc and Vc enhance their firings following pulpitis or periapical periodontitis and play a role in orofacial cutaneous and/or Mass nociception as well as processing tooth pulp or periapical inputs. We hypothesized therefore that Vi/Vc and Vc neurons are involved in masseter muscle hypersensitivity associated with tooth pulp and periapical inflammation.

Extracellular signal-regulated protein kinase (ERK) is a member of mitogen-activated protein kinase family that can be activated by calcium influx within 10 min after noxious stimulation [11]. Phosphorylated ERK-immunoreactive (pERK-IR) cells are known to be distributed in Vc with somatotopic organization, and the number of pERK-IR cells increased in an intensity-dependent manner in the Vc [12]. Previous studies indicated that C-fiber but not A-fiber stimulation accelerates ERK phosphorylation in dorsal root ganglion and spinal dorsal horn (SDH) neurons [13]. These findings indicate that ERK phosphorylation in Vc neurons could be a reliable indicator of neuronal activation following noxious stimulation of the orofacial regions.

Fos-IR cells have been widely used as a marker of neuronal activation in the SDH following noxious stimulation [14]. Fos expression could be detected 0.5–1 hour after noxious stimulation and lasts for 2–3 hours after stimulation. Recently, we have also reported that many pERK-IR cells show Fos-IR in Vc neurons following noxious mechanical stimulation of the periodontal tissues [15], suggesting that ERK phosphorylation is followed by Fos protein expression after noxious stimulation.

To clarify the central mechanisms underlying Mass hypersensitivity associated with pulpitis or periapical periodontitis following CFA application to the tooth pulp, we studied ERK phosphorylation and Fos expression in Vi/Vc and Vc neurons in tooth pulp- or periapical inflamed rats.

Materials and Methods

This study was approved by the Animal Experimentation Committee at the Nihon University (Animal protocol AP10D001). All surgery and animal care were conducted in accordance with the National Institutes of Health Guide for the Care and Use of Laboratory Animals and the guidelines for Institutional Animal Care, and the guidelines of the International Association for the Study of Pain [16]. Male Sprague-Dawley rats (n = 152) weighing 250–450 g were used in this study. The rats were housed under 12 h light/dark cycle conditions and had free access to food and water except during the test period. To minimize animal suffering, the number of animals used was based on the minimum required for statistically valid results. Immunohistochemical and Electrophysiological analysis were carried out in a blind manner.

Pulpal or periapical inflammation

Rats were lightly anesthetized with 2% isoflurane (Mylan, Canonsburg, PA), then deeply anesthetized with intraperitoneal (i.p.) application of sodium pentobarbital (50 mg/kg; Schering Plough, Whitehouse Station, NJ), and placed on a warm mat (37°C) in a dorsal recumbent position. To allow for application of CFA (n = 4, Sigma-Aldrich, 50% CFA was diluted in saline) or vehicle (n = 4, isotonic physiological saline) to the right maxillary first molar (M1) tooth pulp, the rats' mouth was gently opened and the dental pulp was exposed by means of low-speed dental drill with a round tungsten carbide bur (No. 1-4: JOTA, Tokyo) under water cooling. CFA or vehicle was applied to the tooth pulp by a small piece of dental paper point (diameter, 0.15 mm; length, 1.5 mm; PIERCE ABSORBENT POINTS, #15) soaked with CFA or vehicle. After CFA or vehicle application with dental points, the cavity was tightly sealed with dental cement (GC Fuji I, Tokyo). The bone loss around the tooth apex was evaluated using in vivo Micro X-ray CT System R_mCT (R_mCT, Rigaku, Tokyo). There were no any abnormal animal behaviors such as grooming, locomotion and feeding. The rats did not lose weight during experimental period.

The sagittal CT images for tooth apex were obtained at 300 μm intervals, and then the bone loss around tooth apex was drawn using Neurolucida (Micro-Brightfield Inc., Colchester, VT). The drawn images were integrated and 3D image of the periapical bone loss was constructed. The change in the volume was calculated by the Neuroexplore software (Micro-Brightfield Inc., Colchester, VT). Furthermore, on day 3 or week 6 after CFA application to upper molar tooth pulp, rats were anesthetized with sodium pentobarbital (80 mg/kg, i.p.) and perfused with 4% paraformaldehyde. Maxillar bone and M1 were removed and decalcified overnight and 15 mm serial sections were cut. Then sections were stained with hematoxylin and eosin and coverslipped.

pERK and Fos immunohistochemistries

For double immunofluorescence histochemistry for pERK and NeuN, sections were rinsed in PBS, 10% normal goat serum in PBS for 1 h, and then incubated in rabbit antiphospho-p44/42 MAP Kinase Antibody (1:200, Cell Signaling Technology) for 72 h at room temperature. Then the sections were incubated in mouse anti-neuronal nuclei monoclonal Antibody (1:500, Chemicon, Temicula, CA) for 2 h at room temperature. Next, the sections were incubated in Alexa Fluor 488 anti-rabbit IgG (1:200 in 0.01 M PBS; Invitrogen, Paisley) and in Alexa Fluor 568 anti-mouse IgG (1:200 in 0.01 M PBS; Invitrogen) for 2 h at room temperature. After rinsing with 0.01 M PBS, sections were coverslipped in mounting medium (Thermo Fisher Scientific, Fremont, CA) and examined under a fluorescence microscope and analyzed using a BZ-9000 system (Keyence, Osaka).

At 3 days and 6 weeks after CFA or vehicle application to M1 (n = 6 each), rats were deeply anesthetized with 2% isoflurane, and a 26 G needle with a Hamilton syringe was inserted into the ipsilateral Mass. After 30 min rest period, capsaicin was applied to the ipsilateral Mass, and at 5 minutes after capsaicin application, rats were transcardially perfused with isotonic saline followed by a fixative containing 4% paraformaldehyde in 0.1 M phosphate buffer (pH 7.4). The whole brain including medulla and upper cervical cord was removed and post-fixed in the same fixative for 3 days at 4°C. The tissues were then transferred to 20% sucrose (w/v) in 0.01 M phosphate-buffered saline (PBS) for several days for cryoprotection. Thirty-micron-thick sections were cut with a freezing microtome, and every fourth section was collected in PBS. Free-floating tissue sections were washed in PBS and rinsed in 1% hydrogen peroxide with 0.75% Triton X-100 (Sigma, St. Louis, MO) in PBS for 1 hour. After washing in PBS, the sections were incubated in 10% normal goat serum in PBS, and then incubated in polyclonal rabbit anti-Fos antibody (c-Fos ab-5, 1:5,000 dilution; Oncogene, Cambridge, MA) for overnight at 4°C. Next, the sections were incubated in biotinylated goat anti-rabbit IgG (1:600; Vector Labs, Burlingame, CA) for 2 h at room temperature. After washing in PBS, the sections were incubated in peroxidase-conjugated avidin-biotin complex (1:100; ABC, Vector Labs) for 2 h at room temperature. After washing in 0.05 M Tris Buffer (TB), the sections were incubated in 0.035% 3,3-diaminobenzidine-tetra HCl (DAB, Sigma, St. Louis, MO), 0.2% nickel ammonium sulfate and 0.05% peroxide in 0.05 M TB (pH 7.4). After washing in PBS and incubated in 10% normal horse serum in PBS, the sections reacted with Fos antibody were incubated in mouse anti-phospho-p44/42 MAP Kinase Antibody (pERK, 1 1000, Cell Signaling Technology) for 72 h at 4°C. The following immunohistochemical procedures were similar to those of c-Fos immunohistochemistry. The reaction products of biotinylated horse anti-mouse antiserum and avidin-conjugated horseradish peroxidase were visualized with 0.035% DAB and 0.05% hydrogen peroxide without nickel.

The sections were washed in PBS, serially mounted on gelatin-coated slides, dehydrated in alcohols and cover slipped. The pERK-IR, Fos protein-IR and double-labeled neurons were drawn under the light microscope using Neurolucida drawing tube. The neurons stained with DAB as brown in the nuclei and cytoplasm were determined as pERK-IR cells. The neurons stained with DAB as black in the nuclei were determined as Fos-IR cells. The number of pERK-IR, Fos protein-IR neurons was counted from every 8th section. The total number of IR neurons from 3 of every 8th section was calculated, and the mean number of those cells (3 sections/rat) was obtained from each animal.

Digastric electromyographic recording after capsaicin application into the Mass

On day 3 or week 6 after CFA or vehicle application to the M1 tooth pulp (n = 6 each), rats were anesthetized with 2% isoflurane and a pair of bipolar wire electrodes (enamel-coated stainless steel wire, inter-polar distance: 5 mm) was inserted into the digastric muscle on the side ipsilateral to the tooth. After that, a 26G needle connected with a Hamilton syringe was gently inserted into the ipsilateral Mass.

The digastric electromyographic (d-EMG) activity was continuously monitored before, during and after the application of capsaicin, dissolved in 100% ethanol and 7% Tween 80 in saline (3 μM, 100 μl), into the Mass. Before capsaicin application, baseline of d-EMG activity was monitored for 20 min, and d-EMG activity was continuously monitored for an additional 20 min. Then, the d-EMG activity was amplified, rectified and integrated, and the area under the curve of d-EMG activity was calculated by the Spike 2 software (CED, Cambridge). The area under the curve of d-EMG activity was measured for every 1 min before and after capsaicin application, and mean d-EMG activity was calculated in each time period. The calculated d-EMG value more than 2 standard deviation of the baseline after capsaicin application was selected and evaluated.

PD98059 administration

Rats were anesthetized with 2% isoflurane and placed in a stereotaxic apparatus. After a midline skin incision, an opening was made in the caudal part of the skull with a dental drill to insert intrathecally (i.t.) a soft polyethylene tube (PE45, ID, 0.58 mm; OD, 0.96 mm; Natsume, Tokyo, Japan) [17]. The tube was connected to a mini-osmotic pump (Alzet model 2001, Alzet, Cupertino, CA, USA; total volume, 200 μL) filled with the drug and embedded subcutaneously in the dorsal portion of the body. Thus, the MEK1 inhibitor PD98059 was intrathecally applied for 7 days (1.0 μL/h). The dosage and duration of the drug (0.1 μg/μL) for pump infusion was chosen primarily based on previous reports [18–21]. For the rats with periapical periodontitis, CFA was applied into the M1 at 35 days before PD98059 or saline administration, and then capsaicin was applied to the Mass on 7 days after PD98059 administration. For the rats with pulpitis, CFA was applied into the M1 at 4 days after PD98059 or saline administration, and then capsaicin was applied into the Mass at 3 days after CFA application. The d-EMG activity was continuously monitored before and after capsaicin application (n = 6 each).

For pERK and Fos immunohistochemistries, capsaicin was applied into the Mass in CFA-treated rats on day 7 after PD98059 or saline administration (n = 6 each). At 5 minutes after capsaicin application, the rats were perfused, and the pERK and Fos immunohistochemistries were performed.

All subsequent d-EMG recording and staining steps and counting analysis were the same as described above. All d-EMG recording and immunohistochemical experiments were conducted on animals without any obvious neurological deficits. Also, the Alzet pump was removed at the end of each experiment, and the amount of the drug remaining in the pump was checked. If there was still residual drug in the pump, the data from that rat were excluded from the final analysis.

Statistical analysis

Data were expressed as mean ± SEM. Statistical analyses were performed by Student's t-test, one-way or two-way repeated-measures analysis of variance (ANOVA) followed by Turkey or Dunnet test appropriately. A value of $p<0.05$ was considered as significant.

Results

1. The effect of CFA on tooth and periapical tissues

The application of CFA to the M1 tooth pulp induced inflammation in the tooth pulp on day 3 and in the periapical tissues on week 6 (Fig. 1). The detail tooth structures of M1 were indicated in Fig. 1A–C. In naive rats or the rats with CFA application to the M1 tooth pulp on day 3, periapical bone loss was not observed (Fig. 1A, B), indicating that the CFA-induced inflammation is limited within the pulp or at the apex region of the tooth. The periapical bone loss was clearly detected at 3 weeks after CFA application to the pulp, as shown by formation of granuloma in the periapical periodontitis (Fig. 1C–I). The bone loss was gradually increased and peaked at 6 weeks after CFA application (Fig. 1J). The volume of bone loss measured by 3D micro-CT imaging analysis software was significantly greater in CFA-treated rats compared with vehicle-treated rats from 3 weeks after CFA application ($p<0.05$, Fig. 1J).

2. Change in d-EMG activities following tooth pulp or periapical inflammation

We observed significant increase in the d-EMG activity within 1 min after capsaicin application into the Mass in pulpal CFA-applied rats ($p<0.01$, Fig. 2A, B). On the other hand, the duration of d-EMG activities after pulpal-CFA or pulpal-vehicle application was about 2 minutes, and no significant difference was observed between CFA and vehicle groups (Fig. 2C).

The d-EMG activities elicited by capsaicin application into the Mass at 6 weeks after pulpal-CFA application were shown in Fig. 2D. Compared with the pulpal-vehicle applied rats, the d-EMG activity was significantly increased (Fig. 2E) and the duration of the d-EMG activity was significantly lasted (Fig. 2F)

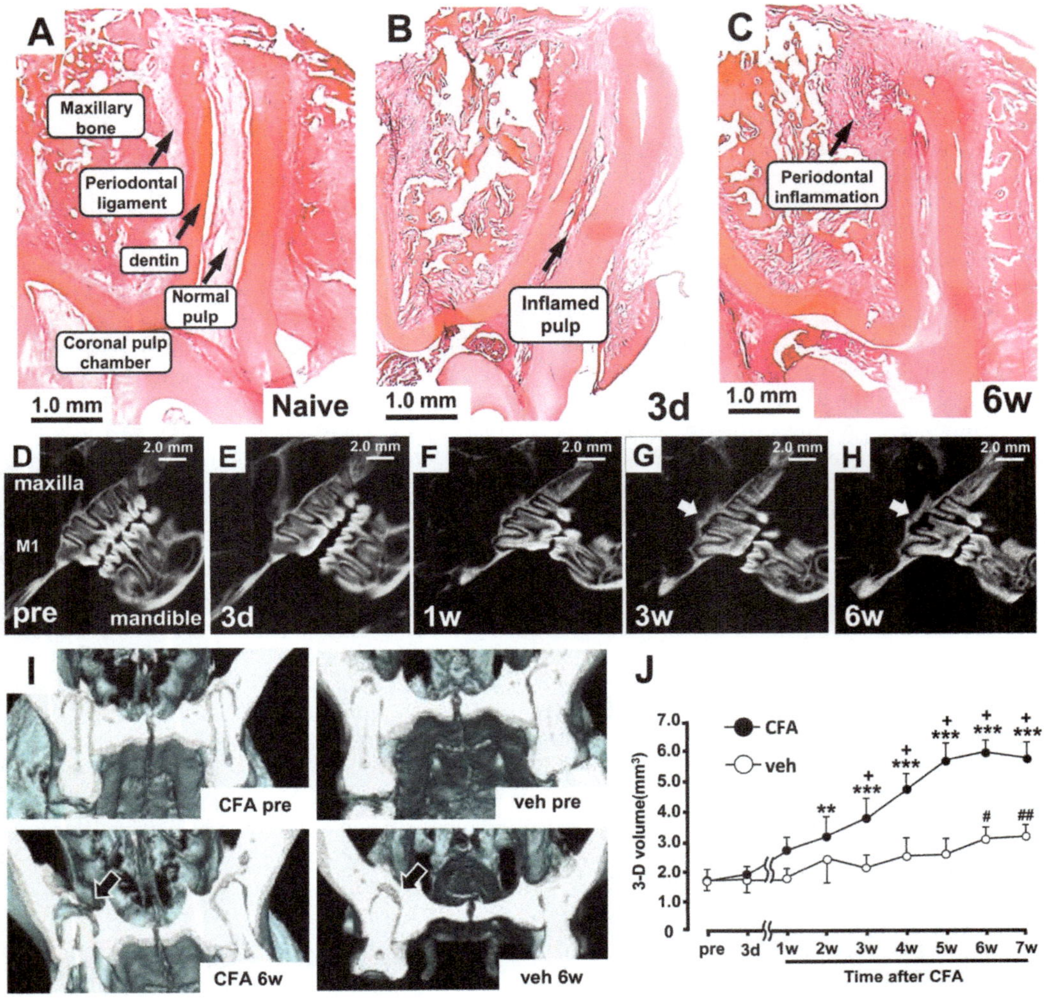

Figure 1. The change in the apical periapical tissues after CFA application to M1 tooth pulp. A, B and C: Photomicrographs of periapical tissues of the naive rats (A) and the rats on day 3 (B) and week 6 (C) after CFA application to the pulp. D–H: Lateral views of 3D X-lay photographs of periapical tissues of pre-CFA application (D), on day 3 (E), on 1 week (F), 3 week (G) and 6 week (H) after CFA application. I: Sagittal views of X-lay micro-CT images of the periapical tissues before and at 6 week after CFA or vehicle application to the pulp. J: Time course change in the size of the bone loss at the periapical tissues after CFA application to the M1 pulp (n = 4 each). Solid arrows in A-C indicate detail tooth and periapical structures. White arrows in G and H, and black arrow in I indicate periapical bone loss. veh: vehicle in this and following figures. *: Pre vs. post (CFA), #: Pre vs. post (veh), +: CFA vs. veh, +, #: $p<0.05$, ##, **: $p<0.01$, ***: $p<0.001$.

after capsaicin application into the Mass at 6 weeks after pulpal CFA application.

3. pERK-IR and Fos-IR cells and Rostral-caudal distribution in Vi/Vc or Vc

To examine the effect of M1 pulpitis or periapical periodontitis on the neuronal excitability, the ERK phosphorylation and Fos expression were studied in Vi/Vc and Vc neurons following unilateral capsaicin application into the Mass. A number of pERK-IR cells in the Vi/Vc and Vc induced by capsaicin at 3 days or 6 weeks after pulpal CFA application were double-stained with NeuN, a neuronal marker (Fig. 3A–C). However, some of the pERK-positive cells lacked NeuN staining. These results suggest that ERK phosphorylation occurs in grail cells as well as neurons. A large number of pERK-IR and Fos-IR cells were observed in the ventral portion of the Vi/Vc and in the dorsal portion of the Vc after capsaicin application into the Mass on day 3 or week 6 after CFA application into the M1 tooth pulp (Fig. 3G and 4A). Though we observed a few cells double-stained (Fig. 3F) with Fos (Fig. 3D) and pERK (Fig. 3E) antibodies, there are no double-stained cells in the Vi/Vc and Vc.

Rostral-caudal distribution of pERK-IR and Fos-IR cells in the medulla and upper cervical spinal cord were shown in Fig. 3G, H and Fig. 4A and B. A large number of pERK-IR and Fos-IR cells were observed in the Vi/Vc and Vc following capsaicin application into the ipsilateral Mass on day 3 or week 6 after pulpal CFA application (Fig. 3H and 4B). The total number of cells in Vc and Vi/Vc region indicated by red squares in Fig. 3H and 4B were calculated and the results of statistical analysis were shown in Fig. 3I and Fig. 4C, respectively. Blank indicate a lack of significant difference. The total number of pERK- or Fos-IR cells in the Vi/Vc or Vc in each group was compared respectively (Fig. 3I and Fig. 4C).

On day 3 (Fig. 3I), the number of Fos-IR cells was significantly larger in M1 CFA/Mass veh and M1 CFA/Mass cap rats compared to M1 veh/Mass cap rats in the ipsilateral Vi/Vc. The number of Fos-IR cells was significantly larger in M1 CFA/Mass

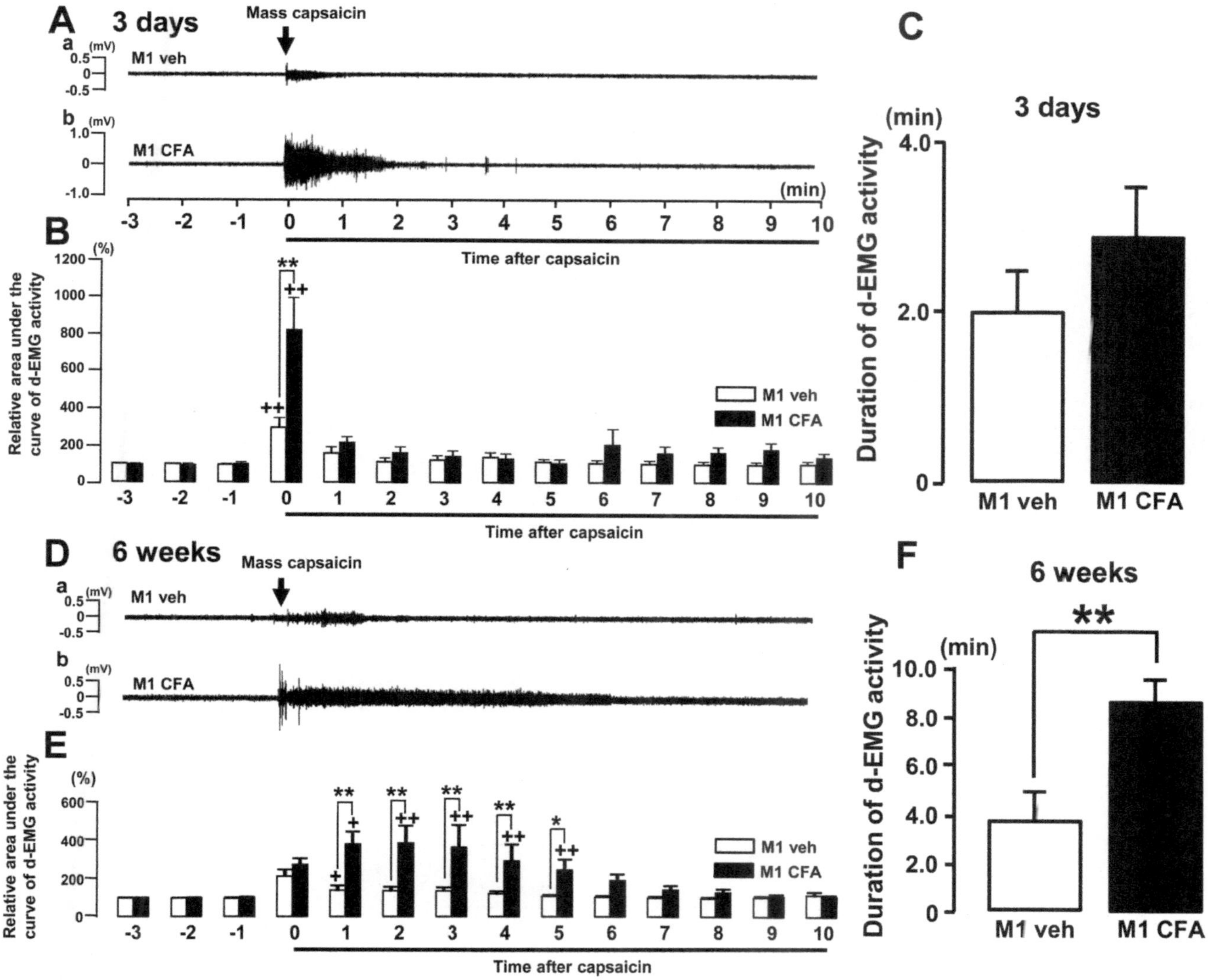

Figure 2. The d-EMG activities after tooth pulp or periapical inflammation. The capsaicin was applied into the Mass in the rats with CFA or vehicle application to the tooth pulp on day 3 and week 6. A: The d-EMG activity following capsaicin application into the Mass in the rats with pulpal-vehicle or pulpal-CFA application on day 3. B: Relative d-EMG activity following capsaicin application into the Mass in the rats with pulpal-vehicle or pulpal-CFA application. C: Mean duration of d-EMG activity following capsaicin application into the Mass in the rats with pulpal-vehicle or pulpal-CFA application. D: The d-EMG activity following capsaicin application into the Mass in the rats with pulpal-vehicle or pulpal-CFA application on week 6. E: Relative d-EMG activity following capsaicin application into the Mass in the rats with pulpal-vehicle or pulpal-CFA application. F: Mean duration of d-EMG activity following capsaicin application into the Mass in the rats with pulpal-vehicle or pulpal-CFA application. +: vs. −1 min, *: veh vs. CFA, +, *: $p<0.05$, ++, **: $p<0.01$.

capsaicin rats compared to M1 veh/Mass veh rats in the contralateral Vi/Vc and Vc.

Furthermore, the numbers of pERK-IR cells was significantly larger in M1 veh/Mass cap and M1 CFA/Mass cap rats compared to M1 veh/Mass veh rats and M1 CFA/Mass veh in the ipsilateral Vi/Vc or Vc, respectively. In the contralateral side to injections, the number of pERK-IR cells was significantly larger in M1 veh/Mass cap compared to M1 CFA/Mass veh in the Vi/Vc.

On week 6 (Fig. 4C), the number of Fos-IR cells was significantly larger in M1 CFA/Mass veh or M1 CFA/Mass cap rats compared to M1 veh/Mass cap rats in the ipsilateral Vi/Vc, respectively. The number of pERK-IR cells was also significantly larger in M1 CFA/Mass cap rats compared to M1 veh/Mass veh, M1 veh/Mass cap or M1 CFA/Mass veh rats in the ipsilateral Vi/Vc. Furthermore, the number of pERK-IR cells was significantly larger in M1 veh/Mass cap or M1 CFA/Mass cap rats compared to M1 CFA/Mass veh rats in the ipsilateral Vc. In the contralateral side to M1 injections, the number of pERK-IR cells was significantly larger in M1 CFA/Mass cap compared to M1 CFA/Mass veh in the Vi/Vc.

4. Comparison of pERK-IR and Fos-IR cells on day 3 and week 6

To examine the difference for the expression of pERK-IR and Fos-IR cells on day 3 and week 6, the ERK phosphorylation and Fos expression were studied in Vi/Vc and Vc neurons following unilateral saline or capsaicin application into the Mass.

In the rats with saline application into the Mass, the number of Fos-IR cells was significantly larger in M1 veh/Mass veh rats in the ipsilateral Vi/Vc or in M1 CFA/Mass veh rats in the ipsi- and

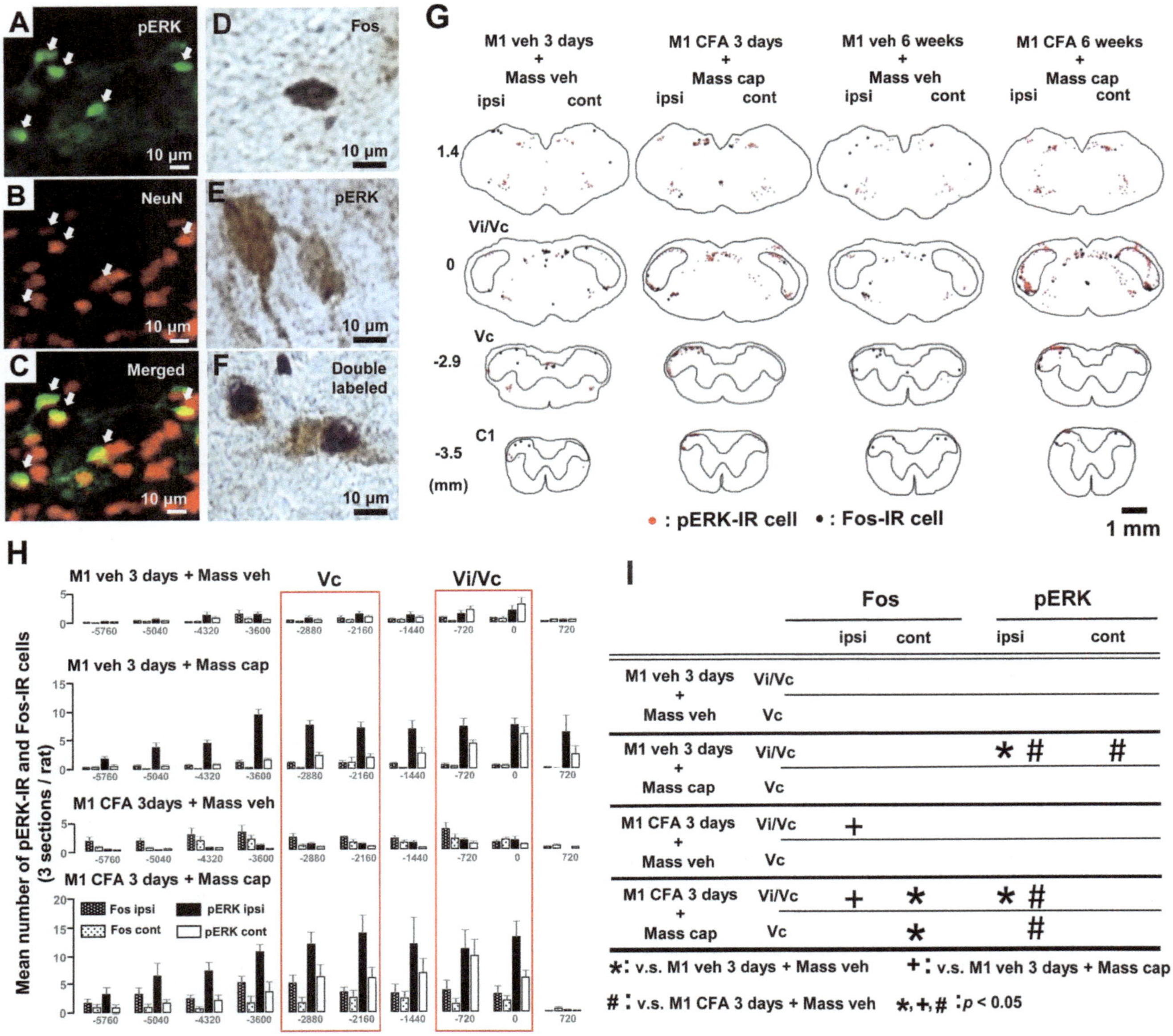

Figure 3. Photomicrographs and Rostral-caudal distribution for pERK-IR cells and Fos-IR cells after tooth pulp inflammation in Vi/Vc and Vc. A: pERK-IR cells. B: NeuN-IR cells. C: A merged with B. D: Fos-IR cell stained with nickel-conjugated DAB. E: pERK-IR cell stained with DAB. F: double stained cells (black: Fos-IR, brown: pERK-IR). G: Neurolucida drawings of pERK-IR (red and triangle dots) and Fos-IR cells (black and round dots) in the Vi/Vc and Vc. H: Rostral-caudal distribution of pERK-IR and Fos-IR cells in the Vi/Vc and Vc. I: *, + and # signs indicate significant expression of pERK-IR or Fos-IR cells compared to each region in M1 veh/Mass veh, M1 veh/Mass cap and M1 CFA/Mass veh on day 3, respectively. Arrows in A indicate pERK-IR cells, those in B indicate NeuN-IR cells and those in C are pERK-IR cells merged with NeuN-IR cells. The negative numbers on the left in G indicate the distance caudal to the obex (0 mm). cap: capsaicin, veh: vehicle, ipsi: ipsilateral, cont: contralateral.

contralateral Vi/Vc and ipsilateral Vc on week 6 compared to those in M1 veh/Mass veh rats on day 3 ($p<0.05$). The number of pERK-IR cells was also significantly larger in M1 CFA/Mass veh rats on week 6 compared to M1 veh/Mass veh on day 3, M1 veh/Mass veh on week 6 or M1 CFA/Mass veh rats on day 3 in the ipsilateral Vi/Vc ($p<0.05$).

In the rats with capsaicin application into the Mass, the number of Fos-IR cells was significantly larger in M1 CFA/Mass cap rats on week 6 compared to M1 veh/Mass cap rats on day 3 or M1 veh/Mass cap rats on week 6 in the ipsilateral Vi/Vc ($p<0.05$).

5. The effect of PD98059 in the Vi/Vc and Vc neurons

We further examined the effect of MEK1 inhibitor PD98059-pretreatment for the Mass hypersensitivity in the rats with M1 pulpitis or periapical periodontitis. We observed significant decrease in the d-EMG activity within 1 minute after capsaicin application into the Mass in the PD98059 i.t.-pretreated rats compared with saline i.t.-pretreated rats on day 3 after M1 CFA application ($p<0.01$, Fig. 5A, B).

On the other hand, the durations of d-EMG activities after capsaicin application were about 2 minutes, and no significant difference was observed between PD98059- or saline-pretreated rats on day 3 after M1 CFA application (Fig. 5C).

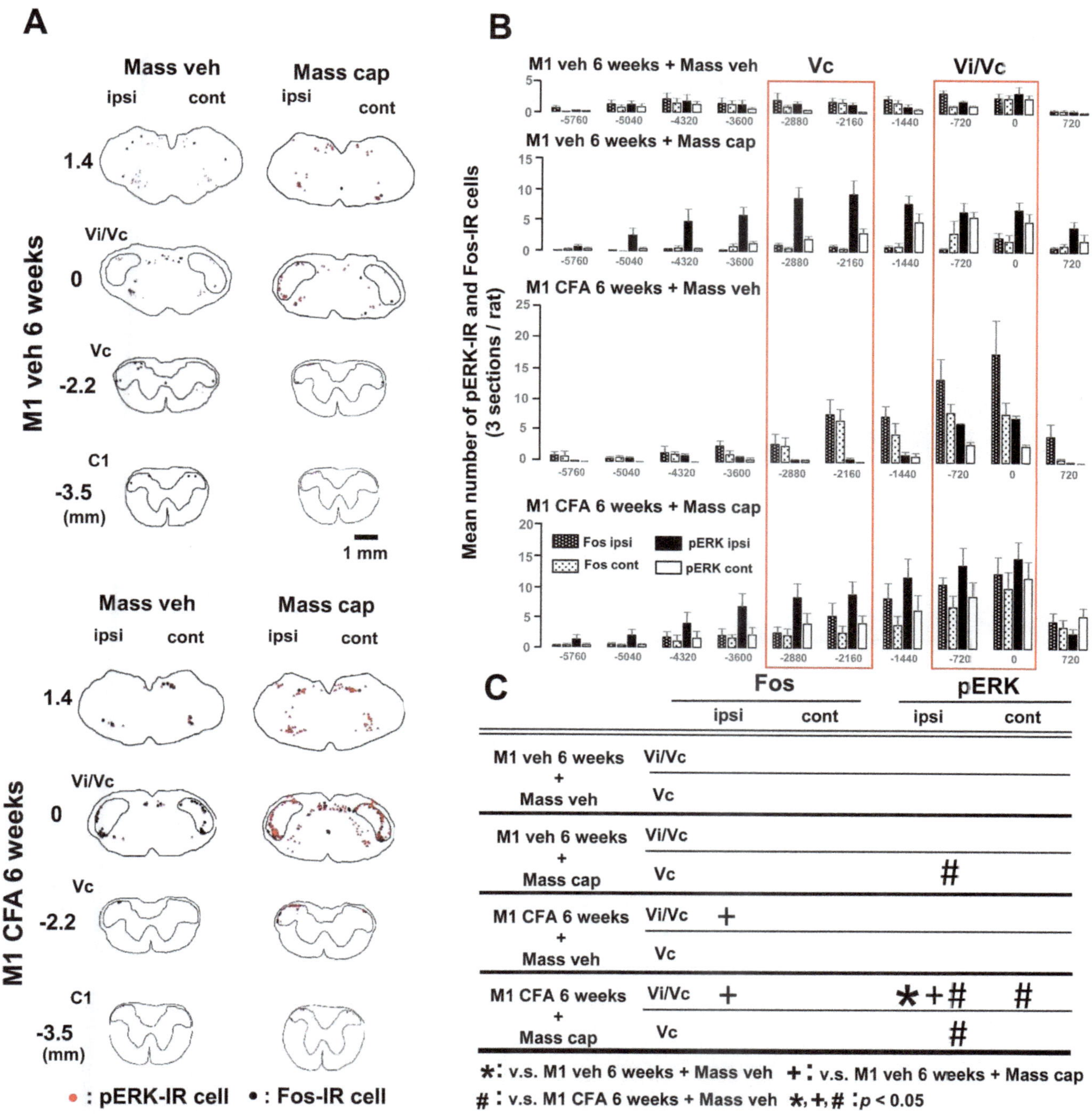

Figure 4. Rostral-caudal distribution for pERK-IR cells and Fos-IR cells after periapical inflammation in Vi/Vc and Vc. The capsaicin was applied into the Mass in the rats with CFA or vehicle application to the tooth pulp on week 6. A and B: Neurolucida drawings (A) and Rostral-caudal distribution (B) of pERK-IR and Fos-IR cells in the Vi/Vc and Vc. C: *, + and # signs indicate significant expression of pERK-IR or Fos-IR cells compared to each region in M1 veh/Mass veh, M1 veh/Mass cap and M1 CFA/Mass veh on day 3, respectively.

We observed significant attenuation in the d-EMG activity with in 2 minute after capsaicin application into the Mass in the PD98059 i.t.-pretreated rats compared with saline i.t.-pretreated rats on week 6 after M1 CFA application ($p<0.01$, Fig. 5D, E).

Furthermore, the mean duration of d-EMG activities after capsaicin application was significantly decreased in the PD98059-pretreated rats compared with saline-pretreated rats on 6 week after M1 CFA application ($p<0.01$, Fig. 5F).

To examine the effect of PD98059 on ERK phosphorylation caused by M1 pulpitis or periapical periodontitis, the change in the number of ERK-IR cells following pretreatment with PD98059 was studied in Vi/Vc and Vc following capsaicin application into the Mass (Fig. 6A and B).

On day 3 and week 6, the number of pERK-IR cells after Mass-capsaicin application was significantly decreased following PD98059 i.t. administration compared to saline i.t. administration in the ipsilateral Vi/Vc and Vc of the M1 CFA rats. Furthermore, the number of Fos-IR cells was not altered after the pretreatment of PD98059 or saline on day 3 or week 6 in the rats with M1 CFA/Mass cap (Fig. 6C).

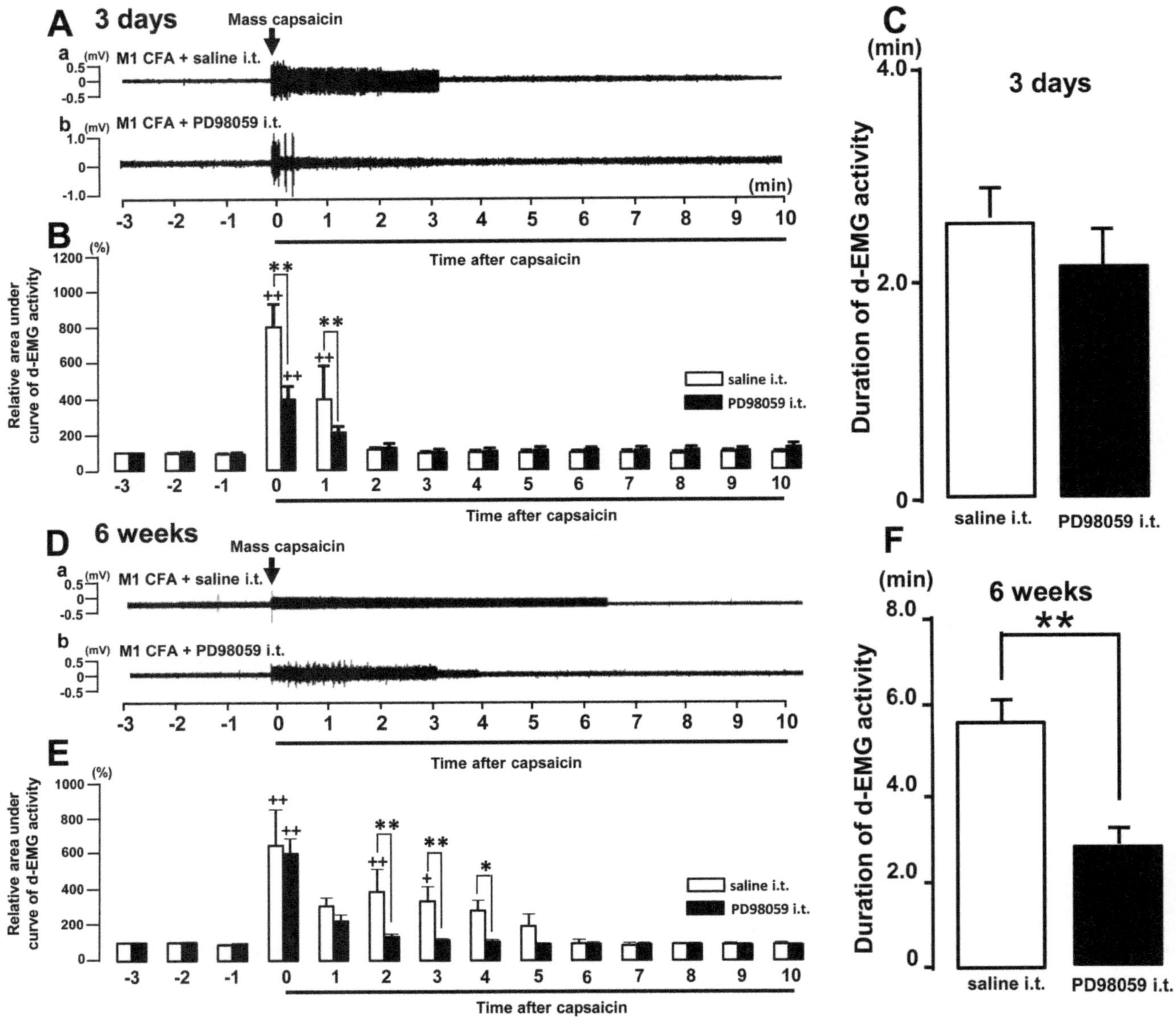

Figure 5. The effect of PD98059 on the d-EMG activities after tooth pulp or periapical inflammation. The capsaicin was applied into the Mass after pretreatment of PD98059 in the rats with M1 CFA application on day 3 and week 6. A: The d-EMG activity following capsaicin application into the Mass after pretreatment of PD98059 or saline in the rats with M1 CFA application on day 3. B: Relative d-EMG activity following capsaicin application into the Mass after pretreatment with PD98059 or saline in the rats with M1 CFA application. C: Mean duration of d-EMG activity following capsaicin application into the Mass after pretreatment with PD98059 or saline in the rats with M1 CFA application. D: The d-EMG activity following capsaicin application into the Mass after pretreatment of PD98059 or saline in the rats with M1 CFA application on week 6. E: Relative d-EMG activity following capsaicin application into the Mass after pretreatment with PD98059 or saline in the rats with M1 CFA application. C: Mean duration of d-EMG activity following capsaicin application into the Mass after pretreatment of PD98059 or saline in the rats with M1 CFA application. +: vs. −1 min, *: saline i.t. vs. PD98059 i.t., +,*: $p<0.05$., ++, **: $p<0.01$.

Discussion

Periapical inflammation frequently causes referred pain in the orofacial cutaneous tissue and/or muscle as well as tooth pulp [22]. It is well known that inflammation within the tooth pulp often extends into the periapical tissues after pulpal inflammation, resulting in pulpal necrosis and periapical inflammation. At the early stage of periapical inflammation, severe persistent pain occurs in the apex region of the tooth [23]. Eventually, periapical pain could change its' quality from an acute to a chronic state. Chronic periapical pain is dull and persistent, lasts for a long period, and also causes referred pain in the orofacial skin and/or muscles. The orofacial referred pain originated from the periapical inflammation is difficult to diagnose and treat [3]. Despite increasing necessity of the clarification of the pathogenesis for the odontogenic referred pain in the orofacial region, it is still unclear on the mechanisms underlying extraterritorial orofacial persistent pain associated with periapical inflammation. In the present study, therefore, we examined the excitability of the Vi/Vc and Vc neurons in a rat model of experimental pulpitis/periodontitis and its' involvement in the enhancement of d-EMG activity.

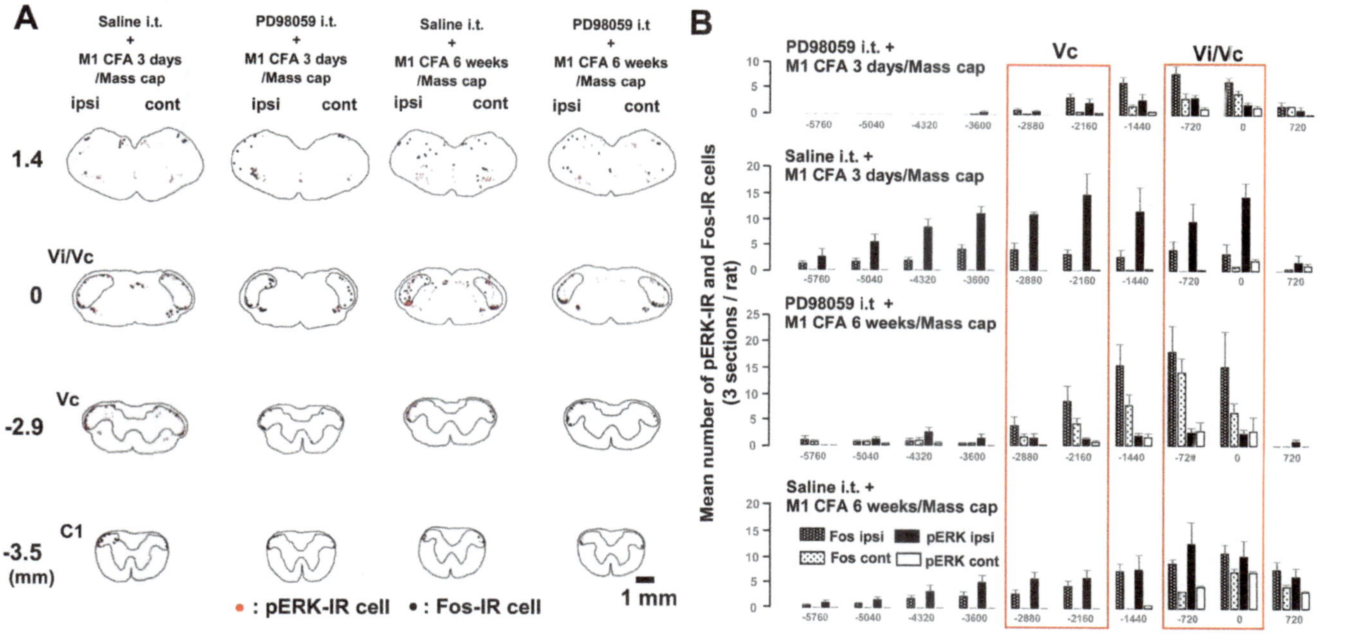

C

		3 days				6 weeks			
		Fos		pERK		Fos		pERK	
		ipsi	cont	ipsi	cont	ipsi	cont	ipsi	cont
PD98059 i.t. + M1 CFA/Mass cap	Vi/Vc			*				*	
	Vc			*				*	

*: v.s. Saline i.t. + M1 CFA/Mass cap *: $p < 0.05$

Figure 6. The effect of PD98059 on ERK phosphorylation in Vi/Vc and Vc neurons after tooth pulp or periapical inflammation. The capsaicin was applied into the Mass after PD98059 i.t. administration in the rats with M1 CFA on day 3 or week 6. A and B: Neurolucida drawings (A) and Rostral-caudal distribution (B) of pERK-IR and Fos-IR cells in the Vi/Vc and Vc. C: * indicates significant decrease in the number of pERK-IR or Fos-IR cells. Each region in each model was compared with M1 CFA/Mass cap rats with saline i.t. on day 3 or week 6, respectively.

1. Rat model of periapical inflammation

It is well known that periapical bone loss is observed during development of the periapical inflammation, suggesting that the periapical bone loss could be one of the reliable indicators for the periapical inflammation [24]. Thus, we analyzed the time-course change in the bone loss using X-ray micro-CT imaging to quantify the periapical inflammation. The advantage of this technique is that the size of bone loss can be measured in same rats throughout the experimental period. Periapical bone loss was detected at 3 weeks after pulpal application of CFA, and the largest bone loss was observed at 6 weeks after CFA application to the pulp, indicating that chronic phase characterized by lesion stabilization was commenced from 6 weeks after CFA application. The time-course of bone loss we observed in this study is similar to that of previous study [24], suggesting that this model can be used as a reliable animal model with experimental periodontitis following long lasting pulpal inflammation.

2. Changes in the Vi/Vc and Vc neuronal activities following pulpal or periapical inflammation

The d-EMG activity elicited by noxious stimulation is known as a good indicator of the noxious responses in the trigeminal system [25]. We observed significant increase in the d-EMG activity after capsaicin application into the Mass on day 3 and week 6 after pulpal-CFA or pulpal-vehicle application. Furthermore, the d-EMG activity elicited by Mass-capsaicin application was significantly higher in M1 CFA-applied rats compared with M1-vehicle applied rats. The number of Fos-IR cells in the Vi/Vc was significantly larger in M1 CFA applied rats compared with M1 vehicle-applied rats on day 3 and week 6. On the other hand, ERK phosphorylation in the Vi/Vc and/or Vc neurons significantly increased in Mass-capsaicin applied rats compared with Mass-vehicle applied rats both in pulpal CFA- or vehicle applied rats. These indicate that noxious stimulus to the Mass induces the enhancement of noxious responses in the orofacial region following pulpal or periapical inflammation. It is strongly suggested that the increase in d-EMG activities and pERK expression in Vi/Vc and Vc neurons are the result of enhancement of Vi/Vc and/or Vc neuronal activities following pulpal or periapical inflammation. Taken together, the EMG activities and pERK expression were significantly enhanced after capsaicin application into the Mass on day 3 and week 6 after pulpal CFA application, suggesting that pathogenesis of pulpal or periapical inflammation might induce pain hypersensitivity in remote organs or tissues in the orofacial region.

We also observed that the duration of EMG activity was significantly longer at 6 weeks after pulpal CFA application compared with that of pulpal vehicle application. The enhancement of EMG activity and the increased duration were significantly reversed following i.t. administration of PD98059. These results indicate that periapical inflammation may induce and maintain pain hypersensitivity in the remote organs or tissues in orofacial region, whereas pulpal inflammation may only induce pain hypersensitivity. Furthermore, the ERK phosphorylation in Vi/Vc and Vc neurons has a pivotal role in the maintenance and/ or modulation of pain processing in remote regions after tooth pulp or periapical inflammation.

3. Involvement of the Vi/Vc and Vc neurons in Mass hypersensitivity

Fos protein expression in SDH neurons following noxious stimulation of the peripheral structures is known to be caused 1–2 hours and lasted 24 hours after noxious stimulation [26], and therefore Fos protein expression in SDH neurons is thought to be a good marker of the excitation of nociceptive neurons [27]. The ventral portion of the Vi/Vc is known to have a various functions in trigeminal nociception [28]. Many Vi/Vc neurons are known to express Fos-IR products following CFA application into the Mass or noxious stimulation of the cornea [29,30]. Many of them were also observed on both sides of the Vi/Vc following unilateral noxious stimulation.

It has been reported that the number of pERK-IR cells increases unilaterally in the Vc following increase in noxious stimulus intensity [31]. In the trigeminal system, ERK can be phosphorylated in a large number of dorsal horn neurons in the Vc and C1-C2 within 5 min after noxious stimulation to various orofacial regions; these pERK-IR neurons are somatotopically organized in Vc and C1-C2, and the number of pERK-IR neurons increases following increases in the noxious stimulus intensity [12,20], indicating that ERK phosphorylation in Vc and C1-C2 neurons is a reliable marker of excitable neurons following orofacial noxious stimulation.

We observed that pERK expression was significantly enhanced after capsaicin application into the Mass both in M1 CFA- and vehicle-applied rats compared with Mass-vehicle applied rats in both Vi/Vc and Vc on day 3 and week 6. Furthermore, on day 3 after pulpal application, we observed a large number of Fos-IR cells in the bilateral Vi/Vc in pulpal CFA-applied rats. Meanwhile, on week 6 after pulpal-CFA application, we observed a large number of Fos-IR cells just in the ipsilateral Vi/Vc in pulpal CFA-applied rats, and the number of them was also significantly larger in CFA-applied rats compared with vehicle-applied rats. These findings suggest that nociceptive neurons in the Vi/Vc and Vc may have important roles for orofacial pain hypersensitivity associated with tooth pulp inflammation and periapical inflammation.

Furthermore, we could not observe significant change in the number of Fos-IR cells in these two areas between Mass-capsaicin and vehicle applied rats, suggesting that Fos expression may be mainly due to the CFA application to the tooth pulp but not Mass-capsaicin application.

Conclusions

The present findings revealed that the Vi/Vc and Vc neurons was involved in the enhancement of Mass nociception under acute pulpal-inflamed state as well as chronic periapical inflammation, suggesting that nociceptive neurons in these areas are involved in pain hypersensitivity for orofacial muscle associated with acute pulpal and chronic periapical inflammation.

Author Contributions

Conceived and designed the experiments: KS. Performed the experiments: KS KM NN SM KO KH KD TW HK YT. Analyzed the data: KS KM NN SM KO YN YT. Contributed reagents/materials/analysis tools: BO. Wrote the paper: KS KI. Contributed to discussion and reviewed/edited the manuscript: MS KI BO.

References

1. Ertekin C, Secil Y, Yuceyar N, Aydogdu I (2004) Oropharyngeal dysphagia in polymyositis/dermatomyositis. Clin Neurol Neurosurg 107: 32–37.
2. Grushka M, Sessle BJ (1984) Applicability of the McGill Pain Questionnaire to the differentiation of 'toothache' pain. Pain 19: 49–57.
3. Bender IB (2000) Pulpal pain diagnosis–a review. J Endod 26: 175–179.
4. Wright EF (2008) Pulpalgia contributing to temporomandibular disorder-like pain: a literature review and case report. J Am Dent Assoc 139: 436–440.
5. Iwata K, Takahashi O, Tsuboi Y, Ochiai H, Hibiya J, et al. (1998) Fos protein induction in the medullary dorsal horn and first segment of the spinal cord by tooth-pulp stimulation in cats. Pain 75: 27–36.
6. Sessle BJ (1987) The neurobiology of facial and dental pain: present knowledge, future directions. J Dent Res 66: 962–981.
7. Sessle BJ, Hu JW, Amano N, Zhong G (1986) Convergence of cutaneous, tooth pulp, visceral, neck and muscle afferents onto nociceptive and non-nociceptive neurones in trigeminal subnucleus caudalis (medullary dorsal horn) and its implications for referred pain. Pain 27: 219–235.
8. Shimizu K, Asano M, Kitagawa J, Ogiso B, Ren K, et al. (2006) Phosphorylation of Extracellular Signal-Regulated Kinase in medullary and upper cervical cord neurons following noxious tooth pulp stimulation. Brain Res 1072: 99–109.
9. Wang H, Wei F, Dubner R, Ren K (2006) Selective distribution and function of primary afferent nociceptive inputs from deep muscle tissue to the brainstem trigeminal transition zone. J Comp Neurol 498: 390–402.
10. Amano N, Hu JW, Sessle BJ (1986) Responses of neurons in feline trigeminal subnucleus caudalis (medullary dorsal horn) to cutaneous, intraoral, and muscle afferent stimuli. J Neurophysiol 55: 227–243.
11. Shoda E, Kitagawa J, Suzuki I, Nitta-Kubota I, Miyamoto M, et al. (2009) Increased phosphorylation of extracellular signal-regulated kinase in trigeminal nociceptive neurons following propofol administration in rats. J Pain 10: 573–585.
12. Noma N, Tsuboi Y, Kondo M, Matsumoto M, Sessle BJ, et al. (2008) Organization of pERK-immunoreactive cells in trigeminal spinal nucleus caudalis and upper cervical cord following capsaicin injection into oral and craniofacial regions in rats. J Comp Neurol 507: 1428–1440.
13. Dai Y, Iwata K, Fukuoka T, Kondo E, Tokunaga A, et al. (2002) Phosphorylation of extracellular signal-regulated kinase in primary afferent neurons by noxious stimuli and its involvement in peripheral sensitization. J Neurosci 22: 7737–7745.
14. Harris JA (1998) Using c-fos as a neural marker of pain. Brain Res Bull 45: 1–8.
15. Hasegawa M, Kondo M, Suzuki I, Shimizu N, Sessle BJ, et al. (2012) ERK is involved in tooth-pressure-induced Fos expression in Vc neurons. J Dent Res 91: 1141–1146.
16. Zimmermann M (1983) Ethical guidelines for investigations of experimental pain in conscious animals. Pain 16: 109–110.
17. Terayama R, Omura S, Fujisawa N, Yamaai T, Ichikawa H, et al. (2008) Activation of microglia and p38 mitogen-activated protein kinase in the dorsal column nucleus contributes to tactile allodynia following peripheral nerve injury. Neuroscience 153: 1245–1255.
18. Gasparini F, Lingenhohl K, Stoehr N, Flor PJ, Heinrich M, et al. (1999) 2-Methyl-6-(phenylethynyl)-pyridine (MPEP), a potent, selective and systemically active mGlu5 receptor antagonist. Neuropharmacology 38: 1493–1503.
19. Honda K, Kitagawa J, Sessle BJ, Kondo M, Tsuboi Y, et al. (2008) Mechanisms involved in an increment of multimodal excitability of medullary and upper cervical dorsal horn neurons following cutaneous capsaicin treatment. Mol Pain 4: 59.
20. Honda K, Noma N, Shinoda M, Miyamoto M, Katagiri A, et al. (2011) Involvement of peripheral ionotropic glutamate receptors in orofacial thermal hyperalgesia in rats. Mol Pain 7: 75.
21. Kobayashi A, Shinoda M, Sessle BJ, Honda K, Imamura Y, et al. (2011) Mechanisms involved in extraterritorial facial pain following cervical spinal nerve injury in rats. Mol Pain 7: 12.
22. Sessle BJ (1978) Oral-facial pain: old puzzles, new postulates. Int Dent J 28: 28–42.
23. Morse DR (1977) Immunologic aspects of pulpal-periapical diseases. A review. Oral Surg Oral Med Oral Pathol 43: 436–451.
24. Stashenko P, Yu SM, Wang CY (1992) Kinetics of immune cell and bone resorptive responses to endodontic infections. J Endod 18: 422–426.

25. Sunakawa M, Chiang CY, Sessle BJ, Hu JW (1999) Jaw electromyographic activity induced by the application of algesic chemicals to the rat tooth pulp. Pain 80: 493–501.
26. Hunt SP, Pini A, Evan G (1987) Induction of c-fos-like protein in spinal cord neurons following sensory stimulation. Nature 328: 632–634.
27. Williams S, Evan GI, Hunt SP (1990) Changing patterns of c-fos induction in spinal neurons following thermal cutaneous stimulation in the rat. Neuroscience 36: 73–81.
28. Ren K, Dubner R (2011) The role of trigeminal interpolaris-caudalis transition zone in persistent orofacial pain. Int Rev Neurobiol 97: 207–225.
29. Bereiter DA, Hathaway CB, Benetti AP (1994) Caudal portions of the spinal trigeminal complex are necessary for autonomic responses and display Fos-like immunoreactivity after corneal stimulation in the cat. Brain Res 657: 73–82.
30. Imbe H, Dubner R, Ren K (1999) Masseteric inflammation-induced Fos protein expression in the trigeminal interpolaris/caudalis transition zone: contribution of somatosensory-vagal-adrenal integration. Brain Res 845: 165–175.
31. Ji RR, Baba H, Brenner GJ, Woolf CJ (1999) Nociceptive-specific activation of ERK in spinal neurons contributes to pain hypersensitivity. Nat Neurosci 2: 1114–1119.

22

Validation of Self-Reported Information on Dental Caries in a Birth Cohort at 18 Years of Age

Alexandre Emidio Ribeiro Silva[1]*, Ana Maria Baptista Menezes[1], Maria Cecília Formoso Assunção[1], Helen Gonçalves[1], Flávio Fernando Demarco[1], Fabiana Vargas-Ferreira[1], Marco Aurélio Peres[2]

1 Postgraduate Programme in Epidemiology, Federal University of Pelotas, Pelotas, Rio Grande do Sul, Brazil, **2** Australian Research Centre for Population Oral Health, School of Dentistry, University of Adelaide, Adelaide, Austrália

Abstract

Objective: Estimate the prevalence of dental caries based on clinical examinations and self-reports and compare differences in the prevalence and effect measures between the two methods among 18-year-olds belonging to a 1993 birth cohort in the city of Pelotas, Brazil.

Method: Data on self-reported caries, socio-demographic aspects and oral health behaviour were collected using a questionnaire administered to adolescents aged 18 years (n = 4041). Clinical caries was evaluated (n = 1014) by a dentist who had undergone training and calibration exercises. Prevalence rates of clinical and self-reported caries, sensitivity, specificity, positive and negative predictive values, absolute and relative bias, and inflation factors were calculated. Prevalence ratios of dental caries were estimated for each risk factor.

Results: The prevalence of clinical and self-reported caries (DMFT>1) was 66.5% (95%CI: 63.6%–69.3%) and 60.3% (95%CI: 58.8%–61.8%), respectively. Self-reports underestimated the prevalence of dental caries by 9.3% in comparison to clinical evaluations. The analysis of the validity of self-reports regarding the DMFT index indicated high sensitivity (81.8%; 95%CI: 78.7%–84.7%) and specificity (78.1%; 95%CI: 73.3%–82.4%) in relation to the gold standard (clinical evaluation). Both the clinical and self-reported evaluations were associated with gender, schooling and self-rated oral health. Clinical dental caries was associated with visits to the dentist in the previous year. Self-reported dental caries was associated with daily tooth brushing frequency.

Conclusions: Based on the present findings, self-reported information on dental caries using the DMFT index requires further studies prior to its use in the analysis of risk factors, but is valid for population-based health surveys with the aim of planning and monitoring oral health actions directed at adolescents.

Editor: Peter M. Milgrom, University of Washington, United States of America

Funding: The cohort study was funded by Wellcome Trust. The initial phases of the cohort were funded by the European Union and the Brazilian agencies National Programme for Centres of Excellence (PRONEX), National Research Council (CNPq) and the Ministry of Health. The providers of funding played no role in the study design, data collection and analysis, decision to publish or preparation of the manuscript.

Competing Interests: The authors have declared that no competing interests exist.

* Email: emidio3@ig.com.br

Introduction

Self-reported health status is considered a valid, acceptable method for the assessment of the prevalence of diseases in the general population, such as hypertension and diabetes [1], as well as risk factors, such as poor diet and lack of physical activity [2]. In the field of dentistry, self-reported information is an economically feasible option for measuring oral health conditions in population-based multidisciplinary surveys and diminishes the need for time-consuming clinical exams [3]. Moreover, self-reports have the potential to be a useful method for monitoring oral health conditions and trends over time, which is important to the planning and evaluation of public health policies. For instance, the Centers for Disease Control and Prevention in the United States of America use health information acquired from telephone surveys [4].

Health inquiries involving self-reported information indicate that characteristics related to socio-demographic aspects [5] and past disease experience [6] have a direct influence on the knowledge of individuals regarding their health, producing greater or lesser agreement between self-reports and clinically determined data. In the field of oral health, studies indicate an underestimation of periodontal disease in self-reported information. [2,7,8]. A systematic review on this issue demonstrates that the use of self-reported data is inadequate for information on gingivitis, but other self-reported measures of periodontal disease have proven to be valid [1], such as the occurrence of periodontal pockets. However, standardisation is required regarding the different methods used for the acquisition of self-reported information.

The literature demonstrates greater validity in self-reported information related to the use of dentures and the number of teeth in the oral cavity [2,4,5,9–11]. However, some studies indicate a slight underestimation [2] or overestimation [2,7] regarding the number of teeth. For measures related to tooth decay, an underestimate of the number of teeth with carious tissue has been found in self-reports [2] and reports of missing teeth should be used with the proper corrections [10]. However, with regard to the presence/absence of dental caries, studies involving adults indicate a lack of agreement with clinical measures, mainly because individuals are often unable to recognise caries [2,6].

Few studies have been conducted on the validity of self-reported information regarding dental caries in 18-year-olds in countries of low to middle income. Therefore, the aims of the present study were to estimate the prevalence of dental caries based on clinical examinations and self-reports and compare differences in the prevalence and effect measures between the two methods among 18-year-olds belonging to a 1993 birth cohort in the city of Pelotas, Brazil.

Materials and Methods

Description of 1993 Pelotas birth cohort

This was the second birth cohort in the city of Pelotas (southern Brazil) and was separated from the first cohort study by 11 years. The aim was to allow the comparison of mother/child characteristics of the population and changes in the main health indicators as well as to evaluate the influence of factors related to birth and early childhood on health throughout the life cycle. Moreover, it is one of the few population-based studies to investigate oral health.

All live births recorded at hospitals in the city of Pelotas in 1993 from mothers residing in urban areas were included in this cohort. Among the 5265 women who had children in the period, 5249 (99.7%) agreed to participate in the study. Subsamples were revisited when the members of the cohort were 1, 3, and 6 months of age as well as 1, 3, 6, and 9 years of age. In 2004, when the members were 11 years of age, the entire cohort was evaluated; the same occurred in 2008 (15 years of age) and 2011 (18 years of age). The last visit (18 years of age) occurred between September 2011 and April 2012 and all members of the cohort were asked to appear at the Federal University of Pelotas for a clinical examination and the administration of questionnaires. Descriptions of the methods employed during past visits to the members of the cohort are found in previous studies [12,13].

Oral health subsamples of 1993 Pelotas birth cohort

The oral health follow up evaluations were performed with subsamples at six, 12 and 18 years. The subsample at six years was obtained from the follow up of the cohort performed when the children were one year of age, in which all underweight children were included. The oral health subsample at six years involved 359 members of the cohort, including 28.7% of underweight children. This information was weighted to represent the true proportion of live births of underweight children. Another home follow up was performed at 12 years, when 339 members of those visited at six years were located. The description of the oral health follow-up methods at six and 12 years is found in a previous publication [14].

The third follow up occurred at 18 years in a clinical setting during morning and afternoon shifts from Monday to Saturday from September 2011 to March 2012. The oral health subsample at 18 years was formed by adolescents who appeared for evaluations during the four predefined appointments (two in the morning and two in the afternoon) throughout the week, which were scheduled in a randomised fashion. Besides the adolescents who appeared for the predefined appointments, attempts were made to examine all 359 member members of the cohort that had been evaluated in the previous oral health subsamples. The oral health subsample of the final follow up evaluation consisted of 1014 adolescents, 307 of whom had been part of the subsample at six years of age and 301 of whom had been part of the subsample at 12 years of age.

Oral health exams at 18 years of age

At the 2012 follow up, the oral health exam was performed by a single examiner who had undergone training and calibration exercises using the diagnostic criteria of the World Health Organization [15]. Two calibration exercises were conducted (August and December 2011) with the participation of the researcher of the study and three dentists. The aim of the two exercises was to maintain the reproducibility of the exams, as the fieldwork occurred over approximately eight months. Weighted Kappa coefficients were calculated. The lowest values during the two calibration exercises were 0.78 and 0.83 for intra-examiner and intra-examiner agreement, respectively.

Outcome – Dental Caries

1. **Clinical dental caries.** A World Health Organization (WHO) periodontal probe and mouth mirror were used for the clinical detection of dental caries based on the WHO criteria [15]. The distal, vestibular, mesial, and lingual/palatine surfaces of the anterior teeth were examined. These same surfaces plus the occlusal surface were examined on the posterior teeth. The overall decayed, missing, and filled teeth (DMFT) index and each of its components were calculated for each participant. The prevalence of dental caries was determined based on the proportion of adolescents with DMFT $\geq$1.
2. **Self-reported dental caries.** For the self-reported data on dental caries, a 24-item questionnaire (Figure 1) was administered by trained interviewers to 4041 adolescents of the overall cohort. This questionnaire was first tested on individuals with a similar age to those in the cohort. The aim of obtaining self-reported information was to identify the individuals' knowledge regarding the number of decayed, missing and filled teeth. Based on the findings, the DMFT index was calculated for each participant. As with the clinical exam, the prevalence of dental caries was determined based on the proportion of adolescents with DMFT $\geq$1.

Exploratory variables

A questionnaire addressing socioeconomic and demographic variables, visits to the dentist, tooth brushing habits, and self-rated oral health was administered to all adolescents in the cohort by the same interviewers who administered the questionnaire on self-reported dental caries. The demographic and socioeconomic variables analysed were gender, adolescent's schooling in number of completed years of study (categorised as $\leq$4, 5 to 8, 9 to 11, and $\geq$12), and household income in the previous month (sum of the monthly income of all members of the household in Brazilian currency [Real – R$], converted to a figure based on the minimum Brazilian wage and categorised in tertiles).

Variables related to oral health (visits to the dentist, daily tooth brushing frequency, and self-rated oral health) were obtained from the following questions: 1) Have you visited the dentist since <month> of last year (yes or no); 2) How many times a day do you brush your teeth? (categorised as <2 times a day and $\geq$2 times

THE FOLLOWING QUESTIONS ARE ABOUT THE NUMBER OF TEETH YOU HAVE IN THE UPPER PART AND LOWER PART OF YOUR MOUTH.

1. **We have a maximum of 16 natural teeth in the upper part of the mouth, counting both wisdom teeth. How many natural teeth do you have in the upper part of your mouth?**
16 15 14 13 12 11 10 9 8 7 6 5 4 3 2 1 0

IF LESS THAN 16 TEETH:
2. **Were any teeth pulled because of cavities?**
(0) No → *GO TO QUESTION 4* (1) Yes
IF YES: 3. **How many teeth in the upper part of your mouth were pulled because of cavities?** ___ ___ teeth [00=IGN]

4. **Do you have any natural tooth with an untreated cavity or hole in the upper part of your mouth?**
(0) No → *GO TO QUESTION 6* (1) Yes
IF YES: 5. **How many natural teeth with an untreated cavity or hole in the upper part of your mouth do you have?** ___ ___ teeth [00=IGN]

6. **Do you have any natural tooth with a restoration or filling in the upper part of your mouth?**
(0) No → *GO TO QUESTION 8* (1) Yes
IF YES: 7. **How many natural teeth with a restoration or filling in the upper part of your mouth do you have?** ___ ___ teeth [00=IGN]

8. **Do you have bridges or partial denture in the upper part of your mouth?**
(0) No → *GO TO QUESTION 10* (1) Yes
IF YES: 9. **How many natural teeth have been replaced with a bridge or partial denture in the upper part of your mouth?** ___ ___ teeth [00=IGN]

10. **Do you have any fixed bridge in the upper part of your mouth?**
(0) No → *GO TO QUESTION 12* (1) Yes
IF YES: 11. **How many natural teeth have been replaced with a fixed bridge in the upper part of your mouth?**
___ ___ teeth. [00=IGN]

NOW WE ARE GOING TO TALK ABOUT THE LOWER PART OF YOUR MOUTH

12. **We have a maximum of 16 natural teeth in the lower part of the mouth, counting both wisdom teeth. How many natural teeth do you have in the lower part of your mouth?**
16 15 14 13 12 11 10 9 8 7 6 5 4 3 2 1 0

IF LESS THAN 16 TEETH:
13. **Were any teeth pulled due to cavities?**
(0) No → *GO TO QUESTION 15* (1) Yes
IF YES: 14. **How many teeth in the lower part of your mouth were pulled because of cavities?** ___ ___ teeth [00=IGN]

15. **Do you have any natural tooth with an untreated cavity or hole in the lower part of your mouth?**
(0) No → *GO TO QUESTION 17* (1) Yes
IF YES: 16. **How many natural teeth with an untreated cavity or hole in the lower part of your mouth do you have?** ___ ___ teeth [00=IGN]

17. **Do you have any natural tooth with a restoration or filling in the lower part of your mouth?**
(0) No → *GO TO QUESTION 19* (1) Yes
IF YES: 18. **How many natural teeth with a restoration or filling in the lower part of your mouth do you have?** ___ ___ teeth [00=IGN]

19. **Do you have bridges or partial denture in the lower part of your mouth?**
(0) No → *GO TO QUESTION 21* (1) Yes
IF YES: 20. **How many natural teeth have been replaced with a bridge or partial denture in the lower part of your mouth?** ___ ___ teeth [00=IGN]

21. **Do you have any fixed bridge in the lower part of your mouth?**
(0) No → *GO TO QUESTION 23* (1) Yes
IF YES: 22. **How many natural teeth have been replaced with a fixed bridge in the lower part of your mouth?**
___ ___ teeth. [00=IGN]

IF YOUTH HAS NO TEETH IN UPPER ARCH: 23. **Do you wear a complete denture on the upper part of your mouth?**
(0) No (1) Yes

IF YOUTH HAS NO TEETH IN LOWER ARCH: 23. **Do you wear a complete denture on the lower part of your mouth?**
(0) No (1) Yes

Figure 1. Self-reported survey of dental caries. Pelotas, Rio Grande do Sul, Brazil, 2012.

a day); and 3) How would you rate the health of your teeth today? (very good, good, fair, poor, and very poor [subsequently categorised as very good/good, fair, and poor/very poor]).

Statistical analysis

The data were analysed with the aid of the Stata 12.0 program. The chi-square test was used to compare the participants in the subsample at 18 years of age with all members of the original cohort. Descriptive analysis was then performed of the DMFT index as well as the individual decayed, missing, and filled components, with the calculation of mean values and 95% confidence intervals (CI). The following were also calculated: intraclass correlation coefficient (ICC) for the DMFT index as well as the individual decayed, missing, and filled components; prevalence of clinically determined dental caries (gold standard); prevalence of self-reported dental caries; estimates of sensitivity, specificity, and positive and negative predictive values; absolute bias (prevalence of self-reported caries minus gold standard prevalence); relative bias (percentage of underestimation of true prevalence = absolute bias/gold standard prevalence × 100); and inflation factor (gold standard prevalence/self-reported prevalence) [16]. Estimates of sensitivity, specificity, and positive and negative predictive values were stratified by gender and schooling (12 or more years of study *versus* 4 years or less). Prevalence ratios for clinically determined and self-reported dental caries were calculated for risk factors using Poisson regression models with robust variance [17].

Ethical aspects

This study received approval from the Human Research Ethics Committee of the Federal University of Pelotas (Brazil) under process number 67/11. All participants received clarifications regarding the objectives and procedures and agreed to participate by signing a statement of informed consent.

Results

A total of 1014 members of the cohort were evaluated with regard to oral health at 18 years of age, 526 (51.9%) of whom were male and 386 (41.7%) had mothers with five to eight years of schooling. Regarding household income, the first, second, and third tertiles corresponded to less than two times the Brazilian minimum wage, between two and four times the minimum wage, and more than four times the minimum wage, respectively. Table 1 displays the characteristics of the original cohort (n = 5248) and oral health subsample (n = 1014). Statistically significant differences were found regarding gender, mother's schooling, and household income, with an increase in the proportion of male subjects, mean mother's schooling, and household income in the subsample.

Both the clinical and self-reported DMFT indices had a median value of 1 decayed, missing or filled tooth and an interquartile interval (Q3–Q1) of 3 DMFT. Regarding the mean values, the clinical DMFT was 2.06, and the self-reported DMFT was 1.75. All mean values of the DMFT components demonstrated the underestimation of self-reported information in comparison to the clinical evaluation. In the analysis of the ICC, which allowed measuring the concordance or reliability of the tools used to compare the clinical and self-reported DMFT and its components, the lowest degree of reliability was found for the decayed component (ICC = 0.43) and the highest was found for the missing component (ICC = 0.61) (Table 2).

Table 3 displays the prevalence rates of dental caries and estimates of sensitivity, specificity, positive and negative predictive values, absolute bias, relative bias, and inflation factor. Self-reports underestimated the prevalence of dental caries by 9.3% in comparison to the clinical evaluation. The results indicate high sensitivity (81.8%) and specificity (78.1%). The positive predictive value of 88% indicates that, among those identified with dental caries, the majority actually had the condition. The negative predictive value indicates that, among those identified as not having dental caries, only 68.6% were confirmed as actually not having the condition. The inflation factor for self-reported dental caries was 1.10.

Table 4 displays the estimates of sensitivity, specificity, and positive and negative predictive values stratified by gender, greater (12 or more years of study) or less schooling (4 years or less), lower (1st tertile) or higher (3rd tertile) household income, and visit to the dentist in the previous year among the adolescents. Sensitivity was higher for female subjects (87.3%), adolescents with a greater level of schooling (82.6%), those with a lower household income (84.5%) and those who visited the dentist in the previous year (81.9%). Specificity was higher for male subjects (84.1%), adolescents with a greater level of schooling (92.6%), those with a higher household income (83.5%) and those who did not visit the dentist in the previous year (78.2%). The confirmation of the diagnosis of dental caries (measured by the positive predictive value) was also higher among male subjects (89.5%), adolescents with a greater level of schooling (90.5%), those with a higher household income (89.3%) and those who visited the dentist in the previous year (89.8%). The confirmation of the absence of the condition (measured by the negative predictive value) was greater among female subjects (71.6%), adolescents with a greater level of schooling (86.2%), those with a lower household income (69.7%) and those who did not visit the dentist in the previous year (72.5%).

Table 5 displays the prevalence ratios according to the independent variables evaluated for the binary DMFT (0/≥1) based on the clinical and self-reported assessments. Higher prevalence ratios were found for the majority of variables when considering clinically detected dental caries. Adolescent's schooling and household income were inversely associated with clinically detected dental caries. Self-rated oral health was positively associated with both the clinical and self-reported measures of dental caries. Clinically determined dental caries was positively associated with visits to the dentist in the previous year. The self-reported measure of dental caries was inversely associated with daily tooth brushing frequency.

Discussion

The findings of the present study indicate adequate validity in self-reported data regarding dental caries in adolescents in relation to the clinical measure using the DMFT index. Self-reported measures exhibited high sensitivity and specificity.

To adjust the prevalence of self-reported dental caries (which was underestimated by 9.3% in comparison to the clinical evaluation in the present study), the literature proposes the use of correction factors, such as the inflation factor [16], for health surveys that assess self-reported information regarding periodontal disease [18].

Moderate agreement was found between self-reported and clinically determined tooth decay in the present study. Studies on the validation of self-reported oral health information have indicated low agreement regarding the comparison of the decayed component [2]. This may be related to the fact that laypersons are unable to recognise dental caries [2,6] or only perceive the

Table 1. Characteristics of original 1993 birth cohort and oral health subsample of cohort members at 18 years age, Pelotas, Rio Grande do Sul, Brazil, 2012.

	Original cohort		Subsample at 18 years of ages		
	N	% (95%CI)	N	% (95%CI)	p-value *
Gender					
Male	2603	49.6 (48.3; 50.9)	526	52.2 (49.8; 55.3)	<0.001
Female	2645	50.4 (49.1; 51.8)	487	47.8 (44.6; 50.9)	
Mother's schooling (years)					
≤4	1468	28.0 (26.8; 29.2)	228	24.6 (21.8; 27.4)	
5–8	2424	46.24 (44.9; 47.6)	386	41.8 (38.5; 44.9)	<0.001
9–11	923	17.60 (16.6; 18.6)	261	28.4 (25.5; 31.4)	
≥12	427	8.1 (7.4; 8.9)	48	5.3 (3.8; 6.8)	
Household income (based on minimum wage)					
1st tertile	2226	43.3 (41.9; 44.7)	339	32.7(29.9; 35.7)	
2nd tertile	1445	28.1 (26.9; 29.4)	335	33.2(30.2; 36.2)	<0.001
3rd tertile	1466	28.5 (27.3; 29.8)	336	34.0(31.0; 37.0)	

*chi-square test.

presence of the condition when it affects their social relations or when they experience pain [19].

Stronger agreement is described regarding reports of the number of missing and filled teeth [20]. The literature states that the number of self-reported missing teeth in adults and elderly individuals differs from the number determined clinically [10] because individuals have difficulties remembering treatment received years ago. Moreover, the loss of the first permanent molar may have occurred early in life, which further hinders the recollection of such an event. The stronger agreement in the present study regarding the number of missing teeth may be explained by the fact that adolescents are more likely to remember adverse oral conditions in their life. Moreover, missing teeth is a rare occurrence in this group. Indeed, the most recent national oral health surveys in Brazil [21,22] report that adolescents between 15 and 19 years of age have an increasingly fewer number of decayed teeth, which is the main cause of tooth loss in this age group. This decrease in the prevalence of caries is directly related to an improved socioeconomic status, which allows the population access to fluoridated toothpaste, a fluoridated water supply and oral healthcare services [23].

The findings for the filled teeth component are in agreement with those reported in a previous study [2]. The greater agreement between the self-reported and clinical assessments regarding restored teeth is likely related to the aforementioned reduction in the prevalence of dental caries as well as the change in the oral healthcare model adopted in Brazil, which was previously directed more toward surgical and restorative procedures and currently involves a health vigilance model [24]. This aspect may have contributed to the fact that the adolescents analysed had an average of less than one tooth with carious tissue.

The similar prevalence rates between clinically determined and self-reported dental caries measured by the DMFT index in the present study were likely due to the fact that the clinical exam for dental caries based on the WHO criteria for epidemiological surveys identifies more advanced stages of tooth decay. Another aspect that diminished the possibility of error in self-reported information on DMFT was the fact that all participants were informed regarding the maximum number of teeth in the upper and lower arches, which differs from methods reported in previous studies [2,5,6].

The high sensitivity and specificity in the present investigation differ from findings reported in a study carried out in the United States involving individuals in different age groups (19 to 78 years), but the prevalence rate of dental caries was similar (63.8%) [2]. It should be stressed that the study cited only compared the decayed component, whereas the present investigation involved the entire DMFT index. Nonetheless, the difference between studies is likely

Table 2. Description and correlation of clinically determined and self-reported Decayed, Missing and Filled Teeth (DMFT) index of members of 1993 birth cohort at 18 years of age, Pelotas, Rio Grande do Sul, Brazil, 2012.

	Clinical Mean (95% CI)	Self-reported ean (95% CI)	Intraclass correlation coefficient	p-value
DMFT	2.06 (1.92; 2.21)	1.75 (1.68; 1.82)	0.50	<0.001
Decayed component	0.79 (0.71; 0.88)	0.63 (0.59; 0.67)	0.43	<0.001
Missing component	0.33 (0.29; 0.38)	0.28 (0.25; 0.30)	0.61	<0.001
Filled component	0.94 (0.84; 1.04)	0.84 (0.79; 0.89)	0.58	<0.001

Table 3. Prevalence of clinically determined and self-reported dental caries (DMFT ≥1) with estimates of sensitivity, specificity, positive predictive value, negative predictive value, absolute bias, relative bias and inflation factor for members of 1993 birth cohort at 18 years of age, Pelotas, Rio Grande do Sul, Brazil, 2012.

Prevalence of dental caries						
Clinical % (95% CI)		**Self-reported % (95% CI)**			**p-value[1]**	
66.5(63.6; 69.3)		60.3(58.8; 61.8)			0,001	
Dental caries determined by clinical (gold standard) and self-reported methods						
Sensitivity % (95% CI)	**Specificity % (95% CI)**	**PPV[2] % (95% CI)**	**NPV[3] % (95% CI)**	**Absolute bias[4]**	**Relative bias[5]**	**Inflation factor[6]**
81.8(78.7; 84.7)	78.1(73.3; 82.4)	88(85.2; 90.5)	68.6(63.7; 73.2)	−6.2	9.3	1.1

[1]chi-squared test.
[2]positive predictive value.
[3]negative predictive value.
[4]absolute bias = tested prevalence - gold standard prevalence.
[5]relative bias = underestimated true prevalence = absolute bias/gold standard prevalence X 100.
[6]inflation factor = gold standard prevalence/tested prevalence.

due to the age groups analysed, which may have exerted an influence on the quality of the self-reported information, as discussed previously. Sensitivity is dependent on the prevalence of a disease [20]. Moreover, socioeconomic issues and health-related behaviour exert an influence on the quality of self-reported information regarding the health of a population and consequently affect the degree of sensitivity. The positive predictive value is affected by these same factors. In the analysis of adolescent's schooling, higher sensitivity and positive predictive values were found among those with a greater level of schooling and those who visited the dentist in the previous year. Thus, different results can be found in different socioeconomic contexts, indicating that the findings of the present study should be analysed with caution, considering the socioeconomic profile of Brazil.

In the analysis of the unadjusted prevalence ratios for socio-demographic aspects and oral health habits, some variables were only associated with the clinical determination of caries and others were only associated with self-reported caries. This indicates that self-reported information should be used with caution in epidemiological studies with the aim of establishing significant associations between risk factors and dental caries. None of the studies consulted in the literature performed such comparisons, with the exception of studies addressing self-reported information on periodontal disease [18].

The advantage of using self-reported information for knowledge on the situation of dental caries in adolescents resides in the fact that the data collection questionnaire can be administered by any trained interviewer and does not require a dental professional. For oral health professionals, especially those linked to public health-care services, such information is of extreme importance to the planning and monitoring of oral health policies and actions.

The quality of the information obtained in the present study should be stressed, as the data came from a sample from a cohort study, with due methodological care taken to confer a high degree of reliability to the information obtained.

Table 4. Estimates of sensitivity, specificity, positive predictive value and negative predictive value for clinically determined and self-reported dental caries (DMFT ≥1) according to gender, adolescent's schooling, household income and visit to dentist in previous year in 1993 birth cohort at 18 years of age, Pelotas, Rio Grande do Sul, Brazil, 2012.

	Sensitivity % (95% CI)	**Specificity % (95% CI)**	**PPV[1] % (95% CI)**	**NPV[2] % (95% CI)**	**Accuracy**
Female	87.3 (83.2; 90.7)	70.7(62.7; 77.8)	86.8 (82.7; 90.2)	71.6 (63.6; 78.7)	82.1
Male	76.4 (71.5; 80.9)	84.1 (78.1; 89.0)	89.5 (85.4; 92.8)	66.8 (60.4; 72.8)	78.2
Lesser schooling of adolescent (≤4 years of study)	75.0 (56.8; 88.5)	65.0 (40.8; 84.6)	77.4 (58.9; 90.4)	61.9 (38.4; 31.9)	71.1
Greater schooling of adolescent (≥12 years of study)	82.6 (61.2; 95.0)	92.6 (75.7; 99.1)	90.5 (69.6; 98.8)	86.2 (68.2; 96.1)	88.0
Lower household income (1st tertile)	84.5 (79.8; 88.5)	75.4 (67.2; 82.4)	87.9 (83.4; 91.5)	69.7 (61.5; 77.0)	83.9
Higher household income (3rd tertile)	78.0 (71.3; 83.8)	83.5 (74.9; 90.1)	89.3 (83.4; 93.6)	68.3 (59.4 76.3)	80.0
Visited dentist in previous year	81.9 (77.6; 85.6)	78.0 (70.7; 84.2)	89.8 (86.1; 92.8)	64.6 (57.4; 71.3)	80.7
Did not visit dentist in previous year	80.8 (75.9; 86.0)	78.2 (71.4; 84.0)	85.9 (81.3; 89.8)	72.5 (65.7; 78.7)	80.4

[1]positive predictive value.
[2]negative predictive value.

Table 5. Prevalence ratios (95% CI) for exploratory variables of clinically determined and self-reported dental caries (DMFT ≥1) in 1993 cohort at 18 years of age, Pelotas, Rio Grande do Sul, Brazil, 2012.

	Clinical DMFT	Self-reported DMFT
Gender	**p = 0.003**	**p<0.001**
Male	1.0	1.0
Female	1.2 (1.1; 1.4)	1.25 (1.2; 1.4)
Adolescent's schooling (years of study)	**p<0.001**	**p<0.001**
≤4	2.1 (1.2; 3.6)	1.0 (0.9; 1.3)
5–8	2.5 (1.6; 4.0)	1.3 (1.1; 1.6)
9–11	1.8 (1.2; 3.6)	1.3 (1.0; 1.7)
≥12	1.0	1.0
Household income (based on minimum wage)	**p = 0.05**	**p = 0.27**
1st tertile	1.2 (1.0; 1.5)	1.2(1.0; 1.4)
2nd tertile	1.1 (0.9; 1.3)	1.1 (0.9; 1.3)
3rd tertile	1.0	1.0
Visit to dentist in previous year	**p = 0.001**	**p = 0.098**
No	1.0	1.0
Yes	1.3 (1.2; 1.5)	1.1 (1.0; 1.3)
Daily tooth brushing frequency	**p = 0.81**	**p = 0.007**
<2 times	1.1 (0.7; 1.6)	1.3 (1.1; 1.6)
≥2 times	1.0	1.0
Self-rated oral health	**p<0.001**	**p<0.001**
Very good/good	1.0	1.0
Fair	1.4 (1.2; 1.6)	1.7 (1.4; 1.9)
Poor/very poor	2.1 (1.8; 2.6)	(2.6; 3.8)

Based on the present findings, self-reported information on dental caries using the DMFT index requires further studies prior to its use in the analysis of risk factors, but is valid for population-based health surveys with the aim of planning and monitoring oral health actions directed at adolescents without the need to submit the population to clinical exams for the diagnosis of dental caries.

Author Contributions

Conceived and designed the experiments: AERS AMBM MAP MCFA HG FFD. Performed the experiments: AERS AMBM MAP MCFA HG FFD. Analyzed the data: AERS AMBM MAP FVF. Contributed reagents/materials/analysis tools: AERS MCFA HG FFD. Contributed to the writing of the manuscript: AERS MCFA HG FFD FVF.

References

1. Blicher B, Joshipura K, Eke P (2005) Validation of self-reported periodontal disease: A Systematic Review. J Dent Res 84: 881–890.
2. Pitiphat W, Garcia RI, Douglass CW, Joshipura KJ (2002) Validation of self-reported oral health measures. J Public Health Dent 62: 122–128.
3. Joshipura KJ, Pitiphat W, Douglass CW (2002) Validation of Self-reported periodontal measures among health professionals. J Public Health Dent 62: 115–121.
4. Taylor GW, Borgnakke WS (2007) Self-Reported periodontal disease: validation in an epidemiological survey. Periodontol 78: 1407–1420.
5. Axelsson G, Helgadottir S (1995) Comparison of oral health data from self-administered questionnaire and clinical examination. Community Dent Oral Epidemiol 23: 365–8.
6. Pinelli C, Loffredo LCM (2007) Reproducibility and validity of self-perceived oral health conditions. Clin Oral Invest 11: 431–437.
7. Heloe LA (1972) Comparison of dental health data obtained from questionnaires, interviews and clinical examination. Scand J Dent Res 80: 495–499.
8. Reisine ST, Bailit HL (1980) Clinical oral health status and adult perceptions of oral health. Soc Sci Med Med Psychol Med Sociol 14A: 597–605.
9. Kononen M, Lipasti J, Murtomaa H (1986) Comparison of dental information obtained from self-examination and clinical examination. Community Dent Oral Epidemiol 14: 258–260.
10. Palmqvist S, Soderfeldt B, Arnbjerg D (1991) Self-assessment of dental conditions: validity of a questionnaire. Community Dent Oral Epidemiol 19: 249–51.
11. Gilbert GH, Duncan RP, Kulley AM (1997) Validity of self-reported tooth counts during a telephone screening interview. J Public Health Dent 57: 176–180.
12. Araújo CL, Menezes AMB, Vieira MFA, Neutzling MB, Gonçalves H, et al. (2010) The 11-year follow-up of the 1993 Pelotas (Brazil) birth cohort study: methods. Cad Saúde Pública 26: 1875–186.
13. Victora CG, Hallal PC, Araujo CL, Menezes AM, Wells JC, et al. (2008): Cohort profile: the 1993 Pelotas (Brazil) birth cohort study. Int J Epidemiol. 37: 704–9.
14. Peres MA, Barros AJ, Peres KG, Araújo CL, Menezes AMB, et al. (2010) Oral health follow-up studies in the 1993 Pelotas (Brazil) birth cohort study: methodology and principal results. Cad Saúde Pública 26: 1990–1999.
15. World Health Organization (1997) Oral Health Surveys: Basic Methods. Geneva: World Health Organization. 66p.
16. Albandar JM (2011) Underestimation of periodontitis in NHANES surveys. J Periodontol 82: 337–341.
17. Barros AJ, Hirakata VN (2003) Alternatives for logistic regression in cross-sectional studies: An empirical comparison of models that directly estimate the prevalence ratio. BMC Med Res Methodol 3: 21.
18. Peres MA, Peres KG, Cascaes AM, Correa MB, Demarco FF, et al. (2012) Validity of Partial Protocols to Assess the Prevalence of Periodontal Outcomes and Associated Sociodemographic and Behavior Factors in Adolescents and Young Adults. J Periodontol 83: 369–378.
19. Gooch BF, Dolan TA, Bourque LB (1989) Correlates of self-reported dental health status upon enrollment in the Rand Health Insurance Experiment. J Dent Educ. 53: 629–637.
20. Szklo M, Javier Nieto F (2004) Epidemiology: Beyond the Basics. Sudbury, MA: Jones and Bartlett Publishers. 309 p.
21. Brasil. Ministério da Saúde. Departamento de Atenção Básica: Condições de Saúde Bucal da População Brasileira 2002–2003. Disponível: http://dtr2001.

saude.gov.br/editora/produtos/livros/pdf/05_0053_M.pdf. Acessado 25 de março de. 2012.

22. Brasil. Ministério da Saúde. Departamento de Atenção Básica: SB Brasil 2010-Pesquisa Nacional de Saúde Bucal. Disponível: http://189.28.128.100/dab/docs/geral/projeto_sb2010_relatorio_final.pdf. Acessado 25 de março de 2012.

23. Costa SM, Martins CC, Bonfim MLC, Zina LG, Paiva SM, et al. (2012) A Systematic Review of Socioeconomic Indicators and Dental Caries in Adults. Int. J Environ Res Public Health 9: 3540–74.

24. Moreira RSM, Nico LS, Tomita NE, Ruiz T (2005) Oral health of Brazilian elderly: a systematic review of epidemiologic status and dental care access. Cad Saúde Pública 21: 1665–1675.

23

Dental Status of New Caledonian Children: Is There a Need for a New Oral Health Promotion Programme?

Hélène Pichot[1,2], Martine Hennequin[1,3*], Bernard Rouchon[2], Bruno Pereira[3], Stéphanie Tubert-Jeannin[1,3]

1 Clermont University, University of Auvergne, EA 4847, Centre de Recherche en Odontologie Clinique, BP 10448, Clermont-Ferrand, France, 2 Sanitary and Social Agency of New Caledonia, Nouméa, New Caledonia, 3 CHU Clermont-Ferrand, Clermont-Ferrand, France

Abstract

Background: Before implementing a new oral health promotion program in the French overseas territory of Nouvelle Calédonie, the health authorities needed recent data about dental status of the New Caledonian child population.

Objectives: This study aimed to describe the dental status of 6, 9 and 12-yr-old New Caledonian children and to investigate the environmental and behavioural risk factors related to oral health.

Methods: A randomly selected sample of 2734 children (744 6-yr-olds, 789 9-yr-olds, and 1201 12-yr-olds) was examined clinically by seven calibrated investigators and participants responded to a questionnaire. The main variables were objective criteria about dental status and subjective criteria about experience of dental care, dental fear, self-perception of oral health, cultural or ethnic identity and environmental and behavioural risk factors.

Results: Overall, most of the children had infectious oral diseases: more than 50% had gingivitis, and 60% of 6- and 9 yr-olds had at least one deciduous or permanent tooth with untreated caries. The mean 12-yr-old number of decayed missing and filled teeth (DMFT) was 2.09±2.82. The number of carious lesions was related to the unfavourable lifestyle, deprived social status and no preventive dental care. Kanak, Polynesians and Caledonians (respectively 27%, 18% and 45% of the study sample) were more affected by caries than metropolitan French and Asian children. Children with many untreated carious lesions had negative perceptions of their oral health; they complained of chewing difficulty and had higher scores for dental anxiety.

Conclusion: This study highlights the need for new strategies aimed at improving oral health and at reducing inequalities in New Caledonia. An oral health promotion program would need to be developed in connection with other health programmes using the common risk factor approach within the context of the local environment.

Editor: Peter M. Milgrom, University of Washington, United States of America

Funding: The Regional Public Health Services of New Caledonia, the Sanitary and Social Agency of New Caledonia, the University of Auvergne, Clermont-1, France, and the University Hospital of Clermont-Ferrand, France, financed this study. The funders had no role in study design, data collection and analysis, decision to publish, or preparation of the manuscript.

Competing Interests: The authors have declared that no competing interests exist.

* Email: martine.hennequin@udamail.fr

Introduction

Although oral health has improved in many industrialised countries, the World Health Organization (WHO) recently emphasised that dental caries remains a major health problem in disadvantaged and poor population groups in both developing and developed countries [1]. New Caledonia (pop. 245 580 persons) is a French overseas territory with extensive administrative autonomy. The population is a mix of 40% Kanak people (the original inhabitants of New Caledonia), 30% White European people (Caledonians and Metropolitan Frenchmen), 10% Polynesian people (Wallisians essentially), South-East Asian people and people from Vanuatu. There is little in the literature about the oral health of the New Caledonian population. The last national study was conducted in 1996 and concerned the dental status of 12-yr-old children only [2]. Furthermore, this national study only reported DMF scores and no other aspects of children's dental status. Since then, some local studies have been conducted but they had methodological flaws and did not include adults or other child age groups.

Considering the lack of information about children's dental status in 2011, the New Caledonian health authorities required more complete and recent oral health data. Several aspects of New Caledonia had to be considered during the conception of this study. In New Caledonia, health and educational services are administrated separately in three regions: the North, the Islands and the South. The population varies according to the region, with more Kanak people in the North and the Islands and more

Polynesians, white Europeans and Asians in the South. Three quarters of the population live in the South, where economic activity is concentrated, and 39% of the total population lives in Nouméa, the administrative capital. The mean income per inhabitant places New Caledonia within the richest countries of the South Pacific area but there are strong social and economic disparities within the population. The aim of this study was to provide epidemiological data on the dental status of a representative sample of 6-, 9- and 12-yr-old children in New Caledonia. To provide a more comprehensive view of oral health, we also explored the relationships existing between dental status, health behaviours and socioeconomic status (SES) and the children's perceptions of their oral health and dental anxiety.

Population and Methods

Study population

The study population included children aged 6, 9 and 12 years (born in 2005, 2002 and 2000), who were pupils in New Caledonian schools between July 2011 and September 2012.

Sample size

The desired sample size was calculated using the formula $N = 1.96 \times P(1-P)/i2$ with dental caries prevalence (P) as the main indicator, a precision (i) of 5% according to a previous study from New Caledonia [4] and the first species risk (α) was fixed at 0.05. Caries prevalence was estimated for 12-yr-olds using previous New Caledonian data [2] and for 6- and 9-yr-olds, from a French study which was conducted under the same conditions [3]. The desired sample size was 300 for each 6- and 9-yr-old groups and 400 for 12-yr-olds. The sample size was adjusted to take into account a cluster effect (1+ (m-1)*ICC) with m = 24 being the mean number of children per classroom and an Intra-Class Coefficient (ICC) of 0.05 estimated from data of a previous survey [3] and a participation rate >75%. Finally, the number of children to be selected was set at a minimum of 800 at age 6 and 9 years and 1100 at age 12 years.

Sampling method

Children were randomly selected using a computerised cluster sampling method (cluster = school) with a probability proportional to size [4,5]. The pool of NC schools (217 public and 107 private) was stratified according to the area (South/North/Island) and the type of school (public/private). Seventy-six schools were selected. All the children aged 6 and 9 years in 2011 (40 public schools and 16 private; 14 in the North region, 32 in South and 10 in Islands) and 12 years in 2012 (10 public schools and 10 private; 6 in the North region, 9 in South and 5 in Islands), were included in the study. The total sample size was 3138 children (911 6-yr-olds, 923 9-yr-olds and 1304 12-yr-olds).

Ethical concerns

In the absence of a single New Caledonian ethical committee, ethical approvals were obtained from the New Caledonian educational institutions (Evangelical Alliance for School Education (ASEE), Protestant federation for education (FELP), Diocesan Directorate for Catholic Education (DDEC), Directorate for education in South (DES), Directorate for youth, education, training and integration (DEFIJ), Directorate for education in Islands (DEPIL), New Caledonian directorate for education (DENC), New Caledonian Vice Rectory) and from the New Caledonian health authorities (Directorate for community actions and health in Islands (DACAS), Directorate for health and social affairs and of social problems in northern province (DASSPS-Nord), Directorate for sanitary and social action of southern province (DPASS-Sud), Sanitary and Social Agency of New Caledonia (ASSNC), Directorate of health and social affairs of New Caledonia (DASSNC). Schools were approached through local educational authorities. Explanatory letters and consent forms were sent to parents a few days prior to the dental examinations and those children whose parents returned written consent were examined.

Study variables and health indicators

Pertinent indicators were identified through a literature review and after interviews with professional experts in epidemiology and paediatric dentistry. The children's dental status was evaluated during the clinical examination.

Dental caries was diagnosed at the threshold level (D3) for deciduous and permanent teeth, and at the enamel threshold level (D1) for the first permanent molars [6]. For caries experience, five indices were recorded: (1) numbers of decayed deciduous and permanent teeth (d3t, D3T), (2) numbers of decayed or filled deciduous teeth (d3ft), (3) numbers of decayed, missing or filled permanent teeth (D3MFT), (4) numbers of decayed first permanent molars (D1M), (5) numbers of decayed, missing or filled first permanent molars (D1MFM). Additionally, the significant caries index, which is the mean number of decayed, missing or filled permanent teeth for the third of the subjects having the highest D3MFT values, was calculated [7]. Radiographs were not used. The Gingival Index of Löe & Silness [8] was used to express the gingival status, and the scores were dichotomised: without gingivitis (score 0 for all sextants) or with gingivitis (score >0 for at least one sextant). Chewing efficiency was evaluated by recording the number of functional dental units (PFU). It has been demonstrated that the number of PFU measured clinically is a pertinent and discriminant criterion that independently influences nutritional status in adults [9–11]. The relationship between PFU and orofacial dysfunctions in children is being investigating: firsts results indicate that is it a good indicator of masticatory performance in children too [12]. The presence of at least one dental sealant on a permanent molar and at least one discoloured permanent tooth or non-carious dental structural defect were also recorded.

Socio-demographic variables (gender, date of birth, region of residence, public or private school) were recorded from the school register. Socioeconomic variables (type of health insurance and father's or mother's employment status) were recorded only for 6- and 9-yr-olds by school managers. Additionally, children responded to questions relating to their lifestyle (frequency of tooth brushing, daily consumption of sweet drinks), dental attendance (had never visited a dentist or had already visited a dentist) and dental fear (VAS scale from 0, no fear, to 10, severe fear) [13]. The children' self-perceptions of oral health (has no oral health problem or has oral health problems) were recorded for 9- and 12-yr-olds and the self-perception of chewing difficulties (can bite or chew every food item or type of food, difficult to bite or chew, or some types of food impossible to bite or chew) and smoking habits (had never smoked, had already smoked) were recorded for 12-yr-olds only. Finally, at age 12 yr, children were asked to which main cultural or ethnic group (Kanak/Polynesian/Caledonian/European, Asian/Other) they felt they belonged. A detailed list of the initials and acronyms is given Table 1.

Investigators and Calibration

Seven general dental practitioners performed the children's examinations. They were recruited through an email announcement delivered by the local dentists' registration authority.

Table 1. Description of the abbreviations and acronyms.

dt	Number of deciduous teeth with at least one carious lesion
DT	Number of permanent teeth with at least one carious lesion
dmft	Number of decayed, missing and filled deciduous teeth
DMFT	Number of decayed, missing and filled permanent teeth
DM	Number of first permanent molars with at least one carious lesion
DMFM	Number of decayed, missing and filled first permanent molars
SiC Index	Mean DMFT of the one third of the study group with the highest caries score for 12 years old children [7].
D_3	Dentine threshold for carious lesions according to the Ekstrand classification [6]
D_1	Enamel threshold for carious lesions according to the Ekstrand classification [6]
PFU	Posterior Functional Unit: pair of antagonist post-canine teeth having at least one occlusal contact
DF-VAS	Dental fear-Visual analogic scale
SES	Socio-Economic Status
CI	Confidence Interval
AMG	Aide Médicale Gratuite (Free Medical Assistance)
OHP	Oral Health Promotion
WHO	World Health Organization

Examiners were assigned to one or several schools, depending on feasibility criteria that were mostly depending on geographical locations. Children from the same school or the same grade were not systematically examined by the same investigator. Prior to the start of the study, all the investigators underwent a two-day training course consisting of projection of pictures illustrating clinical situations and explaining the data collection process. This training method has been described in a previous study [14]. The investigators were subjected to a test-retest procedure within a one-month period in order to check their reliability for the main study variables (D_3T, d_3t). Re-examining ten children for each examiner allowed intra-examiner reliability to be assessed. Inter-examiner reproducibility was evaluated using photographs illustrating various clinical situations for the study variables. Intra- and inter-examiner agreements were evaluated using Cohen's Kappa and varied from 0.46 to 0.92 and from 0.69 to 1, depending on the clinical cases.

Data collection

In the 6-yr-old and 9-yr-old groups, children answered questions during a personal interview with an investigator. For the 12-yr-old children, the questionnaire was self-administrated. Children of all groups were examined while seated facing the examiner either in the school dispensary or in a classroom. For the oral examination, investigators used disposable gloves and mouth mirrors and a portable light. Probing was not permitted but debris could be removed with cotton rolls, if necessary. To count functional units (PFU), examiners used blue articulating paper of 200 μm thickness (Bausch) [15]. The children were asked to bite on the paper and the number of posterior mandibular teeth that had at least one coloured mark was counted.

Data analysis

Data entry was duplicated and errors were corrected on Microsoft ACCESS software before analysis. The statistical analyses were performed using the Statistical Package for the Social Sciences (SPSS, Inc. Chicago, IL, USA, version 16.0) and Stata software (version 13, Stat/SE, StataCorp, College Station, US). To describe the dental status of Caledonian children (national epidemiological survey), all statistical analyses were conducted separately for each age group as participants were stratified by age. Results were expressed with 95% confidence intervals (CI). According to literature [16–19], mixed models were used, including the school and examiner parameters as random effects [20]. Indeed, due to the correlation of observations within a school, the usual tests were invalid and inter-cluster variances were inflated. Moreover, the number of examiners was high and despite the calibration process, an examiner effect was expected. The examiner effect was integrated throughout the analysis because it differed from the school effect and was significant in the South Region. Carious status was explained using explanatory variables following two steps, firstly with a bivariate analysis and then with a multiple random-effects regression. Factors significantly associated with d3t and D3T in bivariate analyses were entered in the regression models if $p<0.1$. Non-significant parameters considered as being clinically relevant were maintained in the analyses (sex, region, type of school, frequency of tooth brushing, consumption of sweet drinks and dental sealants) taking into account variability between and within cluster and examiner [21]. The mean numbers of carious lesions on deciduous teeth (d3t) or permanent teeth (D3T) were not normally distributed (even with a normality transformation), thus a log transformation was used. Chi-squared tests were used to study the interrelationships between oral health variables. The interactions between factors were tested and the results were reported using regression coefficients, 95% confidence intervals (CI) and P-values (P). The level of significance (type I error α) was set at 0.05.

Results

Sample description

Of the children initially selected, 87% participated in the study; 2734 children were thus examined and interviewed (744 6-yr-olds, 789 9-yr-olds and 1201 12-yr-olds). The variables age, sex, area and type of school had similar distributions in the sample and in the study population. Among the participants, 52% were boys, > 70% of the children attended public schools, 10% lived in the Islands area, 20% in the northern and 70% in the southern region.

Table 2. Subjective oral health, social and behavioural characteristics of the studied population.

	Age 6 yr		Age 9 yr		Age 12 yr	
	N	%	*N*	%	*N*	%
Gender	*744*		*789*		*1201*	
Male		52.1		51.8		51.8
Female		47.9		48.2		48.2
Type of school	*744*		*789*		*1201*	
Public		69.9		76.2		74.8
Private		30.1		23.8		25.2
Region of Residence	*744*		*789*		*1201*	
Islands		10.3		10.1		9.2
North		18.7		21.2		20.7
South		71.0		68.7		70.1
Cultural or Ethnic group	NI		NI		*1161*	
Kanak						27.3
Polynesian						18.2
Caledonian						45
European, Asian and others						9.5
Mother's employment status	*509*		*505*		NI	
Unemployed		29.5		42.6		
blue collar, tradesman		32.0		20.6		
Management, executive		38.5		36.8		
Father's employment status	*479*		*485*		NI	
Unemployed		10.2		9.9		
blue collar, tradesman		59.7		49.1		
Management, executive		30.1		41.0		
Type of health insurance	*508*		*508*		NI	
Basic insurance only		22.8		20.1		
State aid supplemental (AMG)		26.8		33.1		
Private supplemental		50.4		46.8		
Usual drinks when thirsty	*741*		*789*		*1199*	
Water		69.6		64.9		64.6
Sweet drinks		30.4		35.1		35.4
Smoking habits	NI		NI		*1201*	
Never smoked						88.3
Has smoked						11.7
Frequency of tooth brushing	*739*		*789*		*1196*	
<1 weekly		25.6		37.5		20.2
≥1 weekly		8.1		6.7		24.5
≥1 daily		66.3		55.8		55.3
Dental attendance	*730*		*785*		*1189*	
Had never visited a dentist		49.7		22.0		16.9
Had visited a dentist		50.3		78.0		83.1
Dental fear (VAS scale from 0 (no fear) to 10 (severe fear))	*739*		*780*		*1201*	
DF-VAS 0–3		77.7		61.1		64.6
DF-VAS 4–6		11		23.2		19.2
DF-VAS 7–10		11.3		15.7		16.2
Self-perception of oral health	NI		*687*		*1092*	
No oral health problem				41.2		50.9
Oral health problems				58.8		49.1
Chewing difficulties	NI		*NI*		*1011*	

Table 2. Cont.

	Age 6 yr		Age 9 yr		Age 12 yr	
	N	%	*N*	%	*N*	%
Food impossible to chew						16.7
Food difficult to chew						14.6
No difficulties						68.6

N: Numbers; %: Proportion; NI: not investigated.

Among the 12 yr-old group, 45% of children saw themselves as Caledonian, 27% Kanak, 18% Polynesian, 9% European or Asian or other communities and 3% did not want to answer the question (Table 2).

Socioeconomic status

Data about socioeconomic status was missing in more than 30% of children. Unemployment was approximately 10% for fathers, and varied from 29% to 43% for mothers, depending on age group. More than 20% of the 6-yr-old and 9-yr-old children were covered by the basic compulsory health insurance alone; 27% of the 6-yr-olds and 33% of the 9-yr-olds benefited from a state aid supplemental insurance dedicated to economically disadvantaged families (Table 2).

Lifestyle and experience of dental care

Negative dental behaviours were noticed for some children; more than 30% of the children consumed sweet drinks regularly, almost 12% of the 12-yr-olds had already smoked and more than one third of the children did not brush their teeth daily (Table 2).

In the study sample, half of the 6-yr-old children had already attended a dentist and this proportion rose to 83% for 12-yr-olds. Dental fear varied slightly by age; older children tended to have higher scores and more than 15% of the 9- to 12-yr-olds had high scores (DF-VAS >6). Almost 60% of the children at age nine yr and 50% of the children at age 12 yr considered that they had oral health problems and more than 30% of the 12-yr-olds reported having chewing difficulty (Table 2).

Dental status

Data on dental status are gathered in Tables 3 and 4. More than 50% of the children had poor oral hygiene indicated by gingivitis and 12-yr-olds were more affected by gingivitis than younger children. At age six yr, 58% had at least one untreated carious lesion (d_3t or D_3T >0) and the mean d_3t was 2.58 (±3.40) teeth. The prevalence of untreated carious lesions in the mixed dentition was high at age nine yr (60%) with a mean D_3T of 0.53 (±1.04) teeth. At age 12 yr, 47% of the children had at least one untreated carious deciduous or permanent tooth and the mean D_3T was 1.49 (±2.39) teeth and one third of the most affected children had 5.37 (±2.80) teeth with at least one carious lesion. The number of permanent first molars affected by initial or dentinal carious lesions increased with age, from D_1M of 0.24(±0.64) teeth among 6-yr olds to D_1M of 0.84 (±1.11) teeth in 12-yr-olds.

The carious components (d_3t, D_3T and D1M) were predominant within the global components of caries experience (d_3ft, D_3MFT and D1MFM), indicating that dentinal carious lesions remained mostly untreated. The mean number of sealed permanent molars was also very low (fewer than one) in all age groups.

Fifteen per cent of the 9-yr-olds had fewer than four functional units but this proportion was lower at age 12 yr (2.7%). The proportion of children with enamel or dentinal defects on permanent teeth was high (>14%), particularly in 9-yr-old children (25%), but the type of defect was not specified.

Inter-relationships between oral health problems

Infectious oral health problems were inter-related in all age groups, with a higher number of carious lesions in children with gingivitis (Chi-squared test, $P<0.0001$).

Risk factors related to caries experience

Caries experience varied substantially depending on socioeconomic status, environment and culture. Six yr-old children with the state aid dental insurance and children at age six and nine yr whose mothers were jobless had more untreated carious teeth compared with other children. On the other hand, children in public schools had less untreated dental caries than children attending private schools in the 6-yr-old group. In the 12-yr-old group, the mean number of untreated carious teeth was higher among Kanak, Polynesian and Caledonian children when compared with European and Asian children. It also appeared that 6-yr-old children living in the Islands had more untreated dental caries (Table 5).

Caries experience was significantly related to the children's lifestyle and their access to preventive dental care. Indeed, six and 12-yr-old children who used sweet drinks daily and 12-yr-olds who had already smoked had higher caries scores than others. A higher number of decayed teeth was also observed for children who reported they did not brush their teeth daily at ages nine yr and 12 yr. In all groups, dental status did not differ, whether or not a child had already been to the dentist, but 9- and 12-yr-old children who had benefited from preventive dental care (with dental sealants) had less caries experience than others (Table 5).

Children's dental status was associated with dental anxiety, perceptions about their own oral health and children's oral functioning. At age 12 yr, children with lower levels of dental fear (DF-VAS<3) had less caries experience than children with higher DF-VAS levels (DF-VAS >6). Moreover, nine and 12-yr-old children who reported having no oral health problems and 12-yr-olds who reported they had no difficulties for chewing had better dental status than others. Nine yr-old children with fewer untreated carious lesions had significantly more functional units (PFU) than other children (Table 5).

Multidimensional analysis

All the variables, which were significantly related to caries experience in the bivariate analyses, were included in the model.

Table 3. Prevalence of oral diseases.

	Age 6 yr		Age 9 yr		Age 12 yr	
Oral status	*N*	**% [95%CI]**	*N*	**% [95%CI]**	*N*	**% [95%CI]**
Caries	*744*		*789*		*1201*	
No carious lesion (d_3t or $D_3T=0$)		42.3 [38.8;46.0]		40.1[36.6;43.6]		53.1[50.3;56.0]
At least one carious lesion (d_3t or $D_3T>0$)		57.7 [54.0;61.2]		59.9[56.4;63.4]		46.9[44.0;49.7]
Gingival status	*731*		*787*		*1201*	
No gingivitis		46.9 [43.3;50.6]		40.4[37.0;43.9]		37.8[35.1;40.6]
Gingivitis on one or more sextants		53.1 [49.4;56.7]		59.6[56.1;63.0]		62.2[59.4;64.9]
Number of posterior Functional units	NI		*754*		*1201*	
<4 PFU				15.1[12.6;17.9]		2.7[1.9;3.8]
4 to 6 PFU				43.1[39.5;46.7]		17.0[14.9;19.2]
>6 PFU				41.8[38.2;45.4]		80.3[77.9;82.5]
Dental structure of permanent teeth	*740*		*787*		*1198*	
No structural defect		85.6[82.8;88.0]		74.6[71.4;77.6]		80.0[77.6;82.2]
At least one structural defect		14.4[12.0;17.2]		25.4[22.4;28.6]		20.0[17.8;22.4]

N: Number; %: Proportion; NI: not investigated; CI: confidence interval.

The variables gender, region, type of school were included in the model even if no significant relationship with dental status was observed in the bivariate analysis. Table 6 gives the regression coefficients only for the explanatory variables that were significant for at least one age group.

The multidimensional random effects model showed a significant influence of the type of health insurance, cultural background, oral hygiene, consumption of sugared drinks and dental preventive care on dental caries experience (Table 6). In six yr-olds, the type of health insurance and the consumption of sweet drinks significantly influenced the number of carious lesions. In 9 and 12-yr-olds, frequency of tooth brushing and presence of dental sealant also showed a significant association with the number of carious lesions. When compared with the Kanak 12-yr-olds, Europeans and Asians had fewer carious lesions (Table 6).

On the other hand, significant associations were found between lower numbers of carious lesions, a high number of functional units and no perception of oral health problems. Nine yr-old children with more than 6 PFUs were significantly less affected by dental caries than children with fewer than 4 PFUs and 12-yr-olds who reported that they had no oral problems had fewer carious lesions. Moreover, perception of chewing difficulties by 12 years old children was related to the number of carious teeth (Table 6).

Discussion

This survey aimed to evaluate the dental status of children at age six, nine and twelve years old in New Caledonia. The participation rate was high; 2734 children were examined. In the study sample, more than half of the children were affected by gingivitis and the prevalence of untreated dental caries was almost 60% among 6- and 9-yr-olds and about 50% among 12-yr-olds. Caries experience is unevenly distributed in the population, with one third of 12-yr-olds having more than five teeth with at least one carious lesion. Dental caries experience was particularly high

Table 4. Dental status and caries experience (Mean ± standard deviation).

	Age 6 yr	Age 9 yr	Age 12 yr
	N=744	*N=789*	*N=1201*
Number of Permanent teeth	4.61±3.51	15.87±4.19	25.74±3.13
Number of Deciduous teeth	16.87±2.82	7.35±4.26	0.68±1.77
D_3MFT	0.09±0.44	0.76±1.29	2.09±2.82
D_3T	0.07±0.36	0.53±1.04	1.49±2.39
d_3ft	3.01±3.56	2.26±2.17	0.95±1.16
d_3t	2.58±3.4	1.72±1.99	0.73±1
SiC Index	NA	NA	5.37±2.80
D_1MFM	0.33±0.82	1.70±1.53	1.92±1.59
D_1M	0.24±0.64	1.06±1.24	0.84±1.11
Number of sealed molars	0.11±0.53	0.39±0.95	0.32±0.95

N: Number; NA: not applicable.

Table 5. Bivariate analysis: relationship between caries experience (d_3t, D_3T) and environmental or behavioural variables.

	Age 6 yr			Age 9 yr			Age 12 yr		
	N	d3t[+]	*p**	N	D3T	*p*	N	D3T	*p*
Gender	724		*Ns*	789		*ns*	1201		*ns*
Male		2.6 (3.5)			0.51 (1)			1.38 (2.1)	
Female		2.55(3.3)			0.55 (1.1)			1.6 (2.6)	
Type of school	743		*<0.05*	789		*ns*	1201		*ns*
Public		2.41 (3.3)			0.54 (1)			1.4 (2.3)	
Private		3.02 (3.5)			0.5 (1)			1.73 (2.5)	
Region	743		*<0.05*	789		*ns*	1201		*ns*
Islands		4.06 (3.3)			0.57 (1)			1.46 (1.8)	
North		2.39 (3)[a]			0.35 (0.7)			1.82 (2.6)	
South		2.43 (3.5)[a]			0.58 (1.1)			1.39 (2.4)	
Cultural or Ethnic group	NI			NI			1161		*<0.01*
Kanak								1.58 (2.4)	
Caledonian								1.64 (2.4)	
Polynesian								1.56 (2.7)	
European, Asian and others								0.45 (1.3)[a, b, c]	
Mother's employment status	509		*<0.05*	505		*<0.05*	NI		
Unemployed		3.44 (3.9)			0.69 (1.1)				
Blue collar, tradesman		2.67 (3.3)			0.36 (0.8)[a]				
Management, executive		1.9 (3)[a]			0.44 (0.9)[a]				
Father's employment status	479		*ns*	485		*<0.01*	NI		
Unemployed		3.26 (4.4)			0.44 (0.9)				
Blue collar, tradesman		2.74 (3.3)			0.66 (1.1)				
Management, executive		1.96 (3.2)			0.41 (1)[b]				
Type of health insurance	508		*<0.001*	508		*ns*	NI		
State aid supplemental		3.5 (3.5)			0.49 (1)				
Basic insurance only		3.26 (3.8)			0.63 (1.2)				
Private supplemental		1.8 (2.9)[a, b]			0.42 (0.8)[b]				
Usual drinks when thirsty	740		*<0.05*	789		*ns*	1199		*<0.05*
Sweet drinks		2.96 (3.5)			0.56 (1.1)			1.74 (2.45)	
Water		2.42 (3.3)			0.5 (1)			1.35 (2.3)	
Smoking habits	NI			NI			1139		*<0.01*
Has smoked								2.16 (2.8)	
Never smoked								1.39 (2.2)	
Frequency of tooth brushing	729		*ns*	789		*<0.01*	1173		*<0.001*

Table 5. Cont.

	Age 6 yr			Age 9 yr			Age 12 yr		
	N	**d3t[+]**	*p**	**N**	**D3T**	*p*	**N**	**D3T**	*p*
<1/day		3.01 (3.4)			0.73 (1.2)			1.93 (2.5)	
≥1/day		2.35 (3.4)			0.37 (0.8)			1.11 (2.1)	
Dental attendance	730		*ns*	785		*ns*	1189		*Ns*
Had never visited a dentist		2.6 (3.4)			0.5 (1)			1.34 (2.1)	
Had already visited a dentist		2.6 (3.4)			0.53 (1.1)			1.51 (2.4)	
Dental sealants on permanent molars	593		*ns*	789		*<0.001*	1201		*<0.001*
Absence of dental sealants		2.68 (3.4)			0.58 (1.1)			1.64 (2.5)	
At least one sealant		2.45 (2.5)			0.32 (0.7)			0.57 (1.3)	
Dental Fear-Visual Analogue Scale	738		*ns*	780		*ns*	1201		*<0.01*
DF-VAS <3		2.5 (3.4)			0.52 (1)			1.39 (2.3)	
DF-VAS 3-6		2.86 (3.8)			0.49 (1)			1.42 (2.39)	
DF-VAS>6		2.95 (3)			0.62 (1.1)			1.92 (2.5)[a, b]	
Self-perception of oral health	NI			687		*<0.05*	1092		*<0.001*
No problem					0.35 (0.8)			1.04 (1.8)	
Oral health problems					0.66 (1.2)			1.94 (2.8)	
Chewing difficulties	NI			NI			1011		*<0.05*
Food impossible to chew								1.81 (2.4)	
Food difficult to chew								1.57 (2.2)	
No difficulties								1.36 (2.3)[a]	
Number of posterior functional units (PFU)	NI			754		*<0.001*	1201		*Ns*
PFU<4					0.94 (1.2)			1.78 (3.8)	
4≤PFU<6					0.63 (1.1)[a]			1.32 (2.1)	
PFU≥6					0.33 (0.8)[a, b]			1.51 (2.4)	

N: Number; NI: not investigated; ns: not significant
[+]Mean (Standard deviation), * p value
[a]p<0.05 vs 1st modality, [b] p<0.05 vs 2nd modality and [c] p<0.05 vs 3rd modality

Table 6. Regression coefficients derived from regression: Caries experience (d_3t, D_3T) as dependent variable and environmental or behavioural risk factors as independent variables.

	Age 6 yr *(N=744)*			**Age 9 yr** *(N=789)*			**Age 12 yr** *(N=1201)*		
	d_3t			**D_3T**			**D_3T**		
	RC	**95% CI**	*p*	**RC**	**95% CI**	*p*	**RC**	**95% CI**	*P*
Type of health insurance							NI		
State aid									
Basic	0.59	−0.43 1.62	*ns*						
Private	−1.02	−1.99–0.05	*<0.05*						
Frequency of tooth brushing									
≥1/day vs <1/day				−0.34	−0.56 −0.13	*<0.01*	−0.35	−0.64 −0.05	*<0.05*
Usual drinks when thirsty									
Sugared drinks vs water	0.76	0.02 1.52	<0.05						
Cultural or Ethnic group	NI			NI					
Kanak									
European, Asian and others							−0.79	−1.35 −0.24	*<0.01*
Caledonian							−0.02	−0.57 0.16	*ns*
Polynesian							−0.23	−0.68 0.22	*ns*
Dental sealants on permanent molars									
At least one sealant vs Absence							−1.10	−1.50 −0.70	*<0.001*
Self-perception of Oral Health	NI								
Oral health problems vs No problem							0.68	0.42 0.95	*0.001*
Number of posterior functional units (PFU)	NI								
PFU<4									
4≤PFU<6				−0.30	−0.62 0.02	*ns*			
PFU≥6				−0.51	−0.84 − 0.18	*<0.01*			
Chewing difficulties	NI								
Food impossible to chew									
Food difficult to chew							−0.43	−0.91 0.05	ns
No difficulties							−0.42	−0.80 −0.35	*<0.05*

Other non-significant variables included in the models were not presented here. These were: for the 6 yrs group: sex, region, type of school, mother employment status; for the 9 yrs group: sex, region, type of school, mother and father employment status; for the 12 yrs group: sex, region, type of school, dental fear, smoking status.
N: Number, CI: confidence interval, NI: not investigated, ns: not significant

in socially deprived children, those who had an unfavourable lifestyle or who had not benefited from preventive dental care. The presence of a high number of untreated carious lesions had a negative impact on the children's perceptions of their oral health and the number of functional dental units

The dental status of children has largely improved since the last epidemiological survey was conducted in New Caledonia in collaboration with the WHO in 1996 [2]. The mean D_3MFT at age 12 yr has decreased from 4.09 teeth in 1996 to 2.09 teeth in 2012. This decline has been observed all around the world in developed countries over recent decades. The evolution is mainly attributed to changes in living conditions, lifestyles and improved self-care practices including the effective use of fluorides [1,22,23]. The disease has not been totally eradicated, but is controlled to a certain degree by retarding the initiation of carious lesions to a later age, or totally preventing the condition [1].

According to the "2003 World Oral Health Report", the current dental status of 12-yr-olds in New Caledonia is similar to that observed in other developed countries such as the USA ($D_3MFT = 3.0$) or Europe ($D_3MFT = 2.6$) [23,24]. For 9-yr-olds, the same observation can be made with similar caries experience levels as in the present study and in a French region in 2006 (respectively $D_3MFT = 0.76$ and 0.85) [3]. Greater improvement could be achieved for the youngest New Caledonian children. The prevalence of dental caries in the mixed dentition remains high in the New Caledonian 6-yr-olds (58%) when compared with that observed in a group of 6-yr-old French children (33%) examined in 2009 [25]. Important disparities were found in the present study, with high caries burden in children with unfavourable health behaviours, deprived social background, low access to preventive dental care or from the Kanak culture. The association of oral health with social or cultural determinants is well known, in France and in other countries [3,26–28]. In New Caledonia, such inequalities are particularly noticeable.

The present study has also shown that the weight of the D component of the DMFT and DMFM was very high in all age groups, while the relative weight of the F and M components were weak. Moreover, the number of untreated carious lesions did not decrease for children who had already visited a dentist. It is thus suggested that the dental care on offer is not in accordance with the population's needs. Three actors are involved in the care delivering: the children, the parents and the practitioners. As shown in a previous French study, children with anxiety about dental care were more affected by dental caries [29], however this study did not explore the relationship between dental anxiety and dental care distribution in NC. Parental social deprivation and low education are often involved as barriers for children's dental treatment. In New Caledonia, per capita income is high and the whole population is covered by basic public medical and dental insurance with a supplemental state subsidised insurance for low income families. Nevertheless, there is no comprehensive, free of charge public dental service for children as health services in schools. Moreover, as in many other countries, dentistry in New Caledonia uses a patient-centred curative approach. Even when dental services are available at no charge, other barriers to care may exist [27]. Socially deprived populations and ethnic minorities are sometimes reluctant to consult dentists because of previous negative experience, communication barriers and ignorance of their rights. They also perceive oral health in a way that strongly influences their treatment preferences and explains low and selective use of dental services [30–33]. This study did not explore the practitioner-related barriers for NC children's dental care. Further approaches are required to solve the problem of dental care access for children with high dental needs and deprived social backgrounds [34,35].

The study has some limitations. The sample size and the population's geographical spread made the enrolment of seven examiners necessary. To minimize the limitations of this methodological concern, the inter- and intra-examiner variability was limited by thoroughly calibrating the examiners. A moderate to very good level of agreement was obtained, depending on the examiner pair. Furthermore, a mixed model was used for all the statistical comparisons, which treated the cluster and examiner parameters as random effects. These methodological and statistical precautions prevented our results from being highly biased by this parameter.

The second limitation of our study is that some variables were recorded using a questionnaire completed by the school managers. Several reminders were sent to the non-responding schools but only 80% of the questionnaires were returned. Despite this non-response rate (some families may not have wanted to give personal information about their socioeconomic status), the final sample remained representative of the study population in terms of gender, region and type of school attended. Thus, we could reasonably assume that the non-responses were not linked to specific variables and had not reduced the quality of our results.

The third limitation is the non-inclusion of children with disabilities in the study sample due to the lack of demographic information on children with disabilities living at home, attending ordinary schools or living in educational institutions. However, data on oral health condition of this population are necessary to elaborate a fair comprehensive oral health programme, aiming to reduce inequalities in oral health. Consequently a further survey in special schools is needed, as has been undertaken in France [36].

In conclusion, this study highlights the need for new strategies aimed at improving oral health and at reducing inequalities. An alternative approach is needed, based on the principles of oral health promotion (OHP) such as those developed in the WHO's Ottawa Charter [37]. The development of healthy environments and the adoption of health promoting behaviours would be particularly suited for schools and the collaboration with local populations would probably facilitate improvements in children's dental health, as in the health promoting schools programs [38]. OHP programs, with culturally relevant interventions for the populations most concerned with oral diseases, and multidisciplinary collaborative networks also need to be developed. A reorientation of dental services towards preventive interventions and fewer operative treatments would be desirable. An OHP program would need to be developed in connection with other health programs in New Caledonia, namely programs related to the prevention of other chronic diseases as rheumatic heart disease or obesity. The common risk factor approach would need to be used in order to address risk factors common to those chronic conditions within the context of the local environment.

Acknowledgments

Clinical parts of the study were assisted by Drs R Cagliero, JP Cassagne, P Lefèvre, G Niquet, O Moyon, and K Tran Ba, whom the authors thank. The authors would like to thank Prof Paul Riordan (Write2Publish; http://correction-home.fr) for correction of the English manuscript.

Author Contributions

Conceived and designed the experiments: ST MH HP. Performed the experiments: HP MH ST. Analyzed the data: BP ST HP MH. Contributed reagents/materials/analysis tools: BR MH ST. Wrote the paper: HP ST MH.

References

1. Petersen PE, Bourgeois D, Ogawa H, Estupinan-Day S, Ndiaye C (2005) The global burden of oral diseases and risks to oral health. Bull World Health Organ 83: 661–669.
2. Bourgeois D, Gaillard P, Doury J (1996) Caries prevalence in 12-year-old schoolchildren in New Caledonia. Community Dent Health 13: 93–95.
3. Enjary C, Tubert-Jeannin S, Manevy R, Roger-Leroi V, Riordan PJ (2006) Dental status and measures of deprivation in Clermont-Ferrand, France. Community Dent Oral Epidemiol 34: 363–371.
4. Kerry SM, Bland JM (2001) Unequal cluster sizes for trials in English and Welsh general practice: implications for sample size calculations. Stat Med 20: 377–390.
5. Guittet L, Ravaud P, Giraudeau B (2006) Planning a cluster randomized trial with unequal cluster sizes: practical issues involving continuous outcomes. BMC Med Res Methodol 6: 17.
6. Ekstrand KR, Kuzmina I, Bjørndal L, Thylstrup A (1995) Relationship between external and histologic features of progressive stages of caries in the occlusal fossa. Caries Res 29: 243–250.
7. Bratthall D (2000) Introducing the Significant Caries Index together with a proposal for a new global oral health goal for 12-year-olds. Int Dent J 50: 378–384.
8. Loe H, Silness J (1963) Periodontal disease in pregnancy. I. Prevalence and severity. Acta Odontol Scand 21: 533–551.
9. Godlewski AE, Veyrune JL, Nicolas E (2008) [Obesity and oral health: risk factors of obese patients in dental practice]. Odontostomatol Trop 31: 25–32.
10. Decerle N, Nicolas E, Hennequin M (2013) Chewing Deficiencies in Adults with Multiple Untreated Carious Lesions. Caries Res 47: 330–337.
11. El Osta N, Hennequin M, Tubert-Jeannin S, Abboud Naaman NB, El Osta L, et al. (2014) The pertinence of oral health indicators in nutritional studies in the elderly. Clin Nutr 33: 316–321.
12. Pichot H, Nicolas E, Hennequin M (2010) Relationship between area of occlusal contact and orofacial dysfunction in children. J Disabil Oral Health 11.
13. Plutzer K, Spencer AJ (2008) Efficacy of an oral health promotion intervention in the prevention of early childhood caries. Community Dent Oral Epidemiol 36: 335–346.
14. Catteau C, Mishellany A, Faulks D, Lassauzay C, Hennequin M (2011) Oral health status of persons with disabilities attending special establishments. First results of the national health education programme "Oral Health and Autonomy". Bull Group Int Rech Sci Stomatol Odontol 50: 15–18.
15. Millstein P, Maya A (2001) An evaluation of occlusal contact marking indicators. A descriptive quantitative method. J Am Dent Assoc 132: 1280–1286; quiz 1319.
16. Snijders T, Bosker R (1999) Multilevel analysis: An introduction to basic and advanced multilevel modeling. London: Sage Publications. 266 p.
17. Verbeke G, Molenberghs G (2000) Linear mixed models for longitudinal data. New York: Springer. 568 p.
18. Hox J (2002) Multilevel analysis, techniques and applications. Mahwah, New Jersey: Lawrence Erlbaum Associates.
19. Goldstein H (2003) Multilevel statistical models. 3rd edition. London: Edward Arnold.
20. Donald A, Donner A (1987) Adjustments to the Mantel-Haenszel chi-square statistic and odds ratio variance estimator when the data are clustered. Stat Med 6: 491–499.
21. Burt BA, Eklund SA, Landis R, Larkin FA, Guire KE, et al. (1982) Diet and dental health, a study of relationships: United States, 1971–74. Vital Health Stat 11: 1–85.
22. Marthaler TM (2004) Changes in dental caries 1953-2003. Caries Res 38: 173–181.
23. Adam C, Eid A, Riordan PJ, Wolikow M, Cohen F (2005) Caries experience in the primary dentition among French 6-year-olds between 1991 and 2000. Community Dent Oral Epidemiol 33: 333–340.
24. Petersen PE (2003) The World Oral Health Report 2003: continuous improvement of oral health in the 21st century–the approach of the WHO Global Oral Health Programme. Community Dent Oral Epidemiol 31 Suppl 1: 3–23.
25. Joseph C, Velley AM, Pierre A, Bourgeois D, Muller-Bolla M (2011) Dental health of 6-year-old children in Alpes Maritimes, France. Eur Arch Paediatr Dent 12: 256–263.
26. Wigen TI, Wang NJ (2010) Caries and background factors in Norwegian and immigrant 5-year-old children. Community Dent Oral Epidemiol 38: 19–28.
27. Guarnizo-Herreño CC, Watt RG, Pikhart H, Sheiham A, Tsakos G (2013) Socioeconomic inequalities in oral health in different European welfare state regimes. J Epidemiol Community Health 67: 728–735.
28. Zander A, Sivaneswaran S, Skinner J, Byun R, Jalaludin B (2013) Risk factors for dental caries in small rural and regional Australian communities. Rural Remote Health 13: 2492.
29. Nicolas E, Bessadet M, Collado V, Carrasco P, Rogerleroi V, et al. (2010) Factors affecting dental fear in French children aged 5–12 years. Int J Paediatr Dent 20: 366–373.
30. Bolden AJ, Henry JL, Allukian M (1993) Implications of access, utilization and need for oral health care by low income groups and minorities on the dental delivery system. J Dent Educ 57: 888–900.
31. Bedos C, Brodeur J-M, Benigeri M, Olivier M (2004) [Social inequalities in the demand for dental care]. Rev Epidemiol Sante Publique 52: 261–270.
32. Shi L, Stevens GD (2005) Disparities in access to care and satisfaction among U.S. children: the roles of race/ethnicity and poverty status. Public Health Rep 120: 431–441.
33. Marshman Z, Porritt J, Dyer T, Wyborn C, Godson J, et al. (2012) What influences the use of dental services by adults in the UK? Community Dent Oral Epidemiol 40: 306–314.
34. Azogui-Lévy S, Lombrail P, Riordan PJ, Brodin M, Baillon-Javon E, et al. (2003) Evaluation of a dental care program for school beginners in a Paris suburb. Community Dent Oral Epidemiol 31: 285–291.
35. Baelum V (2011) Dentistry and population approaches for preventing dental diseases. J Dent 39 Suppl 2: S9–S19.
36. Hennequin M, Moysan V, Jourdan D, Dorin M, Nicolas E (2008) Inequalities in oral health for children with disabilities: a French national survey in special schools. PLoS ONE 3: e2564. doi:10.1371/journal.pone.0002564.
37. Petersen PE, Kwan S (2011) Equity, social determinants and public health programmes–the case of oral health. Community Dent Oral Epidemiol 39: 481–487. doi:10.1111/j.1600-0528.2011.00623.x.
38. Kwan SYL, Petersen PE, Pine CM, Borutta A (2005) Health-promoting schools: an opportunity for oral health promotion. Bull World Health Organ 83: 677–685.

Permissions

All chapters in this book were first published in PLOS ONE, by The Public Library of Science; hereby published with permission under the Creative Commons Attribution License or equivalent. Every chapter published in this book has been scrutinized by our experts. Their significance has been extensively debated. The topics covered herein carry significant findings which will fuel the growth of the discipline. They may even be implemented as practical applications or may be referred to as a beginning point for another development.

The contributors of this book come from diverse backgrounds, making this book a truly international effort. This book will bring forth new frontiers with its revolutionizing research information and detailed analysis of the nascent developments around the world.

We would like to thank all the contributing authors for lending their expertise to make the book truly unique. They have played a crucial role in the development of this book. Without their invaluable contributions this book wouldn't have been possible. They have made vital efforts to compile up to date information on the varied aspects of this subject to make this book a valuable addition to the collection of many professionals and students.

This book was conceptualized with the vision of imparting up-to-date information and advanced data in this field. To ensure the same, a matchless editorial board was set up. Every individual on the board went through rigorous rounds of assessment to prove their worth. After which they invested a large part of their time researching and compiling the most relevant data for our readers.

The editorial board has been involved in producing this book since its inception. They have spent rigorous hours researching and exploring the diverse topics which have resulted in the successful publishing of this book. They have passed on their knowledge of decades through this book. To expedite this challenging task, the publisher supported the team at every step. A small team of assistant editors was also appointed to further simplify the editing procedure and attain best results for the readers.

Apart from the editorial board, the designing team has also invested a significant amount of their time in understanding the subject and creating the most relevant covers. They scrutinized every image to scout for the most suitable representation of the subject and create an appropriate cover for the book.

The publishing team has been an ardent support to the editorial, designing and production team. Their endless efforts to recruit the best for this project, has resulted in the accomplishment of this book. They are a veteran in the field of academics and their pool of knowledge is as vast as their experience in printing. Their expertise and guidance has proved useful at every step. Their uncompromising quality standards have made this book an exceptional effort. Their encouragement from time to time has been an inspiration for everyone.

The publisher and the editorial board hope that this book will prove to be a valuable piece of knowledge for researchers, students, practitioners and scholars across the globe.

List of Contributors

Robert J. Losey, Erin Jessup and Tatiana Nomokonova
Department of Anthropology, University of Alberta, Edmonton, Alberta, Canada

Mikhail Sablin
Zoological Institute, Russian Academy of Science, Saint-Petersburg, Russia

Cecilia Young
Private Practice, Hong Kong

Kin Yau Wong
Department of Biostatistics, University of North Carolina at Chapel Hill, Chapel Hill, North Carolina, United States of America

Lim K. Cheung
The University of Hong Kong, Hong Kong

Antoine Popelut and Philippe Bouchard
Department of Periodontology, Service of Odontology, Hôtel-Dieu Hospital, AP-HP, Paris 7 - Denis Diderot University, U.F.R. of Odontology, Paris, France

Fabien Valet
Department of Biostatistics, Institut Curie, Paris, France

Olivier Fromentin
Department of Prosthetic Dentistry, Service of Odontology, Hôtel-Dieu Hospital, AP-HP, Paris

Aurélie Thomas
Library of Odontology, Paris 7 - Denis Diderot University, U.F.R. of Odontology, Paris, France

Marco Scazzocchio
Istituto dei Sistemi Complessi Udr "La Sapienza", Roma, Italy

Antonio Scala
Istituto dei Sistemi Complessi Udr "La Sapienza", Roma, Italy
London Institute of Mathematical Sciences, London, United Kingdom

Pietro Auconi
Istituto dei Sistemi Complessi Udr "La Sapienza", Roma, Italy
Private Practice of Orthodontics, Rome, Italy

Lorenzo Franchi
Department of Orthodontics and Pediatric Dentistry, School of Dentistry, The University of Michigan, Ann Arbor, Michigan, United States of America
Department of Orthodontics, The University of Florence, Florence, Italy

Guido Caldarelli
Istituto dei Sistemi Complessi Udr "La Sapienza", Roma, Italy
London Institute of Mathematical Sciences, London, United Kingdom
NATWORKS Unit for the Study of Natural Networks, IMT Lucca Institute for Advanced Studies, Lucca, Italy

James A. McNamara
Department of Orthodontics and Pediatric Dentistry, School of Dentistry, The University of Michigan, Ann Arbor, Michigan, United States of America
Department of Cell and Developmental Biology, School of Medicine, The University of Michigan, Ann Arbor, Michigan, United States of America
Center for Human Growth and Development, The University of Michigan, Ann Arbor, Michigan, United States of America
Private Practice of Orthodontics, Ann Arbor, Michigan, United States of America

Jörg Eberhard, Wieland Heuer and Meike Stiesch
Department of Prosthetic Dentistry and Biomaterials Science, Hannover Medical School, Hannover, Germany

Karsten Grote, Maren Luchtefeld, Harald Schuett, Dimitar Divchev and Bernhard Schieffer
Department of Cardiology and Angiology, Hannover Medical School, Hannover, Germany

Ralph Scherer
Department of Medical Statistics, Hannover Medical School, Hannover, Germany

Ruth Schmitz-Streit and Daniela Langfeldt
Institute for Microbiology, Christian-Albrechts-University Kiel, Kiel, Germany

Ingmar Staufenbiel
Department of Operative Dentistry and Periodontology, Hannover Medical School, Hannover, Germany

Mohammad Khursheed Alam, Muhammad Asyraf Hamza and Muhammad Aizuddin Khafi
Orthodontic Unit, School of Dental Science, Universiti Sains Malaysia, Kota Bharu, Kelantan, Malaysia

Shaifulizan Abdul Rahman and Ramizu Shaari
Oral and Maxillofacial Surgery Unit, School of Dental Science, Universiti Sains Malaysia, Kota Bharu, Kelantan, Malaysia

Akram Hassan
Periodontology Unit, School of Dental Science, Universiti Sains Malaysia, Kota Bharu, Kelantan, Malaysia

Hitoshi Miyachi and Kazuo Shimozato
Department of Maxillofacial Surgery, School of Dentistry, Aichi-Gakuin University, Nagoya, Aichi, Japan

Yujiro Higashi
Department of Perinatology, Institute for Developmental Research, Aichi Human Service Center, Kasugai, Aichi, Japan

Peter Jezewski
Department of Periodontology, University of Alabama at Birmingham School of Dentistry, Institute of Oral Health Research, Birmingham, Alabama, United States of America

Atsuo Nakayama
Department of Embryology, Institute for Developmental Research, Aichi Human Service Center, Kasugai, Aichi, Japan

Masashi Kimura, Akio Shibata, Tadashi Tatematsu and Yoshihito Tokita
Department of Maxillofacial Surgery, School of Dentistry, Aichi-Gakuin University, Nagoya, Aichi, Japan
Department of Perinatology, Institute for Developmental Research, Aichi Human Service Center, Kasugai, Aichi, Japan

Junichiro Machida
Department of Maxillofacial Surgery, School of Dentistry, Aichi-Gakuin University, Nagoya, Aichi, Japan
Department of Oral and Maxillofacial Surgery, Toyota Memorial Hospital, Toyota, Aichi, Japan

Seishi Yamaguchi
Department of Maxillofacial Surgery, School of Dentistry, Aichi-Gakuin University, Nagoya, Aichi, Japan
Department of Dentistry and Oral Surgery, Aichi Children's Health and Medical Center, Obu, Aichi, Japan
Department of Perinatology, Institute for Developmental Research, Aichi Human Service Center, Kasugai, Aichi, Japan

Peter Durand Skottrup, Grete Sørensen and Erik Riise
Biomolecular Interaction Group, Department of Drug Design and Pharmacology, Faculty of Health and Medical Sciences, University of Copenhagen, Copenhagen, Denmark

Miroslaw Ksiazek
Department of Microbiology, Faculty of Biochemistry, Biophysics and Biotechnology, Jagiellonian University, Krakow, Poland

Jan Potempa
Department of Microbiology, Faculty of Biochemistry, Biophysics and Biotechnology, Jagiellonian University, Krakow, Poland
Oral Health and Systemic Diseases Research Group, University of Louisville, School of Dentistry, Louisville, Kentucky, United States of America

Yvonne Jockel-Schneider, Imme Haubitz, Stefan Fickl, Martin Eigenthaler and Ulrich Schlagenhauf
Department of Periodontology, University Hospital Wuerzburg, Wuerzburg, Germany

Inga Harks
Department of Periodontology, University Hospital Muenster, Muenster, Germany

Johannes Baulmann
Clinic of Internal Medicine II, University Hospital Schleswig-Holstein, Luebeck, Germany

Adrien Boillot, Bechara El Halabi, Hélène Range and Philippe Bouchard
Department of Periodontology, Service of Odontology, Rothschild Hospital, AP-HP, Paris 7 - Denis Diderot University, U.F.R. of Odontology, Paris, France

George David Batty
Department of Epidemiology and Public Health, University College London, London, United Kingdom

Sébastien Czernichow
Department of Nutrition, Ambroise Paré Hospital, University Versailles St-Quentin, Boulogne-Billancourt, France
INSERM, U1018, Centre for Research in Epidemiology and Population Health, Villejuif, France

Saadika Khan
Department of Restorative Dentistry, University of the Western Cape, Cape Town, South Africa

Alfred Musekiwa
Centre for Evidence-Based Health Care, Faculty of Medicine and Health Sciences, Stellenbosch University, Cape Town, South Africa

Usuf M. E. Chikte
Department of Interdisciplinary Health Sciences, Stellenbosch University, Cape Town, South Africa

Ridwaan Omar
Head ofProsthodontics, Faculty of Dentistry, Kuwait University, Safat, Kuwait

Eduardo Bernabé
King's College London Dental Institute at Guy's, King's College and St. Thomas' Hospitals, Division of Population and Patient Health, London, United Kingdom

Aubrey Sheiham
Department of Epidemiology and Public Health, University College London, London, United Kingdom

Wicher J. van der Meer
Assistant professor, Department of Orthodontics, University Medical Centre Groningen, University of Groningen, Groningen, The Netherlands

Frank S. Andriessen
Postgraduate, Section of Oral Implantology, Academic Centre for Dentistry Amsterdam, Amsterdam, The Netherlands

Daniel Wismeijer
Professor and chair, Department of Oral Function and Restorative Dentistry, Head of the Section of Oral Implantology and Prosthodontics, Academic Centre for Dentistry Amsterdam, Amsterdam, The Netherlands

Yijin Ren
Professor and chair, Department of Orthodontics, University Medical Centre Groningen, University of Groningen, Groningen, The Netherlands

Charles E. Shelburne, P. Sandra Shelburne, Vishnu M. Dhople and Dennis E. Lopatin
Department of Biologic and Materials Sciences, The University of Michigan School of Dentistry, Ann Arbor, Michigan, United States of America

Domenica G. Sweier
Department of Cariology, Restorative Sciences and Endodontics, The University of Michigan School of Dentistry, Ann Arbor, Michigan, United States of America

William V. Giannobile and Janet S. Kinney
Department of Periodontics and Oral Medicine and The Michigan Center for Oral Health Research, The University of Michigan School of Dentistry, Ann Arbor, Michigan, United States of America

Wilson A. Coulter and Brian H. Mullally
Centre for Oral Research, Queen's University, Belfast, Northern Ireland

Georgios Papantonopoulos
Center for Research and Applications of Nonlinear Systems, Department of Mathematics, University of Patras, Patras, Greece

Keiso Takahashi
Department of Conservative Dentistry, School of Dentistry, Ohu University, Fukushima, Japan

Tasos Bountis
Laboratory of Nonlinear Systems and Applied Analysis, Department of Mathematics, University of Patras, Patras, Greece

Bruno G. Loos
Department of Periodontology, Academic Center for Dentistry Amsterdam (ACTA), University of Amsterdam and VU University, Amsterdam, The Netherlands

Véronique Moysan and Martine Dorin
Caisse Nationale de l'Assurance Maladie des Travailleurs Salariés (CNAMTS), Paris, France

Didier Jourdan
Institut Universitaire de Formation des Maîtres, JE 2432, Clermont-Ferrand, France

Martine Hennequin and Emmanuel Nicolas
University of Auvergne (Clermont 1) EA 3847, Clermont-Ferrand, France
CHU de Clermont-Ferrand, Clermont-Ferrand, France

Virginia M. Barnes, Fotinos Panagakos, William Devizio and Harsh M. Trivedi
Colgate Palmolive Technology Center, Piscataway, NJ, United States of America

Adam D. Kennedy, Thomas Jönsson and Lining Guo
Department of Oral Biology, School of Dental Medicine, University at Buffalo, State University of New York, Buffalo, NY, United States of America

Shannon Cervi and Frank A. Scannapieco
Metabolon, Durham, NC, United States of America

Hai Ming Wong and Yi Feng Wen
Paediatric Dentistry & Orthodontics, Faculty of Dentistry, The University of Hong Kong, Hong Kong

Nigel M. King
Paediatric Dentistry, School of Dentistry, University of Western Australia, Perth, Australia

Colman P. J. McGrath
Dental Public Health, Faculty of Dentistry, The University of Hong Kong, Hong Kong

Si-Min Peng
Paediatric Dentistry & Orthodontics, Faculty of Dentistry, The University of Hong Kong, Hong Kong
Department of Paediatric Dentistry, Guanghua School of Stomatology, Hospital of Stomatology, Sun Yat-sen University, Guangzhou, China

Tanmoy Sarkar and Parimal Das
Centre for Genetic Disorders, Faculty of Science, Banaras Hindu University, Varanasi, Uttar Pradesh, India

Rajesh Bansal
Faculty of Dental Sciences, Institute of Medical Sciences, Banaras Hindu University, Varanasi, Uttar Pradesh, India

Xingxing Wang, Xu Han, Xiaolong Luo and Dalin Wang
Department of Stomatology, Changhai Hospital, The Second Military Medical University, Shanghai, China

Xiaojing Guo
Department of Health Statistics, The Second Military Medical University, Shanghai, China

Shingo Matsuura, Kinuyo Ohara, Hiroki Komiya and Tetsuro Watase
Department of Endodontics, Nihon University School of Dentistry, Tokyo, Japan

Yuka Nakaya
Department of Oral Diagnosis, Nihon University School of Dentistry, Tokyo, Japan

Kohei Shimizu, Bunnai Ogiso and Keisuke Hatori
Department of Oral Diagnosis, Nihon University School of Dentistry, Tokyo, Japan
Divisions of Advanced Dental Treatment, Dental Research Center, Nihon University School of Dentistry, Tokyo, Japan

Kunihito Matsumoto
Department of Radiology, Nihon University School of Dentistry, Tokyo, Japan
Divisions of Advanced Dental Treatment, Dental Research Center, Nihon University School of Dentistry, Tokyo, Japan

Noboru Noma
Department of Oral Diagnosis, Nihon University School of Dentistry, Tokyo, Japan
Divisions of Clinical Research, Dental Research Center, Nihon University School of Dentistry, Tokyo, Japan

Yoshiyuki Tsuboi and Masamichi Shinoda
Department of Physiology, Nihon University School of Dentistry, Tokyo, Japan

Division of Functional Morphology, Dental Research Center, Nihon University School of Dentistry, Tokyo, Japan

Koicho Iwata
Department of Physiology, Nihon University School of Dentistry, Tokyo, Japan
Division of Functional Morphology, Dental Research Center, Nihon University School of Dentistry, Tokyo, Japan
Division of Applied System Neuroscience Advanced Medical Research Center, Nihon University Graduate School of Medical Science, Tokyo, Japan

Alexandre Emidio Ribeiro Silva, Ana Maria Baptista Menezes, Maria Cecília Formoso Assunção, Helen Gonçalves, Flávio Fernando Demarco and Fabiana Vargas-Ferreira
Postgraduate Programme in Epidemiology, Federal University of Pelotas, Pelotas, Rio Grande do Sul, Brazil

Marco Aureélio Peres
Australian Research Centre for Population Oral Health, School of Dentistry, University of Adelaide, Adelaide, Austrália

Bernard Rouchon
Sanitary and Social Agency of New Caledonia, Nouméa, New Caledoni

Bruno Pereira
CHU Clermont-Ferrand, Clermont-Ferrand, France

Hélène Pichot
Clermont University, University of Auvergne, EA 4847, Centre de Recherche en Odontologie Clinique, BP 10448, Clermont-Ferrand, France
Sanitary and Social Agency of New Caledonia, Nouméa, New Caledoni

Martine Hennequin and Stéphanie Tubert-Jeannin
Clermont University, University of Auvergne, EA 4847, Centre de Recherche en Odontologie Clinique, BP 10448, Clermont-Ferrand, France
CHU Clermont-Ferrand, Clermont-Ferrand, France

Index

R

S

T